A MANUAL OF
LABORATORY &
DIAGNOSTIC
TESTS

A MANUAL OF
LABORATORY & DIAGNOSTIC TESTS

FRANCES TALASKA FISCHBACH, RN, BSN, MSN
Associate Clinical Professor of Nursing
Department of Health Restoration
School of Nursing
University of Wisconsin—Milwaukee
Milwaukee, Wisconsin

FOURTH EDITION

J. B. Lippincott Company   *Philadelphia*
New York   London   Hagerstown

Sponsoring Editor: Diana Intenzo
Coordinating Editorial Assistant: Doris Wray
Project Editor: Lorraine D. Smith
Manuscript Editor: Diane Lamsback
Indexer: Betty Herr Hallinger
Design Coordinator: Doug Smock
Cover Designer: Louis Fuiano
Production Manager: Helen Ewan
Production Coordinator: Maura Murphy
Compositor: Bi-Comp, Incorporated
Printer/Binder: R. R. Donnelley & Sons Company
Cover Printer: Lehigh Press

Library of Congress Cataloging in Publications Data

Fischbach, Frances Talaska.
    A manual of laboratory & diagnostic tests / Frances Talaska
Fischbach. — 4th ed.
        p.   cm.
    Rev. ed. of: A manual of laboratory diagnostic tests. 3rd ed.
© 1988.
    Includes bibliographical references and index.
    ISBN 0-397-54831-1
    1. Diagnosis, Laboratory—Handbooks, manuals, etc. I. Fischbach,
Frances Talaska. Manual of laboratory diagnostic tests. II. Title.
III. Title: Manual of laboratory and diagnostic tests.
    [DNLM: 1. Diagnosis, Laboratory.   QY 25 F528m]
RB38.2.F57   1992
616.07'5—dc20
DNLM/DLC
for Library of Congress   91-32475
                                                                    CIP

Any procedure or practice described in this book should be applied by the
health-care practitioner under appropriate supervision in accordance with
professional standards of care used with regard to the unique circumstances
that apply in each practice situation. Care has been taken to confirm the
accuracy of information presented and to describe generally accepted
practices. However, the author, editors, and publisher cannot accept any
responsibility for errors or omissions or for any consequences from
application of the information in this book and make no warranty, express or
implied, with respect to the contents of the book.

Every effort has been made to ensure drug selections and dosages are in
accordance with current recommendations and practice. Because of ongoing
research, changes in government regulations and the constant flow of
information on drug therapy, reactions and interactions, the reader is
cautioned to check the package insert for each drug for indications, dosages,
warnings and precautions, particularly if the drug is new or infrequently
used.

To Christopher, Matthew, Joseph, and Michael Jonathan

CONTRIBUTORS

Barbara Barron, MT (ASCP)
Supervisor of Serology
Department of Pathology
Clement Zablocki VA Medical
  Center
Milwaukee, Wisconsin

Gloria Boge, RN, BSN, MSN
Professor of Nursing
City College
San Francisco, California

Carol Colosacco, CT (ASCP), CMIAC
Cytotechnologist
Department of Pathology
Howard Young Medical Center
Woodruff, Wisconsin

Bernice Gestaut DeBoer, RN, BSN
Communication Specialist
St. Joseph's Hospital
Milwaukee, Wisconsin

Marshall B. Dunning, BS, MS, PhD
Associate Professor of Medicine
Department of Medicine
Division of Pulmonary and Critical
  Care
Medical College of Wisconsin
Milwaukee, Wisconsin

Mary Kay Feeney, RN, BSN, MSN
Medical Specialist
Northwestern Mutual Life
  Insurance Co.
Milwaukee, Wisconsin

Dolaine Genthe, RN, BSN, MSN
Education and Research Specialist
West Bend, Wisconsin

Former Associate Professor
Medical College of Wisconsin
Milwaukee, Wisconsin

Member, Society for Peripheral
  Vascular Nursing

William Genthe, BS, MS, PhD
Chairman
Metriflow Medical Systems, Inc.
Milwaukee, Wisconsin

Teri Geszvain, EdM, RD, CHE
Associate Professor of Diatetics
Program Coordinator
Mount Mary College
Milwaukee, Wisconsin

Michael Kenneth Kaplon, MD
Chief of Hematology, Oncology
Clement Zablocki VA Medical
  Center
Milwaukee, Wisconsin

Assistant Professor
Medical College of Wisconsin
Milwaukee, Wisconsin

Donna Soik Karweik, MT (ASCP)
Microbiology Specialist
Department of Pathology
Clement Zablocki VA Medical Center
Milwaukee, Wisconsin

Elouise Benford Kemp, REEgT
Supervisor, Neurodiagnostic
Studies
St. Joseph's Hospital
Milwaukee, Wisconsin

David La Gosh, RT (ASCP), CNMT
Supervisor of Nuclear Medicine
St. Francis Hospital
Milwaukee, Wisconsin

Mark S. Lubinsky, MD
Associate Professor
Department of Pediatrics
Birth Defects Center
Medical College of Wisconsin

Director of Genetic Services
Children's Hospital of Wisconsin
Milwaukee, Wisconsin

Barbara Niemczycki, MT (ASCP)
Former Supervisor, Serology
Section
Department of Pathology
Milwaukee County Medical
Complex
Milwaukee, Wisconsin

**Richard Nuccio, MAT, MBA, CNMT, RT
(ASCP)**
Instructor in Nuclear Medicine
Education Coordinator
St. Mary's Hospital
Milwaukee, Wisconsin

Mary Ellen Paisley, MT (ASCP)
Blood Banking and Pre-transfusion
Testing
Department of Pathology
Milwaukee County Medical
Complex
Milwaukee, Wisconsin

Linda Pohl, RN, RVJT
Head Nurse, Vascular Laboratory
Clement Zablocki VA Medical
Center
Milwaukee, Wisconsin

Patricia Pomohac, MT (ASCP)
Supervisor, Immunology
Department of Pathology
Milwaukee County Medical
Complex
Milwaukee, Wisconsin

Roger Ready, RN
Endoscopist
Mayo Clinic
Rochester, Minnesota

**Mary Pat Haas Schmidt, BS, MT
(ASCP)**
Elm Grove Medical Associates
Instructor, Medical Technology
Milwaukee, Wisconsin

Jean M. Schultz, BS, RT, RDMS
Instructor in Radiology and
Ultrasound
St. Luke's Medical Center
Milwaukee, Wisconsin

**Corrinne Strandell, RN, BSN, MSN,
PhD**
Nursing Research and Education
Specialist
West Allis, Wisconsin

PREFACE

In this era of high technology, professionals in the medical field demand and use the sophisticated information made available to them to deliver expert health care. Thus, we live in an age that bears witness to the impact of diagnostic components of patient care upon health care delivery. However, in the present financial reimbursement climate, a number of health care reform issues that deal with the use of some of these diagnostic tests and procedures are being brought to the forefront.

One of these issues relates to defining what constitutes *necessary* care. Some reformers would like to cut 15 percent to 30 percent of those medical tests and procedures believed to be of little medical or diagnostic benefit. On the other hand, physicians continue to make most care consumption decisions, including the use of tests and treatments, as diagnostic adjuncts. Medicine, like other health care professions, is an art as well as a science. Moreover, it is not always an "exact" science. Consequently, what appears unnecessary on statistical charts may indeed be necessary when treating the individual patient. Despite the proposals for change, there is disagreement about what changes to pursue, except for consensus that the use of technology represents one of the largest cost components of health care today.

The technology involved in diagnostic testing is no exception. For example, just those procedures developed since 1975—which include but are not limited to total body and brain scanners, PET (Positron Emission Tomography), updated ultrasound and nuclear medicine procedures, genetic studies and oncology testing—now account for major portions of monies spent on health care. Advancements and refinements in technology, by their very nature, expand what the health care market can offer. Consequently, diagnostic care, even while facilitating accurate diagnoses to provide safer and more refined treatments, continues to add to the increased cost of health care. Still, if one views this in perspective, costs can be less. For example, pinpointing a problem through the use of a magnetic resonance imagery (MRI) scanner rather than through exploratory surgery is a fast, painless, safe, and accurate diagnostic tool. Moreover, the procedure costs less per patient than the expense involved in operative intervention, convalescence, lost work days, and treatment of possible complications. Other trends affecting decisions about the use of diagnostic testing relate to government regulations and company policies. For instance, many companies and agencies now routinely require their employees to participate in drug screen testing as a condition of employment.

Consequently, this updated fourth edition of *A Manual of Laboratory & Diagnostic Tests* is presented at a time when comprehensive knowledge of classic, traditional, and contemporary technologies is demanded by health care professionals, students, and bedside clinicians. This group includes practicing nurses, physicians, dentists, medical and x-ray technologists, chiropractors, and nursing and medical students. Those individuals employed in ambulatory care settings and testing laboratories and people who perform their life's work on the perimeter of the patient care environment should also benefit from this information. Specifically, persons employed in medical records and utilization review, or management, financial, and administrative positions, as well as those engaged in the practice of law, should find this manual a comprehensive resource and reference tool.

The teaching and learning of diagnostic test processes is a crucial element in many health care education programs. Therefore, this textbook should provide an up-to-date resource for all levels of students. Likewise, the experienced practitioner may appreciate the concise, consistent outline format and easily retrieved information.

Ultimately, the purpose of this text is to promote the delivery of responsible and safe care for patients undergoing diagnostic tests and procedures by providing information to facilitate use of the nursing and medical problem-solving processes. It provides necessary and detailed information for individualized patient assessment, adequate care analysis and planning, appropriate interventions, patient education, and timely evaluation of patient outcomes. Several unique features make this possible. Each chapter is arranged so that the introductory statements highlight the main topics of the chapter. Descriptions of testing modalities include background information, explanations of tests, interfering factors, procedures for collection of specimens and/or completion of tests, patient involvement, clinical implications, patient preparation, patient aftercare, and clinical alerts.

The book is organized into 16 chapters. All chapters have been revised to correspond to standards of the 1990s. Throughout the text the normal values now include age-related values, with clinical considerations of the newborn, and those in infancy, childhood, adolescence and old-age groups, where appropriate. Appendices to supplement chapters have also been expanded. Tables of vitamins and minerals, conversion tables for conventional units to international units, infection control data, and examples of informed consent forms for AIDS testing are available in this edition.

All bibliographies have been updated. They represent a composite of selected references from the fields of medicine, nursing, physiology, psychology, medical technology, x-ray technology, ultrasound and nuclear medicine technology, and other special methodologies such as magnetic resonance scanning, noninvasive vascular testing, and endoscopic examination.

The material for this book has been gathered and adapted from many and varied sources. The content/research process has made use of extensive personal interviews and library and literature studies. As in other editions, all new methodologies that directly involve patient participation have been personally observed by the author, research assistants, and/or contributors.

My hope is that this text will help students, clinicians, technologists, and other health care professionals to provide humane, knowledge-based care in the pre- and post-test phases as well as direct care during the procedure. If my words and ideas assist students and professional caregivers to provide necessary patient education and follow-up care, if they benefit both clinicians and students, helping them to recognize the significance of proper pre- and post-diagnostic care, and if they provide a unifying knowledge and communication model for learning and applying diagnostic test information to patient care, then I will have achieved the goal I wished to reach.

Frances Talaska Fischbach, RN, BSN, MSN

ACKNOWLEDGMENTS

I want to give special thanks and recognition to Jack Fischbach, my research assistant, to Frances Talaska for information management, and to Kathie Gordon and Margaret Fischbach Haag for typing the manuscript.

I would also like to acknowledge the expert contributors to this fourth edition and the following persons for providing information and help in manuscript preparation: Ronald C. Arndorfer, Sally Creegan, Henry J. DeBoer, Rod Doering, James Cooper, Sharon Flesch, and Irene Schreck. This work would not have been complete without the help and information provided by the librarians and staff of the Todd Wehr Library of the Medical College of Wisconsin and the Murphy Library of the Milwaukee County Medical Complex.

Appreciation is also due those persons who helped with the first, second, and third editions, especially Timothy Philipp, Charles Kerr, Theresa Philipp, Julie Erickson, Mary Fischbach Johnson, Dick Johnson, Margaret Fischbach Haag, Marshall B. Dunning, Barbara Niemczycki, Randle Pollard, M.D., Rod Doering, Dolaine Genthe, and Corrinne Strandell.

Gratefully remembered is Victor Buendia who helped with the first, second, and third editions and who has since died.

Many special thanks to Diana Intenzo, Mary Murphy, Doris Wray, and Lorraine Smith of the J. B. Lippincott Company for their editorial support and guidance.

CONTENTS

A MANUAL OF

LABORATORY &
DIAGNOSTIC
TESTS

CARE-GIVERS' RESPONSIBILITIES

Introduction

In this era of high technology, health care delivery involves so many different personnel and specialties that the care-giver must have an understanding and working knowledge of other professional endeavors, including the role of diagnostic evaluation. Basically, laboratory and diagnostic tests are tools. By and of themselves, they are not therapeutic. In conjunction with a pertinent history and a physical examination, however, these tests may confirm a diagnosis or provide valuable information about a patient's status and response to therapy.

Because health care consumers expect to be more involved in decision making and are more knowledgeable about diagnosis and treatment, informed consent becomes an important issue. Informed consent implies that the patient understands the following:

1. The reason for performing the test or procedure
2. Benefits and risks involved in performing or not performing the tests
3. The impact of data collected upon the overall treatment program

Preparing patients for diagnostic or therapeutic procedures and providing follow-up care have long been accepted parts of professional practice. Professionals today need to have expertise in developing meaningful care plans and in helping patients to adjust their daily activities to meet the test requirements. The responsibility of the care-giver can be divided into two phases: the pretest phase and the posttest phase of diagnostic care.

Pretest Phase
Basic Knowledge
1. Know test terminology, purpose, and procedures.
2. Know admission test results. The plan of care is developed or changed on the basis of these test results.
3. Be alert to critical laboratory test values that have immediate life or death significance to the patient, and report these findings to the attending physician immediately. Know institutional policy regarding prompt reporting and appropriate filing of these results.
4. Know how to gather diagnostic information from charts. Look at the most recent laboratory data first to determine the current status; then work backward to note trends and changes in data.

History and Assessment
1. Obtain a relevant health history and an individualized assessment.
2. Identify conditions that could interfere with test outcomes (*e.g.*, pregnancy or diabetes)

(a) The history should identify contraindications to testing, allergies to contrast substances such as iodine, and previous testing procedures

(b) Assessment should include the patient's need for information and methods of coping

3. Identify patients who are afraid or who are disturbed by confined spaces, because some procedures require this.
4. Be alert to the possibility that a patient may not disclose drug or alcohol usage.
5. In summary, document appropriate data and note patient concerns and questions. This information then forms a data base for inclusion into the medical and nursing process problem-solving methodologies.

Correct Procedures

1. Order correct tests. Use appropriate forms. Information should be complete, accurate, and legible.
2. When appropriate, ensure that all specimens are correctly obtained, preserved, handled, labeled, and delivered to the correct department. For example, it is not generally acceptable to draw blood from an extremity with an intravenous line infusing. Use infection control precautions for patients placed in isolation.

Proper Coordination of Activities

1. Coordinate patient activities and testing to avoid conflicts with meal times, medications, lengthy treatments, and other diagnostic tests.
2. Be mindful of patients who are not allowed to receive anything orally (NPO).
3. Know when to give medications prior to specific tests: Schedule tests needing contrast substances in such a manner as not to invalidate succeeding tests.
4. Take measures to minimize stress, anxiety, fear, nausea, and vomiting.

Minimizing Interference

1. Care-giver actions that affect or interfere with accurate test results include the following

Incorrect specimen collection handling, labeling

Wrong preservative or lack of necessary preservative

Delayed delivery of a collected specimen to the laboratory

Incorrect or incomplete patient preparation

Hemolysis of blood samples

Incomplete collection, especially of timed samples

Old specimens that may contain destroyed cells that may alter test results

2. Patient factors that affect or interfere with accurate test results include the following:

Diet preparation
Current drug history
Illness
Plasma volume
Position or activity at time specimen was obtained
Postprandial status (time patient last ate)

Time of day
Pregnancy
Age and sex
Lack of patient knowledge/ understanding
Stress
Nonadherence or noncompliance with instructions
Undisclosed drug or alcohol usage

Avoiding Errors
Knowledge and communication are the keys to prevention of diagnostic testing error.

1. The primary care-giver should be aware of how the test is performed and should have a basic understanding of how the results are obtained and measured.
   a. Patients and their families (when appropriate) should also be informed about tests as well as what is expected of them in preparation for the exams.
   b. Dietary restrictions or the collection process for multiple or timed specimens should be communicated to the patient and to staff.
2. The other side of the coin is that personnel in the diagnostic departments do not always coordinate their activities for the benefit of the patient. Technologists complain that specimens are not marked correctly, are lost, or are ineptly handled by the nursing or medical staff. Patients are not always correctly or completely prepared for the examination. Sometimes, testing personnel are not informed of changes in orders.

Proper Preparation of the Patient
Prepare the patient correctly.

1. Be alert to clinical considerations and needs of special patients such as ostomy patients, those with diabetes, children, and the elderly.
2. Be aware that patient preparation may well affect the outcome of tests. For example, patients need to know when they can eat and drink or what they are permitted to eat before certain tests.
3. Realize that fear or apprehension may be experienced by patients undergoing diagnostic procedures. Help the patient use imagery and relaxation techniques to reduce anxiety during the examination.

4. When giving a patient information, be sure the person can read written materials and can hear instructions (hearing aid adjusted, eyeglasses available).
5. Assess for language and cultural barriers. Be aware of and understand that each patient behaves according to personal value systems, beliefs, tradition, culture, and ethnicity.
6. Document care-giving activities performed in the pretest phase.

Patient Education

1. Educate patient and family about tests. Record information given to the patient and family.
   (a) Patients need both sensory and objective information about the purpose and the process of testing so that they can create an image of what is going to occur. Descriptions that are clear and well thought out enable patients to form a realistic schema of what they can expect. Avoid medical jargon, and teach according to the patient's level of understanding.
   (b) Sensory information helps the patient interpret a situation that is completely different from anything experienced in the past. Subjective features include physical sensations. Objective features characterize such things as equipment used or length of procedure. Sensations should be discussed so that the person is less apt to misinterpret and to conclude falsely that something has gone wrong.
2. Encourage questions, and allow the patient to verbalize fears and concerns. Do not minimize or invalidate the patient's anxiety by making remarks such as "Don't worry." Develop a "listening ear." Be aware of nonverbal cues (body language) that indicate a patient may not fully understand the testing process or may be very frightened by the process. Above all, be nonjudgmental!
3. Make chart entries about the specific manner in which information is given and the patient's response to that information. Because something is "taught" does not necessarily mean that it was "learned." The specific names of audiovisual or reading materials and handouts need to be documented correctly for audit purposes.

Protocols

1. Develop protocols for testing that encompass comprehensive pretest and follow-up care. Guidelines for giving patients necessary information should be developed and used consistently.
2. Prepare patients for those aspects of the procedure that are noticed by the majority of patients. Care-givers can collaborate to develop a pattern of response by using a list (when testing is completed) to determine what things most patients noticed and what words they used to describe their sensations.

Patient Independence

1. Plan care so the patient maintains as much control of the diagnostic phase as possible to reduce stress.

   (a) Patients should be included in decision making as much as possible. Because anxiety is usually higher during the diagnostic period, the person may not fully assimilate instructions and explanations. Therefore, the patient's understanding must be validated.

2. Inform the patient of the diagnostic plan, of the time frames for conducting the tests, and how the patient can comply to ensure reliable and successful test results.

Test Results
The meaning of normal or reference values is vital knowledge.

1. Be aware that normal ranges in published materials vary to some degree from laboratory to laboratory. Theoretically, "normal" can refer to normal health, to the ideal health state, to the average value, or to types of statistical distribution.

2. Keep in mind that the reported reference range for a test varies with the method used for testing as well as with the population tested. Each laboratory must provide its own normal range for the particular testing method it uses and for the special population for which the set of values is described.

SI Values

1. Scientific publications and a number of professional organizations are in the process of changing the reporting of clinical laboratory data from conventional units to Système International (SI) units. Currently, much clinical laboratory data are reported in conventional units with SI units placed in parentheses. After a transition period, SI units may be the only reference values used.

2. The SI system uses seven dimensionally independent units of measurement. These units are intended to provide a logical and consistent system of measurement.

   (a) In laboratory reports given in SI, the concentration is written as amount per volume (moles or millimoles per liter) rather than as mass per volume (grams, milligrams, or milli equivalents per deciliter, 100 milliliters, or liter)

   (b) Sometimes numerical values differ between systems; other times, they are the same. For example, chloride is the same—95 to 105 mEq/liter (conventional) and 95 to 105 mmol/liter (SI) (Tables 1–1 and 1–2 and Appendix).

Margins of Error

1. Know that if a patient has a battery of chemistry tests such as sequential multiple analyzers (SMAC) or multiple sequential

TABLE 1–1.
Seven Fundamental Units of SI

Physical Quantity/Property	Base Unit	SI Symbol
Length	Meter	m
Mass	Kilogram	kg
Time	Second	s
Amount of substance	Mole	mol
Thermodynamic temperature	Kelvin	K
Electric current	Ampere	A
Luminous intensity	Candela	cd

screening panel (MSSP), the possibility exists that some tests will be abnormal owing purely to chance. This occurs because a significant margin of error arises from the arbitrary setting of limits.

2. We know that if a laboratory test is considered normal up to the 95th percentile, then 5 times out of 100, the test will show an abnormality even though a patient is not ill. If the patient has a second test performed, the probability that both will be within the normal range is 0.95×0.95 or 90.25%. This means that 9.75 times out of 100 a test will show an abnormality even though the person has no underlying health disorder. With three tests, the probability that all three will have results within the normal range is $0.95 \times 0.95 \times 0.95$ or 85.7%. The point here is that if the patient has a group of tests performed on one blood sample, the possibility that some of the tests will be abnormal, due purely to chance, is not an uncommon occurrence.

Legal Implications

1. Be aware of the legal implications of diagnostic testing. These considerations include the patient's right to information, properly

TABLE 1–2.
Seven Representative Derived Units of SI

Derived Unit	Name and Symbol	SI Symbol
Area	Square meter	m^2
Volume	Cubic meter	m^3
Force	Newton (N)	$kg\ m\ s^{-2}$
Pressure	Pascal (Pa)	$kg\ m^{-1}\ s^{-2}$ (N/M^2)
Work, energy	Joule (J)	$kg\ M^2\ s^{-2}$ (N/M)
Density	Kilogram per cubic meter	kg/m^3
Frequency	Hertz (Hz)	s^{-1}

signed and witnessed consent forms, and explanations to patient or significant other regarding risks inherent in such tests as angiography or amniocentesis.

2. The patient must possess full use of cognitive and reasoning faculties in order to sign a valid consent legally.

    (a) This also means that the patient may not legally give consent to a procedure while under the immediate influence of sedation, anesthetic agents, or certain classes of analgesics and tranquilizers.

    (b) In the event the patient cannot validly and legally sign a consent form, an appropriately qualified individual may give consent for the patient.

3. A team approach to diagnostics is essential for responsible patient care.

    (a) It is the role of the attending physician to inform the patient about test results, as well as alternatives and medical and surgical actions for follow-up care.

    (b) It is the purview of all other care-givers to provide information and clarification, and to give support to patient and family, especially when test results are abnormal.

Ethical Considerations

1. Situations such as confidentiality of information, reporting of infectious diseases, or the dehumanizing effects of some diagnostic procedures reflect basic ethical considerations.

2. Patients and family need to and have the right to know both the benefits and the risks of testing. They also need to recognize their right to consent to or to refuse diagnostic tests.

Infection Control Issues

1. Care-givers have the right to know the diagnoses of the patients they care for so that they can obtain and handle diagnostic specimens properly in order to minimize risks to themselves.

2. Proper protective clothing and devices must be worn, and procurement and disposal of specimens according to OSHA standards must be adhered to.

3. The term *universal precautions* refers to a system of disease control that presupposes that each direct contact with body fluids is infectious and that every employee exposed to these fluids needs to be protected. It is a method of preventing infections in certain classes of health care workers. Consequently, health care workers need to be conscientious about adhering to infection control guidelines. Moreover, they must be scrupulous about proper handwashing (see Appendix).

Post-test Care
Abnormal Test Results
1. It is important to be able to recognize abnormal test results and to have some idea of the implications upon the patient's health state. For example, know when test results indicate serious disease or shortened life span.
2. Help the patient and the family understand what a positive or a negative test result might mean for them.
3. Recognize "panic values" that reflect life-threatening situations.

   Note: Critical lab values need to be reported to the attending physician and to be documented immediately.

4. Clinical laboratories will need to tabulate their own "panic values," which are expressed in conventional or SI units.

False Results
Know the meaning of false-positive and false-negative test results.

1. Certain drugs frequently produce negative or positive results.
2. Sometimes the testing methods can actually cause positive or negative results. For example, in the Venereal Disease Research Laboratories (VDRL) test for syphilis, certain persons may receive positive test results even though they do not have syphilis.
3. On the other hand, false negatives also occur. For example, the electrocardiogram (ECG) is not sensitive to coronary disease *before* a myocardial infarction. In other words, coronary disease is not detected or predicted by this particular test. A person may have a normal ECG one day and develop a myocardial infarction the next.
4. Extreme negative psychological and social consequences can result from being identified as having a serious disease like acquired immunodeficiency syndrome (AIDS) or syphilis because of false-positive test results. Major alterations in life-styles and relationships can be a consequence of these clinical aberrations.

Safety Measures
Detection and prevention of complications should promote patient safety and well-being.

1. Post-test assessments should include evaluation of patient's behavior and appearance relative to abnormal test results and the patient's response (acceptance or nonacceptance) of the test results. For example, patients with chemical or electrolyte imbalances may sustain decreased mental alertness or sensorial disturbances. Consequently, they need to be protected from possible injury to themselves or others. Also, patients who have taken barium need to know the importance of completely evacuating this contrast medium.

2. Closer observation may be necessary for older persons and children after certain diagnostic studies.
3. Infection control measures and aseptic technique should be used after invasive diagnostic methods such as cardiac catheterization or in the presence of infectious disease processes. This information needs to be permanently documented.

Follow-up Care

Follow-up care should be consistent and should include discharge instructions based upon test results and infection control measures. Instruction about site care after cardiac catheterization is an example of this.

1. Make sure the patient understands medical and surgical management and "jargon."
2. Allow time for listening, support, and discussion. Clarify the meaning of test results, if necessary. A patient who has just been diagnosed with anemia or diabetes has vastly different concerns and problems than the patient with a diagnosis of cerebral aneurysm or bone cancer.
3. Deal with each patient problem in a highly individualized manner. Make sure that information is consistently and accurately recorded.

Documentation

1. Document the diagnostic processes used. This is as important as other record entries because it has legal, budgetary, reimbursement, and diagnostic related grouping (DRG) implications.
2. Note the following examples of documentation content:
   (a) Entries should include allergies and a recorded history and physical assessment to support indications and contraindications to testing as well as the patient's or family's need for this information.
   (b) The health care record should indicate that the patient has been informed about the purpose and any effects from the test and has been offered an explanation (when appropriate) of the value, risks, and expected results from the test as well as alternative methods available.
   (c) Nursing preparations (*e.g.*, enemas) should be charted.
   (d) The length of time the testing procedure takes, as well as an assessment of the patient's response to the test, needs to be documented.
   (e) Specimens obtained, together with their disposition, must be entered into the record.
   (f) Follow-up care and instructions given for patient well-being and safety should also be included.

(g) It is most important to record and to report any adverse effects or complications from either the test or the contrast media.

(h) Record, in the patient's own words if possible, any refusal to be tested.

3. Much of the foregoing information will be obtained and used during implementation of the medical and nursing processes and development of the care plan. Where applicable, include diagnostic test information as a component of discharge planning.

Disclosure Guidelines

1. The issues of ethical standards as well as the role of the professional nurse as patient advocate can be potential sources of conflict and anxiety. Development of accepted guidelines for informing a patient about test results (how much to reveal and how to reveal the diagnosis) can resolve some of this uncertainty.

2. Guidelines are as follows:

(a) The physician is ultimately responsible for providing initial information to the patient. The nurse or other designated individuals can arrange and facilitate communication between patient, doctor, family, and nurse. Normally, the patient has the right to information about test results.

(b) Explanations to the patient about the diagnosis, the illness, and the approach to treatment seem to be the most acceptable methods of dealing with disclosure issues.

(c) Disclosure can prevent a "conspiracy of silence" from developing.

(d) The most effective method of revealing the diagnosis may be to tell the patient and the family together. Question the assumption and insistence that the patient "cannot take the truth."

Patient Response to Outcome

1. Develop appropriate crisis intervention skills in the event that they are called for. For example, informing a patient that she or he has AIDS has been graphically described as "an amputation of the future" for the person involved. Accordingly, many persons whose diagnostic tests confirm cancer experience sheer terror. They have reported that their "whole lives passed before them" during the immediate confirmation stage.

2. Encourage the patient to take as much control of the situation as possible.

3. Recognize and be attuned to initial patient responses to learning the diagnosis of those diseases that threaten their life-style and self-image. Typically, the immediate pattern of response lasts several days. It is then followed by a secondary response that may last several weeks.

Immediate Response	*Secondary Response*
Acute emotional turmoil, shock, disbelief about diagnosis	Insomnia, anorexia, difficulty in concentration, depression, difficulty in performing work-related responsibilities
Feelings of anxiety will usually last several days as the person assimilates the information.	Depressed feelings may last several weeks as the person begins to incorporate the information and to participate realistically in a treatment plan.

Comfort Measures

1. Give those comfort measures that seem appropriate to the situation, especially if outcome reveals a chronic or a life-threatening disease.
2. Help patient work through anxiety and depression. Point out that concerns and fears related to the diagnosis are normal and expected.
3. Provide positive interventions such as helping the patient and the family cope with necessary alterations in life-style and self-concept.
4. Emphasize that some risk factors associated with certain disorders can be reduced. These include overweight, unrelieved stress and worry, lack of exercise, poor sleep habits, poor nutrition, and excessive alcohol intake.

Expected Outcomes

Expected outcomes include the following:

1. The patient demonstrates the ability to define the purpose of the test, the test procedure, and the preparation necessary to complete the test.
2. The patient is physically and mentally able, with assistance if necessary, to follow through with appropriate pretest preparation.
3. The patient properly performs those activities expected of the patient in order to complete the testing process correctly.
4. Based upon test outcomes and recommendations, the patient makes appropriate life-style changes.
5. Complications either do not occur or are satisfactorily resolved.
6. The patient does not feel or exhibit undue anxiety or fear during the testing process.

Conclusion

As professionals, we need to maintain the perception that we are dealing with people not so unlike ourselves in many ways. These individuals come to us with their perceptions of what the diagnostic process and their illness means to them and their loved ones, what strategies they use to cope, what resources are available for their use, and what knowledge they have about themselves. As care-givers and patient advocates, then, we have to be willing to try to "take on the mind" of another—to identify with that patient's point of view. In other words, we must be willing to show empathy. Once we reach that point, we can then begin to understand each other and to communicate with one another.

BIBLIOGRAPHY

Aller RD: New directions in interpretive test reporting. MLO 21(4):26–33, April 1989

American Hospital Association Committee on Health Care for the Disadvantaged: Statement on a patient's bill of rights. Chicago, American Hospital Association, 1975

American Medical Record Association: Position statement on confidentiality of patient health information. J Am Med Rec Assoc 1–11: December 1985

Applebaum P et al: Informed Consent: Legal Theory and Clinical Practice. New York, Oxford University Press, 1987

Axneck KJ, Yarbrough M: Infection Control: An Integrated Approach. St. Louis, CV Mosby, 1984

Benner P, Wrubel J: The Primacy of Caring: Stress and Coping in Health and Illness. Menlo Park, CA, Addison Wesley, 1989

Blair RE et al (eds): Damon Clinical Laboratories Handbook. Stow, OH, Lex i-comp, 1989

Cotton P: Furor looms over workplace drug tests. Med World News: 76–77, October 13, 1986

Fischbach FT: Documenting Care—Communication; Nursing Process; Documentation Standards. Philadelphia, FA Davis, 1991

Fuller SS, Endress MP, Johnson JE: The effects of cognitive and behavioral control on coping with an aversive health examination. J Human Stress 4:18–25, 1978

Garner BC: Guide to changing lab values in elders. Geriatr Nurs 10(3):144–145, May/June 1989.

Garner JS, Simmons BP: CDC guidebook for isolation precautions in hospitals. Infection Control 4(4):July/August, 1983

Hadley A: The anxieties of endoscopy. Nurs Mirror 158(4):26–28, January 25, 1984

Johnson JE, Leventhal H: Effects of accurate expectations and behavioral instructions in reactions during a noxious medical examination. J Pers Soc Psychol 29:710–718, 1974

Johnson J, Louver D: Alternative explanation of coping with stressful experiences associated with physical illness. Advances in Nursing Science 11:39–52, 1989

Kohles MK et al: Clinical laboratory and nursing personnel: Collaboration in improving patient care. J Nurs Qual Assur 3(2):1–10, February 1989

LaFontaine P: Alleviating patients' apprehensions and anxieties. Gastroenterol Nurs 11(4):256–257, Spring, 1989

Lewis MA, Warden CD: Have a Care: Law and Ethics in the Medical Office, Including Bioethical Issues, 2nd ed. Philadelphia, FA Davis, 1988

McHugh NG, Christman NJ, Johnson JE: Preparatory information: What helps and why. Am J Nurs 82:780–782, 1982

Miller SM, Morgan CE: Interacting effects of information and coping style in adapting to gynecologic stress: Should the doctor tell all? J Pers Soc Psychol 45(1):223–236, 1983

Misiano DR et al: Current and future directions in the technology related to bedside testing of critically ill patients. Chest 97(5):204S–214S, May 1990

Monroe D: Will your patient survive that trip to X-ray? RN 52(4):40–44, April 1989

Moren JD: Private genes and public ethics. Hastings Center Report 13(5), 1983

O'Bannon RH: The effects of improper specimen handling on lab tests. MLO 20(11):42–47, November 1988

Purvis A: Unbelieveable blood tests: Laboratory reports are often misleading or downright mistaken. Time 135(11):79, March 12, 1990

Ravel R: Clinical Laboratory Medicine: Clinical Application of Laboratory Data, 5th ed. Chicago, Year Book Medical Pub, 1989

Shulkin DJ et al: When the laboratory tests are abnormal and the patient feels fine. Hosp Pract 25(7):85–86, 89–90, 92, July 15, 1989

Soloway HB: Should the public have direct access to lab services? MLO 22(6):26–28, June 1990

Thrasher SB: What I didn't know really hurt me. RN 52(9):49–50, September 1989.

Young DS et al: A hospital-wide task force to reduce lab utilization. MLO 21(10):31–32, 34, 36, October 1989

BLOOD STUDIES

2

Introduction

Composition

The average person has about 5 L of blood (5 to 6 qt) that may be separated into 3 L of plasma and 2 L of cells. The plasma is a liquid derived from the intestines and organs of the body, and the cells compose the solids formed mainly by the bone marrow. The normal adult's blood volume is estimated at one thirteenth of his total body weight.

The blood can be thought of as a tissue serving many functions. Without plasma, cells cannot circulate, and without cells, the vascular fluid alone cannot maintain life.

The cells normally found in blood are classified as white cells (leukocytes), red cells (erythrocytes), and platelets (thrombocytes). White cells are further divided into granulocytes, lymphocytes, and monocytes.

A. Erythrocytes (red blood cells)
B. Leukocytes (white blood cells)
   1. Granulocytes (polymorphonuclear leukocytes)
      (a) Neutrophils
      (b) Eosinophils
      (c) Basophils
   2. Nongranulocytes
      (a) Lymphocytes
      (b) Monocytes
C. Platelets or thrombocytes

The cells vary in size, with the white cells being the largest, the red cells next, and the platelets the smallest. Red cells greatly predominate; for every 500 red cells, there are approximately 30 platelets and only one white cell.

Blood Disorders

Red Blood Cell Disorders

Disorders of the red blood cells (RBCs) are grouped into *anemias* (severe reductions in circulating red blood cells due to blood loss, production and destruction disorders) and *polycythemias* (abnormal increases in circulating red cells).

Leukocyte Disorders

Disorders of the leukocytes are termed either as *leukocytosis* (an increased number of cells) or *leukopenia* (a decreased number of cells). Because there are numerous types of white blood cells (WBCs), variations in the counts of the different types of cells may reflect a wide range of disorders, including infection, leukemia, agranulocytosis, or granulocytopenia.

Platelet Disorders
A decreased number of platelets is called *thrombocytopenia*, which can become manifest in hemorrhage. An increased number of platelets is known as *thrombocytosis*. Thrombocytosis can be due to a primary bone marrow disorder or may be a reaction to some other underlying disorder. In thrombocytosis due to a bone marrow disorder, the platelets may not function properly, putting the patient at risk for either abnormal bleeding or clotting.

Disorders of Blood Cell Function
In addition to disorders that affect the number of cells in the blood, there are abnormalities that affect the function of the cells.

The production of red cells, platelets, and white cells is referred to as *hematopoiesis* and occurs mainly in bone marrow. Under normal conditions, only mature cells enter the bloodstream from the bone marrow. In pathologic states, a variety of immature cells can be found in the circulating blood.

Determining Blood Disorders
Therefore, examination of the blood and bone marrow constitutes the major means of determining certain types of blood disorders. The procedures involved in obtaining the specimens are skin puncture of finger, toe, or heel, venipuncture, and bone marrow aspiration.

COLLECTION PROCEDURES

Proper collection of specimens is very important and takes into account both timing of the sample collection and careful techniques.

Skin Puncture

Capillary blood is preferred for a peripheral blood smear.

1. Capillary blood is obtained from
   (a) The tip of a finger or earlobe in adults
   (b) The great toe or heel in infants
   (c) The tip of the finger in infants over 1 year old
2. Puncture site is washed with disinfectant (70% alcohol), dried with sterile gauze, and skin is punctured no deeper than 2 mm with a sterile disposable lancet. If povidone–iodine (Betadine) is used, it must be allowed to dry thoroughly to be effective.
3. First drop of blood is wiped away with sterile gauze, and subsequent drops are collected in a microtube and slides.

> **Clinical Alert**
>
> Avoid squeezing the extremity to obtain blood, because doing this will alter the composition of the blood.

Venipuncture

Venipuncture is a procedure necessary for most tests that require anticoagulation and large quantities of blood. It is the puncturing of a vein with a needle attached to a syringe for the purpose of obtaining a blood sample.

1. Venous blood is usually obtained from the antecubital vein, although veins in other sites may be chosen. There is no variation in blood values if specimens are obtained from different veins.
2. A tourniquet is placed and tightened on the upper arm to cause venous congestion and prevent venous return.

   Note: A blood pressure cuff that is inflated to a level between systolic and diastolic pressure can be used as a tourniquet.
3. The patient is asked to make a fist and to open and close his or her hand several times.
4. The puncture site is cleansed with 70% alcohol and dried with sterile gauze. If povidone–iodine (Betadine) is used, it must be allowed to dry thoroughly.
5. The vein is cleanly punctured with either a sterile needle and syringe or a Vacutainer system.

   Note: The size of needle and syringe is determined by the amount of blood needed as well as the size and integrity of the vein to be used. Furthermore, many hospitals use the Vacutainer system because it is cheaper. The Vacutainer system consists of a vacuum tube (Vacutainer tube), a holder, and a multisample collecting needle.
6. After the vein is entered, blood will fill the vacuum tubes of the Vacutainer system. However, if a needle and syringe are used, gentle suction with the syringe is needed to obtain the specimen. Excessive suction can collapse the vein.
7. Remove needle and apply sterile gauze with pressure to stop bleeding. Cover puncture site with an adhesive bandage.
8. The anticoagulant needed is dependent on the test to be performed. In general, most hematology tests use ethylene diamine tetraacetic

acid (EDTA) anticoagulant. The tests are done on well-mixed whole blood. Even slightly clotted blood invalidates the test.

Clinical Alert

1. If oozing from the puncture site is difficult to stop, elevate area and apply a pressure dressing. Stay with the patient until bleeding stops.
2. Never draw blood for any laboratory test from the same extremity that is being used for intravenous medications, intravenous fluids, or blood.
3. In patients with leukemia or agranulocytosis and in others with lowered resistance, the finger-stick and earlobe puncture are more likely to cause infection and bleeding than venipuncture. If a capillary sample is necessary in these patients, the cleansing agent should remain in contact with the skin for at least 7 to 10 minutes. Alcohol is not bactericidal; povidone–iodine is the cleansing agent of choice on patients with leukemia.

If a povidone–iodine swab is used, the skin is scrubbed, allowed to dry (this can take up to 2 minutes), and then wiped off with alcohol and dried with sterile gauze.

4. If difficulty is encountered in obtaining blood
   (a) Warm the extremity (this must be done for all blood gases).
   (b) Allow the extremity to remain in a hanging position for some time.
5. Hematomas can be prevented by
   (a) Using good technique
   (b) Releasing the tourniquet before the needle is removed
   (c) Applying sufficient pressure over the puncture site after completion of the procedure

---

Prolonged use of a tourniquet causes stasis of blood, produces hemoconcentration, and causes other changes that make the blood unsuitable for blood gases, blood count, blood pH, and some clotting.

Bone Marrow Aspiration

Normal Appearance
Rust-red color; thick, fluidlike consistency with visible amounts of fatty material; and pale gray white marrow fragments

Explanation of Test

Bone marrow is that organ located within cancellous bone and in cavities of long bones. A smear is made from a bone marrow aspiration or biopsy to see if the bone marrow is performing its function of manufacturing normal red and white cells and platelets. The developmental stages of the most immature cells, relative to those ready to be released into the circulating blood, can be seen (Table 2–1).

Indications for Test

A bone marrow examination is important in the evaluation of a number of hematologic disorders. At times, bone marrow is sampled for

TABLE 2–1.
Bone Marrow Normal Range

Formed Cell Elements	Normal (Mean %)	Range (%)
Undifferentiated cells	0.0	0.0–1.0
Reticulum cells	0.4	0.0–1.3
Myeloblasts	2.0	0.3–5.0
Promyelocytes	5.0	1.0–8.0
Myelocytes		
Neutrophilic	12.0	5.0–19.0
Eosinophilic	1.5	0.5– 3.0
Basophilic	0.3	0.0– 0.5
Metamyelocytes		
Neutrophilic	25.6	17.5–33.7
Eosinophilic	0.4	0.0– 1.1
Basophilic	0.0	0.0– 0.2
Segmented granulocytes		
Neutrophilic	20.0	11.6–30.0
Eosinophilic	2.0	0.5– 4.0
Basophilic	0.2	0.0– 3.7
Monocytes	2.0	1.6– 4.3
Lymphocytes	10.0	3.0–20.7
Megakaryocytes	0.4	0.0– 3.0
Plasma cells	0.9	0.1– 1.7
Erythroid series		
Pronormoblasts	0.5	0.2 – 4.2
Basophilic normoblasts	1.6	0.25– 4.8
Polychromatic normoblasts	10.4	3.5 –20.5
Orthochromatic normoblasts	6.4	3.0 –25
Promegaloblasts	0	0
Basophilic megaloblasts	0	0
Polychromatic megaloblasts	0	0
Orthochromatic megaloblasts	0	0
Myeloid : erythroid ratio (M : E) ratio of WBC to nucleated RBC	3.0–4.1	6.1–2.1

(Platt WR: Color Atlas and Textbook of Hematology. Philadelphia, JB Lippincott, 1969)

cultures in patients with suspected infectious diseases. However, a bone marrow examination does not always provide specific or even relevant information and is not diagnostically sufficient in and of itself. The presence or the suspicion of a blood disorder is not always an indication of the need to study the bone marrow. The decision to employ this procedure is made for each patient on the basis of the history, physical examination, and examination of his or her peripheral blood and consideration of how the results of the bone marrow examination will affect the management of patient care. Bone marrow aspiration alone or aspiration and biopsy may be necessary depending upon the suspected disorder.

Procedure

1. Patient is positioned on his or her back or side according to site selected. The posterior iliac crest is the preferred site in all patients over the age of 12 to 18 months. Other sites include the anterior iliac crest, sternum, spinous vertebral processes T10 through L4, ribs, and tibia in children.

    The sternum usually is not used in children because the cavity is too shallow, danger of mediastinal and cardiac perforation is too great, and observation of procedure is associated with apprehension and lack of cooperation.
2. The area is shaved, if necessary, cleansed, and draped as for any minor surgical procedure.
3. A local anesthetic of procaine or lidocaine is injected. The infiltration of the medication is accompanied by pain from needle insertion and a burning sensation.
4. A short, rigid, sharp-pointed needle with stylet is introduced through the periosteum into the marrow cavity. The stylet is removed from the needle and 0.2 to 0.5 ml. of marrow fluid is aspirated.

    When the bone marrow is entered, a feeling of pressure is experienced. Moderate discomfort, which only lasts a few seconds, *may* be felt when aspiration is done, especially if the iliac crest is the chosen site. There is no way to prevent or lessen this discomfort.
5. If a biopsy is to be performed, the Jameshedi needle is commonly used. The Westerman–Jensen modification of the Vim–Silverman needle may also be used. An incision (3 mm) is often made in the skin.
6. The needle with the stylet in place is passed through the incision, subcutaneous tissue, and cortex of the bone.
7. With the stylet removed, the biopsy needle is advanced with a twisting motion toward the anterior superior iliac spine.
8. After adequate penetration of the base (3 cm), the needle is rotated several times in both directions. The needle may also be rocked

back and forth in an attempt to free the specimen from its attachment in the marrow space. The needle is then slowly withdrawn.
9. The biopsy specimen is pushed out "backwards" and may be used to make touch preparations or immediately placed in fixative.
10. After the needle is removed, pressure is applied to the site until any bleeding ceases and a small sterile dressing is applied to the puncture site. Slides are usually smeared at the bedside.
11. Total procedure time is approximately 20 to 30 minutes.
12. Label specimen container with patient's name, date, and room number, and take it immediately to the laboratory.

Clinical Implications
1. A specific and diagnostic bone marrow picture is associated with many diseases. The report indicates the presence, absence, and ratio of cells that are characteristic of the suspected disease. However, bone marrow interpretation is a complicated task and requires considerable training and experience. Only a highly trained hematologist can be expected to evaluate a marrow specimen accurately.
2. Bone marrow examination may reveal the following abnormal cell patterns (not meant to be all-inclusive):
   (a) Leukemia or multiple myeloma
   (b) Deficiency states, including vitamin B_{12}, folic acid, iron, and pyridoxine
   (c) Toxic states producing marrow depression or destruction
   (d) Neoplastic diseases in which the marrow is invaded by tumor cells
   (e) Agranulocytosis (a decrease in the production of certain types of white cells). This occurs when the bone marrow activity is severely depressed, usually as a result of radiation therapy and drugs used in cancer therapy, and it means that the patient can be in danger of death due to overwhelming infection.
   (f) Platelet disorders
   (g) Some types of infectious diseases
   (h) Deficiency of body iron stores

Patient Preparation
1. A legal permit must be signed.
2. Instruct the patient about the procedure, purpose, benefits, and risks of the test.
3. Reassure the patient that many persons are extremely fearful about this test, especially if they have had it done previously.
4. Advise the patient that analgesics or sedatives may be ordered.
5. If the iliac crest is the site used, prepare the patient for pain by having him or her hold a pillow and bite into it if pain is experienced.

Patient Aftercare

1. Observe for bleeding at the puncture site and continued pain, which may indicate fracture.
2. Recommend bed rest for 30 minutes; then normal activities may be resumed.
3. Administer analgesics or sedatives if necessary. Slight soreness over the puncture site area for 3 to 4 days after procedure is normal and is no cause for alarm.

Clinical Alert

1. Bone marrow aspiration is usually contraindicated in patients with hemophilia and other bleeding dyscrasias. However, the importance of further information that could be obtained by this method should be weighed against the risks.
2. Complications include bleeding and sternal fractures. Osteomyelitis and death due to injury to heart or great vessels are rare but do occur if the sternum is used.
3. Pressure over the puncture site will control excessive bleeding that sometimes occurs in patients with thrombocytopenia and other bleeding disorders.

Hemogram

A hemogram includes platelet count, white blood count (WBC), red blood count (RBC), hematocrit (HCT), and indices. Complete blood count (CBC) is a hemogram plus differential count.

BASIC BLOOD TESTS
Complete Blood Count (CBC)

Explanation of Test

The CBC is a basic screening test in all patients and is one of the most frequently ordered laboratory procedures. The significant findings in the CBC give valuable information about the patient's diagnosis, prognosis, response to treatment, and recovery. The CBC consists of

White blood count (WBC)
Differential white cell count (Diff)
Red blood count (RBC)

Hematocrit (HCT)
Hemoglobin (Hgb)
Red blood cell indices
    Mean corpuscular volume (MCV)
    Mean corpuscular hemoglobin (MCH)
    Mean corpuscular hemoglobin concentration (MCHC)
Stained red cell examination (film or peripheral blood smear)
Platelet count (often included in CBC)

These tests will be described in detail in the following pages.

The White Blood Cell (Leukocyte)

Leukocyte Function

The main function of leukocytes is to fight infection, defend the body by phagocytosis against invasion by foreign organisms, and to produce, or at least transport and distribute, antibodies in the immune response. Behaving as separate yet related systems, the various types of leukocytes serve different functions. These functions will be discussed in detail in subsequent test descriptions.

Types of Leukocytes

Leukocytes, or white blood cells, are divided into two main groups: granulocytes and agranulocytes. These are further classified as follows:

Granulocytes		*Nongranulocytes*	
Band neutrophils	0%–5%	Lymphocytes	20%–40%
Neutrophils	60%–70%	Monocytes	2%–6%
Eosinophils	1%–4%		
Basophils	0.5%–1%		

    The granulocytes receive their name from the granules that are present in the cytoplasm of neutrophils, basophils, and eosinophils. However, each of these cells also contains a multilobed nucleus, which accounts for their also being called *polymorphonuclear leukocytes*. In laboratory terminology, they are often called "polys" (PMNs)
    The nongranulocytes, which consist of the lymphocytes and monocytes, do not contain granules and have nonlobular nuclei. They are not necessarily spherical; thus, the term *mononuclear leukocytes* is applied to these cells.

Leukocyte Formation

Because granulocytes and monocytes are formed in the red bone marrow, all of these cells can be considered myelogenous. The lymphocytes are formed in the bone marrow and in the lymphatic tissue, which includes the spleen, thymus, and tonsils. After formation, they are transported in the blood to the different regions, organs, or tissues of the body where they are needed. Vitamins, folic acid, and amino acids are used by the body in the formation of the leukocytes.

The endocrine system is an important regulator of the number of leukocytes in the blood. Hormones affect production of the leukocytes in the blood-forming organs, their storage and release from the tissue, and their disintegration. A local inflammatory process exerts a definite chemical effect on the mobilization of the leukocytes.

The life span of leukocytes varies from 13 to 20 days, after which the cells are destroyed in the lymphatic system; many are excreted from the body in fecal matter.

Granulocyte Development
Granulocytes develop through the following progression:

1. Myeloblasts (immature cells normally found in bone marrow); increased numbers found in granulocytic leukemia
2. Promyelocytes (immature cells normally can be found in blood in granulocytic [myelocytic] leukemia)
3. Myelocytes (found in the bone marrow)
4. Metamyelocytes (cells found in granulocytic [myelocytic] leukemia or severe infection)
5. "Bands" (neutrophils in early stages of maturity; increased numbers found in blood when leukocyte count is elevated [stabs])
6. "Polys" (mature cells sometimes referred to as "segs" [segmented neutrophils])

Staining Properties
Neutrophils, basophils, and eosinophils are distinguished from one another by the staining properties of the granules in their cytoplasm.

Neutral staining reaction: Neutrophils
Acid stain reaction: Eosinophils
Basic stain reaction: Basophils

Nongranulocyte Development
Nongranulocytes develop through the following progression:

Lymphocytes
1. Lymphoblast (immature cell found in lymphocytic leukemia)
2. Prolymphocyte (immature cell found in lymphocytic leukemia)
3. Lymphocyte (mature cell)

Monocytes
1. Monoblasts
2. Promonocytes (immature cells seen in monocytic leukemia)
3. Monocyte (mature cell)

White Blood Cell Count (WBC) (Leukocyte Count)

Normal Values
$5-10^3/\mu l$ or $5-10^9/L$

Explanation of Test
Measurement of the total number of circulating leukocytes is an important procedure in the diagnosis and prognosis of the disease process. Specific patterns of leukocyte response can be expected in different types of diseases. It is known that certain diseases are accompanied by a specific type of white blood cell increase or decrease that is proportional to the severity of the signs and symptoms of the disease.

Because leukocytes are affected by so many diseases, the leukocyte count serves as a useful guide to the severity of the disease process. The differential count (count of the numbers of different types of leukocytes; see pp. 30–31) will identify certain persons with increased susceptibility to infection. A leukocyte function test may be done to determine the white blood cells' ability to phagocytize and destroy bacteria.

Leukocytes and differential counts by themselves are of little value as aids to diagnosis unless the results are related to the clinical condition of the patient; only then is a correct and useful interpretation possible. Serial examinations have diagnostic and prognostic value. Disorders of the WBC are often associated with changes in the red blood cells and platelet counts. The stained red cell examination is done with the differential count. The same blood slide is examined to detect variations in structure, size, shape, color, and content of the red blood cells.

Procedure
1. A venous anticoagulated EDTA blood sample of 7 ml or a fingerstick sample is obtained.
2. The time when specimen was obtained is recorded (*e.g.*, 7:00 AM).
3. Blood is processed either manually or in an automated piece of equipment such as the Coulter counter. Results obtained by such methods are reported.

Clinical Implications
A. *Leukocytosis* (white blood cell count above $10,000/\mu l$)
   1. Leukocytosis is usually due to an increase of only *one* type of white cell and is given the name of the type of cell that shows the main increase.
      (a) Neutrophilic leukocytosis or neutrophilia
      (b) Lymphocytic leukocytosis or lymphocytosis
      (c) Eosinophilic leukocytosis or eosinophilia

  (d) Monocytic leukocytosis or monocytosis

  (e) Basophilic leukocytosis or basophilia

2. An increase in circulating leukocytes is rarely due to a proportional increase in leukocytes of all types. When it occurs, it is usually due to hemoconcentration.

3. In certain diseases (such as measles, pertussis, and sepsis), the increase of leukocytes is so great that the blood picture suggests leukemia. *Leukocytosis of a temporary nature* must be distinguished from leukemia. In leukemia, the leukocytosis is permanent and progressive. Associated abnormalities in the red blood cell count and platelet count may not distinguish severe infection from acute leukemia. A bone marrow examination may be necessary.

4. Leukocytosis occurs in acute infections in which the degree of increase of white cells depends on

  (a) The severity of the infection

  (b) The patient's resistance

  (c) The patient's age

  (d) Marrow efficiency and reserve

5. Other causes of leukocytosis include

  (a) Hemorrhage

  (b) Trauma or tissue injury as occurs in surgery

  (c) Malignant disease, especially of the gastrointestinal tract, liver, bone, and metastasis

  (d) Toxins, uremia, coma, eclampsia, thyroid storm

  (e) Drugs, especially ether, chloroform, quinine, adrenalin, colony stimulating factors

  (f) Serum sickness

  (g) Circulatory disease

  (h) Tissue necrosis or inflammation

  (i) Leukemia (in acute leukemia there is an increase in the total WBC with a decrease in normal-appearing cells)

6. Occasionally leukocytosis is found when there is no evidence of clinical disease. Such findings suggest the presence of one of the following:

  (a) Occult disease

  (b) Physiologic leukocytosis due to excitement, exercise, pain, cold or heat, anesthesia

7. Steroid therapy modifies the leukocyte response.

  (a) When ACTH is given to a healthy person, leukocytosis occurs.

  (b) When ACTH is given to a patient with severe infection, the infection can spread rapidly without producing the expected leukocytosis; thus, what would normally be an important sign is obscured.

8. Hematologic disorders; recovery from marrow suppression, hemolysis, asplenia, myeloproliferative disorders
9. Cigarette smoking

B. *Leukopenia* (a decrease of white blood cells below 4000)
Occurs during and following
1. Viral infections
2. Hypersplenism
3. Bone-marrow depression due to
   (a) Drugs
       (1) Antimetabolites
       (2) Barbiturates
       (3) Benzine
       (4) Antibiotics
       (5) Antihistamines
       (6) Anticonvulsives
       (7) Antithyroid drugs
       (8) Arsenicals
       (9) Cancer chemotherapy (causes a decrease in leukocytes; leukocyte count is used as a link to disease)
       (10) Cardiovascular drugs
       (11) Diuretics
       (12) Analgesics and anti-inflammatory drugs
   (b) Heavy metals
   (c) Radiation
4. Primary bone marrow disorders
   (a) Leukemia
   (b) Myeloma
   (c) Aplastic anemia
   (d) Myelodysplastic syndromes
   (e) Congenital disorders
       (1) Kostmann syndrome
       (2) Reticular agenesis
       (3) Cartilage—hair/hypoplasia
       (4) Shwachman–Diamond syndrome
       (5) Chédiak–Higashi syndrome
5. Immune-associated neutropenia
6. Marrow-occupying diseases—fungal infection, metastatic tumor

Clinical Alert

1. White blood cell count below 500 (<500 WBC) represents a panic value

2. Agranulocytosis (marked neutropenia and leukopenia) is extremely dangerous and is often fatal because the body is unprotected against invading agents. Patients who exhibit this disorder must be protected from infection by means of reverse isolation techniques with strictest emphasis on handwashing technique.

Clinical Considerations
In prolonged severe granulocytopenia,

1. Give no fresh fruits or vegetables because the kitchen, especially in a hospital, may be a source of food contamination. When leukocytes are low, a person can get pseudomonas or fungal infection from fresh fruits and vegetables.
2. Use minimal bacteria diet or commercially sterile diet. All food must be served from a single serving or a new package.
3. Consider leukemia diet. See dietary department for restrictions such as cooked food only and careful food preparation.
4. Do not give intramuscular injections.
5. Do not take rectal temperatures.
6. Do not give medicines by suppository.
7. Do not give aspirin or nonsteroidal anti-inflammatory drugs (produce abnormal platelet dysfunction).
8. Watch carefully for any signs or symptoms of infection. Without white cells to produce inflammation, serious infections can present very subtle findings. Often patients will have only a fever.

Interfering Factors
1. Hourly rhythm: There is an early-morning low level and late-afternoon high peak.
2. Age: In newborns and infants, the count is high (10,000–20,000) and gradually decreases in children until the adult values are reached at about age 21.

Differential White Blood Cell Count (Diff)
(Differential Leukocyte Count)

Normal Values

	Relative Values	Absolute Values (No/μl)
Neutrophils	60%–70% (56% average)	3000–7000
Eosinophils	1%–4% (2.7% average)	50–400

	Relative Values	*Absolute Values (No/µl)*
Basophils	0.5%–1% (0.3% average)	25–100
Lymphocytes	20%–40% (34% average)	1000–4000
Monocytes	2%–6%	100–600

Explanation of Test

The total leukocyte count of the circulating white blood cells is differentiated according to the five types of leukocyte cells, each of which performs a specific function.

Cell	*These Cells Function to Combat*
Neutrophils	Pyogenic infections
Eosinophils	Allergic disorders and parasitic infestations
Basophils	Parasitic infections
Lymphocytes	Viral infections (measles, rubella, chickenpox, infectious mononucleosis)
Monocytes	Severe infections, by phagocytosis

The differential count is expressed as a percentage of the total number of white cells. The distribution of the number and type of cells and the degree of increase or decrease are diagnostically significant.

The differential count expressed in percent is the *relative* number of each type of leukocyte in the blood. The absolute number of each type of leukocyte is obtained mathematically by multiplying the percentile value of one type of leukocyte by the total leukocyte count.

Formula

$$\underset{\text{WBC/mm}^3}{\text{Absolute value}} = \underset{(\%)}{\text{Relative value}} \times \underset{(\text{cells/mm}^3)}{\text{Total WBC count}}$$

The differential count alone has a limited value; it must always be interpreted in relation to the total leukocyte count. The reason for this interpretation can be explained in the following way: If the percentage of one type of cell is increased, it can be inferred that cells of that type are relatively more numerous than normal, but it is not known if this reflects an absolute decrease in cells of another type or an actual absolute increase in the number of cells that are relatively increased. On the other hand, if the relative percentile values of the differential are known and if the total leukocyte count is known, it is possible to calculate absolute values that are not subject to misinterpretation.

Segmented Neutrophils (Polymorphonuclear Neutrophils, PMNs, "Segs," or "Polys")

Normal Values
50%–60% of total white cell count
3000–7000/mm.³
0%–3% of the total count of stabs or band cells

Background
The neutrophils are the most numerous and most important type of white cells in the body's reaction to inflammation. They constitute a primary defense against microbial invasion through the process of phagocytosis. These cells can also cause some damage to body tissue by their release of enzymes and endogenous pyrogens.

In their immature stage of development, they are referred to as "stab" or "band" cells. The term *band* stems from the appearance of the nucleus that has not assumed the lobed shape of the mature cell.

Clinical Implications
A. *Neutrophilia*, or neutrophilic leukocytosis, is an increased percentage of circulating neutrophils. The previously stated causes of leukocytosis include the causes of neutropenia.
   1. The following are instances when the presence of early and immature neutrophils is the only indication that infection is present:
      (a) In elderly persons or in instances when the infection is overwhelming, there can be an increase in immature neutrophils with little or no leukocytosis (degenerative shift to the left).
      (b) On the other hand, absence of severe infection indicates a poor prognosis.
      (c) In pernicious anemia and chronic morphine addiction, only adult or mature hypersegmented neutrophils are associated with increased neutrophils.
   2. *Shift to the Right*
      An increase in mature cells (known as a "shift to the right," as in liver disease and megaloblastic anemia due to vitamin B_{12} or folic-acid deficiency) can occur
      (a) In hemolysis
      (b) With drugs such as digitalis, mercury, ACTH, sulfonamides, arsenicals, potassium chlorate, benzene, venoms
      (c) With tissue breakdown as in burns, myocardial infarction, tumors, gangrene, or pus formation; hemolytic transfusion reactions, after surgery, after cancer of liver, GI tract, and bone marrow
      (d) With allergies

3. *Shift to the Left*
    1. Any stimulus that causes an increase in neutrophils also causes early and immature neutrophils to be released into the blood. An increase in these cells is known as a "shift to the left" and is an indication of a regenerative response.
B. *Morphologic Alterations of Neutrophils*
    1. Toxic granulation–dark blue granules in cytoplasm indicative of severe infection or other toxic conditions
    2. Döhle bodies–light blue inclusions in cytoplasm found in severe infections
    3. May–Hegglin anomaly—large blue inclusion bodies found along with giant platelets
    4. Pelger–Huët anomaly—hereditary, autosomal dominant condition involves failure of normal segmentation of neutrophils—all neutrophils are "band"- or "dumbbell"-shaped
    5. Chédiak–Higashi syndrome—autosomal recessive disorder, characterized by large granules in neutrophils

---

Clinical Alert

A neutropenia of less than 500 increases dramatically a patient's susceptibility to bacterial infections. If this occurs, institute necessary measures to protect the patient.

Interfering Factors
1. Age
    (a) Children respond to infection with a greater degree of neutrophilic leukocytosis than adults.
    (b) Some elderly patients respond weakly or not at all, even when the infection is severe.
2. Resistance
    (a) People of any age who are weak and debilitated may fail to respond with a significant neutrophilia.
    (b) When an infection becomes overwhelming, the patient's resistance is exhausted and as death approaches, the number of neutrophils decreases greatly.
3. Steroids
    Tissue resistance is weakened when ACTH is given to a person suffering from a severe infection, so that the expected neutrophilia does not occur.
4. Myelosuppressive chemotherapy
5. Marrow efficiency and reserve

Eosinophils

Normal Values
1%–4% of total leukocyte count (relative value) or
50–250/mm³ (absolute value) or
50–250 10⁶/L

Background
Although not too much is known about its function, the eosinophil is capable of phagocytosis. Eosinophils become active in the later stages of inflammation and ingest antigen–antibody complexes. These cells are also active in allergic reactions and parasitic infections. The number of eosinophils in the blood is increased in these conditions.

Explanation of Test
1. Used to diagnose allergic infections, severity of infestations with worms and other large parasites, and the response to treatment
2. Also the basis for the Thorn test, which is used to evaluate the adrenal response to ACTH.

Procedure
1. Note the time the blood sample is obtained (*e.g.*, 3:00 PM).
2. If the count is done separately, a blood sample of 7 ml is obtained.
3. A manual WBC is performed, 100 cells counted, and the percentage of eosinophils is reported.

Clinical Implications
A. *Eosinophilia*—an increase of circulating eosinophils greater than 5% or more than 500
   1. Causes
      (a) Allergies
      (b) Parasitic disease such as trichinosis and tapeworm
      (c) Addison's disease
      (d) Tumors, including Hodgkin's disease and lymphoma, brain tumors, myeloproliferative disorders
      (e) Chronic skin infections such as psoriasis, pemphigus, and scabies
      (f) Polycythemia
      (g) Subacute infections
      (h) Familial eosinophilia (rare)
      (i) Polyarteritis nodosa
      (j) Gastrointestinal diseases, such as ulcerative colitis, Crohn's disease
      (k) L-tryptophan ingestion

B. *Eosinopenia*—a decrease in the amount of circulating eosinophils
  1. Usually due to an increased adrenal steroid production that accompanies most conditions of bodily stress
  2. Associated with
     (a) Infectious mononucleosis and other acute infections
     (b) Congestive heart failure
     (c) Cushing's syndrome
     (d) Use of certain drugs such as ACTH, epinephrine, thyroxine, prostaglandins
     (e) Infections with neutrophilia
     (f) Any disorder associated with neutropenia
  3. Eosinophils disappear early in pyogenic infections when there is a leukocytosis with a marked shift to the left (increase in immature white cells).
C. *Eosinophilic myelocytes*
  In the differential count, all the eosinophils are placed in one group, except the eosinophilic myelocytes, which are counted separately because they have a greater significance, being found only in leukemia or leukemoid blood pictures.

Interfering Factors
1. Hourly rhythm
   (a) The normal eosinophil count is lowest in the morning, then rises from noon until after midnight.
   (b) For this reason, serial eosinophil counts should be repeated at the same time in the afternoon each day.
2. Stress
   Stressful situations, such as in burns, postoperative states, lupus erythematosus, electroshock, eclampsia, and labor will cause a decreased count.
3. Steroid therapy
   (a) Eosinophilia can be masked by steroid use; infections can be fatal.
   (b) It is not clear why eosinophils disappear promptly from the blood following injection of ACTH.

Basophils

Normal Values
0.5%–1.0% of the total leukocyte count or
25–100/mm^3

Background

Basophils constitute a small percentage of the total leukocyte count—about 0.5%. Their function is not clearly understood, although they are considered to be phagocytic and to contain heparin, histamines, and serotonin. Tissue basophils are also called *mast cells;* like basophils, they store and produce heparin, histamine, and serotonin. Normally, mast cells are not found in peripheral blood and are rarely seen in healthy bone marrow.

Explanation of Test

Basophil counts are used to study allergic reactions. There is a positive correlation between high basophil counts and high concentrations of blood histamines, although this correlation does not imply cause and effect.

Clinical Implications

A. *Increased count* (basophilia)
   1. Associated most commonly with granulocytic and basophilic leukemia and myeloid metaphasia
   2. Associated less commonly with
      (a) Inflammation or allergy
      (b) Polycythemia vera
      (c) Chronic hemolytic anemia
      (d) Following splenectomy
      (e) Following radiation
      (f) Endocrine problems such as myxedema diabetes
      (g) Infections, including tuberculosis, smallpox, chickenpox, influenza
      (h) Iron deficiency
B. *Decreased count*
   Associated with
   1. Allergic reactions
   2. Hyperthyroidism
   3. Stress reactions such as myocardial infarction and bleeding peptic ulcer
   4. Following prolonged steroid therapy
   5. Hereditary absence of basophils
C. *Presence of numbers of tissue mast cells*
   Associated with
   1. Rheumatoid arthritis
   2. Urticaria
   3. Anaphylactic shock
   4. Hypoadrenalism
   5. Lymphoma
   6. Macroglobulinemia
   7. Mast cell leukemia
   8. Lymphoma invading bone marrow
   9. Urticaria pigmentosa
   10. Asthma
   11. Chronic liver and renal disease
   12. Osteoporosis
   13. Systemic mastocytosis

Monocytes (Monomorphonuclear Monocytes)

Normal Values
2%–6% of total leukocyte count relative value or
100–600/mm^3

Background
These agranulocytes, the monomorphonuclear monocytes, are the body's second line of defense against infection and are the largest cells of normal blood. A histiocyte is a *fixed tissue macrophage.* Histiocytes, which are large macrophagic phagocytes, are classified as monocytes in a differential leukocyte count. Histiocytes and monocytes are thought to be capable of reversible transformation from one to the other.

These phagocytic cells of varying size and mobility remove injured and dead cells, microorganisms, and insoluble particles from the circulatory blood. Monocytes escaping from the upper and lower respiratory tracts and the gastrointestinal and genitourinary organs perform a scavenger function, clearing the body of debris. These phagocytic cells are able to produce the antiviral agent called *interferon.*

Monocytes are known to circulate in certain conditions in which their macrophagic properties act specifically—tuberculosis, leprosy, lipid storage disease, and subacute bacterial endocarditis (infectious leukocytosis).

Procedure
A blood sample of 7 ml is obtained.

Clinical Implications
A. *Monocytosis*—an increase in the number of monocytes
  1. Present during recovery stage from acute infections—a favorable sign
     (a) Present in tuberculosis—unfavorable
  2. Viral infections
     (a) Infectious mononucleosis, cytomegalovirus
     (b) Chickenpox, mumps
  3. Subacute bacterial endocarditis
  4. Parasitic infections
     (a) Malaria
     (b) Amebic dysentery
  5. Rickettsial infections
  6. Collagen diseases
  7. Hematologic disorders
     (a) Acute and chronic myelogenous leukemia
     (b) Polycythemia vera
     (c) Lymphoma—Hodgkin's disease
     (d) Multiple myeloma

8. Any nonhematologic malignancy
9. Phagocytic monocytes (macrophages) may be found in small numbers in the blood in many conditions, including the following:
   (a) Severe infections
   (b) Lupus erythematosus
   (c) Hemolytic anemias
   (d) Agranulocytosis
   (e) Thrombocytopenic purpura

B. *Decreased monocyte count* (not usually identified with specific diseases)
   1. Prednisone treatment
   2. Hairy cell leukemia
   3. Rheumatoid arthritis
   4. HIV infection

Lymphocytes (Monomorphonuclear Lymphocytes)

Normal Values
20%–40% of total leukocyte count (relative value) or
1000–4000/mm^3

Explanation of Test
These agranulocytes are small, motile cells that migrate to areas of inflammation in both the early and late stages of the inflammation process. They may possibly convert to tissue macrophages and plasma cells. These cells are the source of serum immunoglobulins and of cellular immune response and play an important role in immunologic reactions. It is believed that lymphocytes are responsible for the storage of immunologic memory. This means that a second contact with an antigen elicits an accelerated and increased response. The cells are found in the blood in infectious leukocytosis at the recovery stage of disease.

Procedure
Lymphocytes are counted as part of the differential count.

Clinical Implications
A. *Lymphocytosis* (an increase in the amount of circulating lymphocytes)
   1. Above 9000/mm^3 in infants and young children

   Above 7000/mm^3 in older children
   Above 4000/mm^3 in adults
   2. *Conditions causing or associated with lymphocytosis*
      (a) Infectious lymphocytosis (as high as 100,000/mm^3)
         (1) Occurs mainly in children
         (2) 95% are small, mature lymphocytes
      (b) Infectious mononucleosis
         (1) Caused by Epstein–Barr virus
         (2) Most common in adolescents and young adults
         (3) Characterized by atypical lymphocytes—Downey cells—large, deeply indented, with deep blue (basophilic) cytoplasm
         (4) Differential diagnosis—positive heterophil test
      (c) Cytomegalovirus infection and other viral infections
      (d) Most viral upper respiratory infections, atypical pneumonia
      (e) Other viral diseases, such as mumps, rubella, rubeola
      (f) Infectious hepatitis
      (g) Some bacterial infections such as tuberculosis, brucellosis and syphilis, pertussis
      (h) Acute and chronic lymphocytic leukemia, lymphoma
      (i) Toxoplasmosis
      (j) Graves' disease
B. *Lymphopenia* (a decrease in the amount of circulating lymphocytes) Occurs
      (a) In Hodgkin's disease
      (b) In lupus erythematosus
      (c) After administration of ACTH and cortisone
      (d) After burns or trauma
      (e) In chronic uremia
      (f) In Cushing's syndrome
      (g) In early acute radiation syndrome
      (h) Many congenital immunodeficiency states
      (i) Acquired immunodeficiency syndrome
      (j) Aplastic anemia
      (k) Tuberculosis

Clinical Alert

A decreased lymphocyte count of less than 500 means that a patient is dangerously susceptible to infection, especially viral infections. *Institute measures to protect patient from infection.*

The Red Blood Cell (Erythrocyte)

Background
Red Cell (Erythrocyte) Function
The main function of the red blood cell or erythrocyte is to carry oxygen from the lungs to the body tissue and to transfer carbon dioxide from the tissues to the lungs. This process is achieved by means of the *hemoglobin* in the red cells that combines easily with oxygen and carbon dioxide. The combination of hemoglobin and oxygen gives arterial blood a bright red appearance. Because venous blood has a low oxygen content it appears dark red.

To enable the maximum amount of hemoglobin to be utilized, the red cell is shaped like a biconcave disk, which affords more surface area for the hemoglobin to combine with oxygen. The cell is also able to change its shape when necessary to allow for passage through the smaller capillaries.

Red Cell (Erythrocyte) Formation
Red blood cells are formed in the red bone marrow (erythropoiesis). Normally the mature erythrocyte, without nucleus, is the major cell released into the circulation. Frequently, when the hematopoietic (blood forming) system is faced with a heavy demand for red blood cell replacement (due to hemorrhage or disease), immature blood cells are released into the blood system. This would include nucleated red blood cells.

The mature erythrocyte, once released into the circulation, has a life span of about 120 days. When worn out, it is removed from the circulation by phagocytes in the spleen, liver, and red bone marrow (reticuloendothelial system).

Millions of red blood cells are destroyed daily, while millions are formed to replace them. To maintain health, the number of erythrocytes and the amount of hemoglobin they contain must remain fairly constant.

If the number of red cells in the blood is reduced, the normal bone marrow can increase its rate of production. The trigger of this increased production is the decrease of oxygen in the body system, which stimulates the production of erythropoietin, a hormone that in turn stimulates the production of red blood cells.

Many tests look at the red blood cells: their number, size, amount of hemoglobin, rate of production, percent composition of the blood. These various tests and their use are discussed in the sections that follow.

The red blood cell count (RBC), hematocrit (Hct), and hemoglobin (Hgb) are closely related but different ways to look at the adequacy of red blood cell production. The same conditions cause respective rise and fall in each of these indicators. Values will vary according to age and individual laboratory standards. Selected hematologic values in normal individuals of various ages appear below.

Age	Red Blood Cell Count ($\times 10^6$ cells/ul or $\times 10^{12}$ cells/L)	Hematocrit % or volume fraction (mean) $\times$ 0.01	Hemoglobin g/dl or $\times$ 10 g/L
1 mo	3.3–5.3	33–55	10.7–17.1
12 mo	4.1–5.3	33–41	11.3–14.1
1–2 yr	3.8–4.8	32–40	11.0–14.0
12–14 yr			
Male	4.1–5.2	35–45	12.0–16.0
Female	3.8–5.0	34–44	11.5–15.0
18–44 yr			
Male	4.3–5.7	39–49	13.2–17.3
Female	3.8–5.1	35–45	11.7–15.5
45–64 yr			
Male	4.2–5.6	39–50	13.1–17.2
Female	3.8–5.3	35–47	11.7–16.0
65–74 yr			
Male	3.8–5.8	37–51	12.6–17.4
Female	3.8–5.0	35–47	11.7–16.1

Red Blood Cell Count (RBC) (Erythrocyte Count)

Normal Values
Men: 4.2–5.4 $\times 10^6/\mu$l (average 4.8) or 4.2–5.4 $\times 10^{12}$/L
Women: 3.6–5.0 $\times 10^6/\mu$l (average 4.3) or 3.6–5.0 $\times 10^{12}$/L

Explanation of Test
The RBC determines the total number of red blood cells or erythrocytes found in a cubic millimeter of blood. It is an important measurement in the determination of anemia or polycythemia.

Procedure
Automated electronic devices are generally used to determine the number of red blood cells.

Clinical Implications
A. *Decreased RBC Values*
　　1. Anemia, a condition in which there is a reduction in the number of circulating RBCs, in the amount of hemoglobin, and/or in the volume of packed cells (hematocrit).
　　　　(a) Is associated with many factors such as cell production and destruction, blood loss, dietary insufficiency of iron and certain vitamins which are essential in the production of RBCs.

See pages 53 and 56 for classification of anemias based upon the underlying mechanisms of anemia and for the discussion of the purpose and the clinical implications of the reticulocyte count (pp 51–52).
(b) Disorders such as:
   (1) Hodgkin's disease
   (2) Multiple myeloma
   (3) Leukemia
   (4) Lupus erythematosus
   (5) Addison's disease
   (6) Rheumatic fever
   (7) Subacute endocarditis
   (8) List not meant to be all-inclusive

Clinical Alert

1. Refer to pages 00 and 00 for a discussion of the composite of the clinical implications of *decreased* RBC count, hematocrit, and hemoglobin values (closely related but different ways to look at the adequacy of RBC production). The same underlying conditions will cause a decrease in each of these three tests of red blood cell production.

B. *Increased RBC Values*
1. Polycythemia, a condition in which there is an increase in the number of red blood cells above normal.
  (a) The term polycythemia means many blood cells and usually refers to increased red cell mass. A better term is erythremia or erythrocytosis.
  (b) Is associated with many factors such as overproduction of RBCs and decrease in plasma value.
  (c) Conditions such as:
    (1) Dehydration
    (2) Acute poisoning
    (3) Severe diarrhea
    (4) Pulmonary fibroses
    (5) During and immediately following hemorrhage

Clinical Alert

Please refer to page 48 for discussion of the combined clinical implications of *increased* RBC count, hematocrit, and hemoglobin values (as stated above, closely related but different ways to look at the adequacy of RBC production). The same underlying conditions will cause an increase in each of these three tests of red blood cell production.

Interfering Factors
Physiological Variation
1. Posture: When blood sample is obtained from a healthy person in a recumbent position, the count is lower than normal. (If the patient is anemic, the count will be even lower.)
2. Exercise: Extreme exercise and excitement produce higher counts than those obtained under basal conditions. Counts obtained under these conditions are of doubtful clinical value.
3. Dehydration: Hemoconcentration in dehydrated adults due to severe burns, untreated intestinal obstruction, and severe, persistent vomiting may obscure significant anemia.
4. Age: The normal RBC of a newborn is higher than that of an adult with a rapid drop to the lowest point in life at 2 to 4 months. The normal adult level is reached at age 14 and is maintained until old age, where there is a gradual drop. (See page 41.)
5. Altitude: The higher the altitude, the greater the increase in RBC. Decreased oxygen content of the air stimulates the RBC to rise (erythrocytosis).
6. Pregnancy: There is a normal decrease in RBC when the body fluid increases in pregnancy with the normal number of erythrocytes becoming more diluted.
7. There are many drugs that may cause *reduced* RBCs.
8. Among the drugs that may cause *increased* RBCs are gentamicin and methyldopa.

Hematocrit (HCT); Packed Cell Volume (PCV)

Normal Values
Men: 40%–54% packed red cell volume (varies widely) or 0.40–0.54 volume fraction
Women: 37%–47% or 0.37–0.47
Newborn (both genders): 50%–62% or 0.50–0.62

Microhematocrit (done on small amount of blood, usually drawn from finger prick)
Men: 45%–47% packed red cell volume or 0.45–0.47 volume fraction
Women: 42%–44% or 0.42–0.44
Infants: 44%–62% or 0.44–0.62

Explanation of Test

The purpose of this test is to determine the red blood cell mass by measuring space occupied by packed red blood cells. The results are expressed as the percentage of red cells in a volume of whole blood. The word *hematocrit* means "to separate blood," which underscores the mechanism of the test, because the plasma and blood cells are separated by centrifugation. It is an important measurement in the determination of anemia or polycythemia.

Procedure

The tube used in this test is a capillary hematocrit tube, which is two thirds filled with venous blood to which an anticoagulant has been added. The tube is then centrifuged to separate the cellular elements from the plasma. The height of the packed cells in the tube indicates the hematocrit. The measure is recorded in terms of the volume of cells found in 100 ml of blood and is expressed as a percentage of the total amount of blood centrifuged.

Clinical Implications

1. *Decreased hematocrit values* are an indicator of anemia, a condition where there is a reduction in the hematocrit (volume of packed cells), amount of hemoglobin, and the number of circulating RBCs.
    (a) An hematocrit of 30 or less means the patient is moderately to severely anemic.
    (b) Leukemia
    (c) Hyperthyroidism
    (d) Cirrhosis
    (e) Acute, massive blood loss
    (f) Hemolytic reaction—This condition may be found in
        (1) Transfusion of incompatible blood
        (2) Reaction to chemicals or drugs
        (3) Reaction to infectious agents
        (4) Reaction to physical agents, *e.g.,* severe burn or prosthetic heart valves
2. The hematocrit may or may not be reliable immediately after even a moderate loss of blood and immediately after transfusions. For example, even though Hgb and Hct are accepted ways of monitoring how a patient is coming along after treatment, they can be considered unreliable if the patient is continuing to lose blood; however, Hct is a good indicator of how much blood has been lost up to the time the blood sample is obtained.
3. Hematocrit may be normal following acute hemorrhage. During the recovery phase, the Hct and RBC will drop markedly.
4. Usually, the hematocrit parallels the RBC when the cells are of a normal size. As the number of normal-sized erythrocytes increases, so does the hematocrit.

(a) However, for the patient with microcytic or macrocytic anemia, this relationship does not hold true.
(b) If a patient has an iron-deficiency anemia with small red cells, the hematocrit decreases because the microcytic cells pack to a smaller volume. The RBC, however, may be normal.

Clinical Alert

Please refer to pages 49–50 for a discussion of the combined clinical implications of *decreased* hematocrit, hemoglobin, and RBC count (closely related but different ways to look at the adequacy of RBC production. The same underlying conditions will cause a decrease in each of these three tests' values).

1. *Increased hematocrit.*
    (a) Polycythemia, an increase in the number of RBCs that is based upon the hematocrit and hemoglobin values
    (b) Erythrocytosis
    (c) Severe dehydration
    (d) Shock, when hemoconcentrates rise considerably

Clinical Alert

Please refer to pages 48–49 for a discussion of the combined clinical implications of *increased* hematocrit and hemoglobin (closely related tests done to determine RBC mass).

Interfering Factors
People living in high altitudes will have high values, the same as in Hgb.

1. Normally, the value slightly decreases in the physiologic hydremia of pregnancy.
2. The normal values for the hematocrit vary with the age and sex of the individual. The normal value for infants is higher because the newborn has many macrocytic red cells. Hcts in females are usually slightly lower than in males.
3. There is also a tendency toward lower values in men and women after age 50, corresponding to lower values for erythrocyte counts in this age group.

Hemoglobin (Hgb)

Normal Values
Women: 12–16 g/dl or 1.86–2.48 nmol/L
Men: 13.5–17.5 g/dl or 2.09–2.71 nmol/L
Newborn (both genders): 14–20 g/dl

Varies widely according to the standard used.

Background
Hemoglobin, the main component of erythrocytes, serves as the vehicle for the transportation of oxygen and carbon dioxide. It is composed of (1) amino acids that form a single protein called *globin*, and (2) a compound called *heme*, which contains iron atoms and the red pigment porphyrin.

The iron pigment is that portion of the hemoglobin that combines readily with oxygen and gives blood its characteristic red color.

Each gram of hemoglobin can carry 1.34 ml of oxygen. The oxygen-combining capacity of the blood is directly proportional to the hemoglobin concentration rather than to the RBC, because some red cells contain more hemoglobin than others. This is why hemoglobin determinations are more important in the evaluation of anemia than the RBC.

Although oxygen transport is the main function of hemoglobin, it also serves as an important buffer in the extracellular fluid. In tissue, the oxygen concentration is lower, and the carbon dioxide level and hydrogen ion concentration are higher. At a lower pH, more oxygen dissociates from hemoglobin. The unoxygenated hemoglobin binds to hydrogen ion, thus raising the pH. As carbon dioxide diffuses into the red cell, carbonic anhydrase converts carbon dioxide to bicarbonate and protons. As the protons are bound to hemoglobin, the bicarbonate ions leave the cell. For every bicarbonate ion leaving the cell, a chloride ion enters. The efficiency of this buffer system depends upon the ability of carbon dioxide or bicarbonate to be eliminated in the lungs and kidneys, respectively.

Explanation of Test
The hemoglobin determination test is used to

1. Screen for disease associated with anemia
2. Determine the severity of anemia
3. Follow the response to treatment for anemia
4. Evaluate polycythemia

Procedure
A venous blood EDTA sample of 2 ml is obtained. Automated electronic devices are generally used to determine the Hgb; however, a manual colorimetric procedure is also widely used.

Clinical Implications
A. *Decreased levels of hemoglobin* found in
1. Anemia states (a condition when there is a reduction of hemoglobin, hematocrit, and/or RBC numbers). It is difficult to say explicitly what hemoglobin level represents the presence of anemia *per se*, because of the variable adaptability and efficiency of the body in response to blood hemoglobin concentrations.
An arbitrary level of 12 g is acceptable.
   (a) This level must be evaluated along with the erythrocyte count and the hematocrit.
2. Hyperthyroidism
3. Cirrhosis of the liver
4. Severe hemorrhage
5. Hemolytic reactions due to
   (a) Transfusions of incompatible blood
   (b) Reactions to chemicals and drugs
   (c) Reactions to infectious agents
   (d) Reactions to physical agents (severe burns and artificial heart valves)
   (e) Various systemic diseases
      (1) Hodgkin's disease
      (2) Leukemia
      (3) Lymphoma
      (4) Systemic lupus erythematosus
      (5) Carcinomatosis
      (6) Sarcoidosis
      (7) Renal cortical necrosis
      (8) List not meant to be all inclusive.

Clinical Alert

Please refer to pages 49–50 for a discussion of the combined clinical implications of *decreased* hemoglobin, hematocrit, and RBC count (closely related but different ways to look at the adequacy of RBC production. The same underlying conditions will cause a decrease in each of these test values).

B. *Increased levels of hemoglobin* found in
1. Hemoconcentration of the blood (any condition such as polycythemia and severe burns in which the number of circulating erythrocytes rises above normal)
2. Chronic obstructive pulmonary disease
3. Congestive heart failure

C. *Variance in levels of hemoglobin*
   1. After transfusions, hemorrhages, burns. (Hgb and Hct are both high during and immediately after hemorrhage.)
   2. Hgb and Hct give valuable information in an emergency situation if interpreted not in an isolated fashion but in conjunction with other pertinent laboratory data. There are very few tests in laboratory medicine that can be regarded as diagnostic all on their own.

Clinical Alert

Please refer to pages 48–49 for a discussion of the combined clinical implications of an *increased* hemoglobin, increased hematocrit, and RBC numbers (closely related tests done to determine the RBC mass).

Interfering Factors
1. People living at high altitudes will have increased values, as in hematocrit values.
2. Excessive fluid intake will cause a decreased value.
3. Normally, the value is higher in infants before active erythropoiesis begins.
4. Hemoglobin levels are normally decreased in pregnancy.
5. Drugs that may cause *increased* levels of hemoglobin include gentamicin and methyldopa.
6. There are many drugs that may cause *decreased* levels of hemoglobin.

Clinical Alert

Panic value is <5.0 g/dl; leads to heart failure and death.

Clinical Implications: *Polycythemia, Increased RBC Count, Hematocrit, and/or Hemoglobin Values*
A. Polycythemia is the term used to describe an increase in the number of red blood cells above normal. While there are a number of tests to determine the red blood cell mass, these tests are expensive and somewhat cumbersome. For screening purposes, we rely on the hematocrit and hemoglobin to evaluate polycythemia.

B. *Classification of Polycythemias**
1. Relative—an increase in hemoglobin or hematocrit caused by a decrease in the plasma volume.
   a. Dehydration
   b. Spurious (stress or smoker) erythrocytosis
2. Absolute or true polycythemia
   a. Primary
      (1) Polycythemia vera
      (2) Erythremia/erythrocytosis
   b. Secondary
      (1) Appropriate—an appropriate bone marrow response to physiological conditions
         (a) Altitude
         (b) Cardiopulmonary disorder
         (c) Increased affinity for oxygen
      (2) Inappropriate—an overproduction of red cells not necessary to deliver oxygen to the tissues
         (a) Renal tumor or cyst
         (b) Hepatoma
         (c) Cerebellar hemangioblastoma
   c. Essential

Clinical Implications: *Anemia, Decreased RBC Count, Hematocrit, and Hemoglobin Values*

A. Anemia is the term used to describe a condition in which there is a reduction in the number of circulating RBC, in the amount of hemoglobin, and/or in the volume of packed cells (hematocrit). A pathophysiologic classification of anemia based upon the underlying mechanisms of anemias follows. Anemias are further explained on pages 53–56.
B. Classification of Anemias†
   1. Hypoproliferative anemias—inadequate production of red blood cells
      (a) Marrow aplasias
      (b) Myelophthistic anemia
      (c) Anemia with blood dyscrasias
      (d) Anemia of chronic disease
      (e) Anemia with organ failure

---

* Adapted from Williams WJ, Beulter E, Erslen AJ, and Lechtman MA (eds): Hematology, 4th ed. New York, McGraw–Hill, 1990
† (Adapted from Wyngaarden JB and Smith LH: Cecil's Textbook of Medicine, 18th ed. Philadelphia, WB Saunders, 1988)

(1) Renal failure   (3) Hypothyroidism
(2) Hepatic failure   (4) Hypopituitarism

2. Maturation defect anemias
   (a) Cytoplasmic—hypochromic anemias
   (b) Nuclear—megaloblastic anemias
   (c) Combined—myelodysplastic syndromes
3. Hyperproliferative anemias—decrease in the hemoglobin or hematocrit in spite of an increased production of RBCs.
   (a) Hemorrhagic—acute blood loss
   (b) Hemolytic—a premature accelerated destruction of the RBCs
       (1) Immune hemolysis   (6) Toxic hemolysis—physical–chemical
       (2) Primary membrane
       (3) Hemoglobinopathies   (7) Traumatic or microangiopathic hemolysis
       (4) Hypersplenism
       (5) Enzymopathies   (8) Parasitic infections
4. Dilutional anemias
   (a) Pregnancy
   (b) Splenomegaly

Reticulocyte Count

Normal Values
Men: 0.5%–1.5% of total erythrocytes or 0.005-0.015
Women: 0.5%–2.5% or 0.005–0.025
Children: 0.5%–4% of total erythrocytes or 0.005–0.040
Infants: 2%–5% of total erythrocytes or 0.020–0.050
Reticulocyte index = 1.0
Absolute reticulocyte count = % reticulocytes × erythrocyte count
25–85 × 10^3 cells/μl or 25–85 × 10^9 cells/L

Background
A *reticulocyte* is a young, immature, nonnucleated cell of the erythrocyte series formed in the bone marrow. As an immature red cell, it contains reticular material (from organelles in the cytoplasm) that will stain a gray blue when tested in the laboratory. Reticulum is present in newly released blood cells and lasts 1 to 2 days before the cell reaches its full mature state. Normally a small number of these cells is found in the circulating blood (about 0.5%–1.5% of the total red blood count; see the normal value). The number of reticulocytes per 100 erythrocytes yields the reticulocyte count.

In order for the reticulocyte count to be meaningful, it must be viewed in relation to the total number of erythrocytes.

Explanation of Text

A reticulocyte count is used

1. To differentiate anemias due to bone marrow failure from those due to hemorrhage or hemolysis (red cell destruction)
2. To check the effectiveness of treatment in pernicious anemia and the recovery of bone marrow function in aplastic anemia
3. To determine the effects of radioactive substances on exposed workers

Procedure

A small blood sample is mixed with a supravital stain such as brilliant cresyl blue. After the stain is allowed to react with the blood (the reticulum can be stained only while the cells are viable), a blood smear is prepared with this mixture and scanned under a microscope.

Clinical Implications

A. *Increased levels*

An increased count (reticulocytosis) means that hyperactive erythrocyte production is occurring as the bone marrow replaces cells lost or prematurely destroyed. Identifying reticulocytosis may lead to the recognition of an otherwise occult disease such as hidden chronic hemorrhage or unrecognized hemolysis (sickle cell anemia and thalassemia). Increased levels are observed in the following conditions:

1. Hemolytic anemias
   (a) Immune
   (b) Primary RBC membrane problems
   (c) Hemoglobinopathic and sickle cell disease
   (d) RBC enzyme deficits
   (e) Toxin exposure
   (f) Traumatic or microangiopathic
   (g) Hypersplenism
   (h) Parasitic infections
2. Three to four days following hemorrhage
3. Following treatment of anemias (therapeutic–diagnostic test)
   (a) Increase may be used as an index of the effectiveness of treatment.
   (b) After adequate doses of iron in iron-deficiency anemia, the rise in reticulocytes may exceed 20%.
   (c) There is a proportional increase when pernicious anemia is treated by transfusion or vitamin B_{12} therapy.

B. *Decreased levels*

A decreased reticulocyte count means that bone marrow is not producing enough erythrocytes.

Found in
1. Iron-deficiency anemia
2. Aplastic anemia (a persistent deficiency of reticulocytes suggests a poor prognosis)
3. Untreated pernicious anemia
4. Chronic infection
5. Radiation therapy
6. Endocrine problems
7. Tumor in marrow
8. Myelodysplastic syndromes

Interfering Factors
The reticulocyte count is normally increased in pregnancy and in infants.

Red Blood Cell Indices

Background
The red blood cell indices are used to define the size and hemoglobin content of the red blood cell. They consist of the mean corpuscular volume (MCV), mean corpuscular hemoglobin (MCH), and mean corpuscular hemoglobin concentration (MCHC).

Explanation of Test
The red blood cell indices are used as an aid in differentiating anemias. When these are used together with an examination of the red cells on the stained smear, a clear picture of red cell morphology may be ascertained.

On the basis of the red blood cell indices, the erythrocytes can be characterized as normal in every respect, or as abnormal in volume or hemoglobin content. In deficient states, the anemias can be classified by cell size as macrocytic, normocytic, simple microcytic, or by cell size and color as microcytic hypochromic.

Mean Corpuscular Volume (MCV)

Normal Values
87–103 fl/red cell or μm^3/red cell
(Higher values in infants and newborns)

Explanation of Test
This description of individual cell size is the best index for classifying anemias and is based on the visual or electronic counting of erythrocytes. It is an index that expresses the volume occupied by a single red

cell and is a measure in cubic microns of the mean volume. The MCV indicates whether the red blood cell appears normocytic, microcytic, or macrocytic. If the MCV is less than 87 mm³, the red cells are microcytic. If the MCV is greater than 103 mm³, the red cells are macrocytic. If the MCV is within the normal range, the red blood cells are normocytic.

Procedure
The volume of the red blood cells is calculated from the red blood cell count, which measures the number of cells per cubic millimeter of blood, and from the hematocrit, which measures the proportion of the blood occupied by the red blood cells and is expressed as volume rather than percent.

Clinical Implications
The MCV is the basis of classification used in the evaluation of an anemia. Tables 2–2, 2–3, and 2–4 can be used to categorize an anemia and then aid in the orderly investigation of the anemia.

TABLE 2–2.
Classification of Anemias Characterized by Deficient Hemoglobin Synthesis and the Presence of Hypochromic Erythrocytes (RBCs)

Disorders of Iron Metabolism
Iron-deficiency anemia*
Anemia of chronic disease
Hereditary atransferrinemia
Congenital hypochromic-microcytic anemia with iron overload
  (Shahidi–Nathan–Diamond syndrome)

Disorders of Porphyrin and Heme Synthesis: Sideroblastic Anemias
Acquired sideroblastic anemias
  Idiopathic refractory sideroblastic anemia
  Complicating other diseases
  Associated with drugs or toxins—ethanol, INH, lead
Hereditary sideroblastic anemias
  X chromosome-linked
  Autosomal recessive

Disorders of Globin Synthesis
The thalassemias
Hemoglobinophathies characterized by unstable hemoglobins

* *Iron deficiency anemia is the most prevalent worldwide cause of anemia. The major causes of iron deficiency are dietary inadequacy, malabsorption, increased iron loss, and increased iron requirements.*
(Adapted from Wyngaarden JB, Smith LH (eds): Cecil's Textbook of Medicine, 18th ed. Philadelphia, WB Saunders, 1988)

TABLE 2–3.
Classification of the Normocytic Normochromic Anemias
(MCV 87–103 μm^3)

Anemia with Appropriate Marrow Response
Acute posthemorrhagic anemia
Hemolytic anemia (may be macrocytic when there is pronounced
  reticulocytosis)

Anemia with Impaired Marrow Response
A. Marrow hypoplasia
      Aplastic anemia
      Pure red cell aplasia
B. Marrow infiltration
      Infiltration by malignant cells
      Myelofibrosis
      Inherited storage diseases
C. Decreased erythropoietin production
      Kidney disease
      Liver disease
      Endocrine deficiencies
      Malnutrition
      Anemia of chronic disease

(Adapted from Wyngaarden JB, Smith LH (eds): Cecil's Textbook of Medicine, 18th ed. Philadelphia, WB Saunders, 1988

TABLE 2–4.
Etiologic Classification of the Macrocytic Anemias (MCV 103-160 μm^3)

Category	Etiologic Mechanisms
Cobalamin Deficiency	
Decreased ingestion	Poor diet, lack of animal products, strict vegetarianism
Impaired absorption	1. Intrinsic factor deficiency Pernicious anemia Gastrectomy (total and partial) Destruction of gastric mucosa by caustics Anti-IF antibody in gastric juice Abnormal intrinsic factor molecule

	2. Intrinsic intestinal disease
	Familial selective malabsorption
	  (Imerslund's syndrome)
	Ileal resection, ileitis
	Sprue, celiac disease
	Infiltrative intestinal disease
	  (*e.g.*, lymphoma, scleroderma)
	Drug-induced malabsorption

(continued)

TABLE 2–4.
(*continued*)

Category	Etiologic Mechanisms
	3. Competitive parasites Fish tapeworm infestations (*Diphyllobothrium latum*) Bacteria in diverticular of bowel, blind loops
Increased requirement	4. Chronic pancreatic disease Pregnancy Neoplastic disease Hyperthyroidism
Impaired utilization	Enzyme deficiencies Abnormal serum cobalamin binding protein Lack of transcobalamin II Nitrous oxide administration
Folate Deficiency	
Decreased ingestion	Poor diet, lack of vegetables Alcoholism Infancy
Impaired absorption	Intestinal short circuits Steatorrhea Sprue, celiac disease Intrinsic intestinal disease Anticonvulsants, oral contraceptives, other drugs
Increased requirement	Pregnancy, infancy Hyperthyroidism Hyperactive hematopoiesis Neoplastic disease, exfoliative skin disease
Impaired utilization	Folic acid antagonists: methotrexate, triamterene, trimethoprim Enzyme deficiencies
Increased loss	Hemodialysis
Unresponsive to Cobalamin or Folate Therapy	
Metabolic inhibitors	Purine synthesis: 6-mercaptopurine, 6-thioguanine, azathioprine Pyrimidine synthesis: 6-azauridine Thymidylate synthesis: methotrexate, 5-fluorouracil Deoxyribonucleotide synthesis: hydroxy- urea, cytosine arabinoside, severe iron deficiency
Inborn errors	Lesch–Nyhan syndrome Hereditary orotic aciduria Deficiency of formiminotransferase, methyltransferase, etc.

(*continued*)

TABLE 2–4.
(*continued*)

Category	Etiologic Mechanisms
Unexplained disorders	Pyridoxine-responsive megaloblastic anemia
	Thiamine-responsive megaloblastic anemia
	Erythremic myelosis (Di Guglielmo's syndrome)

(Wyngaarden JB, Smith LH (eds): Cecil's Textbook of Medicine, 18th ed. Philadelphia, WB Saunders, 1988)

Mean Corpuscular Hemoglobin Concentration (MCHC)

Normal Values
31–37 g Hgb/dl RBC or 41.81–57.4 mmol Hgb/L RBC

Explanation of Test
This test is a measure of the average concentration of hemoglobin in the red blood cells. For a given MCHC, the smaller the cell, the higher the concentration. The percentage represents grams of hemoglobin per 100 ml of whole blood.

This test is most valuable in evaluating therapy for anemia because the two most accurate hematologic determinations (hemoglobin and hematocrit, not RBC) are used in the calculation of this test.

Procedure
The MCHC is a calculated value. It is an expression of the average concentration of hemoglobin in the red blood cells and as such, it gives the ratio of the weight of hemoglobin to the volume of the red blood cell.

Formulas: $\dfrac{\text{Hgb (g/dl)} \times 100}{\text{Hct (\%)}}$ or % Hgb/cell $\div$ 100

Clinical Implications
A. *Decreased values*
1. A decreased MCHC signifies that a unit volume of packed RBCs contains less hemoglobin than normal, or that hemoglobin has been replaced by erythrocytic stromal material as in
   (a) Iron deficiency
   (b) Macrocytic anemias, chronic blood loss anemia
   (c) Pyridoxine-responsive anemia
   (d) Thalassemia
2. Hypochromic anemia is characterized by an MCHC of 30 or less.

B. *Increased values*
1. An increased MCHC usually indicates spherocytosis.
2. MCHC is not increased in pernicious anemia.
C. *Full saturation*
Occurs at about 30% (greater values are rarely observed)

Mean Corpuscular Hemoglobin (MCH)

Normal Values
26–34 picograms (pg)/cell or 0.40–0.53 fmol/cell
(Normally higher in newborns and infants)

Explanation of Test
The MCH is a measure of the average weight of hemoglobin in the red
blood cell. This index is of value in diagnosing severely anemic patients, but it is not as useful as MCHC because it uses the red cell count
in its calculations, and the red cell count is not always accurate.

The MCH is expressed as picograms of hemoglobin per red blood
cell.

Procedure
The MCH is a calculated value. It is an expression of the average weight
of hemoglobin in the red blood cell.

Clinical Implications
1. An increase of the MCH is associated with macrocytic anemia.
2. A decrease of the MCH is associated with microcytic anemia.
3. Hyperlypidemia will falsely elevate the MCH.
4. Leukocyte counts greater than 50,000/ml will raise the hemoglobin
   value when the hemoglobin is determined electronically.

Red Cell Size Distribution Width (RDW)

Normal Values
8.5–11.5 μm

Explanation of Test
This measurement, determined by automated method, is helpful in the
investigation of some hematologic disorders and in monitoring response to therapy. The RDW is essentially an indication of the degree of
anisocytosis. The size of red cells shows a normal distribution curve.

Procedure
The RDW is determined and calculated by the analyzer using the MCV
and RBC.

Clinical Implications
Changes in coefficients of variation (CV) occur in

1. Pernicious anemia (CV = 12.9%)
2. Posthemorrhagic anemia (CV = 9.9%)
3. Can be helpful in distinguishing uncomplicated heterozygous thalassemia (low MCV, normal RDW) from iron deficiency (low MCV, high RDW).
4. Can be helpful in distinguishing anemia of chronic disease with a low normal MCV (normal RDW) from early iron-deficiency anemia (low normal MCV, elevated RDW)

Stained Red Cell Examination (Film)
(Stained Erythrocyte Examination)

Normal Values
Size: Normocytic (normal size—7–8 μm)
Color: Normochromic (normal)
Shape: Normocyte (biconcave disk)
Structure: Normocytes or erythrocytes (anucleated cells)

Explanation of Test
The stained film examination is the best means of studying the blood to determine variations and abnormalities in erythrocyte size, shape, structure, hemoglobin content, and staining properties. It is useful in diagnosing blood disorders such as anemia, thalassemia, and leukemia. This examination also serves as a guide to therapy and as an indicator of harmful effects of chemotherapy and radiation.

Procedure
A blood sample EDTA of 7 ml is collected. A stained blood smear is studied under a microscope to determine size, shape, and other characteristics of the RBC.

Clinical Implications
A. *Variations in staining, color, and red cell inclusion*
   Normally, the erythrocytes have a tendency to absorb acid stains. The depth of staining is a rough guide to the amount of hemoglobin in the erythrocyte.
   1. *Normochromic cells* are those erythrocytes that are normal in hemoglobin content and color (stains pinkish orange, with a pale central area).
   2. *Hypochromic cells*
      (a) When the amount of hemoglobin is diminished, the central area that is normally pale becomes larger and paler and stains a lighter color.

3. *Basophilic stippling* (the inclusion variation that occurs most frequently)
   (a) Term refers to the fine blue granules enclosed in the cell; they usually represent reticulocytes.
   (b) Basophilic stippling will appear in the stained-film examination of every patient who has symptoms of lead poisoning.
   (c) Except in lead poisoning, basophilic stippling indicates a serious blood disorder, usually related to excessive regeneration of erythrocytes or some impairment of hemoglobin synthesis. It is present in severe pernicious anemia, leukemia, and, less commonly, in other forms of anemia.
4. *Polychromatophilia* (polychromasia)
   (a) Cells that do not take an acid stain, and instead stain with a basic stain to shades of blue; they usually represent reticulocytes.
   (b) Cells that stain in this manner are most numerous in acute blood-loss anemia and hemolytic anemias due to increased erythropoietic activity.
5. *Parasitized RBCs* (malarial stippling)
   (a) Term is applied to the fine granular appearance of erythrocytes that harbor the parasites of tertiary malaria.
   (b) The very fine granules, Schüffner's dots, stain purplish red.
6. *Nucleated RBCs* (normal RBCs do not have a nucleus)
   (a) The variations in structure that are counted and reported as nucleated RBCs (NRBC) per 100 WBCs.
   (b) *Metarubricyte* is another term for a nucleated erythrocyte.
   (c) The presence of NRBCs is an indication of a severe anemia and indicates that the body is making an excessive demand on the blood forming organs to regenerate erythrocytes (increased erythropoietic activity).
7. *Other inclusion variations*
   (a) Howell–Jolly bodies (nuclear remnants, which appear after removal of the spleen, in patients with hemolytic anemias and megaloblastic anemias)
   (b) Cabot rings (ring-like features in the reticulocytes in megaloblastic anemias)
B. *Variations in shape*
   1. *Normocytes* are cells that are normal in size and shape (biconcave disc).
   2. *Poikilocytosis* is the presence of erythrocytes showing abnormal variations and irregularities in shape.
      (a) The cause of abnormally shaped RBCs is defective cell formation, usually due to an irreversible alteration of the cell membrane. It is nonspecific, but it is usually associated with severe anemia and with active erythroid regeneration extra-

medullary hematopoiesis. The hemoglobin content also varies greatly.

(b) Erythrocytes that vary from the normal shape are present in most types of anemia, including severe anemia, and are numerous and most bizarre. Irregularities in shape are especially conspicuous in leukemia and pernicious anemia.

(c) The abnormally shaped cells most commonly seen are

   (1) *Target cells*
      a. Erythrocytes that are thinner than normal with a small amount of hemoglobin in the center (*leptocytes*)
      b. Seen in liver disease, hemoglobin C & S disease, thalessemia, iron deficiency, after splenectomy, and decreased lecithin–cholesterol acetyltransferase (LCAT) activity.

   (2) *Spherocytes*
      a. Erythrocytes that are a little smaller than normal and are round rather than biconcave in shape
      b. Their presence is associated with
         (i)   Hereditary spherocytosis
         (ii) Immune hemolytic anemia
         (iii) Heinz body hemolytic anemia
         (iv) Post-transfusion
         (v)   Water dilution hemolysis

   (3) *Sickle cells*
      a. Erythrocytes that assume a crescent or sickle shape due to the presence of some abnormal hemoglobins, as in sickle cell disease and sickle cell trait disorders: SC disease, SD disorder, and sickle-thalassemia. These sickle cell trait disorders occur when a person has two abnormal hemoglobin genes—one for hemoglobin S and another for hemoglobin C, D, or thalassemia.
      b. They occur in the hemolytic anemias.

   (4) *Schistocytes*
      a. Fragmented erythrocytes with extremely bizarre shapes (triangular or spiral)
      b. They occur in the microangiopathic hemolytic anemias.
         (i)   Thrombotic thrombocytopenia purpura
         (ii) Disseminated intravascular coagulations
         (iii) Vasculitis
         (iv) Glomerulonephritis
         (v)   Renal graft rejection
      c. Severe burns
      d. Associated with artificial heart valves
      e. March hemoglobinuria

C. *Variations in size*
   Normal values: 7–8 μm

   Anisocytosis
   1. Terms used to identify abnormal variations in size of erythrocytes
   2. Degree of anisocytosis measured by RDW (see page 57)

Clinical Alert

Marked abnormalities in size and shape of RBCs without a known cause are an indication for more complete blood studies.

TESTS FOR PORPHYRIA

Tests of blood, urine, and stool are done to diagnose porphyria, an abnormal accumulation of porphyrins in body fluids. These tests are indicated in persons who have unexplained neurologic manifestations, unexplained abdominal pain, or cutaneous blisters and/or the presence of a relevant family history. Test results may identify clinical conditions associated with abnormal heme production. These clinical states include anemia and the genetic (hereditary) or acquired (lead poisoning, alcohol) enzyme disorders associated with abnormal accumulation of the porphyrins (porphyria). Some background information that will clarify the need for testing and the clinical significance of abnormal test results appears below.

Background Information
Porphyrias are a group of diseases caused by a deficit in the enzymes involved in porphyrin metabolism and abnormalities in the production of the metalloporphyrin heme. Heme, a group of molecules that includes vitamin B_{12} and chlorophyll, is required in every cell of the body. Each tissue probably synthesizes its own heme. However, the two major areas of heme synthesis are the bone marrow and the liver. In the bone marrow, heme synthesis leads to the formation of hemoglobin. In the liver, heme synthesis is necessary for production of microsomal cytochromes known as P-450.

The porphyrin precursors of heme are byproducts formed from porphyrinogens. A deficit of any of the enzymes associated with the transformation of porphobilinogen to either heme or coproporphyrin (and the resultant abnormal excretion of heme precursors) can cause accumulation of porphyrinogens and porphyrins and thereby result in porphyria (Leavelle, 1990).

The porphyrias are characterized by the overproduction and excess secretion of porphyrins or the porphyrin precursors, δ aminolevulinic acid (ALA) and porphobilinogen (PBG). Porphyrias can be either hereditary or acquired. Even in hereditary porphyrias, the abnormal porphyrinogenesis is confined primarily to the bone marrow or liver.

Historically, the porphyrias have been separated into erythropoietic and hepatic groups based upon the major organ involved. *Erythropoietic* porphyria (bone marrow group) is characterized by accumulation of excessive quantities of porphyrins in normoblasts and erythrocytes (RBCs) and is associated with congenital erythropoietic porphyria (Gunther's disease) and protoporphyria (erythropoietic or erythrohepatic protoporphyria).

Hepatic porphyria (liver group) is characterized by accumulation of excessive quantities of porphyrins in the feces or urine and is associated with:

Acute intermittent porphyria
Hereditary coproporphyria
Variegate porphyria (South African porphyria)
δ-aminolevulinic aciduria
Porphyria cutanea tarda (symptomatic porphyria)
Toxic porphyria

Accumulation of porphyrins occurs in the blood plasma, serum, erythrocytes, urine, and feces. A discussion of erythrocyte totals and fractionation of erythrocytes and plasma follows. For details of urine, serum, and stool testing for porphyrias, see pages 206 (*Urine*), 242 (*Feces*), and 61–63 (*Serum*). Also, see Uroporphyrinogen in Chapter 6 for other blood testing.

Erythropoietic Porphyrins; Erythrocyte Total

Normal Values
<60 μg/dl packed red cells (normal values reflect heme precursors)

Background
The porphyrins of red blood cells are, in most cases, primarily protoporphyrin and uroporphyrin, and coproporphyrin (occasionally). (See page 61.)

Explanation of Test
The determination is useful in identifying metabolic disorders of the red blood cells, accelerated erythropoiesis, and in detecting and differentiating the porphyrins, along with tests that measure increased porphyrin excretion in urine and feces. Porphyrin disorders, which may be either genetically determined or acquired, result from metabolic de-

fects in heme biosynthesis. Porphyrin disorders are separated into erythropoietic and hepatic types according to the site of the biochemical and pathologic lesion.

Procedure
A venous blood sample is obtained. Washed red blood cells from this specimen are examined.

Clinical Implications
Increased erythrocyte protoporphyrin >75 µg/dl is associated with

1. Protoporphyria
2. Intoxication porphyria that can be caused by heavy metals (lead), halogenated solvents, and many drugs
3. Iron-deficiency anemias

Porphyrins; Fractionation of Erythrocytes and of Plasma

Normal Values
A report is provided in µg/dl
(Normal values reflect heme precursors)

Explanation of Test
Fractionation of erythrocytes is valuable in differentiating congenital erythropoietic coproporphyria from erythropoietic protoporphyria and in confirming a diagnosis of protoporphyria. Plasma fractionation can be used to establish a specific type of porphyria by providing the quantity of a specific porphyrin in plasma. In persons with renal failure, plasma fractionation can help to determine whether the porphyria is due to a deficiency of uroporphyrinogenic dicarboxylase or due to failure of the renal system to excrete porphyrinogens.

Procedure
A venous blood sample is obtained.

Clinical Implications
Increased erythrocyte porphyrins are associated with

1. Protoporphyria
2. Intoxication porphyria
3. Iron-deficiency anemias

Increased plasma porphyrins are associated with

1. Porphyria variegata
2. Coproporphyria
3. Porphyria cutanea tarda

Clinical Alert

1. Caution persons diagnosed with porphyria (with cutaneous manifestations) to avoid sun exposure.
2. Advise persons diagnosed with porphyria (with neurologic symptoms) that attacks can be precipitated by infections, various phases of the menstrual cycle, fasting states, and by certain drugs. A listing of drugs that may precipitate acute attacks follows:

Apronalid	Estrogens	Methsuximide
Barbiturates	Ethanol	Methyldopa
Chlordiazepoxide	Glutethimide	Methyprylon
Chloroquine	Griseofulvin	Novonal
Chlorpropamide	Hydantoins	Sulfonamides
Dichloralphenazone	Imipramine	
Ergot preparations	Meprobamate	

FETAL RED CELLS (FETAL–MATERNAL BLEED)

Normal Values
Negative.

Explanation of Test
A fetal red cell test is done to detect fetal cells in the maternal circulation. The detection of fetal erythrocytes is important in diagnosing anemia of the newborn when it is suspected that a severe loss has occurred from the fetus, but also when there is a serious risk of the mother becoming immunized against the fetal red cell groups, as when an Rh-negative or Du-negative woman delivers or miscarries. In these instances, the mother's blood should be collected immediately after delivery and examined for fetal cells.

Procedure
A venous blood EDTA sample of 5 ml is obtained from the mother. The amount of fetal blood that has escaped into the maternal circulation can be roughly calculated using this formula: milliliters of fetal blood = % HgF cells × 50.

Clinical Implications
1. If the fetal blood loss into the circulation exceeds 35 ml, more than one vial of RhoGAM is required. One vial of RhoGAM will neutralize about 30 to 35 ml of Rh-positive blood.

2. The efficiency of RhoGAM can also be judged by the disappearance of hemoglobin F-containing cells following its administration. If the fetal cells have not disappeared 12 to 24 hours after administration of the first dose, more RhoGAM is required.

IRON TESTS

Iron is an essential element in living cells. Iron can be thought of as being contained in one of several compartments, based on anatomic distribution, chemical characteristics, and function.

Iron Compartments in Man

Compartment	Iron Content (mg)	% Total Body
Hemoglobin iron	2000	67
Storage (ferritin)	1000	27
Myoglobin	130	3.5
Labile pool	80	2.2
Other tissue—enzymes, cytochromes	8	0.2
Transport iron	3	0.08

(Williams WJ, Beulter E, Erslen AJ et al: Hematology, 4th ed. New York, McGraw–Hill, 1990)

Because iron is necessary for the production of hemoglobin, the measurement of iron in one or more of the compartments may be helpful in evaluating an anemic. The most commonly used tests are serum iron, total iron-binding capacity (TIBC), and function.

Transferrin Test; Total Iron-Binding Capacity (TIBC) and Iron

Normal Values
Transferrin: 240–480 mg/dl
TIBC: 240–450 μg/dl
Serum iron (men): 75–175 μg/dl
Serum iron (women): 65–165 μg/dl

Background
Transferrin, a protein and beta globulin, regulates iron absorption and transport in the body. Transferrin (also called *siderophilin*) is believed to contribute in some nonspecific manner to the body's defense against bacterial infection. Serum iron refers to transferrin-bound iron. Iron-

binding capacity reflects the transferrin content of the serum. Serum iron will be highest in the morning and lowest at night.

Explanation of Test

In the laboratory, the quantity of transferrin is measured by the amount of iron with which it can bind. This ability is referred to as the "total iron-binding capacity." In conditions in which the body is deficient in iron, as in pregnancy and iron-deficiency anemia, the TIBC is increased. When the body has an excess of iron, the TIBC is decreased, as in chronic inflammatory states.

Procedure

A venous blood sample of 10 ml is obtained.

Clinical Implications

1. *Increased levels* of transferrin are caused by
   (a) Inadequate dietary iron
   (b) Iron-deficiency anemia due to hemorrhage
   (c) Acute hepatitis
   (d) Polycythemia
   (e) Oral contraceptives
2. *Decreased levels* of transferrin are caused by
   (a) Pernicious anemia
   (b) Thalassemia
   (c) Sickle cell anemia
   (d) Chronic infection
   (e) Cancer
   (f) Hepatic disease
   (g) Uremia
   (h) Rheumatoid arthritis
   (i) Nephrotic syndrome
   (j) Malnutrition
3. *Serum iron decreases are associated with*
   (a) Iron deficiency
   (b) Chronic diseases such as lupus, rheumatoid arthritis, chronic infections
   (c) Third trimester of pregnancy
   (d) Severe physiologic stress such as surgery, infection, myocardial infarction
4. *Serum iron increases are associated with*
   (a) Hemolytic anemias
   (b) Estrogen therapy
   (c) Iron overload syndromes, hemachromatosis, transfusion
   (d) Acute hepatitis
   (e) Recent intramuscular iron

Clinical Alert

A signficant minority of patients with megaloblastic anemias (20%–40%) have co-existing iron deficiency. Megaloblastic anemia can interfere with the interpretation of iron studies; repeat iron studies 1 to 3 months after folate or B_{12} replacement.

Interfering Factors
1. Transferrin is elevated in
   (a) Children 2½ to 10 years of age
   (b) Pregnant women during the third trimester
2. Drugs that may cause increased iron-binding capacity include
   (a) Chloramphenicol
   (b) Fluorides

Ferritin

Normal Values
Men: 15–300 ng/ml or μg/L
Women: 12–150 ng/ml or μg/L

Explanation of the Test
Ferritin is a complex of ferric (Fe^{2+}) hydroxide and a protein, apoferritin. Ferritin is the primary storage form of iron in the body. The plasma ferritin correlates well with total body iron stores.

Procedure
A venous sample of 6 ml is obtained.

Clinical Implications
1. Increased values associated with
   (a) Inflammatory diseases
   (b) Chronic renal disease
   (c) Malignancy
   (d) Hepatitis
   (e) Oral or parenteral iron administration
   (f) Iron overload
2. Decreased values associated with
   (a) Iron-deficiency anemia

OTHER ERYTHROCYTE TESTS

Erythrocyte Fragility (Osmotic Fragility and Autohemolysis)

Osmotic Fragility

Normal Values
Fragility
1. Hemolysis of fresh red blood cells begins at 0.50% saline solution.
2. Hemolysis ends at 0.33% to 0.30% saline solution.

> **Note:** Incubation of red blood cells at 37°C for 24 hours increases the susceptibility of the cells to hemolysis.

Background
A dramatic increase in the rate of RBC destruction can result in anemia. It is important to know if the increased destruction is due to unusual fragility of the erythrocytes, which makes them susceptible to easy damage.

Explanation of Test
Osmotic fragility is determined by exposing red cells to a hypotonic sodium chloride solution, which causes water to enter the cell more rapidly than it leaves. As a result, the cell swells and at some point ruptures, causing the hemoglobin to disperse (hemolysis).

In the fragility test, the red cells are exposed to a hypotonic solution of varying strength, ranging from 0.7% to 0.3%. In each solution, the cells will swell to some extent. The point at which hemolysis begins is noted along with the point at which it is completed. If the cells burst in relatively high salt concentrations, they are identified as having increased fragility. Those that burst in lower salt concentrations have decreased fragility.

Clinical Implications
A. *Increased fragility* (>0.5%) occurs commonly in
1. Hereditary spherocytosis
2. Immune-mediated hemolysis, including hemolytic disease of the newborn

   Rarely in
1. Chemical poisons
2. Burns
3. Spider, bee, and snake venom injury
4. Severe hypophosphatemia

B. *Decreased fragility* (<0.3%) occurs in

1. Obstructive jaundice	5. Polycythemia vera
2. Thalassemia	6. Liver disease
3. Sickle cell anemia	7. Splenectomy (following)
4. Iron-deficiency anemia	

Decreased fragility indicates that red cells have a large surface-to-volume ratio.

Heinz Bodies; Heinz–Ehrlich Body Stain (Beutler's Method)

Normal Values
Negative in healthy individuals

Explanation of Test
These tests are ordered to detect the presence of Heinz–Ehrlich bodies in the red blood cells. Heinz bodies are granules that contain precipitated denatured hemoglobin. Their presence is usually associated with hemolytic anemias and indicates some injury to the erythrocyte due to some type of oxidative activity that interferes with the normal functioning of hemoglobin, such as occurs in patients with glucose-6-phosphate dehydrogenase deficiency (G6PD).

G6PD is an enzyme that accounts for a small portion of glucose metabolized by erythrocytes. When red cells are exposed to an oxidative substance, greater amounts of glucose must be metabolized. A deficiency of G6PD will hamper the ability of the red cells to metabolize the necessary additional glucose and will result in hemolysis of the erythrocyte and formation of Heinz bodies.

Clinical Implications
1. G6PD deficiency is indicated if more than 40% of the cells have five or more Heinz bodies. Affected individuals are often of African, Mediterranean, and Oriental ancestry.
2. Heinz bodies are also found in splenectomized patients who had unstable hemoglobin syndromes or thalassemia prior to surgery.
3. Heinz bodies are associated with acute hemolytic crisis and may be associated with methemoglobinemia.
4. Drugs related to hemolytic anemias
   (a) In hemolytic anemias caused by drug poisoning, 50% to 75% of the erythrocytes may contain Heinz bodies.
   (b) Drugs that have an oxidating activity interfere with the normal functioning of hemoglobin in some individuals.

(c) Drugs that cause this effect include
    (1) Antipyretics and analgesics
    (2) Doxorubicin
    (3) Furazolidone (Furoxone)
    (4) Large doses of vitamin K
    (5) Methylene blue
    (6) Nalidixic acid (NeGram)
    (7) Naphthalene
    (8) Niridazole (Ambilhar)
    (9) Nitrofurans such as Furadantin and Furacin
    (10) Nitrofurantoin (Furadantin)
    (11) Phenazopyridine (Pyridium)
    (12) Phenolhydrazine
    (13) Phenylhydrazine
    (14) Primaquine
    (15) Sulfacetamide
    (16) Sulfamethoxazole (Gantanol)
    (17) Sulfanilamide
    (18) Sulfapyridine
    (19) Sulfonamides
    (20) Thiazole sulfone
    (21) Those used in treatment of malaria
    (22) Tolbutamide
    (23) Toluidine blue
    (24) Trinitrotoluene (TNT)

RED CELL ENZYME TESTS

Glutathione Reductase (GR)

Normal Levels
9–13 U/g of hemoglobin

Explanation of Test
This is one of the red cell enzyme screening tests done to detect the cause of congenital nonspherocytic anemia. A few instances of mild hemolytic anemia have been reported in patients with genetic deficiency in erythrocyte levels of GR. Some have been instances of chronic hemolysis and others have been drug induced (*e.g.*, with primaquine).

Procedure
A venous blood sample of at least 3 ml is obtained. EDTA is added.

Clinical Implications

A *deficiency* of glutathione reductase is associated with

1. Congenital nonspherocytic hemolytic anemia exhibiting either X-chromosome-linked or autosomal-recessive modes of inheritance
2. Panocytopenia
3. Thrombocytopenia
4. Hypoplastic anemia
5. Oligophrenia
6. Gaucher's disease
7. Alpha-thalassemia

Glucose-6-Phosphate Dehydrogenase (G6PD)

Normal Values

Quantitative: 8.34 ± 1.59 IU/g Hgb
Screen: G6PD activity within normal limits; G6PD activity deficient

Explanation of Test

This is one of the tests used to diagnose hereditary enzyme-deficient hemolytic anemia. Hemolytic disease has been associated with deficiencies of nearly 20 erythrocytic enzymes. The most commonly encountered is a deficiency of glucose-6-phosphate dehydrogenase (G6PD). There are more than 50 variants of this sex-linked (X chromosome) condition.

Procedure

A venous blood sample of at least 5 ml is obtained. EDTA is added. A precise assay of G6PD activity of hemolysate involves measuring the rate at which NADP is reduced in the presence of glucose-6-phosphate.

Clinical Implications

1. A *decreased level* is associated with G6PD deficiency, which is a sex-linked disorder. Affected men inherit the abnormal gene from their mothers, who are almost always asymptomatic carriers. In some cases of this disorder, there is lifelong hemolysis, but more commonly the condition is asymptomatic and results only in susceptibility to acute hemolytic episodes that may be triggered by drugs such as primaquine, sulfonamides, and antipyretics, by ingestion of fava beans, or by viral or bacterial infection. (See more complete list under "Heinz Bodies.")
2. The major types of G6PD deficiency are
    (a) Type A, found in blacks
    (b) Mediterranean type, found in both whites and Orientals such as Greeks, Sardinians, and Sephardic Jews
    (c) Rare, congenital nonspherocytic anemia
    (d) Nonimmunologic hemolytic disease of the newborn

3. G6PD levels are *increased* in
   (a) Pernicious anemia
   (b) Idiopathic thrombocyto-
       penic purpura
   (c) Hepatic coma
   (d) Hyperthyroidism
   (e) Myocardial infarction
   (f) Chronic blood loss
   (g) Other megaloblastic ane-
       mias

Pyruvate Kinase (PK)

Normal Values
15.0 + 1.991 IU/g Hgb

Explanation of Test
This is one of the red cell enzyme tests done to determine the cause of hemolytic anemia. Persons with hemolytic anemia due to pyruvate kinase deficiency have no distinguishing clinical features. Deficiency of PK is the most frequent and important form of hemolytic anemia due to deficiency of glycolytic enzymes in the erythrocyte.

Procedure
A venous blood sample of at least 2 ml is obtained, to which EDTA is added. The enzyme activity can be assayed by measuring the ability of hemolysate to form pyruvate from ADP and phosphoenolpyruvate.

Clinical Implications
Pyruvate deficiency may be associated with

1. Congenital inherited nonspherocytic hemolytic anemia with icterus and splenomegaly. These persons will be homozygously affected. The parents of affected patients will be heterozygotes.
2. Acquired type is due to
   (a) Drug ingestion
   (b) Metabolic liver disease
   (c) Myelodysplastic syndromes

2,3-Diphosphoglycerate (2,3-DPG)

Normal Values
Men: 4.2–5.4 μmol/ml of packed cells
        9.2–17.4 μmol/ml of hemoglobin
Women: 4.5–6.1 μmol/ml of packed cells
        8.4–18.8 μmol/g of hemoglobin

Explanation of Test
This measurement is used in the investigation of anemia. An increase in 2,3-DPG decreases oxygen binding capacity of hemoglobin so that increased amounts of oxygen are released and become available to tissues at lower oxygen tensions. The oxygen affinity of red cells is inversely proportional to 2,3-DPG concentration.

Procedure
A venous blood sample of at least 3 ml is obtained.

Clinical Implications
1. *Increased levels* are associated with
   (a) Hypoxia, as in cardiac disease, anemia, and lung disease
   (b) Thyrotoxicosis
   (c) Pyruvate kinase deficiency
   (d) Uremia
   (e) Anemia
2. *Decreased values* are associated with acidosis.

Interfering Factors
1. Increase in value occurs in high altitudes.
2. Decrease in value occurs in stored blood-bank blood.

Erythrocyte Sedimentation Rate (ESR)

Normal Values

Method	Values	
Westergren	Men	0–15 mm/hr
	Women	0–20 mm/hr
	Children	0–10 mm/hr
Cutler	Men	0–8 mm/hr
	Women	0–10 mm/hr
	Children	4–13 mm/hr
Wintrobe	Men	0–9 mm/hr
	Women	0–15 mm/hr
	Children	0–13 mm/hr
Smith	Adults	0–10 mm/hr

Explanation of Test
Erythrocyte sedimentation rate (ESR) is the rate at which erythrocytes settle out of unclotted blood in 1 hour. This test is based on the fact that inflammatory and necrotic processes cause an alteration in blood proteins, resulting in an aggregation of red cells, which make them heavier and more likely to fall rapidly when placed in a special vertical test

tube. The faster the sedimentation rate or settling of cells, the higher the ESR. (As indicated in the listing above, the range of normal values will differ depending on the method or type of tube used.)

Sedimentation is due to the surface changes of the erythrocytes that cause them to clump or aggregate together in a column-like manner (rouleau formation). These changes are related to alterations in the plasma, particularly in the physical state of the plasma proteins.

This test is useful in diagnosing occult disease, in differential diagnosis, and in following individual cases. It is most often used as a gauge for determining the progress of an inflammatory disease, rheumatic fever, rheumatoid arthritis, respiratory infections, and acute myocardial infarction. It is a nonspecific test (not considered diagnostic for any particular disorder).

In many diseases, the ESR rate is normal; in a variety of disease states the rate is rapid, and in some cases it is proportional to the severity of the disease. An abnormal rate indicates a pathologic state rather than a functional disturbance.

Procedure
An anticoagulated venous sample of 7 ml is suctioned into a graduated capillary tube and allowed to settle for 1 hour. The amount of settling is the patient's ESR.

Clinical Implications
A. *Increased values* found in
1. All of the collagen diseases
2. Infections
3. Inflammatory diseases
4. Carcinoma
5. Acute heavy metallic poisoning
6. Cell or tissue destruction
7. Toxemia
8. Syphilis
9. Nephritis
10. Pneumonia
11. Severe anemia
12. Rheumatoid arthritis
B. *Decreased values* found in
1. Polycythemia vera
2. Sickle cell anemia
3. Congestive heart failure
4. Hypofibrinogenemia due to any cause
5. Pyruvate kinase deficiency
6. Hereditary spherocytosis

C. *Varied values* found in
1. Acute disease—The change in rate may lag behind the temperature elevation and leukocytosis for 6 to 24 hours, reaching a peak after several days.
2. Convalescence—The increased rate tends to persist longer than the temperature or the leukocytosis.
3. Unruptured acute appendicitis—Even when suppurative or gangrenous, the rate is normal, but if abscess or peritonitis develops, the rate increases rapidly.
4. Musculoskeletal conditions
   (a) In rheumatic, gonorrheal, and acute gouty arthritis, the rate is significantly increased.
   (b) In osteoarthritis, the rate is slightly increased.
   (c) In neuritis, myositis, and lumbago, the rate is within normal range.
5. Cardiovascular conditions
   (a) In myocardial infarction, the ESR is increased.
   (b) In angina pectoris, the rate is not increased.
6. Malignant diseases
   (a) In multiple myeloma, lymphoma, and metastatic cancer, the rate is very high
   (b) However, there is little correlation between the degree of elevation of the ESR and the prognosis in any one case.

Interfering Factors
1. The blood sample should not be allowed to stand more than 2 hours before the test is started because the rate will increase.
2. In refrigerated blood the sedimentation rate is greatly increased. Refrigerated blood should be allowed to return to room temperature before the test is performed.
3. Factors leading to increased rate include
   (a) The presence of fibrinogen, globulins, and cholesterol
   (b) Pregnancy after 12 weeks until about the fourth week postpartum
   (c) Young children
   (d) Menstruation
   (e) Certain drugs (*e.g.*, heparin and oral contraceptives)
4. The sedimentation rate may be very high (up to 69 mm/hr—Westergren) in apparently healthy women age 70 to 89.
5. Factors leading to reduced rates include
   (a) High blood sugar
   (b) High albumin level
   (c) High phospholipids
   (d) Decreased fibrinogen level in the blood in newborns
   (e) Certain drugs (*e.g.*, steroids, high-dose aspirin)

TESTS FOR HEMOGLOBIN DISORDERS

Normal Values
Hemoglobin A: >95% or 0.95
Hemoglobin A_2: 2.5%–4.0% or 0.025–0.040
Hemoglobin F: <2% or 0.020
No abnormal variants

Hemoglobin Electrophoresis
Normal and abnormal hemoglobins can be detected by electrophoresis, which matches hemolyzed red cell material against standard bands for the various hemoglobins known.

Many different types of hemoglobin result from variations in the amino acid structure of the globin portion of the hemoglobin. The most common form of normal hemoglobin found in the adult is hemoglobin A_1. Two other normal hemoglobins found only in trace amounts in the adult are A_2 and F (fetal hemoglobin).

Of the various types of abnormal hemoglobin (hemoglobinopathies), the best known are hemoglobin S, which is responsible for sickle cell anemia, and hemoglobin C, which may result in a mild hemolytic anemia. The most common abnormality is a significant increase in hemoglobin A_2, diagnostic of α-thalassemia minor. The α-thalassemia trait is in and of itself a harmless condition. A large number of variants (more than 350) of hemoglobin have been recognized. They are identified by capital letters such as HbA or G-Philadelphia.

Interfering Factors
The results may be questionable if a blood transfusion has been given in the preceding 4 months.

Fetal Hemoglobin (Hemoglobin F) (HbF) (Alkali-Resistant Hemoglobin)

Normal Values
Adults: 0%–2% or 0–0.020
Newborns: 60%–90% or 0.60–0.90
Before age 2: 0%–4% or 0–0.040

Explanation of Test
Fetal hemoglobin, also called hemoglobin F, is a normal hemoglobin that is manufactured in the red blood cells of the fetus and infant and composes 50% to 90% of the hemoglobin in the newborn. The remaining portion of the hemoglobin in the newborn is made up of hemoglobin A_1 and A_2, the adult types.

In laboratory testing, hemoglobin F is the only hemoglobin known to be alkali-resistant. Adult hemoglobin does not resist alkali denaturation when analyzed in the laboratory.

Under normal conditions, the manufacture of fetal hemoglobin is replaced by the manufacture of adult hemoglobin during the first year of life. But if hemoglobin F persists and comprises more than 5% of the hemoglobin after 6 months of age, an abnormality should be expected, especially thalassemia. Therefore, determination of hemoglobin F is useful in the diagnosis of thalassemia, an inherited abnormality in the manufacture of hemoglobin, characterized by microcytic, hypochromic anemia.

Procedure
A venous blood EDTA sample of 7 ml is used in determining a patient's hemoglobin type(s). Because the different hemoglobins differ in molecular configuration, they are separated by applying a sample on a cellulose acetate support medium and passing current through this system for a given time. Because of their different molecular configurations, different hemoglobins migrate at different rates.

Clinical Implications
Increased values found in

 1. Thalassemia
 2. Hereditary familial fetal hemoglobinemia
 3. Spherocytic anemia
 4. Sickle cell anemia
 5. Hemoglobin H disease
 6. Anemia, as a compensatory mechanism
 7. Leakage of fetal blood into the maternal blood stream
 8. Aplastic anemia
 9. Acute and chronic leukemia
10. Myeloproliferative disorders
11. Untreated pernicious anemia
12. Metastatic carcinoma to the bone marrow

In *thalassemia minor*, continued production of fetal hemoglobin may occur on a minor scale with values of 5% to 10%. In *thalassemia major*, the values may reach 40% to 90%. This continued production of hemoglobin F leads to a severe anemia. In thalassemia minor, the patient usually lives; in thalassemia major, death usually occurs.

Interfering Factors
If analysis of specimen is delayed for more than 2 to 3 hours, the specimen may falsely appear to have higher quantities of hemoglobin F.

Hemoglobin S (Sickle Cell Test) (Sickledex)

Normal Values
Adult: 0

Background
Sickle cell anemia is caused by an abnormal form of hemoglobin, known as *hemoglobin S*. In this condition, hemoglobin becomes more viscous and tends to precipitate or bond in such a way as to cause the red cells to sickle in shape. The abnormally shaped cells are unable to pass freely through the capillary system, resulting in increased viscosity of the blood and sluggish circulation. This can cause a backup of cells in the capillary system, resulting in a stoppage of blood supply to certain organs.

Sickle cell disorder is genetically transmitted by a recessive gene. When two such genes are present, sickle cell anemia results.

Explanation of Test
This blood measurement is routinely done as a screening test for sickle cell disorder (anemia/trait) or to confirm these disorders. The purpose of the test is to detect the presence of hemoglobin S, an inherited, recessive gene. An examination is made of the erythrocytes for the sickle-shaped forms characteristic of sickle cell anemia or trait. This is done in the laboratory by removing oxygen from the erythrocyte. In erythrocytes with normal hemoglobin the shape is retained, but erythrocytes containing hemoglobin S will assume a sickle shape. However, the distinction between sickle cell trait and sickle cell disease is done by electrophoresis, which identifies a hemoglobin pattern.

Clinical Implications
Positive test
1. Means that great numbers of erythrocytes have assumed the typical sickle cell (crescent) shape
2. Positive tests are 99% accurate.
A. *Sickle cell trait*
1. As an example, definite confirmation of sickle cell trait in a given person by hemoglobin electrophoresis reveals the following A/S heterozygous pattern:
   Hemoglobin S 20%–40%
   Hemoglobin A_1 60%–80%
   Hemoglobin F small amount
2. This means that the patient has inherited a normal hemoglobin A gene from one parent and a hemoglobin S gene from the other.
3. This patient does not have any clinical manifestations of the disease, but some of the children of this patient may inherit the disease if the person's mate has the same recessive gene pattern.

   4. The diagnosis of sickle cell trait does not affect longevity and is not accompanied by signs and symptoms of sickle cell anemia. Sickle cell trait can lead to renal papillary necrosis and hematuria and to an increased risk of pulmonary embolus.
B. *Sickle cell anemia*
   1. Definite confirmation of sickle cell anemia by hemoglobin electrophoresis reveals the following S/S homozygous pattern:
      Hemoglobin S 80%–100%
      Hemoglobin F makes up the rest
      Hemoglobin A_1 0%
   2. This means that an abnormal S gene has been inherited from both parents.
   3. Such a patient has all the clinical manifestations of the disease.

Interfering Factors
1. False negatives occur in
   (a) Infants before 3 months
   (b) Polycythemia
   (c) Protein abnormalities
2. False positives occur up to 4 months after transfusions with RBCs having sickle cell trait.

Clinical Alert

1. A positive Sickledex test must be confirmed by electrophoresis
2. A positive diagnosis of this disorder has genetic implications.
3. A person with sickle cell disease should avoid situations in which hypoxia may occur such as
   (a) Traveling to high-altitude regions
   (b) Traveling in an unpressurized aircraft
   (c) Performing very strenuous exercise
4. Because of general anesthetics and the state of shock-creating hypoxia, surgical or maternity patients with sickle cell disease need very close observation.

Methemoglobin; Sulfhemoglobin; Carboxyhemoglobin

Background
Although abnormalities in the globin portion of the hemoglobin are responsible for hemoglobinopathies such as sickle cell anemia, the ability of the heme portion of hemoglobin to combine with elements

other than oxygen can lead to such complexes as methemoglobin, sulf-hemoglobin, and carboxyhemoglobin.

Note: Hemoglobin *M* is an inherited disorder of the hemoglobin that produces cyanosis. In hereditary methemoglobinemia, the heme moiety is normal, but the enzyme to keep iron in +3 state is deficient → methemoglobinemia Hcbg*M*.

Methemoglobin

Normal Values
2% of total hemoglobin or 0.020
0.06–0.24 g/dl or 9.3–37.2 μmol/L

Explanation of Test
This test is used to diagnose hereditary or acquired methemoglobinemia with the suspected patient having symptoms of anoxia or cyanosis without evidence of cardiovascular or pulmonary disease.

Methemoglobin is formed when the iron in the heme portion of deoxygenated hemoglobin is oxidized to a ferric form rather than a ferrous form. In the ferric form, oxygen and iron cannot combine. The formation of methemoglobin is a normal process and is kept within bounds by the reduction of methemoglobin to hemoglobin. Methemoglobin causes a shift to the left of the oxyhemoglobin dissociation curve.

When a high concentration of methemoglobin is produced in the erythrocytes, it reduces the capacity of the red blood cells to combine with oxygen. Thus, anoxia and cyanosis result. When these symptoms appear without evidence of cardiovascular or pulmonary disease, the erythrocytes are examined in an effort to diagnose methemoglobinemia that may be either hereditary or acquired.

Clinical Implications
A. *Hereditary methemoglobinemia*
   1. The hemoglobin M content may be as high as 40% of the total hemoglobin structure.
   2. Associated with polycythemia (but not with hemolytic anemia)
   3. Possible family history
   4. Treatment includes intravenous methylene blue and oral ascorbic acid.
B. *Acquired methemoglobinemia*
   1. Associated with
      (a) Black water fever
      (b) Paroxysmal hemoglobinuria
      (c) Clostridia infection
      (d) Ingestion of colored wax crayons or chalk
      (e) Exposure to excessive radiation

2. Most common cause is toxic effect of drugs or chemicals

(a) Aniline dyes and deriva- tives	(e) Phenacetin
(b) Sulfonamides	(f) Chlorates
(c) Nitrates and nitrites	(g) Benzocaine
(d) Acetanilid	(h) Lidocaine

3. Exposure to these agents is not always obvious.
   (a) May result from eating Polish sausage and spinach, which are rich in nitrite and nitrate
   (b) Nitrate may also be absorbed from silver nitrate used to treat extensive burns.
   (c) Excessive intake of Bromo-Seltzer is a common cause of methemoglobinemia. (The patient appears cyanotic, but otherwise feels well.)

Clinical Alert

Because fetal hemoglobin is more easily converted to methemoglobin than adult hemoglobin, infants are more susceptible than adults to methemoglobinemia, caused by drinking well water containing nitrites. Bismuth preparations for diarrhea may also be reduced to nitrites by bowel action.

Sulfhemoglobin

Normal Values
Very small amount

Background
Sulfhemoglobin is an abnormal hemoglobin pigment produced by the combination of inorganic sulfides with hemoglobin. Sulfhemoglobinemia presents as a cyanosis. Symptoms are usually not present.

Clinical Implications
1. Once sulfhemoglobin is formed, it remains stable and is irreversible, disappearing with the red blood cells after completion of the 120-day life span of the erythrocyte.
2. Sulfhemoglobin is observed in patients who take oxidant drugs such as phenacetin (excessive intake of Bromo-Seltzer), sulfanamides, and acetanilid.

Carboxyhemoglobin; Carbon Monoxide

Normal Values
0%–2.3% of total hemoglobin or 0–0.023
In heavy smokers: 4%–5% or 0.04–0.05

Background

Carboxyhemoglobin is formed when hemoglobin is exposed to carbon monoxide. The affinity of hemoglobin for carbon monoxide is 218 times greater than for oxygen. Carbon monoxide poisoning causes anoxia because the carboxyhemoglobin formed does not permit hemoglobin to combine with oxygen, and that which does bind is not readily released to the tissues.

Clinical Implications

1. Because carboxyhemoglobin is not capable of transporting oxygen, hypoxia results. A toxic level is greater than 20%.
2. Death may result from anoxia and irreversible tissue changes.
3. Carboxyhemoglobin produces a cherry red or violet color of the blood and skin.
4. The most common cause of carbon monoxide toxicity is automobile exhaust fumes, although smoking is a minor cause.
5. Sixty percent saturation with carbon monoxide is usually fatal.
6. Treatment consists of removal of the patient from the source of carbon monoxide and some form of oxygen therapy. This therapy may be supplemented oxygen at atmospheric pressure or hyperbaric oxygen.

Clinical Alert

1. With values of 10%–20%, the person may be asymptomatic.
2. 20%–30%—headache, nausea, vomiting, loss of judgment
3. 30%–40%—tachycardia, hyperpnea, hypotension, confusion
4. 50%–60%—loss of consciousness
5. 60%—convulsion, respiratory arrest, death

Myoglobin (Mb)

Normal Values

Blood: 30–90 ng/ml or μg/L

Background

Myoglobin is the oxygen-binding protein of striated muscle. It resembles hemoglobin, but it is unable to release oxygen except at extremely low tension. Injury to skeletal muscle will result in release of myoglobin.

Explanation of Test
Blood tests that measure myoglobin are used as an index of damage in myocardial infarction and to detect muscle injury or prediction of disease exacerbation in polymyositis.

Procedure
A venous blood sample of at least 5 ml is obtained.

Clinical Implications
A. *Increased blood values* are associated with
   1. Myocardial infarction
   2. Other muscle injury
   3. Polymyositis
   4. Various muscle enzyme deficiencies
   5. Metabolic stress: carbon dioxide poisoning, hypoglycemia, hypokalemia, or water intoxication
   6. Postinfectious myoglobinuria
   7. Toxin exposure: narcotics, Malayan sea snake toxin

Haptoglobin (Hp)

Normal Values
83–267 mg/dl or 0.83–2.67 g/L

Background
Haptoglobin, a transport glycoprotein synthesized solely in the liver, is structurally similar to hemoglobin. It is the first line of defense for the preservation of iron (located in the heme portion of hemoglobin) in the human body.

Explanation of Test
Measurement of haptoglobin is used primarily as a confirmatory test for the presence of increased intravascular hemolysis. Haptoglobin will increase in any condition that causes tissue damage or repair such as infections and cancer. In this way, it correlates very well with the findings of ESR. On the other hand, a decrease in haptoglobin in most persons with normal liver function is most likely due to an increased consumption. This means that any disease state that can cause an increase in intravascular hemolysis will most likely cause a decrease in haptoglobin. The concentration of haptoglobin is inversely related to the degree of hemolysis as well as the length of time of the hemolytic episode.

Procedure
A venous blood sample of at least 2 ml is obtained, centrifuged, and the serum assayed for haptoglobin by a radial immunodiffusion methodology. A single determination is of limited value.

Clinical Implications
1. *Levels are decreased in acquired disorders* such as
   - (a) Transfusion reactions
   - (b) Erythroblastosis fetalis
   - (c) Systemic lupus erythematosus
   - (d) Autoimmune hemolytic anemia
   - (e) Prosthetic heart valves
   - (f) Malarial infestation
   - (g) Paroxysmal nocturnal hemoglobinuria
   - (h) Hepatocellular disease
   - (i) Thrombotic thrombocytopenic purpura
   - (j) Drug-induced hemolytic anemia (methyldopa)
   - (k) Uremia
   - (l) Hypertension

2. *Levels are also decreased in some inherited disorders* such as
   - (a) Sickle cell disease
   - (b) G6PD deficiency
   - (c) Hereditary spherocytosis
   - (d) Thalassemia and related disorders
   - (e) Hp O-O found in adult blacks

3. *Levels are increased* in
   - (a) Infection (acute and chronic)
   - (b) Neoplasia
   - (c) Biliary obstruction
   - (d) Nephritis
   - (e) Granulomatous disease
   - (f) Adrenal steroid therapy
   - (g) Ulcerative colitis
   - (h) Peptic ulcer
   - (i) Arterial disease
   - (j) Acute rheumatic disease
   - (k) Myocardial infarction (after)

Hemoglobin Bart's

Normal Values
None in children and adults; 0–trace in newborns

Explanation of Test
This test is done to determine the percent of Bart's abnormal hemoglobin in cord blood and to identify α-thalassemia hemoglobinopathies. Bart's is an unstable hemoglobin with high oxygen affinity. There is complete absence of production of the chain of hemoglobin.

Procedure
A sample of cord blood is obtained, and a hemoglobin electrophoresis is performed. There is no hemoglobin A or hemoglobin F.

Clinical Implications
Increased levels are associated with stillborn infants with homozygous α-thalassemia.

Paroxysmal Nocturnal Hemoglobinuria (PNH)

Normal Values
Negative

Background
Paroxysmal nocturnal hemoglobinuria, as the name might suggest, was first described in a patient who noted hemoglobinuria after sleep. In many patients, the hemolysis is quite irregular or occult. Paroxysmal nocturnal hemoglobinuria is commonly considered to be a hemolytic anemia, in which there is also the production of defective platelets and granulocytes. The diagnostic feature of PNH is the increased sensitivity of the erythrocytes to complement-mediated lysis.

Although patients with PNH can present with hemoglobinuria or a hemolytic anemia, they may also present with iron deficiency (because of urinary loss), bleeding secondary to thrombocytopenia, thrombosis, renal abnormalities, or neurologic abnormalities.

Explanation of Tests
These tests are carried out to make a definitive diagnosis of PNH. The basis of these tests is that the cells peculiar to PNH have membrane defects, making them extrasensitive to complement in the plasma. Under certain conditions in the laboratory, osmotic lysis of the cells is demonstrated by activating the serum complement by slightly acidifying the serum (Ham's test) or by means of an osmotic solution of sucrose. Cells from patients with PNH will undergo marked hemolysis after 15 minutes in the laboratory test.

Procedure
1. A venous blood sample of 20 ml is obtained.
2. The patient's red cells are mixed with normal serum and also with the patient's own serum, acidified, incubated at 37°C, and examined for hemolysis. Normally, there should be no lysis of the red cells in this test.

Clinical Implications
1. These tests are almost never positive in any other disease than PNH and are seldom negative in patients with PNH.
2. The tests are performed on patients who have hemoglobinuria, bone marrow aplasia (hypoplasia), or undiagnosed hemolytic anemias. These tests may be useful in the evaluation of patients with unexplained thrombosis or acute leukemia.

Interfering Factors

False-positive results may be obtained when blood contains large numbers of spherocytes and in patients with hereditary erythroblastic multinuclearity associated with a positive acidified serum test (HEM-PAS).

OTHER BLOOD TESTS

Vitamin B_{12} (VB$_{12}$)

Normal Values

Vitamin B_{12}: 160–1300 pg/ml or 118–959 pmol/L
Vitamin B_{12} (unsaturated binding capacity): 1000–2000 pg/ml

Background

Vitamin B_{12}, also known as the antipernicious anemia factor, is necessary for the production of red blood cells. In man it is obtained only from ingesting animal protein and requires an intrinsic factor for absorption. Both vitamin B_{12} and folic acid are dependent on a normally functioning intestinal mucosa for their absorption and are important in the normal adult for the production of red blood cells. Levels of vitamin B_{12} and folate are usually tested in conjunction with one another because the diagnosis of macrocytic anemia requires measurement of both B_{12} and folate.

Transcobalamin is the B_{12} carrier in the blood. Usually, it is only about one fourth saturated with the vitamin. The importance of transcobalamin II was confirmed in two siblings who rapidly developed severe megaloblastic anemia in association with a congenital absence of this protein.

Explanation of Test

This determination is helpful in the differential diagnosis of anemia and conditions marked by high turnover of myeloid cells, as in the leukemias. When binding capacity is measured, it is the unsaturated fraction that is determined. The measurement of unsaturated vitamin B_{12} binding capacity (UBBC) is valuable in distinguishing between untreated polycythemia vera and other conditions in which there is an elevated hematocrit.

Procedure

1. A fasting venous blood sample of at least 5 ml is obtained.
2. The specimen must be obtained before an injection of vitamin B_{12} is administered.

Clinical Implications

1. *Decreased levels* of less than 100 pg/ml of vitamin B_{12} are associated with

(a) Pernicious anemia
(b) Malabsorption syndromes
(c) Fish tapeworm infestation
(d) Primary hypothyroidism
(e) Loss of gastric mucosa as in gastrectomy and stomach cancer
(f) Zollinger–Ellison syndrome
(g) Blind loop syndromes
(h) Vegan diets

2. Decreased unsaturated binding capacity is associated with hepatic cirrhosis and hepatitis.
3. *Increased levels* of greater than 1100 pg/ml of vitamin B_{12} are associated with
   (a) Chronic granulocytic leukemia
   (b) Myelomonocytic leukemia
   (c) Other myeloproliferative diseases such as polycythemia vera
   (d) Liver disease
   (e) Some cases of cancer, especially with liver metastasis
4. Unsaturated binding capacity is also increased in polycythemia vera.

Interfering Factors
Increased values are associated with pregnancy and oral contraceptives.

Patient Preparation
1. Explain purpose and procedure of test.
2. Advise that overnight fasting from food is necessary. Water is permitted.

Clinical Alert

This test is contraindicated in persons who have recently received therapeutic or diagnostic doses of radionuclides.

Folic Acid (Folate)

Normal Values
3–17 ng/ml

Folic acid is needed for the normal function of red and white blood cells and is required for the production of cellular genes. Folic acid is a more potent growth promoter than vitamin B_{12}, although both are dependent on the normal functioning of intestinal mucosa for their absorption. Although fulfilling a different requirement, folic acid, like B_{12}, is required for DNA production. Folic acid is formed by bacteria in the intestines, is stored in the liver, and is present in foods such as eggs, milk, leafy vegetables, yeast, liver, fruits, and other elements of a well-balanced diet.

Explanation of Test
This test is indicated in the differential diagnosis of a hemolytic disorder and in the investigation of folic acid deficiency in altered use. When folic acid absorption is blocked, the liver and body stores of folic acid are depleted, and blood cell production and maturation are affected. If folic acid is deficient, large red cells are produced with shortened life span and impaired oxygen-carrying capacity. Deficiency of folic acid also causes white blood cell abnormalities related to altered DNA or RNA synthesis. It takes several weeks for folate deficiency to develop. The folic acid level must remain at a decreased level for 20 weeks or more before anemia develops. The test is usually done in conjunction with vitamin B_{12} levels.

Procedure
A fasting venous sample of 10 ml is obtained. The specimen must be obtained before any injections of vitamin B_{12} are given.

Clinical Implications
1. The *major* causes of *decreased* folic acid are
   (a) Inadequate intake
   (b) Malabsorption of folic acid
   (c) Excessive utilization of folic acid by the body
   (d) Drugs that are folic antagonists (interfere with nucleic acid synthesis) such as
      (1) Anticonvulsants
      (2) Aminopterin and methotrexate used in leukemia treatment
      (3) Antimalarials
      (4) Alcohol
2. *Decreased* folic acid levels are associated with
   (a) Megaloblastic anemia
   (b) Hemolytic anemia
   (c) Liver disease associated with
      (1) Alcoholism
      (2) Malabsorption syndrome
   (d) Sprue
   (e) Celiac disease
   (f) Idiopathic steatorrhea
   (g) Malignancies

(h) Malnutrition
(i) Drugs mentioned above
(j) Elderly persons with inadequate diets
(k) Hyperthyroidism
(l) Vitamin C deficiency
(m)Febrile states
(n) Chronic dialyses
(o) Pregnancy
(p) Exfoliative dermatitis
3. *Anemias* due to folic acid deficiency include
    (a) Megaloblastic anemia of pregnancy because of fetal requirements for folate
    (b) Nutritional megaloblastic anemia by occurring in
        (1) Infancy
        (2) Early childhood
        (3) Infections
        (4) Old age
            (It occurs more commonly when infections or diarrhea increase folate requirements)
    (c) Macrocytic hemolytic anemia
    (d) Macrocytic anemia due to liver disease associated with alcoholism

Clinical Alert

Elderly persons or those having inadequate diets in this country are known to develop folate-deficient megaloblastic anemia.

Patient Preparation
Instruct patient about fasting from food for 8 hours before testing. Water is permitted.

Sudan Black B Stain (SBB) for Phospholipids

Normal Values
Lymphocytes will not stain with this method. Granulocytic cells will stain with this method. Normal blood is used as a control.

Explanation of Test
This technique is used in the diagnosis of leukemia. The Sudan B Stain is useful in differentiating acute granulocytic leukemia from acute lymphocytic leukemia. Lymphocytes and lymphoblasts (immature lym-

phocytes) do not stain with SBB and are said to be sudanophobic. Cells of the granulocytic and monocytic series contain granules that take the stain and are said to be sudanophilic.

Sudan Black B also stains a wide variety of lipids, including neutral fats, phospholipids, and sterols.

Procedure
A bone marrow aspirate must be taken and a slide prepared from bone marrow. Aspirate is stained with SBB stain and scanned under a microscope.

Clinical Implications
1. Positive staining of primitive cells indicates myelogenous origin of cells.
2. The test is SBB positive in acute granulocytic leukemia.
3. The test is SBB negative in acute lymphocytic leukemia.

Periodic Acid–Schiff Stain (PAS)

Normal Values
No true normal
PAS-positive

Explanation of Test
This staining technique is used to identify reactions to amyloid, a glycoprotein, and to classify immature cells of the blood and bone marrow.

The PAS reaction for glycogen is one of the histologic methods that are helpful in the diagnosis of amyloid diseases such as acute lymphocytic leukemia and erythroleukemia. Amyloidosis is a disease process of unknown cause, characterized by waxy deposits in the liver, kidney, spleen, heart, skin, and alimentary tract. This staining technique is also useful in differentiating erythemic myelosis from sideroblastic anemia.

Methods used other than PAS are metachromatic methyl and crystal violet, thioflavine T, and Congo red.

Procedure
A bone marrow aspirate must be taken and a slide prepared, stained with PAS stain, and scanned under the microscope.

Clinical Implications
1. The test is *positive* in
   (a) Acute lymphocytic leukemia (large blocks of PAS-positive material)

(b) Erythroleukemia
(c) Severe iron-deficiency anemia
(d) Thalassemia
(e) Amyloidosis
(f) Strongly positive lymphocytes in the circulatory blood suggest malignant lymphomas
(g) In some types of myeloid leukemias, numerous small granules are PAS-positive
(h) Megakaryocytic leukemia

Terminal Deoxynucleotidyl Transferase (TDT) Test

Normal Values
0%–2% in bone marrow; negative in peripheral blood or lymph nodes.

Background
Terminal deoxynucleotidyl transferase is an intracellular protein characteristic of certain primitive lymphocytes in the normal thymus and bone marrow. It is believed by some that TDT cells make a special form of DNA, as yet undetected, that plays an important role in the diversification of B and T cells in the immune system.

Explanation of Test
This analysis is a useful tool in the differential diagnosis of leukemia. High levels of TDT are found in some lymphoblastic leukemias and lymphomas. This study may also be helpful in determining prognosis and early diagnosis of relapse. Although no single marker has been found to diagnose acute leukemia, this test is looked upon very favorably by many.

Procedure
1. Heparinized blood (10 ml) and/or heparinized bone marrow aspirate (2 ml) is required for lymphocyte separation.
2. Keep the sample at room temperature.
3. Glass slide smears of blood or bone marrow aspirate, air-dried and stored in a room-temperature desiccator for up to 5 days, can also be used.

Clinical Implications
1. Acute lymphocytic leukemia
2. Lymphoblastic lymphoma
3. Chronic myelogenous leukemia—"blast crisis"

Leukocyte Alkaline Phosphatase Stain (LAP); Alkaline Phosphatase Stain

Normal Values
30–130 units of precipitated dye/neutrophil (each laboratory establishes its own range)

Explanation of Test
This test is usually ordered to differentiate granulocytic leukemia from leukemoid or myeloid reactions. The enzyme, alkaline phosphatase, is present in leukocytes; enzyme activity is represented by granulation in the cytoplasm of neutrophilic granulocytes. High concentrations of this enzyme will be found in normal white blood cells and low to negative concentrations in leukemic leukocytes.

Procedure
A venous blood sample or peripheral finger stick is obtained and a blood smear is prepared. The blood smear is fixed in cold formalin–methanol, then the smears are placed in an incubating solution. At this point, the alkaline phosphatase present in the white cells liberates naphthol, which couples with a special stain to form an insoluble brown black compound. The smear is then counterstained. The degree of reactivity is determined by scoring each neutrophil according to the amount of precipitated dye present.

Clinical Implications
1. In chronic granulocytic anemia, the range is from 0 to 13, meaning that none or little alkaline phosphatase activity is demonstrable.
2. *Values below normal* may be found in
   (a) Acute and chronic granulocytic leukemia
   (b) Paroxysmal nocturnal hemoglobinuria
   (c) Aplastic anemia
   (d) Infectious mononucleosis
   (e) Hereditary hypophosphatasia
   (f) Many infections
   (g) Idiopathic thrombocytopenic purpura
   (h) Sarcoidosis (occasional)
   (i) Granulocytopenia (occasional)
3. *Values above normal* may be found in
   (a) Neutrophilic leukemoid reactions. (A leukemoid reaction is a blood picture that looks like leukemia but is not.)
   (b) Polycythemia vera
   (c) Thrombocytopenia infection
   (d) Myelofibrosis

Interfering Factors
Value is normally increased in pregnancy.

Buffy Coat Smear

The buffy coat smear is not a test per se. This smear is indicated when the white blood cell count is low, and it is done to concentrate the white cells. A buffy coat smear may be used to search for leukemia cells or solid tumor cells in the circulation.

Normal Values
Atypical mononuclear cells ⎫
Megakaryocytes   ⎪ The buffy coat of the blood of
Metamyelocytes and myelocytes ⎬   healthy people contains
Normal white cell components ⎭   these cells.

Procedure
A venous blood sample of 5 ml is obtained, and a finger stick may also be done.

Clinical Implications
Abnormal cells may indicate

1. Leukemia
2. Infiltration of bone marrow by solid tumors or fingers or fibrosis

Tartrate-Resistant Acid Phosphatase (TRAP)

Normal Values
No activity.

Explanation of Test
Hairy cell leukemia is a disease primarily of older men. It is characterized by fatigue, susceptibility to infections, and splenomegaly without peripheral adenopathy. In the peripheral blood, mononuclear cells with hair-like projections may be present. The activity of TRAP is characteristic of these mononuclear cells. This test is done to differentiate hairy cell leukemia from chronic lymphocytic leukemia and lymphomas.

Procedure
A venous blood sample of 5 ml is obtained, and a finger stick may also be done.

Clinical Implications
The activity of TRAP is present in the leukemic cells of most patients with hairy cell leukemia. However, the cells in up to 5% of patients with otherwise typical hairy cell leukemia lack the enzyme. The activity of TRAP can occasionally occur in the malignant cells of patients with lymphoproliferative disorders other than hairy cell leukemia.

Serum Viscosity

Normal Values
1.10–1.22 centipoise
1.4–1.8 relative viscosity

Background
As a flowing liquid, blood is considered a suspension of particles (erythrocytes, leukocytes, and platelets) in plasma. Viscosity of blood is affected by the white blood cell count, the hematocrit, size of red blood cells, and protein composition of plasma. In macroglobulinemia, increased serum viscosity is produced by IgM molecules, which have a high molecular weight and an unusual shape that increases their intrinsic viscosity. Viscosity is further increased by the tendency of IgM molecules to aggregate. Whole blood viscosity may be difficult to measure. Serum viscosity can be more easily measured yet provides useful information.

Explanation of Test
This test is important in the diagnosis of serum hyperviscosity syndromes associated with myeloma or macroglobulinemia. Delayed diagnosis can result in a fatal outcome of a treatable disorder. Because only a few of the many manifestations may be present, this syndrome should be considered in any unexplained coma, bizarre neurologic disorder, hemorrhagic sign, or retinal vein segmentation along with any other classic manifestation of hyperviscosity such as hemorrhage. Also, preoperative measurements of viscosity and volume can be used to avoid complications of surgery in all persons with identified monoclonal gammopathies.

Procedure
A venous blood sample of 10 ml is obtained. The relative viscosity is determined by comparing the time required for a measured amount of serum to flow through a capillary tube to the time required for water to flow through a similar tube. The test is done with the two liquids at 37°C.

Clinical Implications
1. High serum viscosity is associated with uncontrolled multiple myeloma and Waldenström's macroglobulinemia. In a patient with a serum viscosity of 4, symptoms of hyperviscosity *may* appear. These symptoms may include purpuritic and other bleeding, changes in vision, changes in mental status, and other neurologic dysfunction. A relative viscosity between 7 and 8 is **usually** accompanied by symptoms.
2. The relationship between relative viscosity of blood and hematocrit

is nearly linear for hematocrit values above 40%. Above 40%, the relative viscosity becomes progressively greater.

3. The relative viscosity of blood is also affected by the size of the red blood cell. At a given level of red blood cell count, microcytosis decreases and macrocytosis increases the viscosity.

Clinical Alert

Treatment may include chemotherapy of the underlying disorder, or removal of the abnormal protein by plasmaphoresis.

TESTS OF COAGULATION AND HEMOSTASIS
Introduction

A wide variety of laboratory tests are available to determine the nature and extent of coagulation disorders. These tests are generally related to the physiologic response of the body to bleeding disorders, to injury of blood vessels, and to inappropriate activation or localization of the coagulation cascade. Blood flows through a vascular system that is lined by endothelium. When vascular damage occurs, there is immediate reflex vasoconstriction. In large vessels, this vasoconstriction may be the main mechanism of hemostasis. In smaller vessels, vasoconstriction serves to narrow the vessel and to reduce the area that must be occluded by the hemostatic plug. The tissue injury leads to exposure of the subendothelial tissues, and it is to these tissues that the platelet adheres.

Mechanism of Hemostasis and Coagulation
Several mechanisms arrest bleeding: (1) the skin, subcutaneous tissue, and muscle constitute the body's first line of defense and may be considered the extravascular resistance to bleeding; (2) blood vessel walls contract to reduce the quantity of blood flowing through them, and this response is the vascular resistance to bleeding; (3) platelets adhere to each other and to the damaged endothelium and initiate clotting factors; and (4) the clotting factors of the blood react by a cascading mechanism to generate thrombin and to deposit fibrin. Platelet response plus the clotting factor reactions constitute the intravascular resistance to bleeding (Table 2–5).

The entire system of coagulation and fibrinolysis (removal of fibrin clot) is kept in balance by a number of natural inhibitors. Thrombin acts as an activator of platelet aggregation but also attacks Factor V

(*text continues on page 98*)

TABLE 2–5.
The Complex Chain of Reactions Occurring in Coagulation

In the circulating blood, there appears to be a balance between the factors acting to stimulate the formation of thrombin and the forces acting to delay its formation. This balance maintains blood in its fluid state. When the blood vessels are injured or when blood is removed from a vessel, the balance is upset and coagulation occurs. A number of coagulation factors have been identified that are involved in four progressive stages of clotting. The Roman numerals assigned to the coagulation factors identify their order of discovery rather than their involvement in the stages of clot formation.

Stage	Components of Stages	Clotting Factors*
		International Nomenclature
Stage I (3–5 min)		Factor I = Fibrinogen
Phase I—Platelet Activity Platelets serve as a source of thromboplastin.	90% of all coagulation disorders are due to defects in phase I. Platelet counts <1,000,000/mm³ indicate moderate interference with phase I activity.	Factor II = Prothrombin (vitamin K functions in the production of prothrombin)
Phase II—Thromboplastin (Factor III, an enzyme thought to be liberated by damaged cells, is formed by six different factors plus calcium.)	Calcium Factor V Factor VIII Factor IX ⎫ are involved in the formation Factor X ⎬ of tissue thromboplastin Factor XI ⎪ (intrinsic prothrombin Factor XII ⎭ activation)	Factor III = Tissue thromboplastin Factor IV = Calcium ions Factor V = Platelet phospholipids and calcium ions Factor VI = This factor is no longer considered to be a distinct part of coagulation

Stage II (8–15 sec)
Prothrombin, Factor II, is converted to thrombin in the presence of *calcium*.

Factor II	
Factor X	are involved in the conversion
Factor VII	of fibrinogen to fibrin
Factor V	

Stage III (1 sec)
Thrombin interacts with fibrinogen (Factor I) to form the framework of the clot.

At the end of stage III, Factor XIII functions in the stablization of the clot.

Stage IV
Fibrinolytic system (antagonistic system to the clotting mechanism; check and balance system is activated)

Removal of fibrin clot through fibrinolysis Plasminogen is converted to plasmin, which breaks clot into fibrin split products.

Factor VII	=	A coenzyme (stable factor)
Factor VIII	=	Antihemophilic globulin
Factor IX	=	Christmas factor (hemophilia)
Factor X	=	Stuart–Prower factor. Factor X must be activated to convert prothrombin to thrombin
Factor XI	=	Plasma thromboplastin antecedent (PTA)
Factor XII	=	Hageman factor
Factor XIII	=	Fibrin stabilizing factor (FSF)

* Note: The 13 clotting factors of the blood are proteins. They are present in the blood plasma in an inactive form.

and Factor VIII, eventually limiting the coagulation process. A number of antithrombins have been identified—the most important one is probably fibrin itself, which adsorbs thrombin and removes it from the circulation. Antiplasminogen activators and antiplasmins help to control the fibrinolytic activity.

Laboratory diagnostic tests are usually effective in determining the cause of a hemorrhagic disorder. However, judged by the result of laboratory tests, patients can still appear normal and yet have a history of bleeding.

Bleeding does not necessarily indicate a hemorrhagic disorder due to defective hemostasis, nor does the absence of current bleeding rule out an existing hemorrhagic disorder. It is important to remember that the most common cause of hemorrhaging of any sort is thrombocytopenia, the deficiency of platelets. Liver disease, uremia, thrombocytopenia, and disseminated intravascular coagulation disease, as well as the administration of Coumadin (warfarin sodium) and heparin, account for most of the hemorrhagic disorders seen in routine medical practice. Hemophilia is seen infrequently.

Blood clotting is normal when it seals a blood vessel, thereby preventing blood loss and hemorrhage. It is abnormal when it causes inappropriate blood clotting or when clotting is insufficient to stop the flow of blood from the vascular compartment. A bleeding tendency is associated with a delay in clot formation or in premature lysis of clots. Thrombosis is associated with inappropriate activation or localization of blood coagulation. Clotting disorders can be divided into bleeding disorders because of impaired coagulation and hypercoagulability states.

Hypercoagulability States

There are two general forms of hypercoagulability states: (1) hyperreactivity of the platelet system (results in arterial thrombosis), and (2) accelerated activity of the clotting system (results in venous thrombosis). The term hypercoagulability refers to an unnatural tendency to thrombosis. The term thrombus refers to the formation of an insoluble mass (fibrin or platelets) in the bloodstream or chambers of the heart.

Conditions associated with hypercoagulability are summarized below:

Platelet Hyperactivity

Conditions associated with arteriosclerosis

Associated with arterial thrombosis

Diabetes mellitus
Elevated blood lipids and cholesterol
Increased platelet levels
Smoking

Related to (1) disturbances in blood flow and vessel wall changes, and (2) increased sensitivity of platelets to factors that cause platelet adherence and aggregation.

Accelerated Clotting System Activity
Congestive heart failure
Immobility
Oral contraceptives
Pregnancy and postpartum
Postsurgical state
Malignant disease
Obesity and genetic tendency

Associated with venous thrombosis
Related to (1) status of blood flow and (2) alterations in coagulation
Due to an increase in procoagulation factors or a decrease in anticoagulation factors

(Porth C: Pathophysiology, 3rd ed. Philadelphia, JB Lippincott, 1986)

Coagulation and fibrinolysis involve many proteins. As blood coagulation mechanisms are studied in greater depth, the list grows larger. A list of proteins involved in blood coagulation and fibrinolysis is presented in Table 2–6.

Disorders of Hemostasis

A. *Congenital vascular abnormalities*
   Defects of the blood vessel itself are poorly defined and difficult to test. Hereditary telangiectasia is the most commonly recognized. Laboratory studies are all normal, so diagnosis must be made clinically.
B. *Acquired vascular abnormalities*
   1. Schönlein–Henoch purpura in allergic response to infection or drugs
   2. Vitamin C deficiency related to inadequate cementing substance between the muscular endothelial cells
   3. Senile purpura due to loss of elastic tissue
   4. Purpura associated with steroid therapy and easy bruising in females
   5. Vascular damage due to rickettsial diseases, septicemia, or amyloidosis

(*text continues on page 102*)

TABLE 2–6.
Proteins Involved in Blood Coagulation

Proteins	Synonym	Size in Kilodaltons*	Plasma Concentrations in mg/dl (μm)*	Kind of Protein	Function†
Fibrinogen	Factor I	340	300(9)	Structural protein, unique	Gels to form clot
Factor II	Prothrombin	72	15(2)	Vitamin K–dependent zymogen of serine proteinase	Activates I, V, VIII, XIII, protein C, and platelets
Factor V	Proaccelerin	350	2(0.05)	Ceruloplasmin-like binding protein	Supports X_a activation of II
Factor VII	Stable factor	50	0.1(0.02)	Vitamin K–dependent zymogen of serine proteinase	Activates IX and X
Factor VIII	Antihemophilic factor	350	0.1(0.003)	Ceruloplasmin-like binding protein	Supports IX_a activation of X
Factor IX	Christmas factor	57	1(0.2)	Vitamin K–dependent zymogen of serine proteinase	Activates X
Factor X	Stuart–Prower factor	59	1(0.2)	Vitamin K–dependent zymogen of serine proteinase	Activates II
Factor XI	Plasma thromboplastin antecedent	160	0.5(0.03)	Zymogen of serine proteinase	Activates XII and prekallikrein
Factor XII	Hageman factor	75	2(0.2)	Zymogen of serine proteinase	Activates XI and prekallikrein
Factor XIII	Fibrin-stabilizing factor	320	3(0.08)	Zymogen of transglutaminase	Cross-links fibrin and other proteins
von Willebrand factor	Factor VIII–related antigen	800–20,000	2(0.05)	Structural protein, unique	Binds VIII, mediates platelet adhesion
Prekallikrein	—	88	2(0.3)	Zymogen of serine proteinase	Activates XII and prekallikrein, cleaves HMWK

		Size (kd)	Plasma Concentration, mg/dl (μM)*		Function†
High molecular weight kininogen (HMWK)	—	150	2(0.2)	Binding protein, unique	Supports reciprocal activation of XII, XI, and prekallikrein
Fibronectin	—	450	40(1)	Structural protein, unique	Mediates cell adhesion
Major antithrombin	Antithrombin III	60	20(2.5)	Serpin	Inhibits II$_a$, X$_a$, and other proteases; cofactor for heparin
Minor antithrombin	Heparin cofactor II	55	5(0.6)	Serpin	Inhibits II$_a$, cofactor for heparin and dermatan sulfate
Protein C	—	62	0.4(0.06)	Vitamin K–dependent zymogen of serine proteinase	Inactivates V and VIII
Protein S	—	69	3(0.4)	Vitamin K–dependent binding protein	Cofactor for protein Ca, binds C4b-binding protein
Plasminogen	—	86	10(1.2)	Zymogen of serine proteinase	Lyses fibrin and other proteins
Alpha-2-antiplasmin	—	60	3(0.5)	Serpin	Inhibits plasmin
Prourokinase	—	50	—	Zymogen of serine proteinase	Activates plasminogen
Tissue plasminogen activator	TPA	55	—	Serine proteinase	Activates plasminogen
Plasminogen activator inhibitor I	—	52	—	Serpin	Inactivates TPA
Plasminogen activator inhibitor II	—	55	—	Serpin	Inactivates urokinase

* For comparison, the size of albumin is 68 kilodaltons, and the plasma concentration of albumin is 3500 mg/dl (510 μm).

† For zymogens, the function after activation is given.

(Wyngaarden JB, Smith LH (eds): Cecil's Textbook of Medicine, 18th ed. Philadelphia, WB Saunders, 1988)

C. *Quantitative platelet abnormalities*
   1. Thrombocytopenia (decreased platelet count)
      (a) Decreased production
      (b) Increased use or destruction of platelets
      (c) Hypersplenism
   2. Thrombocytosis (elevated platelet level—normal reactive response)
      (a) Hemorrhage
      (b) Iron-deficiency anemia
      (c) Inflammation
      (d) Splenectomy

Clinical Alert

Increased platelets can cause a tendency toward thrombosis.

---

   3. Thrombocythemia (platelet counts greater than 1 million/mm^3)
      (a) Granulocytic leukemia
      (b) Polycythemia vera
      (c) Myeloid metaplasia

Clinical Alert

When platelets are so greatly increased, they do not function properly and can cause hemorrhage episodes.

D. *Qualitative platelet abnormalities*
   1. Glanzmann's thrombasthenia, a hereditary autosomal-recessive disorder that can produce severe bleeding, especially with trauma and surgical procedures.
   2. Platelet factor 3 differences associated with aggregation, adhesion, or release defects
      (a) Storage-pool disease
      (b) Bernard–Soulier syndrome
      (c) May–Hegglin anomaly
      (d) Wiskott–Aldrich syndrome
   3. Conditions and drugs such as
      (a) Dialysis
      (b) Aspirin and other anti-inflammatory agents, dypyridamole, and prostaglandin E

E. *Congenital coagulation abnormalities*
   1. Hemophilia A and B (deficiencies of Factors VIII and IX)
   2. Rare autosomal recessive traits such as hemophilia C
   3. Autosomal dominant traits such as von Willebrand's disease
F. *Acquired coagulation abnormalities*
   1. Circulatory anticoagulant activity
      (a) Hemophilia
      (b) Rheumatoid arthritis
      (c) Immediate postpartum period
      (d) Systemic lupus erythematosus
      (e) Multiple myeloma
   2. Vitamin D deficiency
      (a) Oral anticoagulants
      (b) Biliary obstruction and malabsorption syndrome
      (c) Intestinal sterilization by antibiotics and in newborns
   3. Disseminated intravascular coagulation in which there is continuous generation of thrombin that consumes the other clotting factors and thus causes bleeding
   4. Primary fibrinolysis is the isolated activation of the fibrinolytic mechanism without prior coagulation.
      (a) Streptokinase therapy
      (b) Rarely in electroshock, severe liver disease, and cancer of prostate
   5. Liver disease, in which the extent of coagulation abnormalities depends on the severity of the disease

Disseminated Intravascular Coagulation (DIC)

Disseminated intravascular coagulation (DIC) is a syndrome characterized by uncontrolled formation and deposition of fibrin thrombi. It is an acquired hemorrhagic disease in which there is continuous generation of thrombin that causes depletion "consumption" of the coagulation factors and thus causes bleeding. Fibrinolysis is activated in DIC, which further compounds the hemostatic defect caused by the consumption of clotting factors.

Multiple coagulation test abnormalities found in DIC that cause uncontrolled bleeding include

Prothrombin time (PT) prolonged	Platelet count decreased
Partial thromboplastin time (PTT) or activated PTT prolonged	Fibrinolysin test increased
	Fibrin split products positive
Bleeding time prolonged	
Fibrinogen decreased	

Factor analysis abnormalities found in DIC include

Factors II, V, VIII, X decreased
Fibrinopeptide increased

Disseminated intravascular coagulation is not a primary disease but, rather, a secondary condition caused by another factor. In order to treat DIC, the underlying disease must be uncovered.

The causative factors of DIC include

Septicemia
Malignancies and cancer
Obstetric emergencies (*e.g.*, abruptio placentae)
Cirrhosis of liver
Sickle cell disease
Trauma and crushing injuries
Malaria
Incompatible transfusion
Cold hemoglobinuria and paroxysmal nocturnal hemoglobinuria
Abnormal protein or collagen diseases

In acute DIC, the treatment to stop the uncontrolled bleeding is the use of heparin. Seemingly paradoxically, the heparin blocks thrombin formation, thus blocking consumption of the other clotting factors and causing bleeding to stop. The underlying condition must then be treated to arrest the DIC.

Laboratory Investigation

Generally, a set routine of coagulation studies is followed. Enough blood is collected at one time to provide the specimens needed for the various tests.

1. Usually, at least 20 ml of blood is obtained using the two-syringe technique.
   (a) In the first syringe 5 ml of blood is obtained, and this specimen is discarded.
   (b) In the second syringe 15 to 20 ml of blood is obtained, and this specimen is examined.
2. Coagulation studies, also called *coagulation profiles, coag panels,* or *coagulograms,* are indicated
   (a) In screening of preoperative patients
   (b) With coagulation disorder symptoms such as
      (1) Easy or spontaneous bruising
      (2) Prolonged bleeding
      (3) Heavy or unexplained nosebleeds
      (4) Excessive menstrual flow
      (5) Family history of abnormal heavy bleeding
      (6) Gastrointestinal bleeding

The following sequence of tests is recommended in the investigation of a hemorrhagic disorder (see Table 2–7).

1. Tests for vascular function and platelet function
   (a) Bleeding time
   (b) Capillary fragility test or Rumpel–Leede test
2. Tests of platelet function
   (a) Platelet count
   (b) Bleeding time
   (c) Platelet aggregation studies
   (d) Clot retraction
3. Tests for overall clotting ability
   (a) APTT
   (b) Fibrinogen determination
4. Tests of stage I
   (a) APTT
   (b) Prothrombin consumption
   (c) Platelet function time tests
5. Tests of stage II
   (a) PT
6. Tests of stage III
   (a) Fibrinogen level
   (b) Thrombin time
7. Tests of stage IV
   (a) Euglobulin lysis
   (b) Clot lysis test
   (c) PTT
   (d) Fibrin split products
8. Tests for circulating anticoagulants

The following four primary screening tests are performed in the initial laboratory investigation of suspected coagulation disorders:

1. Platelet count, size, and shape
2. Bleeding time provides information about the ability of platelets to perform their normal function and the ability of the capillaries to constrict their walls.
3. Partial thromboplastin time determines the overall ability of the blood to clot.
4. Prothrombin time measures the activity of second stage clotting factors.

Other commonly ordered tests include

1. Clot retraction
2. Fibrinogen level
3. Factor assays (definitive coagulation studies of a specific factor) such as Factor VIII hemophilia

(*text continues on page 108*)

TABLE 2–7.
Laboratory Tests to Measure Hemostasis

Name of Test	Vascular Function	Platelet Function	Stage 1	Stage 2	Stage 3	Stage 4
Tourniquet test	x	x				
Bleeding time	x	x				
Platelet count		x				
Platelet adhesiveness		x				
Platelet aggregation		x				
Aspirin tolerance		x				
Platelet factor 3 assay		x				
Clot retraction		x				
Prothrombin consumption		x	x			
Lee–White clotting time		x	x			
Siliconized clotting time		x	x			
Activated clotting time		x	x			
Recalcification time		x	x			
Activated recalcification time		x	x			
Partial thromboplastin time			x			
Activated partial thromboplastin			x			
Thromboplastin generation test			x			
Hicks–Pitney test				x		
Prothrombin time—quick						

Thrombotest*	x		
Stypven time*	x		
Circulating anticoagulant factor I.D. substitution	x	x	
Factor assay	x	x	
Thrombin time		x	x
Reptilase time		x	x
Fibrinogen assay		x	
Factor XIII assay		x	
Whole blood clot lysis			x
Dilute blood clot lysis			x
Euglobulin lysis time			x
Fibrin plate lysis			x
Serial thrombin time		x	x
Plasminogen assay			x
Protamine sulfate		x	x
Ethanol gelatin		x	x
TRCH II†			x
Staph clumping			x
Latex agglutination for FSP			x

* Monitors oral and coagulant therapy
† Tanned red cell hemagglutination inhibition immunoassay
These tests measure all facets of hemostasis: vascular function, platelets, and clotting factors.
(Based on table in Kennedy J: Laboratory Investigation of Hemostasis. Dade Monograph. Miami, American Hospital Supply, 1973)

4. Fibrinolysis. When a specific factor has been determined to be low or absent, a factor assay is done in some laboratories. This will give the specific percentage of the factor present. When the problem has been suspected of being in the fibrinolytic system, specific tests provide the most reliable and precise means of establishing an accurate diagnosis. These tests will be performed only in certain laboratories. They are as follows:

(a) Euglobulin clot lysis—identifies increased plasminogen activator activity. (Plasmin is *not* usually present in the blood plasma.)
(b) Factor XIII—fibrin stabilizing factor
(c) Fibrin split products such as protamine sulfate test

The following sequence of tests is performed in the laboratory investigation of thrombotic tendency and thromboembolic disorders. The investigation of hypercoagulable status covers both primary (includes deficiencies of antithrombin III, Protein C and S, Factor XII, and fibrinolytic mechanisms) and secondary (includes acquired platelet disorders and acquired diseases of coagulation and fibrinolytic impairment). There are no ideal screening tests that are sensitive and specific for these states. The most useful tests are of the natural antithrombotic mechamisms as well as the basic studies of the hemostatic and fibrinolytic systems.

a. PT
b. PTT
c. Thrombin–fibrinogen interaction pathways (TCT)
d. Antiplatelet factors such as prostacyclin
e. Anticoagulant factors such as antithrombin III, Protein C and S, and Lupus anticoagulent
f. Fibrinolysis tests such as FDP and Euglobulin lysis time and fibrin monomers

Note: The lupus inhibitor (LI)/lupus anticoagulant (LA) is an antibody (against the phospholipid used in the PT/PTT test) responsible for inhibition of the prothrombin time, partial thromboplastin time, or both. To demonstrate the lupus anticoagulant, one must show an inhibitor is present by mixing one ml of patient's plasma with one ml of normal plasma, followed by a PTT test of the mixture. When an inhibitor of any sort is present, the PTT will not return to normal range. An inhibitor can be shown to be of the lupus type in the laboratory procedure by correction of the PTT by using platelets as a phospholipid source or by demonstrating a characteristic pattern in the PTT that results from sequential dilution of the phospholipid reagent. There is an association of lupus anticoagulants with false positive VDRL reports and another antiphospholipid—the anticardiolipid antibody lipin.

Clinical Alert

Conditions associated with the lupus anticoagulant include:

a. Systemic lupus erythematosus (one third of patients)
b. Other autoimmune diseases
c. Spontaneous abortions with the presence of anticardiolipid autoantibody
d. The presence of this anticoagulant is more often associated with thromboembolism rather than bleeding problems.

Clinical Alert

1. All patients who are known to have hemorrhagic or thrombotic tendencies, or who are being examined through coagulation studies, should be observed closely, and a careful drug history and family history of bleeding and of thromboembolism should be obtained.
2. If multiple vials are being drawn, samples for coagulation studies should be drawn last.

Assessment of Patient

1. Examine skin for bruising on extremities and other parts of the body that patient cannot easily see.
2. Record the appearance of petechiae that may occur after a blood pressure reading or application of tourniquet for venipuncture. These may be the first indication of a bleeding tendency.
3. Note bleeding from the nose or gums.
4. Estimate quantity of blood appearing in vomitus or expectoration, urine, stools, and increased menstrual flow.
5. Record bleeding from injection sites.
6. Intracranial bleeding may develop. Watch for symptoms associated with cerebrovascular disease and increased intracranial pressure.
7. Determine whether the patient has a history of taking coumarin drugs and aspirin in any form.
8. Procedure alert: When a blood sample is obtained for PT, PTT, and TT, sodium citrate is the anticoagulant of choice.

Coagulant Factors (Factor Assay)

Normal Values
Factor VII: 65%–135% of normal or 65–135 Aμ
Factor VIII: 55%–145% of normal or 55–145 Aμ
Factor IX: 60%–140% of normal or 60–140 Aμ
Factor X: 45%–155% of normal or 45–155 Aμ
Factor XI: 65%–135% of normal or 65–135 Aμ
Factor XII: 50%–150% of normal or 50–150 Aμ
Ristocetin–von Willebrand factor: 45%–140% of normal or 45–140 Aμ
Factor XIII Inhibitor: Negative
Factor VIII-Related Antigen: 45%–185% of normal or 45–185 Aμ

Explanation of Test
This test of specific factors of coagulation is done in the investigation of inherited and required bleeding disorders. For example, tests of Factor VIII–related antigen are used in the differential diagnosis of classic hemophilia and von Willebrand's disease in cases in which there is no family history of bleeding and when bleeding times may be borderline or abnormal. A test for ristocetin cofactor is done to help diagnose von Willebrand's disease by determining the degree or rate of platelet aggregation that is taking place.

Procedure
A venous blood sample of 5 ml is obtained. Sodium citrate is the anticoagulant added. Blood is drawn from a normal nonrelated person at the same time to serve as a control.

Clinical Implications
A. *Inherited deficiencies*
    1. All of the specific factors—VII, VIII, IX, X, XI, and XII—may be deficient on a familial basis, for example
        (a) Factor VII is decreased in hypoproconvertinemia (autosomal recessive).
        (b) Factor VIII is decreased in classic hemophilia A and von Willebrand's disease (inherited autosomally).
        (c) Factor IX is decreased in Christmas disease or hemophilia B (sex-linked recessive).
        (d) Factor XI is decreased in hemophilia C, occurring predominantly in Jews, and is autosomal dominant.
B. *Acquired disorders*
    1. Factor VII is also decreased in acquired disorders such as
        (a) Liver disease
        (b) Treatment with coumarin drugs
        (c) Hemorrhagic disease of the newborn
        (d) Kwashiorkor
    2. Factor VIII increases are associated with

(a) Late normal pregnancy
(b) Thromboembolic conditions
(c) Coronary artery disease
(d) Postoperative period
(e) Rebound activity after sudden cessation of coumarin
(f) Hyperthyroidism
(g) Myeloma
(h) Macroglobulinemia
(i) Hypoglycemia
(j) Cushing's syndrome

3. Factor IX levels are decreased in
   (a) Uncompensated cirrhosis (40% of cases)
   (b) Nephrotic syndrome
   (c) Development of circulating anticoagulants against Factor IX
   (d) Normal newborn
   (e) Dicumarol and related anticoagulant drugs cause a decrease after 48 to 72 hours of treatment

4. Factor XI decreased levels are associated with
   (a) Liver disease
   (b) Intestinal malabsorption of vitamin K
   (c) Occasional development of circulatory anticoagulants against Factor IX
   (d) Congenital heart disease
   (e) Paroxysmal nocturnal hemoglobin

5. Factor XII level is decreased in the nephrotic syndrome.

6. Factor VIII inhibitors (anticoagulants capable of specifically neutralizing a coagulation factor and thereby disrupting hemostasis) are associated with
   (a) Hemophilia A
   (b) Immunologic reactions

7. Factor VIII–related antigen is low in von Willebrand's disease and normal in hemophilia.

8. Ristocetin cofactor is decreased in von Willebrand's disease and Bernard–Soulier disease, an intrinsic platelet defect.

9. Factor X is increased during normal pregnancy.

10. Factor XI is decreased in newborns and with use of anticoagulant therapy.

11. Factor XII is decreased in newborns and in normal pregnancy and increased after exercise.

12. Factor XIII levels are decreased in
    (a) Postoperative patients
    (b) Liver disease
    (c) Persistent increased fibrinogen levels
    (d) Myeloma
    (e) Lead poisoning
    (f) Pernicious anemia
    (g) Agammaglobulinemia

Clinical Alert

For meaningful results, avoid Coumadin for two weeks and heparin therapy for two days before testing.

Bleeding Time (Duke and Ivy Methods)

Normal Values
3–10 minutes in most laboratories
Duke method < 8 minutes (usually 1–3 minutes)—earlobe
Ivy method 2–9.5 minutes—forearm

Explanation of Test
Bleeding time measures the primary phase of hemostasis: the interaction of the platelet with the blood vessel wall and the formation of the hemostatic plug. This is one of the four primary screening tests for coagulation disorders. A small stab wound is made in either the earlobe or forearm; the bleeding time is recorded, and a measurement is made of the rate at which a platelet clot is formed. The duration of bleeding from a punctured capillary depends upon the quantity and quality of platelets and the ability of the blood vessel wall to constrict.

The bleeding time test is of significant value in detecting vascular abnormalities and of moderate value in detecting platelet abnormalities or deficiencies. Its principal use today is in the diagnosis of von Willebrand's disease, an inherited defective molecule of Factor VIII, and a type of pseudohemophilia. It has been established that aspirin may cause bleeding in some normal persons, but the bleeding time has not proved to be consistently valuable in identifying such persons. Although the bleeding time is classically recognized as prolonged in thrombocytopenia, the test is an indirect method of identifying the condition. A stained red cell examination and platelet count are more effective than bleeding time in confirming the diagnosis of thrombocytopenia.

Procedure
Two procedures, the Duke method and the Ivy method, are followed.

Duke Method
In the modified Duke method, the area used for puncture is just above the rounded, fatty portion of the earlobe, which is highly vascular.

1. The ear is quickly pierced with a hemolet ("ear sticker") to make a wound 1 to 2 mm deep.

2. A stopwatch is started. Pressure should not be exerted on the ear to initiate bleeding.
3. The blood should be allowed to fall freely on 4″ × 4″ gauze sponges or filter paper.
4. The blood is blotted every 30 seconds until all bleeding has stopped. The wound itself is not disturbed.

Ivy Method
In the Ivy method, the area three finger-widths below the antecubital space is cleansed with alcohol and allowed to dry.

1. A blood pressure cuff is placed on the arm above the elbow and inflated to 40 mm of mercury.
2. A cleansed area of the forearm without superficial veins is selected. The skin is stretched laterally and tautly between the thumb and forefinger.
3. The skin is punctured with a sterile disposable device to a uniform depth of 5 mm and width of 1 mm.
4. A stopwatch is started. The edge of a 4″ × 4″ filter paper is used to blot the blood through capillary action by gently touching the drop every 30 seconds. The wound itself is not disturbed. The blood pressure gauge is removed when bleeding stops spontaneously and a sterile dressing is applied.

The results of both procedures are reported in this way: The end point is reached when blood is no longer blotted from the ear or forearm puncture.

Clinical Implications
1. Bleeding time is prolonged when the level of platelets is decreased or when the platelets are qualitatively abnormal, as in
   (a) Thrombocytopenia
   (b) Platelet dysfunction syndromes
   (c) Decrease or abnormality in plasma factors such as von Willebrand's factor and fibrinogen
   (d) Abnormalities in walls of the small blood vessels
   (e) Vascular defects
   (f) Severe liver disease
   (g) Leukemia
   (h) Aplastic anemia
   (i) DIC disease
2. Bleeding time can be either normal or prolonged in von Willebrand's disease. It will definitely be prolonged if aspirin is administered prior to testing.
3. A single prolonged bleeding time does not prove the existence of hemorrhagic disease because a larger vessel may have been punc-

tured. The puncture should be done twice (on the opposite ear or opposite arm) and the average of the bleeding times taken.
4. Bleeding time is normal in patients with coagulation disorders other than platelet dysfunction or vascular disease

Interfering Factors
1. The normal range may vary when the puncture is not of standard depth and width.
2. Touching the incision during the test will break off any fibrin particles and prolong the bleeding time.
3. Heavy alcohol consumption (as in alcoholics) may cause bleeding time to be increased.
4. Prolonged bleeding time will result from the ingestion of 10 g of aspirin (acetylsalicylic acid) up to 5 days before the test.
5. Other drugs that may cause the bleeding time to be increased include
    (a) Dextran
    (b) Streptokinase–streptodornase (used as fibrinolytic agent)
    (c) Mithramycin
    (d) Pantothenyl alcohol

Patient Preparation
1. Explain the purpose and procedure of the test to patient.
2. Warn patient to take no aspirin or drugs that contain aspirin for at least 5 days before the test.
3. Advise outpatients not to drink alcoholic beverages before coming for test.

Clinical Alert

If the puncture site is still bleeding beyond 15 minutes, the test should be discontinued by applying pressure to area. Report to physician.

Tourniquet Test (Rumpel–Leede Positive-Pressure Test; Capillary Fragility Test; Negative-Pressure Test)

Normal Values
Occasional petechiae or none
   Positive-pressure test—Occasional (5–10) petechiae
   Negative-pressure test—1–2 petechiae or none

Explanation of Test

This test is done to demonstrate a defect of capillary fragility that is due to an abnormality in the capillary walls or thrombocytopenia. Positive or negative pressure is applied to various areas of the body by a blood pressure cuff or a suction cup. The degree of increased capillary fragility is reflected in the number of petechiae (nonraised, round red spots) appearing in a given area of observation.

The forearm, wrists, hands, and fingers are examined for petechiae. The distribution of petechiae is usually irregular, and no effort is made to count the number in a given area. The test is graded 1+ to 4+, depending on whether there are few or many spots.

Procedure

1. In the positive-pressure tourniquet test, a blood pressure cuff is applied to the upper arm and inflated to 70 to 90 mm of mercury or to midway between the patient's systolic and diastolic pressure. The inflated cuff is removed after 5 minutes. The arm, wrist, and hand are then inspected for petechiae.
2. In the negative-pressure test, a lubricated suction cup 2 cm in diameter is applied to the skin of the upper arm. Pressure is applied to the skin for 1 minute. The suction cup is released and 5 minutes later the skin is inspected for petechiae. (This is not commonly done, but a description is included here because it is referred to in the literature about bleeding disorders.)

Clinical Implications

1. Increased petechiae formation occurs most commonly in thrombocytopenia and less commonly in (a) thrombasthenia, (b) vascular purpura, (c) senile purpura, and (d) scurvy.
2. The number and size of petechiae are roughly proportional to the bleeding tendency and possibly to the degree of thrombocytopenia. However, the test can be positive because of capillary fragility in the presence of a normal platelet count.
3. Results will be normal in coagulation disorders and vascular disorders.
4. Positive 1+ is a few petechiae over anterior forearm.
   2+ is many petechiae over anterior forearm.
   3+ is multiple petechiae over the whole arm and top of hand.
   4+ is confluent petechiae in all areas of arm and top of hand.

Interfering Factors

1. Menstruation: Capillary fragility is normally increased before menstruation.
2. Infectious disease: Capillary fragility is increased in measles and influenza.

3. Age: Women over 40 with decreasing estrogen levels may have a positive test that is not indicative of a coagulation disorder.
4. Readministration: Repetition of the test on same arm within 1 week of the first test may lead to error.
5. Variation: Results may vary because of differences in texture, thickness, and temperature of the skin.

Patient Preparation
Explain purpose and procedure of the test.

> **Clinical Alert**
>
> Do not repeat this test on the same arm for at least 1 week because the results will be unreliable. Use the opposite arm for a repeat test.

Thrombin Time; Thrombin Clotting Time

Normal Values
Fifteen seconds or control ±5 seconds. However, there are so many modifications of this test that "normals" vary widely. Check your laboratory values.

Explanation of Test
Stage III defects of fibrinogen abnormalities can be detected by this method. It is a valuable test for detecting hypofibrinogenemia and may also be used for control of heparin therapy. The test measures the time needed for plasma to clot in the laboratory when thrombin is added. Normally, a clot is formed instantly; if not, a fibrinogen deficiency is present (Fig. 2–1).

Procedure
If the test is used to monitor heparin therapy, blood is drawn 1 hour before administration of anticoagulant. A 7 ml venous blood sample is obtained and an anticoagulant, sodium citrate, is added to the syringe.

Clinical Implications
1. No clot will form if afibrinogenemia is present.
2. A small visible clot will form in hypofibrinogenemia, but the thrombin clotting time is prolonged.
3. A thrombin curie can be set up to determine the exact amount of fibrinogen present.

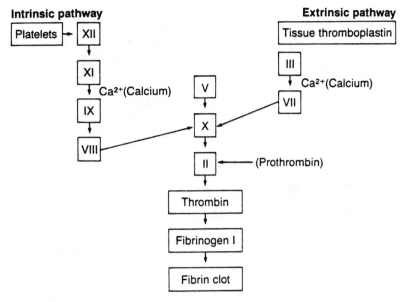

FIGURE 2–1.
Mechanism of fibrin clot formation.

    (a) Normal values—200–400 mg/dl or 2.0–4.0 g/L
    (b) Elevated values occur in pregnancy and inflammation
    (c) Low values found in DIC and liver disease
4. The thrombin time is also prolonged if
    (a) Anticoagulant therapy when heparin is present in the blood
    (b) In the dysproteinemias such as multiple myeloma
    (c) In the presence of breakdown products of fibrin or fibrinogen
    (d) Congenital abnormalities of fibrinogen

Partial Thromboplastin Time (PTT); Activated Partial Thromboplastin Time (APTT)

Normal Values
PTT: 30–45 sec
APTT: 16–25 sec

The basis of this test is fibrin clot formation. Normal ranges vary with phospholipid used.

Explanation of Test

The PTT, which is a one-stage clotting test, is an important and sensitive screening test for coagulation disorders and is of most value in detecting deficiencies of stage II clotting mechanism. Specifically, it is used to detect deficiencies of the components of the intrinsic thromboplastin system. This method will detect not only those abnormalities that are identified by the whole blood clotting time, and some that might be missed by the whole blood clotting time, but will also reveal abnormalities characterized by defects in the second stage of the coagulation mechanism. The PTT is sometimes preferred over the coagulation time test for monitoring heparin therapy.

Note: The PTT and APTT test for the same functions. Deficiency of Factor VII is not measured in this test system. The APTT is a modified PTT that is used frequently to monitor heparin therapy because it is a more sensitive test than PTT.

The APTT is also used to detect circulating anticoagulants. Both classic hemophilia A and hemophilia B can be complicated by the presence of circulating anticoagulants. These circulating anticoagulants are antibodies, most of which are induced in hemophiliacs by the transfusion of plasma from normal persons. The prolonged PTT of hemophiliacs can be corrected by transfusions, but if the anticoagulants (inhibitors of clotting) develop, the PTT again becomes prolonged.

Procedure

1. A venous sample of 7 ml is obtained, using sodium citrate added as an anticoagulant in the syringe. A blue top Vacutainer is used.
2. Do not draw from a heparin lock or heparinized catheter.

   Note: The PTT and APTT are essentially the same test. What applies to one applies to the other. The A = activated. The APTT is slightly more sensitive.

Clinical Implications

A. *APTT*
   1. The APTT is prolonged in all coagulation defects of stage I.
   2. The APTT is usually prolonged in von Willebrand's disease and is accompanied by a consistently diminished Factor VIII level.
   3. The APTT and PT will detect approximately 95% of coagulation abnormalities. When APTT is performed in conjunction with a PT, a further clarification of coagulation defects is possible. For example, a normal PT and an abnormal PTT mean that the defect lies within the first stage of the clotting mechanism.
B. *Causes of prolonged APTT* are
   1. Hemophilia
   2. Vitamin K deficiency

3. Liver disease
4. Presence of circulating anticoagulants
5. DIC disease (chronic or acute)
C. *Shortened APTT occurs*
    1. Extensive cancer, except when the liver is involved
    2. Immediately after acute hemorrhage
    3. Very early stages of DIC
D. *Circulating anticoagulants*
    Usually occur as an inhibitor of a specific factor (*e.g.*, Factor VIII). Most commonly seen in the development of anti–Factor VIII or anti–Factor IX in 5% to 10% of hemophiliacs. Anticoagulants that develop in the treated hemophiliac are detected by prolonged APTT. Circulating anticoagulants also can be detected in some cases.
    1. Following repeated plasma transfusions
    2. Drug reactions
    3. Tuberculosis
    4. Chronic glomerulonephritis
    5. Systemic lupus erythematosus
    6. Rheumatoid arthritis

Clinical Alert

APTT > 100 sec signifies spontaneous bleeding.

E. *Heparin therapy: Protocols and APTT tests*
    1. Heparin combines in the blood with an alpha-globulin (heparin cofactor) for a potent antithrombin.
    2. The intravenous injection of heparin will provide an immediate anticoagulant effect, so it is used when rapid effects are desired.
    3. Because heparin does not remain in the blood very long, the APTT time is measured before each injection.
    4. The APTT is ordinarily maintained at two to two and one half times the normal limit.
    5. To evaluate the effect of heparin, the blood is tested
        (a) Before therapy is started for baseline
        (b) One hour before next dose is administered
        (c) Dependent upon the status of patient (*i.e.*, if there are signs of bleeding); during heparin therapy
    6. Protamine sulfate is the antidote for heparin overdose and hemorrhage.

Prothrombin Time (Pro Time; PT)

Normal Values
10–14 sec or 100% (each laboratory will set its own normals); will vary with type of thromboplastin used.

Explanation of Test
Prothrombin is a protein produced by the liver and is used in the clotting of blood. Production of prothrombin depends on an adequate intake and absorption of vitamin K. During the clotting process, prothrombin is converted to thrombin. The prothrombin content of the blood will be reduced in patients with liver disease.

Prothrombin time is one of the four most important screening tests used in diagnostic coagulation studies. It directly measures a defect in stage II of the clotting mechanism. The clotting ability of five plasma coagulation factors (prothrombin, fibrinogen, Factor V, Factor VII, and Factor X) is measured; this ability is referred to as the "prothrombin time." This test is commonly ordered in conjunction with the management of Coumadin anticoagulant therapy.

Procedure
1. Seven milliliters of venous blood is drawn.
2. A calcium-binding anticoagulant (sodium citrate) is added to the sample or drawn in a blue top Vacutainer.

Oral Anticoagulant Therapy
Oral anticoagulant drugs such as Coumadin and dicumarol (4-hydroxycoumarin) are commonly used to treat blood clots. However, heparin is used first in treatment because it is rapid acting and also because it partially lyses the clot.

1. These drugs act in the liver to delay coagulation by interfering with the action of vitamin K-dependent factors (II, VII, IX, and X). Coumadin is an indirect anticoagulant; heparin is a direct anticoagulant.
2. Drug therapy delays coagulation and causes the PT to increase due to *decreased* Factors II, VII, IX, and X.
3. The usual procedure is to run a PT test every day; after the PT is determined, the dosage of the anticoagulant is adjusted and administered.
4. Coumadin requires 16 to 48 hours to cause a measurable change in the PT.

Drug Therapy and PT Protocols
1. Cardiac patients are usually maintained at a PT of 2 to 2.5 times normal.
2. In the treatment of blood clots, the PT is maintained within the

above range. If the PT drops below this range, the treatment may be ineffective and old clots may expand or new clots may form. If the PT rises above 30 seconds, hemorrhage may occur.

Clinical Implications
1. Conditions accompanied by an increased PT include
   (a) Prothrombin deficiency
   (b) Vitamin K deficiency
   (c) Hemorrhagic disease of the newborn
   (d) Liver disease (*e.g.,* alcoholic hepatitis)
   (e) Anticoagulant therapy
   (f) Biliary obstruction
   (g) Salicylate intoxication
   (h) Hypervitaminosis A
   (i) DIC disease

Interfering Factors
1. Diet: Excessive amounts of green, leafy vegetables will increase the body's absorption of vitamin K.
2. Alcohol: PT is increased due to liver disease.
3. Diarrhea and vomiting: These conditions will increase PT.
4. Quality of venipuncture: It is important that a clean and careful venipuncture is done, otherwise the PT can be shortened.
5. There are many drugs known to cause increases or decreases in PT.

Patient Preparation
1. Explain the purpose and frequency of the test. Patients on long-term anticoagulant therapy must understand the need for regular monitoring through frequent blood testing. *Do not refer to anticoagulants as "blood thinners."* One explanation might be: "Your blood will be tested periodically to determine the pro time, which is an indication of how quickly the blood clots." The dose of the anticoagulant will be increased, decreased, maintained, or discontinued on the basis of this test.
2. Caution the patient to avoid self-medication. Explain that many drugs, including medicines available without a prescription, can either increase or decrease the effect of the anticoagulants and alter the results of the test.
3. Instruct the patient never to start or stop taking any drug without the doctor's permission, for this will affect the PT.

Clinical Alert
1. If PT is excessively prolonged (>40 sec), vitamin K is administered intramuscularly. Ordinarily, intramuscular injections

are contraindicated during anticoagulant therapy because large painful hematomas may form at the injection site. As values get into danger zones (>30) assess carefully for bleeding, including (a) craniotomy checks, (b) lung auscultation, especially of the upper lobes, and (c) occult blood in the urine, using Hemastix (a cellulose strip, saturated with a peroxide and orthotoluidine).

2. Patients who are being monitored by PT for long-term anticoagulant therapy should not take any drugs unless absolutely necessary.
3. When unexpected changes in anticoagulant doses are required to maintain a stable PT, or when there is a consistent change in PT, a drug interaction should be suspected.
4. Blood for PT should be drawn for a baseline and prior to administration of anticoagulants.
5. Protamine sulfate is the antidote for heparin.

Platelet Count

Normal Values
150,000–350,000/mm^3 or 150–350 10^9/L

Phase platelets—the normal value, also as above, can be slightly higher than, or the same as, the standard method. This is the preferred method.

Background
Platelets (or thrombocytes) are the smallest of the formed elements in the blood. These cells are nonnucleated, round or oval, flattened, disk-shaped structures. Platelet activity is necessary for blood clotting.

Function of Platelets
1. Coagulation/clotting of blood
2. Vascular integrity and vasoconstriction
3. Adhesion and aggregation activity in the formation of a platelet plug that occludes (plugs) breaks in small vessels.
4. Ability to take up, store, transport, and release vasoactive amines, platelet factor 3, and thromboxane A$_2$.

Platelet Formation
Platelet (thrombocyte) development takes place primarily in the bone marrow. Thrombocytes are fragments of megakaryocytes, the largest of all bone marrow cells. Megakaryocytes have been found in lungs, spleen, heart, liver, and kidneys. The role of these extramedullary

megakaryocytes is uncertain. The life span of a platelet is approximately 7.5 days. Normally, two thirds of all the body platelets are in the circulating blood and one third are in the spleen.

Explanation of Test

This test is indicated when the platelet count is below normal on a peripheral blood smear. This measurement is helpful in evaluating bleeding disorders that occur in liver disease, thrombocytopenia, uremia, and with anticoagulant therapy. This test is also used in following the course of diseases and disorders associated with bone marrow failure as in leukemia, aplastic anemia, and the use of toxic drugs.

Other tests to study platelet function include

1. Clot retraction—a rough measurement of platelet function
2. Bleeding time—measures activity of platelets, adhesiveness, and platelet factor 3 content or release
3. Prothrombin consumption test—detects a significant decrease of platelet factor 3
4. Special platelet function tests such as platelet aggregation

The platelet count is the most important platelet test because thrombocytopenia is the most common bleeding disease.

Procedure

A venous blood sample of 7 ml is obtained and an anticoagulant (EDTA) is added to the syringe.

Clinical Implications

1. *Abnormally increased numbers* of platelets (thrombocythemia/thrombocytosis) occur in
   (a) Cancer
   (b) Chronic myelogenous and granulocytic leukemia
   (c) Polycythemia vera and primary thrombocytosis
   (d) Splenectomy
   (e) Trauma
   (f) Asphyxiation
   (g) Rheumatoid arthritis
   (h) Iron-deficiency and posthemorrhagic anemia
   (i) Acute infections
   (j) Heart disease
   (k) Cirrhosis
   (l) Chronic pancreatitis
   (m) Tuberculosis
   (n) Recovery from bone marrow suppression

In 50% of those patients who exhibit an unexpected increase in platelets, a malignancy will be found. This malignancy is usually disseminated, advanced, or inoperable.

Clinical Alert

In patients with an extremely elevated platelet count, 1 million/ mm^3, from a myeloproliferative disorder, there may be bleeding because of abnormal platelet function.

2. *Abnormally decreased numbers* of platelets (thrombocytopenia) occur in
   (a) Idiopathic thrombocytopenic purpura
   (b) Pernicious, aplastic, and hemolytic anemias
   (c) After massive blood transfusion
   (d) Pneumonia and other infections
   (e) Allergic conditions
   (f) Exposure to DDT and other chemicals
   (g) During cancer chemotherapy
   (h) HIV Infection
   (i) Lesions involving the bone marrow
   (j) Toxic effects of many drugs

Note: The dose of any drug does not have to be high to have a toxic effect. The development of toxic thrombocytopenia depends on the ability of the body to metabolize and secrete the toxic substance.

   (k) DIC and thrombotic thrombocytopenic purpura (TTC)
   (l) Bernard–Soulier syndrome
   (m)Cavernous hemagioma
   (n) After cardiopulmonary bypass
   (o) Splenic sequestration

Clinical Alert

Panic values—A *decrease in platelets* of <20,000 mm^3 is associated with a tendency to

1. Spontaneous bleeding
2. Prolonged bleeding time
3. Petechiae
4. Ecchymosis

Note: The precise number of platelets necessary for hemostasis is not firmly established. Generally, platelet counts of greater than 50,000 mm^3 are not associated with spontaneous bleeding. Those occasional patients with platelet counts in the 50,000 to 100,000 range will bleed excessively during surgical procedures.

Interfering Factors
1. Normally decreases first day of an infant's life
2. Normally increases at high altitudes
3. Normally increases after strenuous exercise and excitement
4. Normally increases in winter
5. Normally decreases before menstruation

> **Note:** These physiologic variations in the number of platelets in the blood indicate the balance between their production and their utilization, loss, or destruction.

Clinical Alert

Observe patients with serious platelet deficits for signs and symptoms of gastrointestinal bleeding, hemolysis, hematuria, petechiae, vaginal bleeding, epistasis, and bleeding from gums. When hemorrhage is apparent, use emergency measures to control bleeding and notify attending physician.

Mean Platelet Volume

Normal Values
8–10 fL
25 μm in diameter

Explanation of Test
This test provides information about platelet size by an automated method. A stained blood film is also a method of testing that reveals that platelets are of different sizes. This test is done in the investigation of various hematologic disorders such as thrombocytopenic purpura, leukemia, and study of alcoholics under treatment.

Note: Adhesive platelets will be larger than nonadhesive platelets.

Procedure
The mean platelet volume is determined and calculated by an analyzer.

Clinical Implications
1. *Increases* in proportion of platelets exceeding 2.5 μm in diameter occur in
   (a) Idiopathic thrombocytopenic purpura (autoimmune) in apparent remission
   (b) Systemic lupus erythematosus
   (c) DIC

(d) Megaloblastic anemia due to vitamin B_{12} deficiency
(e) Rheumatic heart disease with valve impairment
(f) Diabetes with retinopathy
(g) Prosthetic heart valve plus rheumatic heart disease
(h) Hyperthyroidism
(i) Myeloproliferative disorders
(j) Acute and chronic myelogenic leukemia
2. *Decreases* occur in
    Wiskott–Aldrich syndrome

Clot Retraction

Normal Values
After 1 hour the blood clot appreciably shrinks or retracts from the sides of the test tube and becomes more firm. The clot maintains its molded shape when it is removed from the container in which it has formed. Clot retraction is nearly complete in 4 hours and definitely completed in 24 hours. If clot retraction is normal and complete, approximately half the total volume is clot and the other half is serum.

Explanation of Test
This test is a rough measurement and is used to confirm a platelet problem such as thrombocytopenia.

In this test, blood is allowed to clot in a test tube without an anticoagulant. This test is based on the fact that whole blood that clots normally will retract or recede from the sides of its container, resulting in the separation of transparent serum and the contracted blood clot. Because platelets play a major part in the mechanism of clot retraction, this reaction is impaired when platelets are decreased or function abnormally. This reaction is also influenced by the fibrinogen content of the plasma, the ratio of the plasma volume to red cell mass, and the activity of a retraction-promoting principle in the serum. Results are determined at 1 hour and at 24 hours.

Procedure
1. About 5 ml of venous blood is collected in a tube without anticoagulant.
2. Clot begins separating from tube walls in 30 minutes to 1 hour; clot usually separates completely in 12 to 24 hours.
3. For 72 hours the retracted clot does not change appreciably.

Clinical Implications
There is a distinct parallel between the quality of the clot and the number of platelets. A defective clot is soft and soggy, is readily torn, and, after removal from its container, flattens out as a shapeless mass from which serum continues to ooze.

1. *Poor or decreased clot retraction* occurs in
   (a) Thrombocytopenia
   (b) Von Willebrand's disease when platelets are deficient in quality
   (c) Disorders due to increase in red cell mass
2. *Clot retraction appears to be increased* in severe anemia and hypofibrinogenemia as a result of small clot formation occurring from an increase in plasma volume.

Interfering Factors
1. If the hematocrit is high because of polycythemia or hemocontraction, clot retraction will be decreased.
2. In increased fibrinolysis the clot will lyse in 10 to 30 minutes, and it will appear that no retraction has taken place. Increased fibrinolysis occurs with DIC or alpha$_2$ antiplasmin deficiency.

Plasminogen/Plasmin

Normal Values
6.1 plus or minus 2.3 CTA units (CTA = Committee on Thrombolytic Agents) 2.4 μm (0.2 μg/ml)

Explanation of Test
These measurements of fibrinolysis are done to determine the level of plasminogen, the inactive precursor of plasmin, and of the active enzyme plasmin, which has the ability to dissolve formed fibrin clots. The test is useful during streptokinase therapy in arterial thrombosis.

The concentration of plasminogen is expressed in CTA plasma units.

Procedure
A venous blood sample of 5 ml is obtained. Sodium citrate is added.

Clinical Implications
1. Plasminogen levels fall variably in preeclampsia and eclampsia.
2. Plasmin can activate complement. There is an interrelationship between coagulation, kinin generation, fibrinolysis, and complement activation.
3. Decreased levels of plasminogen or abnormally functioning plasminogen can lead to venous and arterial clotting.

Fibrinolysis/Euglobulin Lysis Time

Normal Values
Euglobulin lysis—no lysis of plasma clot at 37°C for 3 hours. Clot observed for 24 hours.

Explanation of Test

This is one of the tests employed to evaluate a fibrinolytic crisis. No one single test has been universally accepted for the complete diagnosis and management of fibrinolytic states.

Fibrinolysis, without any sign of intravascular coagulation, is extremely rare. Usually seen is secondary fibrinolysis, which follows and occurs simultaneously with intravascular coagulation. This secondary type of fibrinolysis is thought to be a protective mechanism that the body possesses to protect itself against generalized clotting.

Procedure

A venous blood sample of 5 ml is obtained. Sodium citrate is added.

Clinical Alert

A lysis time of less than 1 hour signifies that abnormal fibrinolysis is occurring.

Clinical Implications

1. *Increased fibrinolysis* occurs (with)
   (a) 48 hours after surgery (The fibrinolytic activity continues to increase for the next 6 days.)
   (b) Incompatible blood transfusions
   (c) Cancer of prostate or pancreas
   (d) Cirrhosis (some cases)
   (e) During lung surgery
   (f) Obstetric complications such as antepartum hemorrhage, amniotic embolism, septic abortion, death of fetus, and hydatidiform mole
   (g) Thrombocytopenic purpura
   (h) Extracorporeal circulation
   (i) Leukemia
   (j) Administration of plasminogen activators such as TPA, streptokinase, or urokinase
   (k) Acute trauma or hypoxia
2. *Decreased fibrinolysis* occurs in
   (a) Diabetes
   (b) First 48 hours after surgery
   (c) Premature infants and nonterm infants in the first 2 days after birth.

Interfering Factors

1. Increased fibrinolysis occurs with
   (a) Exercise
   (b) Increasing age

    (c) Hyperventilation

    (d) Steroids and ACTH

2. Decreased fibrinolysis occurs in

    (a) Arterial blood, when compared with venous blood. This difference is greater in arteriosclerosis (especially in young persons)

    (b) Postmenopausal women

    (c) Normal newborns

    (d) On the day after severe unaccustomed exercise by persons out of shape

    (e) Obesity

3. Fibrin degradation products interfere with fibrinolysis.

    (a) False negatives can occur if fibrinolysis is far advanced.

    (b) False positives can be caused by very low fibrinogen levels.

Fibrin Split Products (FSP); Fibrin Degradation Products (FDP)

Normal Values
Negative 4 μg/ml
Normal serum: No fibrinogen on FDP

Explanation of Test
This test is done to determine the degree of consumptive coagulopathy in disorders such as positive tests for DIC, thromboembolic disorders, and renal diseases. When fibrin is split by plasmin, positive tests for fibrin degradation or split products, identified by letters S, Y, D, and E, are produced. These products have an anticoagulant action and inhibit clotting when there is an excess in the circulation.

Procedure
A venous blood sample of at least 4.5 ml is obtained and is placed in a tube containing thrombin and an inhibitor of fibrinolysis (soybean trypsin inhibitor).

Clinical Implications
Increased values are associated with

1. Any condition associated with DIC
2. Venous thrombosis
3. Hypoxia
4. Following thoracic and cardiac surgery and renal transplantation
5. Portacaval shunt
6. Incompatible blood transfusion
7. Acute leukemia
8. Infections

9. Burns
10. Some snake bites
11. Heat stroke
12. Pulmonary embolism
13. Prolonged coma due to hypnotic drugs
14. Late pregnancy
15. Thrombolytic therapy
16. Primary fibrinolysis
17. Falsely elevated with heparin therapy

Interfering Factors
Because all of the laboratory methods are sensitive to fibrinogen as well as FDP, it is essential that no unclotted fibrinogen be left in the serum preparation. Special care must also be taken with blood containing a therapeutic heparin. False-positive reactions could result if any fibrinogen is present.

Clinical Alert

Patients with very high levels of FSP/FDP have blood that does not clot or clots poorly.

D-Dimer

Normal Values
250 mg/ml cross-linked fibrin drivative

Explanation of Test
Fibrin split products are indistinguishable from fibrinogen split products by the previously described tests. D-Dimers are produced by the action of plasmin upon cross-linked fibrin. D-Dimers are not produced by the action of plasmin upon unclotted fibrinogen. Therefore, the D-Dimer test is more specific for DIC than are tests for FSPs.

Procedure
A venous blood sample of 4.5 ml is collected into a tube containing sodium citrate (same tube as for PT/PTT).

Clinical Implications
Increased values are associated with

1. DIC
2. Arterial or venous thrombosis

3. Late in pregnancy
4. Within 2 days of surgery

Interfering Factors

False-positive tests are obtained with high titers of rheumatoid factors.

Platelet Aggregation

Normal Values

The pattern of platelet aggregation depends upon the agonists used and their concentrations. The interpretation of platelet aggregation studies must be made in the context of the patient's history, including medications, and in light of acute medical problems.

Explanation of Test

When the blood vessel walls are injured, a hemostatic platelet plug is formed. This aggregation requires metabolically active platelets—platelet agonists such as epinephrine, adenosine diphosphate, arachidonic acid, collagen or thrombin, and the binding of proteins such as fibrinogen to the platelet surface.

Procedure

A venous sample of 5 ml is obtained. Sodium citrate is the anticoagulant. The sample is kept at room temperature; *never* refrigerate.

When platelets aggregate, the transmission of light through a sample of platelet-rich plasma (PRP) is increased. This increase in light transmission can be used as an index to the aggregation in response to various agonists.

Abnormal platelet aggregation occurs in

A. *Congenital diseases*
    1. Bernard–Soulier syndrome
    2. Glanzmann thrombasthenia
    3. Storage pool diseases
    4. Thrombocytopenia with absent radius
    5. Wiscott–Aldrich syndrome
    6. Albinism
    7. Chédiak–Higashi syndrome
    8. May–Hegglin anomaly
    9. Various connective tissue disorders
B. *Acquired disorders*
    1. Uremia
    2. Antiplatelet antibodies
    3. Cardiopulmonary bypass
    4. Myeloproliferative disorders
    5. Dysproteinemias

6. Drugs and aspirin, some antibiotics, and others
7. Von Willebrand's disease

Fibrinopeptide-A (FPA)

Normal Values
0.6–1.9 mg/ml

Explanation of Test
This measurement is the most sensitive assay done to determine thrombin action. Fibrinopeptide A reflects the amount of active intravascular blood clotting as in subclinical DIC, which is common in patients with leukemia of various types and may be associated with tumor progression. Serial measurements of FPA are used by some researchers to identify a relapse of acute leukemia. Unfortunately, FPA elevations can occur without intravascular thrombosis, decreasing the value of a positive test.

Procedure
A venous blood sample of 9 ml is obtained. Discard sample if not obtained by a clean venipuncture.

Clinical Implications
1. Levels are *increased* in
   (a) DIC
   (b) Leukemic patients at time of initial diagnosis or during relapse after remission
   (c) Early treatment phase of leukemia
   (d) Venous thrombosis and pulmonary embolus
   (e) Infections
   (f) Postoperative patients
   (g) Patients with widespread solid tumors
2. Levels are *decreased* when clinical remission of leukemia is achieved with chemotherapy.

Interfering Factors
1. A traumatic venous puncture results in falsely elevated levels.
2. The biologic half-life is 5 minutes, which imposes limitations on the interpretation of a negative FPA test.

Clinical Alert

Disseminated intravascular coagulation occurs commonly in association with death of tumor cells in acute promyelocytic leukemia. For this reason, heparin is used prophylactically and in association with the initiation of chemotherapy for promyelocytic leukemia. In contrast, DIC less commonly occurs during the treatment of acute myelomonocytic leukemia and acute lymphocyte leukemia. Evidence for DIC should be sought in every patient with leukemia, prior to initiation of treatment.

Fibrinogen

Normal Values
Thrombin time, semiquantitative: 200–400 mg/dl or 2.0–4.0 g/L

Explanation of Test
This test is done to investigate abnormal PT, APTT, and TT (thrombin time) as well as to screen for DIC and fibrin–fibrinogenolysis.

Procedure
A venous blood sample is obtained.

Clinical Implications
1. *Increased values* occur in
   (a) Hepatitis
   (b) Multiple myeloma
   (c) Cancer
   (d) Uremia
   (e) Pregnancy
   (f) Menstruation
   (g) Postsurgery
   (h) Compensated DIC
   (i) Inflammation such as rheumatic fever, pneumonia, tuberculosis, and septicemia
   (j) Nephrosis
   (k) Burns
2. *Decreased values* occur in
   (a) Liver disease
   (b) DIC
   (c) Hereditary afibrinogenemia
   (d) Dysfibrinogenemia

Protein C (PC)

Normal Values
71%–142% of increased functional activity

Explanation of Test
This test is done in the evaluation of patients with severe thrombosis and when there is an increased risk and predisposition to thrombosis

and pulmonary embolism. Protein C is a vitamin K-dependent protein that prevents thrombosis. Protein C is produced in the liver and circulated in the plasma. It functions as an anticoagulant by inactivating Factors V and VIII. Protein C is also a profibrinolytic agent.

Procedure
A venous blood sample is obtained.

Clinical Implications
1. Decreased values are associated with
    (a) Severe thrombotic complications in the neonatal period
    (b) Increased risk of thrombosis
    (c) Coumadin-induced skin necroses (some instances)
    (d) DIC, especially when it occurs with cancer (presumably due to consumption by co-factor thrombin-thrombomodulin-catalyst activities. Thrombomodulin is a potentiator of activation of protein C.)
2. A deficiency of protein C may also be
    (a) Congenital (35%–58%)
    (b) Caused by cirrhosis (13%–25%)
    (c) Due to use of Coumadin (28% to 60%)
    (d) Vitamin K deficiency
    (e) Certain medications (common anticoagulants)

Protein S

Normal Values
61%–130% of functional activity

Explanation of Test
This measurement is indicated for the investigation of hypercoagulable states such as thrombosis. The test may be useful in patients with recurrent or familial thrombosis and may be helpful in genetic counseling for these diseases (Leavelle, 1990). Both protein S and protein C (p. 133) are dependent upon vitamin K for their production and function. The deficiency of either one is associated with a tendency towards thrombosis. Protein S serves as a co-factor to enhance the anticoagulant effects of activated Protein C.

Procedure
A venous blood sample is obtained.

Clinical Implications
1. *Decreased values* are associated with protein S deficiency.
    (a) Familial protein S deficiency is associated with recurrent thrombosis.

(b) Abnormal plasma distribution of protein S occurs in functional protein S deficiency.

   (1) In type I, the free protein S is decreased, although the level of total protein may be normal. In type II, total protein is markedly reduced (Leavelle, 1990).

Antithrombin III (At-III) or Heparin Co-Factor

Normal Values

Immunologic method: 84% to 120% of normal (30% lower in serum than in person)

Functional method: 1–30 days: 26%–61% (premature)
                                    44%–76% (full-term)
                   1–5 months: adult values obtained by 6 months
                   ≥6 months: 77%–122%

Explanation of Test

This test is primarily done to demonstrate a decreased level of antithrombin that is indicative of thrombotic tendency. Only the test of functional activity gives a direct clue to thrombotic tendency. In some families, several members may have a combination of recurrent thromboembolism and reduced plasma antithrombin (30%–60%).

Procedure

A venous blood sample is obtained.

Clinical Implications

1. *Increased values* are associated with
   (a) Acute hepatitis
   (b) Renal transplant
   (c) Inflammation
   (d) Menstruation
   (e) Vitamin K deficiency
2. *Decreased values* are associated with
   (a) Congenital deficiency
   (b) Liver transplant and partial liver removal
   (c) DIC
   (d) Nephrotic syndrome
   (e) Active thrombotic disease (deep vein thrombosis)
   (f) Cirrhosis
   (g) Carcinoma
   (h) Chronic liver failure

(i) Last trimester of pregnancy and early postpartum
(j) Malnutrition
(k) After surgery
(l) Oral contraceptives

Prostacyclin (6-KETO-PG-F$_{1a}$)

Normal Values
72 pg/ml

Explanation of Test
This diagnostic aid is done to detect the presence of prostacyclin (an inhibitor of platelet aggregation and a potent vasodilator). This method is used in the evaluation of several thrombotic diseases such as venous thrombosis, thrombotic thrombocytopenic purpura, angina with occlusion (as opposed to spasm) and acute myocardial infarction (Leavelle, 1990).

Procedure
A venous blood sample is obtained.

Clinical Implications
1. *Decreased levels* occur in
   (a) Hypercoagulability states and thrombotic disease
   (b) Hypertension
   (c) Atherosclerosis
   (d) Diabetes mellitus
2. *Increased levels* occur in
   (a) Congestive heart failure
   (b) Graves' disease (returns to normal during therapy)
   (c) Some tumors of breast and possibly of the prostate
   (d) Dysmenorrhea

BIBLIOGRAPHY

A lab test for pulmonary embolism. Emerg Med 22(11):45–46, June 15, 1990

Bessman JD et al: Improved classification of anemia by MCV and RDW. Clin Pathol 80:322, 1983

Brown Susan: Behind the numbers on the CBC. RN 53(2):46–51, February 1990

Buffone GJ: Transferrin. Brea, CA, Beckman Monograph, Beckman Instruments, 1990

Chuansumrit A, Johnson–Monco MJ, Hattany WE: Heparin cofactor II in adults and infants with thrombosis and DIC. Am J Hematol 31:1109–1113, 1989

Esman CT: The roles of protein C and thrombomodulin in the regulation of blood coagulation. J Biol Chem 264(9):4743–4746, March 25, 1989

Gaedeke–Norris MK: Lab test tips—How to evaluate platelet values. Nursing 91 21(2):20, February 1991

Gralnick HR et al: Collection, transport, and preparation of blood specimens for coagulation testing and performance of coagulation assays. NCCLS Document H21-A. 6(20). Villanova, PA: 1986

Heim CR, DesPrez RM: Pulmonary embolism: A review. Adv Intern Med 39:187–191, 1986

Hirsch DR et al: Bleeding time and other laboratory tests to monitor the safety and efficacy of thrombolytic therapy. Chest 94(4):124S–131S, April 1990

Kee JL: Laboratory and Diagnostic Tests with Nursing Implications. East Norwalk, CT, Appleton and Lange, 1990

Koepke JA (ed): Laboratory Hematology, vol 2. New York, Churchill Livingstone, 1984

Leavelle DE (ed): Interpretive Handbook. Interpretive Data for Diagnostic Laboratory tests. Rochester, MN, Mayo Medical Laboratories, 1990

Pseudohyponatremia: When to question lab values. Emerg Med 21(12):87,90, June 30, 1989

Rice L: Anemia: Using a rational approach to diagnosis. Consultant 30(7):39–40, 43–44, 47–49, July 1990

Schwarz HP et al: Identification and quantification of protein S in human platelets. Blood 66:1452–1455, 1985

Takahashi H et al: Coagulative studies in thrombotic thrombocytopenic purpura, with special reference to von Willebrand factor and protein S. Am J Hematol 30:14–21, 1989

Tietz NB (ed): Clinical Guide to Laboratory Tests, 2nd ed. Philadelphia, WB Saunders, 1990

Wasserman MR et al: Fever, white blood cell count, and culture and sensitivity: Their value in the evaluation of the emergency patient. Top Emerg Med 10(4):81–88, January 1989

Walsh JR: Borderline anemia in old age. Geriatr Med Today 2(3):25, 1983

Williams WJ, Beutler E, Erslen AJ et al: Hematology, 4th ed. New York, McGraw–Hill, 1990

Wyngaarden JB, Smith LH (eds): Cecil's Textbook of Medicine, 18th ed. Philadelphia, WB Saunders, 1988

URINE STUDIES

Introduction

Overview of Urine Formation

Urine, a very complex fluid, is composed of 95% water and 5% solids. It is the end product of the metabolism carried out by billions of cells and results in an average urinary output of 1 to 1.5 L (approximately 1.5 quarts) per day (dependent upon fluid intake). A wide variety of waste products formed in the metabolic processes of the body are carried away in the urine.

The formation of urine takes place in the kidneys, the two small fist-sized organs located outside the peritoneal cavity on each side of the spine, about the level of the last thoracic and upper two lumbar vertebrae. The kidneys, along with the skin and respiratory system, are the chief excretory organs of the body. Each kidney is a highly discriminating organ that maintains the internal environment by selectively excreting or retaining various substances according to specific body needs. The importance of urine formation and excretion as a regulating function is profoundly emphasized when observing situations in which kidney function is suddenly lost. Under these circumstances, death can occur within a few days.

The main functional unit of the kidney is the nephron. There are about 1 million nephrons per kidney, each composed of two main parts: a glomerulus, which is essentially a filtering system, and a tubule through which the filtered liquid passes. Each glomerulus consists of a capillary network surrounded by a membrane called *Bowman's capsule*, which continues on to form the beginning of the renal tubule. The afferent arteriole carries blood from the renal artery into the glomerulus, where it divides to form a capillary network. These capillaries reunite to form the efferent arteriole through which blood leaves the glomerulus. The blood vessels then follow the course of the tubule, forming a surrounding capillary network.

There is a tremendous flow of blood through the kidneys. It is believed that 25% of the blood from the left heart passes through the kidneys. One liter of urine can be thought of as the end result of more than 1000 L of blood passing through the kidneys. The blood enters the glomerulus of each nephron by passing through the afferent arteriole into the glomerular capillaries.

Urine formation begins in the glomerular capillaries, with dissolved substances passing into the proximal tubule as a result of the force of blood pressure in the large afferent arteriole and the pressure in Bowman's capsule. As the filtrate passes along the tubule, more solutes are added by excretion from the capillary blood and secretions from the tubular epithelial cells. Solutes and water pass back into the blood by tubular reabsorption. Urine concentration and dilution take place in the renal medulla. The kidney has the remarkable ability to produce dilute or concentrated urine according to the needs of the individual and to regulate sodium excretion. Blood chemistry, blood pressure, fluid balance, nutrient intake, and state of health are key elements in metabolism. They are also key elements in establishing the character of urine.

Urine contains thousands of dissolved substances, although the three principal constituents are water, urea, and sodium chloride. More solids are excreted from the body in the urine than by any other method. Its composition depends greatly on the quality and the quantity of the excreted waste material. Some constituents of the blood, such as glucose, have a renal threshold; that is, a certain elevated level must be reached in the blood before this constituent will be excreted in the urine. Almost all substances found in the urine are also found in the blood, although in different concentrations. Urea, for example, is present in the blood, but at a much lower concentration than in the excreted urine.

URINE TESTING

Urinalysis is an essential procedure for those individuals undergoing hospital admissions and physical examinations. It is one of the most useful indicators of health and disease, and is especially helpful in the detection of renal or metabolic disorders. It aids in diagnosing and following the course of treatment in diseases of the kidney and urinary system and in detecting disorders in other parts of the body such as metabolic or endocrinologic abnormalities in which the kidneys function normally.

Laboratory Testing

In the laboratory, urinalysis is carried out by technologists who visually examine specimens and test them. Dipsticks are used for a number of tests. Automated instruments are also in use in some laboratories. The Clinitek Reflectance Photometer is an example of a semiautomated instrument for use in routine urinalysis and other tests.

Dipsticks

Although laboratory facilities allow for a wide range of urine tests, modern tablets, tapes, and dipstick tests are available for urinalysis outside the lab setting. They can be read directly by patients, nurses, clinicians, physicians, and technologists.

Similar in appearance to blotter paper, dipsticks are actually miniature laboratories. These chemically impregnated reagent (reactive) strips allow for quick determination of pH, protein, glucose, ketones, bilirubin, hemoglobin (blood), nitrite, leukocyte esterase, and urobilinogen. The tip of the dipstick is impregnated with chemicals that react with specific substances in the urine to produce colored end products. In some tests, the depth of color produced relates to the concentration of the substance in the urine. Color standards are provided against which the actual color can be compared. The reaction rates of the impregnated chemicals are standard for each dipstick, and color changes must be matched at the correct time after each stick is dipped into the urine specimen. These matching methods are included in the instructions that accompany each type of dipstick. When more than one reaction is arranged on a single stick (*e.g.*, pH, protein, glucose), the chemical reagents for each test are separated by a water-impermeable barrier made of plastic.

In addition to dipsticks, there are other reagent strips, chemical tablets, and treated slides for special determinations such as bacteria, PKU, mucopolysaccharide, salicylate, and cystinuria.

Procedure
1. Use fresh urine (within 1 hour of collection or refrigerate).
2. Read directions on the container or brochure.
3. Dip a reagent strip in well-mixed urine, remove, and compare each reagent area with the corresponding color chart on the bottle label at the number of seconds specified on the bottle (*e.g.*, 30 seconds). Hold the strip close to the color blocks and match carefully. Correlate as closely as possible.

Interfering Factors
1. If dipsticks are kept in the urine or urine stream too long, the chemicals impregnated in the cellulose may be overly dissolved. This can result in an inaccurate reading or value.
2. If the chemicals in each impregnated pad become mixed, the readings will be inaccurate.

Clinical Alert

1. Precise timing is essential, or the color change is meaningless. For example, glucose and ketone test areas are so sensitive that overtiming by only 1 to 3 seconds can demonstrate falsely high readings.
2. One must review instructions accompanying bottles of dipsticks frequently because manufacturers change procedures and update substances frequently.
3. When not in use, the container for the tablets, tapes, or dipsticks should be tightly closed to keep the reagents dry. If the dipsticks, tapes, or tablets absorb moisture from the air be-

fore they are used, they will not produce correct results. The desiccant should remain in the container. Store containers in a dry area.

4. Certain drugs give false-positive reactions.
5. Use fresh urine (within 1 hour of collection or refrigerate until examined). Failure to follow this precaution can lead to invalid results (Cella and Watson, 1989) such as the following:
    (a) Glucose level may drop.
    (b) Ketones dissipate.
    (c) Color will deepen.
    (d) Urinary sediment will deteriorate.
    (e) Bacteria (if present) will multiply.
    (f) pH becomes more alkaline.
    (g) Bilirubin and urobilinogen may be oxidized (if exposed to light for long periods of time).

TYPES OF URINE SPECIMENS

During the course of 24 hours, the composition of urine changes continuously. For this reason, various types of urine specimens are collected for urinalysis, such as the following:

Single, random specimen

Timed, short-term specimen

Timed, long-term specimen (12-hr or 24-hr)

Catheterized specimen or specimen from an indwelling catheter

Double-voided specimens (test for sugar and acetone)

Clean-catch mainstream specimen (urine culture and cytologic analyses—see Chap. 7)

Single, Random Specimen

Most testing is done on a random specimen of urine freshly voided by the patient. Because the composition of urine changes over the course of the day, the time of day when the specimen is collected may influence the findings. The first voided morning specimen is particularly valuable, for it is usually concentrated and more likely to reveal abnormalities and formed substances. It is also relatively free of dietary influences and of changes due to physical activity because the specimen is collected after a period of fasting. Because the chemical testing involved in urinalysis measures the concentration of substances, the results will vary according to the time of day the specimen is collected. Significant cellular abnormalities will be missed in dilute urine that is collected later in the day.

Procedure

1. The patient is instructed to void directly into a clean, dry container or into a clean, dry bedpan and then to transfer the specimen directly into an appropriate container. Women should always have a clean, voided specimen if a microscopic examination is ordered (see Chap. 7).
2. Specimens from infants and young children can be collected in a disposable collection apparatus that consists of a plastic bag with an adhesive backing around the opening that can be fastened to the child to permit voiding directly into the bag.
3. All specimens should be covered, labeled properly, and sent immediately to the laboratory.
4. If a urine specimen is likely to be contaminated with vaginal discharge or menstrual blood, then a clean specimen must be obtained using the same procedure as for bacteriologic examination (see collection of specimens for culture in Chap. 7).
5. If a urine specimen is obtained from an individual catheter, it may be necessary to clamp off tubing for about 15 minutes before obtaining the sample with a needle and syringe. Clean the specimen port (in the tubing) with antiseptic prior to aspirating the urine sample.
6. Wear gloves when handling urine.

Interfering Factors

1. Glycosuria appears more often after meals.
2. Proteinuria may occur following strenuous activity or upon assuming an upright position.
3. Hemoglobin may appear in the urine following exertion.
4. The presence of urinary infections and the number of bacteria in the urine vary during the day.
5. Feces, vaginal secretions, and menstrual fluid can contaminate the specimen.
6. If the specimen is kept unrefrigerated for more than 1 hour before analysis, the following changes in composition may occur:
    (a) Bacteria in the urine "split" the urea, converting it to ammonia and producing an alkaline urine.
    (b) Casts decompose in urine after several hours.
    (c) Red blood cells are lysed by hypotonic urine.
    (d) Very low or very high pH may affect cellular components.

Clinical Alert

1. If the specimen is kept for more than 1 hour before analysis, it should be refrigerated to avoid changes in the urine.
2. If the specimen is contaminated by feces or vaginal discharge, a clean voided specimen must be obtained.

Timed, Long-Term Specimen (24-hr)

Explanation of Test

Some diseases or conditions require that a 24-hour urine specimen be collected in order to evaluate the kidney function accurately (see Table 3–1). Substances excreted by the kidney are not excreted at the same rate or in the same amounts during different periods of the day and night; therefore, a random urine specimen might not give an accurate picture of the processes taking place. For measurement of total urine protein, creatinine, electrolytes, and so forth, more accurate information is obtained from urine collected over a 24-hour period. This involves collecting the specimen in a suitable receptacle and either adding a preservative to it or keeping it refrigerated.

Procedure

1. At the beginning of a 24-hour timed urine specimen (or any timed specimen collection), the patient is asked to void. This specimen is *discarded*, and the time noted.
2. The time the test begins and the time the collection should end are labeled.
3. All urine passed over the next 24 hours is collected in a large container (usually made of polyethylene), labeled with the patient's name, and marked for the particular test ordered. It is not necessary to measure urine unless explicitly stated.
4. To conclude the collection, the patient must void 24 hours after the first voiding. Urine from this last voiding must be added to the specimen in the container.

   Note: Because the patient may not always be able to void on command, a last specimen should be obtained as closely as possible to the stated end-time of the test and the exact time marked on the bottle.

TABLE 3–1.
24-Hour Urine Collection Data

Test	Preservative	Notes
Amylase	None	
Calcium	30 ml 6N HCL	
Catecholamines	30 ml 6N HCL	pH 1–3
Chloride	None	Refrigerate
Citrate (citric acid)	30 ml 6N HCL	pH 1–3
Cortisol (Free)	1.0 g boric acid	
Creatinine	None	
Creatinine clearance	None	Refrigerate
Delta-aminolevulinic acid (ALA)	30 ml of 33% glacial acetic acid	Protect/light freeze
Electrolytes (Na,K)	None	Refrigerate
Estrogens (total/non-pregnancy or third trimester)	1.0 g boric acid	Refrigerate
FIGLU	12 ml glacial acetic acid	Refrigerate
5-HIAA (serotonin)	1 g boric acid	
Hydroxyproline	None	
FSH/LH	1.0 g boric acid	
17-Hydroxycorticoste-roids	1.0 g boric acid	pH 4–7
17-Ketogenic steroid (Porter–Silber)	1.0 g boric acid	Do not refrigerate
17-Ketosteroids (total)	1.0 g boric acid	Do not refrigerate
Magnesium	None	
Metanephrine (total)	30 ml 6N HCL	pH 1–3
Oxalate	30 ml 6N HCL	
Phosphorus (inorganic)	None	
Pregnanediol	1.0 g boric acid	
Preganetriol	1.0 g boric acid	
Protein (total)	See Total protein	
Porphobilinogen (quantitative)	None	Refrigerate during collection; protect from light
Potassium (K), sodium (NA)	See Electrolytes	
Porphyrins (uro/copro)	None (preservative added upon receipt in lab)	Protect from light
Total protein	None	Refrigerate
Urea nitrogen	None	
Uric acid	None	
Vanillylmandelic acid	30 ml 6N HCL	pH 1–3

N = Normal

5. Storage
   (a) In the health care facility, nonrefrigerated samples may be kept in a specified area or in the patient's bathroom.
   (b) If refrigeration is necessary, the urine specimen must either be refrigerated immediately after the patient has voided or placed in an iced container.

Clinical Considerations
1. Responsibility for the collection of urine specimens should be specifically assigned.
2. Persons instructing a patient about 24-hour urine collections should make certain that the patient understands that he or she must empty the bladder at the time the 24-hour collection starts and that this specimen must be discarded.
3. Do not predate and pretime the laboratory slips for serial collections. It is difficult for some patients to void at specific times.
4. The marking of exact times the specimens are obtained is crucial to many urine tests.
5. Remind the patient to try to urinate near the end of the collection time period.
6. When a preservative is placed in the collection container (such as the hydrochloric acid preservative used for 24-hour urine collection of vanillylmandelic acid), the patient needs to be warned to take precautions against spilling the contents of the container. Instructions regarding measures to take if spillage does occur need to be addressed at this time.
7. Preservatives used for urine collections will be determined by the substance to be tested. Make sure the proper preservative will be provided before the actual test begins.

Interfering Factors
1. Failure of the patient or attending personnel to comprehend the steps of the procedure is the most common source of error.
   (a) The patient should be given written instructions. If unable to comprehend these, a significant other should be instructed in the process, if possible.
   (b) The proper preservative must be used (see preservative chart on p 146).
2. Toilet paper placed in the collection container may decrease the actual amount of urine available. It may also contaminate the specimen.
3. Feces in the urine specimen may also contaminate the specimen. For this reason, patients who use bedpans should be instructed to void and to have the urine specimen transferred to the collection receptacle before defecating.

Patient Preparation

Most 24-hour urine specimen collections start in the morning. Instruct the patient to do the following:

1. Empty the bladder completely on awakening and then discard this urine specimen. Record the time the voided specimen is discarded (7:08 AM), then begin the test (7:08 AM)
2. Save all urine passed during the rest of the day and night, including the first specimen passed the next morning.
3. The urine voided the next morning (as close to 7:00 AM as possible) is added to the collection container and the 25-hour test is terminated. Write down the time of this last voiding.
4. A bedpan, urinal, or wide-mouth pitcher, or the collection bottle itself can be used for each voiding. It is probably easier for women to void into another receptacle first and then *carefully* transfer the specimen to the collection bottle. Men may find it simpler to void directly into the 24-hour collection container.
5. It is most important that *all* urine be saved and placed in the 24-hour container. Ideally, the container should be stored in the refrigerator or placed in ice.
6. Test results are calculated on the basis of a 24-hour output. Unless all urine is saved, results will not be accurate. Moreover, this test is expensive, complicated, and necessary for the evaluation and treatment of the patient's condition.

ROUTINE URINALYSIS (UA) AND RELATED TESTS

Normal Values

General Characteristics and Measurements	Chemical Determinations	Microscopic Examination of Sediment
Color: pale yellow to amber	Glucose: negative	Casts negative: occasional hyaline casts
Turbidity: clear to slightly hazy	Ketones: negative	Red blood cells: negative or rare
Specific gravity: 1.015–1.025 with a normal fluid intake	Blood: negative	Crystals: negative
pH: 4.5–8.0—average person has a pH of about 5 to 6	Protein: negative	White blood cells: negative or rare
	Bilirubin: negative	Epithelial cells: few
	Urobilinogen: 0.1–1.0	
	Nitrate for bacteria: negative	
	Leukocyte esterase: negative	

Explanation of Test

Urinalysis is the means of determining the various properties of urine: color, odor, turbidity, specific gravity, pH, glucose, ketones, blood, protein, bilirubin, urobilinogen, nitrate, and leukocyte esterase, as well as any abnormal constituents revealed by microscopic examination of the sediment. A 10-ml urine specimen is usually sufficient for conducting these tests.

Specific Gravity (SG)

Normal Values
1.003–1.035 (usually between 1.010 and 1.025) SG
1.025–1.030 + (concentrated urine) SG
1.001–1.010 (dilute urine) SG

Explanation of Test
Specific gravity is a means by which the kidneys' ability to concentrate urine is measured. The test is conducted by comparing the weight of urine against the weight of distilled water, which has a specific gravity of 1.000. Because urine is a solution of minerals, salts, and compounds dissolved in water, the specific gravity is obviously greater than 1.000. The relative difference between the specific gravity of distilled water and the specific gravity of urine reflects the degree of concentration of the urine specimen; specific gravity correlates roughly with osmolality.

The range of urine specific gravity depends on the state of hydration and varies with urine volume and the load of solids to be excreted. When fluid intake is restricted or increased, under standardized conditions, specific gravity measures the concentrating and diluting abilities of the kidney. Loss of these capacities is an indication of renal dysfunction.

Procedure
1. Specific gravity can be tested using a multiple dipstick that has a separate reagent area for specific gravity (most common method).
2. Refractometer
   Specific gravity can be determined with a refractometer or total solids meter. The refractive index is the ratio of light velocity to the specific gravity of the urinometer.
3. Specimen collection
   (a) For regular urinalysis testing, a random specimen is used. One to two milliliters is needed for testing with a refractometer.
   (b) When evaluation of specific gravity is ordered separately from the urinalysis, the patient should fast for 12 hours before the specimen is collected.

Clinical Implications
A. *Normal*
   Specific gravity varies inversely with urine excretion (decrease in volume; increase in specific gravity).

Examples of conditions in which this relationship is not valid are as follows:
1. Diabetes: increased volume; increased specific gravity
2. Hypertension: normal volume; decreased specific gravity
3. Early chronic renal disease: increased volume; decreased specific gravity
B. *Low specific gravity* (1.001 to 1.010)
    1. Diabetes insipidus
        (a) Low specific gravity and large urine volume.
        (b) Due to absence of antidiuretic hormone (ADH). Antidiuretic hormone triggers kidney absorption of water; without it, kidneys produce excessive amounts of urine (sometimes 15 to 20 L a day).
    2. Glomerulonephritis and pyelonephritis (but not in acute disease). Specific gravity can be low in glomerulonephritis when disease occurs.
        (a) Decreased volume; low specific gravity
        (b) Tubular damage affects kidneys' ability to concentrate urine.
    3. Severe renal damage
        Fixed low specific gravity (1.010) that varies little from specimen to specimen
C. *Increased specific gravity*
    1. Diabetes mellitus or nephrosis
        (Abnormally large amounts of glucose and protein increase the specific gravity up to 1.050.)
    2. Excessive water loss (dehydration, fever, vomiting, diarrhea)

Interfering Factors
1. Specific gravity is highest in the morning specimen (this is a normal phenomenon).
2. Specific gravity is elevated whenever there is an excessive loss of water (dehydration).
3. Radiopaque contrast media used in radiographs of urinary tract and dextrin may cause false high specific gravity.
4. Temperature of urine specimens affects specific gravity (when specific gravity is measured in urine removed from the refrigerator, specific gravity will be falsely higher).
5. Highly buffered alkaline urine may also cause a low reading on dipsticks only.
6. Elevated readings may occur in the presence of moderate (100 to 750 mg/dl) amounts of protein.

Concentration

Normal Values
Methods of concentration testing

Fishberg test: specific gravity of 1:024 or higher on one specimen and up to 300 ml of urine

Mosenthal's test: 1.020 and at least a seven-point difference between the lowest and highest specific gravity

Volhard's test: 1.025 or higher with osmolality showing rise above 800 on at least one specimen in the afternoon.

Explanation of Test
This test is carried out in patients with suspected renal disease and measures the kidneys' ability to concentrate urine after liquids have been withheld from the diet for a number of hours. The goal of the test is to see if the kidneys can produce urine with a specific gravity greater than 1.020.

In health, specific gravity normally ranges from 1.003 to 1.035 or higher. When fluids are restricted in accordance with this test, the urine produced is more concentrated and has a specific gravity higher than 1.020 to 1.025. Kidney dysfunction can result in *isothenuria* (urine specific gravity remains consistently at 1.010) or *hyposthenuria* (urine specific gravity is less than 1.008). Whenever a more precise measurement is indicated, osmolality of urine can be determined. Osmolality is a measure of the number of particles in a given weight.

Procedure
A. *Pretest preparation*
   1. All diuretics should be stopped 48 to 72 hours prior to the test and during the test.
   2. An adequate protein diet and normal hydration should be followed for 3 days before the test.
   3. No medications should be given.
B. *Test procedure*
   1. The test begins at 6:00 PM after which time no fluids are permitted until the test is completed ("dry" foods are permitted).
   2. At 10:00 PM, the patient voids, *discards* the specimen, and may retire.
   3. The next morning, urine specimens are collected at 6:00 AM, 7:00 AM, and 8:00 AM. Keep specimens separate. (Normally, kidneys concentrate urine at twice the rate during the night as during waking hours.) If patient voids during the night, save this urine and send it to the laboratory in a separate labeled container.

4. The volume of each urine specimen and total volume of all three specimens are measured and recorded.
5. The specific gravity or osmolality (see pp 149 and 153) of each specimen is measured.

Clinical Implications

1. A specific gravity of less than 1.020 on all specimens indicates renal disease. With severe involvement, the specific gravity is persistently 1.010 or less.
   (a) Total loss of urinary concentrating ability with fixed specific gravity near 1.010 or osmolality between 300 and 400 mOsm/kg is not seen until very late in the course of renal disease.
   (b) Abnormal concentration levels generally reflect progressive inability of the kidneys to increase the osmotic pressure of urine above that of the glomerular filtrate in chronic renal failure.
2. A normal finding does not necessarily rule out active kidney disease.
3. A specific gravity of 1.020 occurs in the following instances:
   (a) Potassium deficiency
   (b) Hypercalcemia due to sarcoidosis
   (c) Bone disease (multiple myeloma; vitamin D intoxication or sensitivity)
   (d) Hyperparathyroidism
   (e) Renal parenchymal disease, such as pyelonephritis, which damages the tubules
   (f) Acute renal disease
4. The urine may be abnormally concentrated for a day or so after injection of dyes used in intravenous pyelograms (IVP)
5. Edema, sweats, diarrhea, and fever interfere with the water tests.
6. Concentration tests are meaningless in patients taking diuretics.
7. Patients who have been markedly overhydrated for several days prior to testing may have impaired concentration if dehydration is then imposed.

Interfering Factors

The test is unreliable when the patient is pregnant, is on low salt or protein diets, or suffers from severe water or electrolyte imbalance, chronic liver disease, edema from renal disease, or heart failure. In these conditions, the tubules may be unable to concentrate urine.

Patient Preparation

1. Explain the purpose and procedure of the test to the patient.
2. Instruct the patient to empty the bladder completely at each voiding.

Clinical Alert

1. The fluid deprivation required in this test may be contraindicated in some patients with heart disease or early renal failure.
2. Accidental or deliberate fluid intake during the night will interfere with the results. Reschedule the test if this occurs.

Osmolality

Normal Values
After 12-hour fluid restriction: 500 to 850 mOsm/kg

Background
Osmolality, a more exact measurement of urine concentration than specific gravity, depends on the number of particles of solute in a unit of solution, whereas specific gravity depends on both the quantity and precise nature of the particles in the unit. Protein, sugar, and intravenous contrasts elevate urine specific gravity disproportionately more than they elevate osmolality.

Explanation of Test
Whenever a more precise measurement than specific gravity is indicated in the evaluation of the concentration and diluting ability of the kidney, this test is done. The measurement of urine osmolality during water restriction is an accurate test of decreased kidney function. It is also used in the differential diagnosis of diabetes insipidus (compulsive water drinking).

Procedure
1. A high protein diet is prescribed for 3 days.
2. On the evening before the test, a dry supper is eaten and no liquids drunk until the test is over.
3. At approximately 6:00 AM, the patient empties the bladder and returns to bed. This urine is not saved.
4. The test urine specimen is collected at 8:00 AM, the sample is labeled and sent to the laboratory, and the proceedings are entered on the patient's record. The test is then completed.

Clinical Implications
1. *Increased* in
   (a) Postsurgery
   (b) Hepatic cirrhosis
   (c) Congestive heart failure
   (d) Addison's disease

      (e) Intravenous sodium   (g) Inappropriate ADH secretion
      (f) High protein diets
2. *Decreased* in
      (a) Aldosteronism   (d) Hypercalcemia
      (b) Diabetes insipidus   (e) Compulsive water drinking
      (c) Hypokalemia   (f) Intravenous 5% dextrose and
                                        water

Patient Preparation

1. Explain the purpose and procedure of the test to the patient.
2. No liquids are to be taken with the evening meal before the test. No food or liquids should be taken after the evening meal until the test is completed.

Patient Aftercare

Provide the patient with foods and fluids as soon as the 8:00 AM urine sample is obtained.

Color

Normal Values

Yellow is the normal color of urine. The specific gravity ranges from 1.011 to 1.019, and the urine output is 1 to 1.5 L/day.

Straw-colored urine is normal and indicates a low specific gravity, usually under 1.010. (The exception is a patient with a 4 + sugar; urine is very light and looks like water, but the specific gravity is high.)

Amber-colored urine is normal and indicates a high specific gravity and a small output of urine. Specific gravity is above 1.020 and output is less than 1 L/day.

Explanation of Test

Urine specimens may vary in color from pale yellow to dark amber. The intensity of the normal amber color may be related directly to the concentration or specific gravity of the urine. The color of normal urine is primarily due to urochrome (pigments that are present in the diet or formed from the metabolism of bile). Owing to the presence of abnormal pigments, the color of urine changes in many disease states.

Procedure

Observe color of urine specimen.

Clinical Implications

1. A nearly *colorless* urine may be due to
      (a) Large fluid intake
      (b) Reduction in perspiration
      (c) Chronic interstitial nephritis

(d) Untreated diabetes mellitus
(e) Diabetes insipidus
(f) Alcohol ingestion
(g) Diuretic therapy
(h) Nervousness
2. An *orange-colored* urine may be due to
    (a) Concentrated urine
    (b) Restricted fluid intake
    (c) Excess sweating
    (d) Fever
    (e) Small quantities of bile pigment
3. A *brownish yellow or greenish yellow* color may indicate bilirubin in the urine.
    (a) However, not all dark urines contain bilirubin.
    (b) Stale urine containing bilirubin may be green owing to an oxidation of the bilirubin to biliverdin.
    (c) Bilirubin crystals in the sediment may cause the urine to have an opalescent appearance.
    (d) *Yellow foam* may be due to biliverdin bile pigment.
    (e) *Green foam* may be due to biliverdin bile pigment.
    (f) Green color may be due to *Pseudomonas*.
4. A *red or reddish dark brown* color may indicate hemoglobinuria and may be due to blood, porphyrins, hemoglobin, or myoglobin.
5. A *port wine* color may be due to porphyrins or a mixture of methemoglobin and oxyhemoglobin.
6. *Dark brown* urine may be due to porphyrias, melanin.
    (a) May indicate a melanotic tumor
    (b) Is sometimes associated with Addison's disease
7. *Brown black* urine may be due to a great deal of hemoglobin, lysol poisoning, or melanin.
8. *Black* urine results from alkaptonuria, a disease of tyrosine metabolism, which causes the urine to turn black on standing.
9. *Smoky* color may be due to red blood cells.

Interfering Factors
1. The color of normal urine darkens on standing. This is due to the oxidation of urobilinogen to urobilin. Decomposition starts in 30 minutes. Many people erroneously call it bilirubin. A trained eye can detect slight increases in urobilinogen.
2. Some foods cause the urine to change color.
    (a) Beets will turn the urine *red.*
    (b) Rhubarb can cause the color to be *brown.*
3. Many drugs cause the urine to change color.
    (a) Cascara and senna laxatives in acid urine will turn the urine *reddish brown;* in alkaline urine, they will turn the urine *red.*

(b) *Orange* may be due to phenazopyridine (Pyridium), amidopyrine, oral anticoagulants.

(c) *Orange to orange red* may be due to Pyridium, ethoxazene.

(d) *Orange to purple red* may be due to chlorzoxazone.

(e) *Orange yellow* in alkaline urine may be due to salicylazosulfapyridine, anisindione, or phenindione.

(f) *Rust yellow to brownish* may be due to sulfonamides or nitrofurantoins.

(g) *Pink to red or red brown* may be due to Dilantin (diphenylhydantoin), Doxidan (dioctyl calcium sulfosuccinate), Ex-Lax (phenolphthalein), and phenothiazine (thiodiphenylamine).

(h) *Magenta* may be due to Ex-Lax.

(i) *Red* may be due to amidopyrine, Pyridium, Neotropin, Prontosil, aniline dyes, PSP and BSP dyes in alkaline urine, phenolphthalein and Pyridium in acid urine, or Desferal (deferoxamine).

(j) *Purple red* may be due to Ex-Lax in alkaline urine.

(k) *Dark brown* may be due to phenolic drugs or phenylhydrazine.

(l) *Brown black* may be due to Jecotofer or cascara.

(m) *Bright yellow* may be due to riboflavin or Pyridium in alkaline urine.

(n) *Blue or green* may be due to methylene blue and amitriptyline.

(o) Urine that *darkens* on standing may be due to antiparkinsonian agents such as levodopa or Sinemet.

(p) *Dark-colored* urine may be due to iron salts.

(q) *Pink to brown* may be due to phenothiazine tranquilizer.

(r) *Pale blue* may be due to Dyrenium (triamterene).

Clinical Alert

If the urine is a red color, do not assume drug causation. Check the urine for hemoglobin.

Odor

The characteristic odor of normal, freshly voided urine is due to the presence of volatile acids.

Normal Values

Fresh urine from most healthy persons has an aromatic odor.

Clinical Implications
1. The sweet smell of acetone can be recognized in diabetic ketosis.
2. Heavily infected urine has a particularly unpleasant odor.
3. An inherited disorder of amino acid metabolism is characterized by the passage of urine in infants that smells like maple syrup. This condition is maple sugar urine disease.

Interfering Factors
1. Some foods, such as asparagus, produce characteristic odors.
2. After urine stands for a long time, ammonia, with its characteristic pungent odor, is formed by bacterial activity and the decomposition of urea in the specimen.

---

*p*H

Normal Values
Average range: 4.6–8
Average *p*H is about 6 (acid).
(The *p*H of normal urine can vary widely.)

Background
The symbol "*p*H" expresses the exact strength of the urine as a dilute acid or a base solution and measures the free hydrogen ion (H^+) concentration in the urine. (The lower the *p*H, the greater the acidity.) *p*H, therefore, is an indication of the renal tubules' ability to maintain normal hydrogen ion concentration in the plasma and extracellular fluid. The kidneys maintain normal acid–base balance primarily through the reabsorption of sodium and the tubular secretion of hydrogen and ammonium in exchange. Secretion of an acid or alkaline urine by the kidneys is one of the most important mechanisms of the body for maintaining a constant body *p*H.

Urine becomes increasingly acidic as the amount of sodium and excess acid retained by the body increases. Alkaline urine, usually containing bicarbonate–carbonic acid buffer, is normally excreted when there is an excess of base or alkali in the body.

Ingestion of different foods and sodium bicarbonate also affects the urinary *p*H. The usual diet, rich in animal protein, produces an acid urine. A diet high in citrus fruits and vegetables produces an alkaline urine.

Control of *p*H
Control of urinary *p*H is important in the management of several diseases, including bacteriuria and renal calculi, and in drug therapy in

which streptomycin or Mandelamine (methenamine mandelate) is administered.

A. *Renal calculi*

Renal stone formation is partially dependent on the *p*H of urine. Patients being treated for renal calculi are frequently given diets or medication to change the *p*H of the urine so kidney stones will not form.

1. Calcium phosphate, calcium carbonate, and magnesium phosphate stones develop in alkaline urine. In such instances the urine must be kept acid.
2. Uric acid, cystine, and calcium oxalate stones precipitate in acid urines. In the treatment of these urinary calculi, the urine should be kept alkaline.

B. *Drug treatment*

1. Streptomycin, neomycin, and kanamycin are effective in genitourinary tract infections provided the urine is *alkaline.*
2. During sulfa therapy, an *alkaline* urine should help prevent formation of sulfonamide crystals.
3. Urine should also be kept persistently *alkaline* in control of salicylate intoxication (excretion is enhanced) and during blood transfusions.

C. *Clinical conditions*

The urine should be kept *acid* in the treatment of urinary tract infections and persistent bacteriuria and in the management of those urinary calculi that develop in alkaline urine.

D. *Diet*

1. A diet that emphasizes citrus fruits and most vegetables, particularly legumes, will help keep the urine alkaline.
2. A diet high in meat and cranberry juice will keep the urine acid.

Explanation of Test

Urine *p*H is an important screening test for diagnosing renal disease, respiratory disease, and certain metabolic disorders. It is also used to monitor specific programs of medication or diet when it is desirable to maintain the urine as acid or alkaline. Keeping the urine at a consistently high or low *p*H requires frequent testing of the urinary *p*H.

Dipstick measurement

1. Multiple reagent strips treated with chemicals provide a spectrum of color changes from orange to green blue in the *p*H range of 5 to 9.
2. The dipstick is dipped into a urine specimen, and the color change is compared to a standardized color chart on the bottle.

Clinical Implications

If urine pH *is to be useful, it is necessary to use the* pH *information in conjunction with other information.* For example, in renal tubular necrosis, the kidney is not able to excrete a urine that is strongly acid. Therefore, if a urine pH of 5 (quite acid) is measured, renal tubular acidosis is eliminated as a possibility.

A. *Acid urine* (pH less than 7)
   1. Found in acidosis, uncontrolled diabetes, pulmonary emphysema, diarrhea, starvation, dehydration
   2. Rarely excreted in severe alkalosis
   3. Found in respiratory diseases in which CO_2 retention occurs and acidosis develops
B. *Alkaline urine* (pH more than 7)
   1. Found in urinary tract infections, pyloric obstruction, salicylate intoxications, renal tubular acidosis, and chronic renal failure
   2. Rarely excreted during severe acidosis
   3. Found in respiratory diseases involving hyperventilation and loss of CO_2 with alkalosis

Interfering Factors
1. On standing, the pH of urine specimens will become alkaline because bacteria split urea, producing ammonia.
2. Alkaline urine specimens tend to cause hemolysis of red cells and the disappearance of casts.
3. High protein diets will cause excessively acid urine (pH less than 6).
4. Ammonium chloride and mandelic acid may produce acid urines.
5. Alkaline urine after meals is a normal response to the secretions of hydrochloric acid in gastric juices.
6. Sodium bicarbonate, potassium citrate, and acetazolamide may produce alkaline urines.

Clinical Alert

1. An accurate measurement of urinary pH can be done only on a freshly voided specimen. If the urine must be kept for any length of time before analysis, it should be refrigerated.
2. Alkaline urine occurs from vegetarian diets, citrus fruits, milk, and other dairy products.
3. Highly concentrated urine, such as that formed in hot, dry environments, is strongly acidic and may be irritating.
4. During sleep, decreased pulmonary ventilation causes respiratory acidosis, and urine becomes highly acid.
5. Chlorothiazide diuretic administration will cause an acid urine to be excreted.
6. Bacteria in urinary tract infection or bacterial contamination of the specimen will result in an alkaline urine. Bacteria in the urine will convert urea to ammonia.

Turbidity

Normal Values
Fresh urine is clear to slightly hazy.

Explanation of Test
The appearance of cloudy urine provides a warning of possible abnormality such as the presence of pus, red blood cells, or bacteria. However, excretion of cloudy urine may not be abnormal because the change in urine pH may cause precipitation within the bladder of normal urinary constituents. Alkaline urine may appear cloudy because of the presence of phosphates, and acid urine may appear cloudy because of urates.

Procedure
Observe the appearance of a fresh urine sample.

Clinical Implications
1. Pathologic urines are often turbid or cloudy, but so are many normal urines. Cloudy urine may result from precipitation of crystals due to rapid cooling of the urine.
2. Urine turbidity may result from urinary tract infections.
3. Abnormal urines may be cloudy owing to the presence of red blood cells, white blood cells, or bacteria.

Interfering Factors
1. After ingestion of food, urates or phosphates may produce cloudiness in normal urine.
2. Vaginal contamination from female patients is a common cause of turbidity.
3. "Greasy" cloudiness may be caused by large amounts of fat.
4. Many normal urines will develop a haze or turbidity after refrigeration or standing at room temperature.

Blood or Hemoglobin (Heme)

Normal Values
Negative.

Explanation of Test
Blood in the urine is usually occult blood that has been hemolyzed or dissolved. Hemoglobin or red blood cells in the urine are not likely to be identified by the naked eye when there is less than one part of the blood per 1000 parts of urine.

The presence of free hemoglobin in the urine is referred to as *hemoglobinuria*. Hemoglobinuria is usually related to conditions outside the urinary tract and occurs when there is such extensive or rapid destruction (hemolysis) of circulating erythrocytes that the reticuloen-dothelial system cannot metabolize or store the excessive amounts of free hemoglobin.

When intact red blood cells are present in the urine, the term *hematuria* is used to indicate bleeding somewhere in the urinary tract. Usually, both red blood cells and hemoglobin mark this disorder. Therefore, hematuria can be distinguished from hemoglobinuria by a microscopic examination of the sediment from a fresh urine specimen.

The use of both urine dipstick and microscopic examination provides a complete clinical evaluation in regard to hemoglobinuria and hematuria. New dipsticks contain a lysing reagent that reads with occult blood urea, and this can detect intact as well as lysed red blood cells.

When urine gives a positive result for occult blood, but no red blood cells are seen in a microscopic examination of the sediment, *myoglobinuria* can be suspected. Myoglobinuria is the excretion of myoglobin, a muscle protein, into the urine as a result of (1) traumatic muscle injury such as may occur in automobile accidents, football injuries, or electric shock, (2) a muscle disorder such as an arterial occlusion to a muscle or muscular dystrophy, or (3) certain kinds of poisoning such as carbon monoxide or fish poisoning. Myoglobin has to be distinguished from free hemoglobin in the urine by chemical tests (see p 218).

Procedure

A. *Hemoglobin in urine—Hemoglobinuria*
   1. Chemical strips are dipped into the urine, and the color change on the dipstick is noted.
   2. The color of the strip is compared with a color chart.
   3. The color blocks indicate negative, moderate, and large amounts of hemoglobin.

B. *Hematuria*
   1. The dipstick method allows detection of intact red blood cells when greater than 10/HPF (high-powered field). The color change appears stippled on the dipstick.
   2. To verify red blood cells, the urine is centrifuged and the sediment is examined microscopically (see p 178).

Clinical Implications

1. *Hematuria* is found in
   (a) Lower urinary tract infection
   (b) Lupus erythematosus
   (c) Polyarteritis nodosa
   (d) Malignant hypertension
   (e) Subacute bacterial endocarditis
   (f) Glomerulonephritis
   (g) Heavy smokers

2. Usually, when blood is present in urine, protein will also be present.
3. *Hemoglobinuria* is found in
   (a) Extensive burns and crushing injuries
   (b) Transfusion reactions to incompatible blood
   (c) Febrile intoxication
   (d) Chemical agents and alkaloids (poisonous mushrooms, snake venom)
   (e) Malaria
   (f) Irrigation of operated prostatic bed with water
   (g) Hemolytic anemias
   (h) Paroxysmal hemoglobinuria (Large quantities of hemoglobin appear in urine at irregular intervals.)

Clinical Alert

One of the early indications of renal disease is the appearance of blood in the urine. This does not mean that blood will be present in every voided specimen in every case of renal disease. It does mean that in most cases of renal disease, occult blood appears in the urine with a reasonable degree of frequency.

Interfering Factors
1. Drugs causing a positive result
   (a) Drugs that are toxic to the kidneys (bacitracin and amphotericin)
   (b) Drugs that cause actual bleeding (coumarin)
   (c) Drugs that cause hemolysis of red blood cells (aspirin)
   (d) Drugs that may give a false-positive result include bromides, copper, iodides, and oxidizing agents.
2. High doses of ascorbic acid may give a false-negative result. (Ascorbic acid may be a preservative for antibiotics such as tetracycline or result from high vitamin C intake.)
3. High specific gravity or elevated protein reduces sensitivity.
4. Myoglobin—false positive.
5. Highly alkaline urine tends to cause hemolysis of red cells.

Protein (Albumin); **Qualitative and 24-hr**

Normal Values
10–140 mg/L in 24 hr or 1–14 mg/dL

Explanation of Test
Detection of protein in urine (proteinuria), combined with a micro-scopic examination of urinary sediment, provides the basis for differen-tial diagnosis of renal disease.

In health, the urine contains no protein or only trace amounts of protein, which consists of albumin (one third of normal urine protein is albumin) and globulins from the plasma. Because albumin is filtered more readily than the globulins, it is usually very abundant in patho-logic conditions. Therefore, the term *albuminuria* is often used synony-mously with *proteinuria*.

Normally, the glomerules prevent passage of protein from the blood to the glomerular filtrate. Thus, the persistent presence of protein in the urine is the single most important indication of renal disease. Therefore, if more than a trace of protein is found in the urine, a quanti-tative 24-hour evaluation of protein excretion is necessary.

Procedure (for Qualitative Protein Collection)
1. Collect urine in a clean container, and test it as soon as possible.
2. Test the specimen with SSA or turbid metric methods. If one of these methods is positive, confirmation by protein electrophoresis is done.

Procedure (for 24-hr Protein Collection)
1. A 24-hour urine container is labeled with the name of the patient, test, and the date.
2. Refrigeration of the specimen is required.
3. General instructions for 24-hour urine collection are on page 146.
4. The exact start and ending of the collection are recorded on the specimen container, and the patient's record (start 7:30 AM 2/6 and end 7:30 AM 2/7).

Clinical Implications
1. Significant proteinuria indicates an abnormally high excretion of protein. Proteinuria is usually the result of increased glomerular filtration of protein because of some kind of glomerular damage. A follow-up of 24-hr urine test for protein is indicated to arrive at a specific diagnosis.
2. Continued proteinuria of any amount in an apparently healthy per-son usually indicates minimal renal disease.
3. In pathologic states, the level of proteinuria is rarely constant, and not every sample of urine will be abnormal in patients with disease.
4. Proteinuria occurs in the following diseases:
   (a) Nephritis/glomerulonephritis
   (b) Nephrosis
   (c) Polycystic kidney
   (d) Tuberculosis and cancer of the kidney

    (e) Venous congestion of kidney
    (f) Pyelonephritis
5. Proteinuria may occur in the following nonrenal diseases and conditions:
    (a) Fever
    (b) Trauma
    (c) Severe anemias and leukemia
    (d) Toxemia, pre-eclampsia of pregnancy
    (e) Abdominal tumors
    (f) Convulsive disorders
    (g) Hyperthyroidism
    (h) Intestinal obstruction
    (i) Cardiac disease
    (j) Ascites
    (k) Liver disease
    (l) Acute infections
    (m)Poisoning from turpentine, phosphorus, mercury, sulfosalicylic acid, lead, phenol, opiates, and drug therapy
6. Large numbers of leukocytes accompanying proteinuria usually indicate infection at some level in the urinary tract. Large numbers of both leukocytes and erythrocytes indicate a noninfectious inflammatory disease of the glomerulus. Proteins with pyelonephritis may have as many red blood cells as white cells.
7. Proteinuria does not always accompany renal disease. Pyelonephritis, obstructions, nephrolithiasis, tumors, and congenital malformations can cause severe illness without protein leakage.
8. Proteinuria is associated with the finding of casts on the sediment examination because protein is necessary for cast formation.
9. Postural proteinuria is the excretion of protein by patients who are standing or moving in the daytime. The proteinuria is intermittent and disappears when the person lies down. Postural proteinuria occurs in 3% to 5% of healthy young adults. It is also known as orthostatic proteinuria.

Collecting the Specimen for Orthostatic Proteinuria
1. The patient is instructed to void at bedtime and discard the urine.
2. The next morning, a urine specimen is collected immediately after the patient awakes and has assumed a standing position.
3. A second specimen is collected after the patient has been standing or walking for a period of time.

Differentiation from other types of proteinuria is done by testing for protein in two urine specimens: one collected before and one collected after the person is erect. In postural proteinuria, the first specimen contains no protein, whereas the second is positive.

Interfering Factors for Qualitative Protein Test

1. Because of renal vasoconstriction, functional, mild, and transitory protein in the urine is associated with
   (a) Violent exercise
   (b) Severe emotional stress
   (c) Cold baths
2. Increased protein in urine occurs
   (a) After eating large amounts of protein
   (b) In pregnancy or immediately following delivery
   (c) In newborn infants
   (d) In premenstrual state
   (e) In orthostatic proteinuria
3. False or accidental proteinuria may be present because of a mixture of pus and red blood cells in urinary tract infections and the menstrual flow.
4. False-positive results can occur from incorrect use and assessment of the color strip test.
   (a) Prolonged dipping or allowing the strip to be held too long in the urine stream
   (b) Failing to match accurately the reactive area with the color chart
5. Alkaline urine can give a false-positive result on the color strip test owing to alkaline, highly buffered urine.
6. A very dilute urine may give a falsely low protein value.
7. Drugs may cause false-positive and false-negative tests for protein.

Patient Preparation for 24-hr Collection

1. Instruct patient about the purpose and collection of the 24-hour specimen. Stress compliance.
2. Food and fluids are permitted. Fluids should not be forced, for a very dilute urine can give a false-negative value.

Bence–Jones Protein

Electrophoresis of urine or turbidimetric methods can be used to demonstrate Bence–Jones protein, a specific low molecular weight protein. The dipstick method does not react very well with globulins; however, albumin reacts very well. This protein is found in the following instances:

50% to 80% of multiple myeloma cases

Amyloidosis
Macroglobulinemia

Tumor metastasis to the bone
Malignant lymphoma

Clinical Alert

If the dipstick is negative for protein and one of the above conditions is suspected, the turbidimetric SSA method should be used and electrophoresis should be performed. It is especially important if the patient is older. This discrepancy also exists with high doses of penicillin and radiographic contrast media. If the dipstick is negative and subsequent tests are positive, this should be reported.

Protein Electrophoresis (PEP), Urine

Normal Values
Interpretive report.

Explanation of Test
This test is done in the investigation of monoclonal gammopathies.

Procedure
1. When a urine PEP is done, a serum specimen must be submitted at the same time.
2. A fresh random or 24-hour refrigerated specimen is required.

Clinical Implications
1. Trace amounts of urine albumin and occasionally trace amounts of both kappa and lambda light chains occur in a 2 : 1 ratio. Variations in this ratio are suggestive of monoclonal gammopathy or light chain urea.
2. Free light chains are found in
   (a) Multiple myeloma
   (b) Renal failure
   (c) Systemic lupus erythematosus
   (d) Lymphoid tumors

Sugar (Glucose)

Normal Values
Random specimen: negative
Quantitative 24-hr specimen: <0.5 g/d or <2.78 mmol/d
1 to 15 mg/dl or 0.1 to 0.8 mmol/L

Explanation of Test

Urine glucose tests are used in (1) screening to detect diabetes, (2) confirming a diagnosis of diabetes, or (3) monitoring the effectiveness of diabetic control.

Normally, urine does not contain a sufficient amount of sugar to react with any of the popular testing methods. Glucose is always present in the glomerular filtrate, but it is reabsorbed by the proximal tubule. However, should the blood glucose level exceed the reabsorption capacity of the tubules, glucose will be spilled into the urine.

The presence of sugar in the urine (*glucosuria* or *glycosuria*), as evidenced by positive tests, is not necessarily abnormal. For example, sugar may appear in urine after a heavy meal is eaten or in conjunction with emotional stress. In addition, for some persons, a low tubular reabsorption rate may account for glycosuria occurring with normal blood glucose levels. This is a benign condition.

In the majority of cases, however, sugar in the urine is abnormal and is usually due to diabetes mellitus. Nonetheless, a positive test for urine sugar is not adequate for a diagnosis of diabetes. A single measurement of postprandial blood sugar gives more meaningful information in diabetes detection programs than does a urine sugar test. A urine sugar test accompanied by a blood sugar test gives more information than does a blood sugar test alone. Also, a postprandial urine sugar test is a more effective test for recognizing diabetes than a fasting urine sugar test.

Types of Glucose Tests

A. *Reduction tests:* Clinitest
  1. Are based on reduction of certain metal ions by glucose. When added to urine, a heat reaction takes place, resulting in precipitation and a change in color of the urine.
  2. Are considered nonspecific for glucose because the reaction can be brought about by other reducing substances in the urine.
     (a) Hypochlorite or chlorine
     (b) Other sugars, such as galactose, lactose, fructose, and maltose
B. *Enzyme tests:* Clinistix, Diastix, Tes-Tape
  1. Are based on interaction between enzymes and glucose. When dipped into urine, the strip changes color according to the amount of glucose in the urine indicated by the manufacturer's color chart.
  2. All are specific for glucose.

Procedure

1. A freshly voided specimen should be used.
2. Directions on the tablet or dipstick container must be followed

exactly and the color reaction compared to the closest matching color on the manufacturer's color chart. Timing must be exact.
3. Results are recorded on the patient's record.
4. If a 24-hour urine specimen should be ordered, the urine must be refrigerated or iced during collection.

Clinical Alert

1. Determine exactly what drugs a diabetic is taking and whether the metabolites of these drugs affect the urine test.
2. Do not encourage patients to drink water between the first and second voidings, because diluted urine may conceal glucose in the urine.
3. Always test for ketone bodies when the urine contains glucose.
4. Be aware that test results are reported as plus (+) or percentages. Reporting results in percentages is more accurate.

Clinical Implications

1. Increased glucose in the urine is found in diabetes mellitus, brain injury, myocardial infarction, and when a lowered renal threshold (positive urine sugar and a normal blood glucose) is present. An elevated blood glucose and negative urine sugar indicate a high renal threshold.
2. A glucose tolerance test is indicated to confirm diabetes mellitus.
3. The greater the concentration of sugar in the urine, the greater the lack of control of the diabetes.

Interfering Factors

Note: Knowledge of the manufacturer's guidelines on drugs known to affect test results must be continually updated.

1. Pregnancy and lactation may cause a false positive in a Clinitest due to lactose or galactose. About 70% of normal pregnant women show a temporary glucosuria that appears to be of no clinical significance.
2. Ascorbic acid, NegGram, Keflin, creatinine in concentrated urine, streptomycin may cause a false-positive Clinitest result; usually it will be only a trace reaction.
3. Stress, excitement, testing after a heavy meal, and following the administration of intravenous glucose may cause false positives of all tests. Usually it is a trace reaction.
4. Ascorbic acid in very large amounts may cause a false negative in the enzyme tests.

5. False negatives may be obtained if deteriorated reagent strips have been used, or if directions are not followed exactly.
6. Large amount of ketones—false negative.

Patient Preparation
1. Instruct the patient about the purpose of the test, the method of testing, and the second voiding technique.
2. Patient voids, tests the specimen, and discards it.
3. The patient voids 30 to 45 minutes later, if possible, and this specimen is tested. The second specimen reflects the immediate state of glucosuria more accurately than the first specimen, which may be urine that has collected in the bladder over a period of hours.

Ketone Bodies (Acetone)

Normal Values
Negative.

Explanation of Test
Ketone bodies, resulting from the metabolism of fatty acid and fat, consist mainly of three substances: acetone, beta-hydroxybutyric acid, and acetoacetic acid. The last two substances readily convert to acetone, making acetone, in essence, the main constituent being tested. However, some test products measure only acetoacetic acid.

In healthy individuals, ketone bodies are formed in the liver and are completely metabolized so that only negligible amounts appear in the urine. However, when carbohydrate metabolism is altered, an excessive amount of ketones is formed (acetosis) on account of fat becoming the predominant body fuel instead of carbohydrates. When the metabolic pathways of carbohydrates are disturbed, carbon fragments from fat and protein are diverted to form abnormal amounts of ketone bodies. The body's alkaline reserves thus become depleted, resulting in acidosis.

The excess production of ketones (ketonuria) in the urine is mainly associated with diabetes. Testing for ketones in the urine of diabetics may provide the clue to early diagnosis of ketoacidosis and diabetic coma.

Indications for Ketone Testing
A. *General*
    Screening for ketonuria is valuable in hospital admissions, presurgical patients, pregnant women, children, and diabetics.
B. *Glycosuria*
    Testing for ketone bodies is indicated in any patients showing greater than normal excretion of sugar.

C. *Acidosis*
  1. Ketone testing is used to judge the severity of acidosis and to follow the effects of treatment.
  2. Blood ketone measurement frequently provides a more reliable estimate of acidosis than urine testing (it is especially useful in emergency room situations).
D. *Diabetes*
  1. Ketonuria may indicate ketoacidosis and possible diabetic coma.
  2. When treatment is being switched from insulin to oral hypoglycemic agents, the development of ketonuria within 24 hours after the withdrawal of insulin usually indicates a poor response to the oral hypoglycemic agents.
  3. The urine of diabetics treated with oral hypoglycemic agents should be tested regularly for glucose and ketones, since oral hypoglycemic agents, unlike insulin, do not control diabetes when acute complications such as infection develop.
E. *Pregnancy*
  In pregnancy, the early detection of ketones is essential because ketoacidosis is an important factor contributing to death in the uterus.

Procedure
1. Dip the reagent strip in fresh urine, tap the strip to remove excess urine, and compare it to the color chart at the time indicated.
2. Follow the manufacturer's directions exactly.
3. Acetest tablets are used to test ketones in blood. (Do not use dipsticks to test blood.)

Clinical Implications
1. Ketosis and ketonuria may occur whenever increased amounts of fat are metabolized, carbohydrate intake is restricted, or the diet is rich in fat.
2. Ketonuria occurs in association with

(a) Fever	(e) Starvation
(b) Anorexia	(f) Prolonged vomiting
(c) Diarrhea	(g) Following anesthesia
(d) Fasting	

3. In nondiabetics, ketonuria will occur frequently in acute illness. Fifteen percent of hospitalized patients will have ketone bodies in their urine even though they do not have diabetes.
4. Children are particularly prone to developing ketonuria and ketosis.
5. Ketone bodies appear in the urine before there is any significant increase of ketone bodies in the blood.

Interfering Factors
1. Carbohydrate-free diets as well as high-protein and fat diets will cause ketonuria.
2. Drugs that may cause a false positive are as follows:

(a) Levodopa	(e) Isopropyl alcohol
(b) Phthalein compound (BSP or PSP)	(f) Metformin
	(g) Paraldehyde
(c) Ether	(h) Pyridium
(d) Insulin	(i) Phenformin

Clinical Implications
1. A test for ketone bodies in the urine is helpful in differentiating between a diabetic coma and an insulin shock.
2. Any stressful situation that distorts the normal regulation of a diabetic can be recognized at any early point by a positive urine ketone test.
3. Urine ketones indicate caution, not a crisis situation, in either a diabetic or a nondiabetic patient.
   (a) In a diabetic patient, the appearance of ketone bodies in the urine suggests that the patient is not adequately controlled, and that adjustments of either the medication or the diet should be made promptly.
   (b) In a nondiabetic patient, ketone bodies indicate a small amount of carbohydrate metabolism and excessive fat metabolism.

Nitrate/Bacteria

Normal Values
Negative for bacteria.

Explanation of Test
Two methods are used to detect bacteria in the urine during routine urinalysis: microscopic examination and clinical testing. The sediment, when examined microscopically, can reveal bacteria when present. Chemical dipstick testing is also done routinely. The nitrite area in the multiple reagent strip is calibrated so that any shade of pink color that develops within 30 seconds indicates an amount of nitrite produced by 10^5 or more organisms per milliliter in the urine specimen.

Procedure
1. A first morning specimen is preferred because urine that has been in the bladder for several hours is more likely to yield a positive nitrite test than a random urine sample that may have been in the

bladder only a short time. A clean-catch or midstream urine is needed to avoid bacterial contamination.
2. Follow the procedure stated in the manufacturer's guidelines *exactly* to achieve reliable test results.
3. Comparison of the reacted reagent area against a white background may aid in the detection of low levels that might otherwise be missed.

Clinical Implications
1. The finding of 20 or more bacteria per high-powered field may indicate a urinary tract infection. Untreated bacteriuria can lead to very serious kidney disease.
2. The presence of only a few bacteria should be interpreted with caution and suggests a urinary tract infection that cannot be confirmed or excluded until more definitive studies, such as culture and sensitivity tests, are performed.
3. A positive result from the nitrite test is a reliable indication of significant bacteriuria and is an indication for urine culture.
4. A negative result should *never* be interpreted as indicating absence of bacteriuria because
    (a) If an overnight sample were not used, there may have been insufficient time for the conversion of nitrate to nitrite to have occurred in the bladder.
    (b) Some urinary tract infections are caused by organisms that do not convert nitrate to nitrite (*e.g.*, staphylococcus or streptococcus).
    (c) Insufficient dietary nitrate is present.

Interfering Factors
1. Azo dye metabolites—false positive
2. Ascorbic acid—false negative
3. High specific gravity—sensitivity reduced false negative

Leukocyte Esterase

Normal Values
Negative.

Explanation of Test
Two methods are used to determine the presence of leukocytes (white blood cells) in the urine: microscopic examination, and chemical testing, using the leukocyte esterase dipstick. The dipstick is calibrated so that any shade of purple that develops in 60 seconds is considered positive for five or more white blood cells per high-powered field. The leukocyte esterase test detects intact leukocytes as well as lysed ones.

Because this test measures the esterase activity of leukocytes, white blood cell casts can also be detected.

Procedure
1. A fresh random specimen is collected. A clean catch or midstream urine is needed to avoid vaginal contamination.
2. Manufacturer's directions must be followed exactly, and timing is critical for accurate results.

Interfering Factors
Vaginal discharge, trichomonas, parasites, and heavy mucus can cause false positives.

Clinical Implications
1. Normal urine gives negative results.
2. Positive results are clinically significant and indicate pyuria.

Clinical Alert

A urine sample that tests positive for both nitrate and leukocyte esterase should be cultured for pathogenic bacteria.

Bilirubin

Normal Values
Negative or 0.02 mg/dl.

Background
Bilirubin is formed in the reticuloendothelial cells of the spleen and bone marrow from the breakdown of hemoglobin and is transported to the liver. Urinary bilirubin excretion will reach significant levels in any disease process that increases the amount of conjugated bilirubin in the bloodstream (see Chemistry Studies, Chap. 6). Normally, there is a small amount of urobilinogen, not bilirubin, in the urine.

Explanation of Test
This test should be done with a routine urinalysis. It is an aid in the diagnosis of hepatitis and liver dysfunction, and it is helpful in monitoring the course of treatment. In persons exposed to toxins and certain drugs, a positive test for bilirubinuria can be an early indication of liver damage.

Bilirubin in the urine is an early sign of hepatocellular disease or intrahepatic or extrahepatic biliary obstruction and should be routinely performed in every urinalysis. Bilirubin may often appear in the urine before other signs of liver dysfunction, such as jaundice or clinical illness, are apparent.

Procedure

1. Examine the urine within 1 hour of collection because bilirubin is not stable in urine, especially when exposed to light.
2. Strip testing:
   (a) A fresh urine specimen is tested with a dipstick according to the manufacturer's directions.
   (b) Close approximation to the color chart is an absolute must. Failure to make a close comparison is an important basis of failure to recognize bilirubin in urine. (Good lighting is necessary).
   (c) The results are interpreted as negative and 1 to 3+ positive or as small, moderate, and large amounts of bilirubin.
3. When it is important to detect very small amounts of bilirubin in the urine, as in the earliest phase of viral hepatitis, Icotest tablets are preferred, because they are more sensitive.
4. When elevated amounts of bilirubin are present in the urine, a blue to purplish color forms. The rapidity and the intensity of the color formation and development are proportionate to the amount of bilirubin in the urine.

Clinical Implications

1. Even trace amounts of bilirubin are abnormal and warrant further investigation. Normally, there is no detectable bilirubin in the urine.
2. *Increased levels* occur in
   (a) Hepatitis and liver diseases due to infectious or toxic agents
   (b) Obstructive biliary tract diseases
3. Urine bilirubin is negative in hemolytic disease

Interfering Factors

1. Drugs may cause false positives and false negatives.
2. Bilirubin rapidly decreases with exposure to light. Urine should be tested immediately.

Urobilinogen (Random, Timed)

Normal Values

2-hour specimen: 0.1–1.0 Ehrlich units/2 hr
24-hour specimen: 1–4 mg/24 hr
Random: 0.1–1 Ehrlich unit/ml

Explanation of Test

This is one of the most sensitive tests used to determine impaired liver function. Although it is usually a 24-hour urine test, a random specimen may be ordered.

Formed from the metabolism of hemoglobin entering the intestine in the bile, bilirubin is transformed through the action of bacteria into urobilinogen. Part of the urobilinogen formed in the intestine is excreted with the feces; another portion is absorbed into the portal bloodstream and carried to the liver, where it is metabolized and excreted in the bile. Traces of urobilinogen that escape removal from the blood by the liver are carried to the kidneys and excreted in the urine, the basis of the urine urobilinogen test. Unlike bilirubin, urobilinogen is colorless.

Procedure

1. General instructions for collection of a 24-hour or 2-hour specimen are followed depending on what has been ordered.
2. The 2-hour timed collection is best done from 1:00 PM to 3:00 PM or 2:00 PM to 4:00 PM. Collect without preservatives. Record total amount of urine voided. Protect from light. Test immediately.
3. If a 24-hour test is ordered, follow general instructions and check with your laboratory for specific protocols.

Clinical Alert

If any specimens are lost during the 24-hour urine collection, the test is nullified and should be restarted immediately. Notify both laboratory and physician if this occurs.

Clinical Implications

1. Urinary urobilinogen is *increased* by any condition that causes an increase in the production of bilirubin and by any disease that prevents the liver from normally removing the reabsorbed urobilinogen from the portal circulation.
    (a) Urobilinogen is *increased* whenever there is excessive destruction of red blood cells as in
        (1) Hemolytic anemias
        (2) Pernicious anemia
        (3) Malaria
    (b) Values above normal also occur in
        (1) Infectious and toxic hepatitis
        (2) Pulmonary infarct
        (3) Biliary disease

      (4) Cholangitis

      (5) Hemolytic jaundice and anemia

      (6) Chemical injury to liver due to chloroform and carbon tetrachloride poisoning

      (7) Cirrhosis

      (8) Congestive heart failure

      (9) Infectious mononucleosis

   (c) An *increased* urobilinogen level is one of the earliest signs of acute liver cell damage.

2. Urinary urobilinogen is *decreased* or absent when normal amounts of bilirubin are not excreted into the intestinal tract. This usually indicates partial or complete obstruction of the bile ducts such as may occur in

   (a) Cholelithiasis

   (b) Severe inflammatory disease

   (c) Cancer of the head of the pancreas

      (1) During antibiotic therapy, suppression of normal gut flora may prevent the breakdown of bilirubin to urobilinogen, leading to its absence in the urine.

      (2) *Decreased* values are also associated with

         (a) Severe diarrhea

         (b) Renal insufficiency

Interfering Factors

1. Drugs that may cause urobilinogen include those that cause cholestasis and those that reduce the bacterial flora in the gastrointestinal tract (*e.g.*, chloramphenicol and neomycin, ammonium chloride, and ascorbic acid).

2. Peak excretion is known to occur from noon to 4:00 PM. The amount of urobilinogen in the urine is subject to diurnal variation.

3. Strongly alkaline urine will show a higher value and strongly acid urine will show a lower level.

4. Intake of foods such as bananas may affect test outcome.

5. False-negative results may be associated with high levels of nitrates in wine.

6. Drugs that may cause *increased* urobilinogen include those causing hemolysis, acetazolamide, and sodium bicarbonate.

7. High carbohydrate meals are associated with increased levels.

MICROSCOPIC EXAMINATION OF SEDIMENT

Background

In health, the urine contains small numbers of cells and other formed elements from the entire length of the genitourinary tract: casts and epithelial cells from the nephron; epithelial cells from the pelvis, ureters, bladder, and urethra; mucous threads and spermatozoa from the prostate; possibly some red or white blood cells and an occasional cast.

In renal parenchymal disease, the urine usually contains increased numbers of cells and casts discharged from an organ that is otherwise accessible only by biopsy or surgery. (See the listing of elements and their significance shown below.)

Urinary sediment provides information useful for both prognosis and diagnosis. It constitutes a direct sampling of urinary tract morphology. The urinary sediment is obtained by pouring 10 ml of well-

---

Significance of Elements Observed in the Urinary Sediment on Microscopic Examination

Urine Sediment	Clinical Significance
Bacteria	Urinary tract infection
Casts	
Broad	Formation in collecting tubules: serious kidney disorder
Epithelial (renal)	Tubular degeneration
Fatty	Nephrotic syndrome
Granular or waxy	Renal parenchymal disease
Hyaline	Acid urine—high salt content
Red cell	Acute glomerulonephritis
White cell	Pyelonephritis
Epithelial Cells	
Renal	Tubular damage
Squamous	Normal or contamination
Erythrocytes (red blood cells)	Most renal disorders; menstruation; severe exercise
Fat bodies (oval)	Nephrotic syndrome
Leukocytes (white blood cells)	Most renal disorders; urinary tract infection; pyelonephritis

Cast width is significant in determining the site of origin and may indicate the extent of renal damage. Cast width is described as narrow (one to two red blood cells in width), medium broad (three to four red blood cells in width), and broad (five red blood cells in width). The broad cast is formed in the collecting tubule and may be of any composition. It usually indicates a marked reduction in the functional capacity of the nephron and suggests severe renal damage or "end-stage" renal disease.

mixed urine into a conical tube and using a centrifuge at a specific speed for 10 minutes. The supernatant is poured off and 1 ml of sediment is mixed in a coverslip on a slide and examined under the microscope.

The sediment collected in the urine can be broken down into cellular elements (red and white blood cells and epithelial cells), casts, crystals, and bacteria.

These may originate anywhere in the urinary tract. When casts do occur in the urine, the indication is one of tubular or glomerular disorders.

Clinical Alert

Microscopic examintion of urine sediment can provide the following information:

1. Provide evidence of renal disease as opposed to lower urinary tract infection.
2. Indicate the type and state of activity of a renal lesion or disease condition.

The microscopic result and urine chemistry result should be checked against each other before reports are issued.

Red Cells and Red Cell Casts

Normal Values
1 or 2/low-powered field
Red blood cells: 0–1/high-powered field
Red cell casts: 0/low-powered field

Explanation of Test
In health, red cells are occasionally found in the urine, but the persistent findings of even small numbers of erythrocytes (red blood cells) should be thoroughly investigated, because these cells come from the kidney and indicate serious renal disease.

Procedure for Urine Microscopic Examination
Urinary sediment is examined microscopically under low and high power. Casts are searched for and enumerated under low power. Red blood cells and white blood cells are searched for and counted under high power. Bacteria are reported per high-powered field: few, moderate, packed, packed solid, or 1t, 2t, 3t, 4t. Crystals and other elements are noted.

Clinical Implications

A. *Red cell casts*

1. Casts composed largely of red blood cells are never found normally and indicate hemorrhage or desquamative conditions of the nephron.
2. Red blood casts indicate acute inflammatory or vascular disorders in the glomerulus.
3. They may be the only manifestation of
   (a) Acute glomerulonephritis
   (b) Renal infarction
   (c) Collagen disease
   (d) Kidney involvement in subacute bacterial endocarditis
4. The usual finding in systemic lupus erythematosus is red blood cell casts and epithelial cell casts.

B. *Red cells*

1. The finding of more than one or two red cells per high-powered field is an abnormal condition and can indicate
   (a) Renal or systemic disease
   (b) Trauma to the kidney
2. Increased red cells occur in
   (a) Pyelonephritis
   (b) Lupus
   (c) Renal stones
   (d) Cystitis
   (e) Prostatitis
   (f) Tuberculosis and malignancies of the genitourinary tract
   (g) Hemophilia
   (h) Malaria
   (i) Polyarteritis nodosa
   (j) Malignant hypertension
3. Red cells in excess of white blood cells indicate bleeding into the urinary tract as may occur in
   (a) Trauma
   (b) Tumor
   (c) Aspirin ingestion
   (d) Anticoagulative therapy
   (e) Thrombocytopenia

Clinical Alert

1. In health, red cells are occasionally found in the urine, but the persistent finding of even small numbers of erythrocytes should be thoroughly investigated.
2. Rule out menstrual contamination in women.

Interfering Factors

1. Increased numbers of red blood cells can be found following a traumatic catheterization and passage of stones.
2. Alkaline urine hemolyzes red cells and dissolves casts.

3. Many drugs can cause increased numbers of red blood cells to appear in the urine.
4. Red cell casts may occur after very strenuous physical activity and contact sports.
5. Heavy smokers have small amounts of red blood cells in urine.

White Cells and White Cell Casts

Normal Values
White blood cells: 0–4/high-powered field
White blood cells casts: none–negative/low-powered field

Background
Leukocytes may come from anywhere in the genitourinary tract. White cell casts always come from the kidney tubules.

Procedure
Urinary sediment is examined microscopically under high power for cells and crystals and under low power for casts.

Clinical Implications
A. *Leukocytes*
1. Large numbers of white cells (50/high-powered field) usually indicate acute bacterial infection in the urinary tract.
2. Increased leukocytes are seen in
   (a) All renal disease
   (b) Urinary tract disease
      (*e.g.* cystitis, prostatitis)
   (c) Fever
   (d) Strenuous exercise
   (e) Chronic pyelonephritis
   (f) Bladder tumors
   (g) Tuberculosis
3. In kidney infections, the white cells tend to be associated with cellular and granular casts, bacteria, epithelial cells, and relatively few red cells.

> **Clinical Alert**
>
> Call for a urine culture (see section on urine cultures in Chap. 7) in presence of increased leukocytes.

B. *White cell casts*
1. White cell casts indicate renal parenchymal infection.
2. They may be found in
   (a) Pyelonephritis—most common cause
   (b) Acute glomerulonephritis
   (c) Interstitial inflammation of the kidney

3. It is very difficult to differentiate between white blood cell casts and epithelial cell casts.
4. Because pyelonephritis may remain completely asymptomatic even though renal tissue is being progressively destroyed, careful examination (using low power) of urinary sediment for leukocyte casts is important.

Interfering Factors
Vaginal discharge can contaminate the specimen. Either a clean-catch specimen or a catheterized specimen should be taken to rule out contamination.

Epithelial Cells and Epithelial Casts

Normal Values
Occasional renal epithelial cell is found.

Background
Renal epithelial cell casts are formed by cast-off tubular cells. Because the tubule is a living membrane, it is always replacing itself. For this reason, the finding of occasional epithelial cells or clumps is not remarkable.

Clinical Implications
Many epithelial casts are found when the following diseases have damaged the tubular epithelium:

1. Nephrosis
2. Amyloidosis
3. Poisoning from heavy metals and other toxins
4. Glomerulonephritis
5. Acute tubular necrosis

Interfering Factors
Squamous epithelium is usually seen when the urine is contaminated with vaginal discharge. Squamous epithelia are large and flat with abundant cytoplasm. They can be readily differentiated from renal epithelial cells.

Hyaline Casts

Normal Values
Occasional hyaline casts per low-power field are found.

Background
Hyaline casts are clear, colorless casts formed when protein (Tamm–Horsfall) within the tubules precipitates and gels. Their appearance

within the urine depends on the rate of urine flow, urine pH, and the degree of proteinuria.

Procedure
Urinary sediment is examined microscopically for casts under low power.

Clinical Implications
1. Hyaline casts indicate possible damage to the glomerular capillary membrane, which is permitting leakage of proteins through the glomerular filter.

   (a) Nephritis   (d) Congestive heart failure
   (b) Malignant hypertension   (e) Diabetic nephropathy
   (c) Chronic renal disease

2. Hyaline casts may be a temporary phenomenon due to the following:

   (a) Fever   (d) Strenuous exercise
   (b) Postural strain   (e) Palpation of the kidney
   (c) Emotional stress

3. When large numbers of hyaline casts appear in the urine along with heavy proteinuria, fine granular casts, fatty casts, or oval fat bodies or fat droplets, nephrotic syndrome may be suggested.
4. Casts may not be found even if proteinuria is heavy because of dilute urine (1.010) or because the pH is alkaline.
5. In cylindruria, large numbers of casts may be counted, but there may not be any protein in the urine.

Granular Casts

Normal Values
Occasional granular casts are found.

Background
In pathologic disease, granular casts result from the disintegration of the cellular material in white and epithelial blood cells into coarse and then fine granular particles. A rare but final step in this process may be the formation of waxy casts when urine flow is reduced and renal failure progresses. Waxy casts may be cell casts, hyaline casts, or renal failure casts. In normal subjects, granular casts probably are the result of irregular precipitation of Tamm–Horsfall protein, and the cast is precipitated the same as cell casts.

Procedure
Urinary sediment is examined microscopically under low power.

Clinical Implications
1. Acute tubular necrosis
2. Advanced glomerulonephritis
3. Pyelonephritis
4. Malignant nephrosclerosis
5. Chronic lead poisoning

Waxy Casts (Renal Failure Casts)

Waxy casts are found in

1. Chronic renal failure
2. Tubular inflammation and degeneration
3. Localized nephron obstruction

Clinical Alert

Broad waxy casts are the most ominous of all casts found in urinary sediment.

Oval Fat Bodies and Fatty Casts

Background
In nephrotic syndrome, fat accumulates in the tubular cells and eventually sloughs off, forming oval fat bodies. This fat is probably a cholesterol esther. Fatty casts are usually composed of individual fat droplets. The presence of fat droplets, oval fat bodies, or fatty casts is the hallmark of the nephrotic syndrome.

Clinical Implications
Fatty casts are found in chronic renal disease and indicate tubular inflammation and degeneration.

Crystals

Background
In a routine urinalysis, the presence of crystals is identified as a normal finding. The type and number of crystals vary with the pH of the urine.

Clinical Implications
A. *Normal findings*
  1. Acid urine
    (a) Amorphous urates
    (b) Uric acid
    (c) Calcium oxalate (if numerous, may indicate hypercalcemia [only in warm, freshly voided urine])
    (d) Sodium acid urates
    A normal specimen may show large numbers of calcium oxalate crystals once the urine cools.
  2. Alkaline urine (increased pH)
    (a) Amorphous phosphates
    (b) Calcium phosphate
    (c) Ammonium biurate
    (d) Triple phosphate crystal (Mg, NH_4, and PO_4 are the most common)
    (e) Calcium carbonate
B. *Abnormal findings*
  1. Cystine
  2. Leucine or tyrosine (indicate protein breakdown)
  3. Cholesterin/cholesterol
  4. Drug crystals (sulfonamides, ampicillin)

Interfering Factors
Specific drugs may cause increased levels of their own crystals.

Shreds

Background
Shreds consist of a mixture of mucus, pus, and epithelial (squamous) cells. They can be seen on gross examination.

Clinical Implications
1. When mucus predominates, the shreds float on the surface.
2. When epithelial cells predominate, the shreds occupy the mid zone.
3. When pus (white blood cells) predominates, the shreds are drawn to the bottom of the specimen.
4. Other findings in urine due to contamination include microscopic yeast, trichomonas, spermatozoa, vegetable fibers, parasites, and meat fibers. They should be reported because they have clinical significance.

DRUG INVESTIGATION SPECIMENS

To screen for an unknown drug, the most valuable samples are (1) urine, (2) gastric specimens, and (3) blood. Urine drug screening is preferred for several reasons.

TABLE 3–2.
Common Urine Drug Tests*†

Amphetamines	Phencyclidine (PCP)
Alcohol	Lysergic acid diethylamide (LSD)
Barbiturates	Analgesics
Benzodiazepines	Sedatives
Cocaine, "Crack"	Major tranquilizers†
Cyanide	Stimulants
Opiates	Sympathomimetics
Marijuana (THC)	

* Many of the above drugs that are detectable in urine are not detectable in blood serum. All drugs detectable in serum are also detectable in urine, except glutethimide.
† Because minor tranquilizers are extensively metabolized, they are not likely to be detected in urine unless an overdose is taken.

1. Specimens are easily procured.
2. It is not an invasive procedure (unless urinary catheterization is involved).
3. Drug concentrations are more elevated in urine or are not detectable in blood (Table 3–2).
4. Drug metabolites are excreted for a longer period of time through urine (shows usage days or weeks ago).
5. Test procedures are more easily done and are more economical.

Note: Blood is the preferred medium for ethyl alcohol testing because drug concentration is more elevated and therefore more reliable (see Chap. 6).

Indications for Toxicology Screening
1. To confirm clinical or after-death diagnosis
2. To differentiate drug-induced disease from other causes such as trauma, metabolic, or infectious disease processes
3. To identify contributing diagnoses such as ethanol, trauma, other drugs, or underlying psychoses
4. Test results used as basis for high-risk interventions such as hemodialysis
5 To test for drug abuse in the workplace, especially where public safety is at risk or concern
6. As pre-employment testing for drug use or abuse.

Clinical Alert

When reporting drug test results for substance abuse, health care workers and patients should be aware of the psychological, social, economic, and legal implications and potential liabilities associated with the reporting or mismanagement of incorrectly reported results. Documented procedures should be established and maintained to ensure that before a result is reported as positive or negative, corroborating evidence exists to support that result or, in the absence of confirmation, that the result is identified as being an "unconfirmed" result. Confirmation of questionable results and values should be done by an equally sensitive and specific methodology that uses a different chemical principle. Keep in mind that problems associated with incorrect test results rise proportionately as the volume of drug abuse testing increases. For example, false-positive results can lead to employment disqualification or unfair dismissal. On the other hand, false-negative reports can fail to detect hazards.

Witnessed Urine Sampling for Suspected Substance Abuse

Procedure
1. The actual procurement or delivery of the sample is witnessed by a trained individual, is collected, and is tagged with a numerical code. A 50-ml random urine sample is obtained.
2. The sample is placed in a plastic heat-sealed sack and marked with a notary-style seal to protect against the possibility of unnoticed tampering.
3. A "chain of custody" document originates at sample collection. The person who provides the urine specimen signs the document, as does every person who handles the sample.
4. After both initial and confirmatory testing, the sample is resealed, marked, and securely stored for a minimum of 30 days.

Clinical Implications
A list of certain drugs that can be detected (based upon the duration of detectability) in urine follows (Pappas, Fody, and Cannon, 1987):

Amphetamines (4 hr duration)
Barbiturates (24 hr to 7 days duration)
Benzodiazapines (3 days duration)
Cannabenoids (21 hr to 3 days)
Cocaine as Metabolites (2 to 3 days duration)
Codeine (4 hr duration)
Methadone (3 days duration)

Methaqualine (7 days duration)
Morphine (4 hr duration)
Phencyclidine (7 days duration)
Proxyplene (6 hr duration)

Interfering Factors
Factors associated with incorrect test results for urine drug screens include the following:

Detergents
Sodium chloride (table salt)
Low specific gravity (dilute urine)
High *p*H (acid urine)
Low *p*H (base or alkaline urine)
Blood in the urine

OTHER URINARY CONSTITUENT TESTS

Chlorides (Cl); **Quantitative** (24-hr)

Normal Values
110–250 mEq/24 hr or 110–250 mmol/L
Vary greatly with salt intake and perspiration.

It is rather difficult to talk about "normal" and "abnormal" ranges. The test findings have meaning only in relation to salt intake and output.

Explanation of Test
The amount of chloride excreted in the urine in a 24-hour period is an indication of the state of electrolyte balance. Chloride is most often associated with sodium and fluid change.

The measurement of urine chloride may be useful as a means of diagnosing dehydration or as a guide in adjusting fluid and electrolyte balance in postoperative patients. It also serves as a means of monitoring the effects of reduced salt diets, which are of great therapeutic importance in patients with cardiovascular disease, hypertension, liver disease, and kidney ailments.

A patient on a restricted salt intake diet will usually not excrete more than 0.6 g/100 ml of NaCl in the urine, whereas a person on a normal salt diet would excrete 0.7 g/100 ml of NaCl or more.

Procedure
1. A 24-hour urine specimen is collected.
2. The exact times to start and complete the collection are recorded on the specimen container and on the patient's record.

3. When the specimen is completed, it should be sent to the laboratory for refrigeration.

> **Clinical Alert**
>
> Because electrolyte and water balance are so closely related, appraise the patient's state of hydration by checking daily weight and accurate intake and output, and by observing and recording skin turgor and the appearance of the tongue and the urine.

Clinical Implications
Results are significant only when considered in relation to other data, such as state of health or illness, salt intake, and urine volume.

A. *Normal findings*
   Urinary excretion of chloride decreases to a very low level whenever the serum level is much below 100 mEq/L.
B. *Decreased levels*
   1. In some conditions, urinary excretion of chloride increases even when the serum level is as low as 85 mEq/L or less. It occurs in Addison's disease when there is a deficiency of adrenal hormone that controls the excretion of sodium and chloride.
   2. Decreased levels associated with
      (a) Malabsorption syndrome   (e) Diaphoresis
      (b) Pyloric obstruction   (f) Congestive heart failure
      (c) Prolonged gastric suction   (g) Emphysema
      (d) Diarrhea
C. *Increased levels*
   Associated with
   (a) Dehydration
   (b) Starvation
   (c) Salicylate toxicity
   (d) Mercurial and chlorothiazide diuretics

Interfering Factors
1. Urinary chloride concentration varies with dietary salt intake and, to some degree, with urine volume.
2. False elevations may result if the patient has taken bromides.

Patient Preparation
Instruct the patient about the purpose of the test and the method for collecting a 24-hour specimen.

Sodium (Na); **Quantitative** (24-hr)

Normal Values
40–220 mEq/L/24 hr or 40–220 mmol/L, diet-dependent

Explanation of Test
This test measures electrolyte balance in the body by determining the amount of sodium excreted in 24 hours. It is indicated in the study of renal and adrenal disturbances and of water and acid–base imbalances.

Sodium is a primary regulator in the body's ability to retain or excrete water and maintain acid–base balance. The body has a strong tendency to maintain a total base content; only slight changes are found even under pathologic conditions. As the main base substance in the blood, sodium helps regulate acid–base balance because of its ability to combine with chloride and bicarbonate. Sodium also helps maintain the normal balance of electrolyte composition in intracellular and extracellular fluids by acting in conjunction with potassium (sodium–potassium pump). Sodium and potassium are important factors in nerve conduction, and they influence the irritability of the muscles, nerves, and heart.

Procedure
1. A 24-hour urine container is labeled with the name of the patient, the test, and the date.
2. Urine must be refrigerated or collected in an iced container.
3. General instructions for 24-hour urine collection are followed.
4. Exact start and ending of the collection are recorded on the specimen container and the patient's record.
5. Send the specimen to the laboratory refrigerator when the test is completed.

Clinical Implications
Results are significant only when considered in relation to other data, such as the state of health or illness, salt intake, and urine volume.
A. *Increased levels*
   1. Caused by
      (a) Dehydration
      (b) Starvation
      (c) Salicylate toxicity
      (d) Adrenal cortical insufficiency
      (e) Mercurial and chlorothiazide diuretics
      (f) Chronic renal failure
      (g) Diabetic acidosis
B. *Decreased levels of sodium* associated with
   (a) Malabsorption syndrome
   (b) Congestive heart failure
   (c) Pyloric obstruction
   (d) Diarrhea

(e) Diaphoresis
(f) Acute renal failure
(g) Pulmonary emphysema
(h) Aldosteronism
(i) Cushing's disease

C. *Decreased levels*
Often accompanied by an equivalent loss of chloride

Interfering Factors
1. Dietary salt intake
2. Altered kidney function

Patient Preparation
1. Instruct the patient about the purpose of the test, collection, and refrigeration of 24-hour urine specimen. Give a written reminder.
2. Food and fluids are permitted and encouraged.

Clinical Alert

Because electrolyte and water balance are so closely related, determine the patient's state of hydration by checking daily weight, accurate intake and output, observation and recording of skin turgor, and appearance of tongue and urine.

Potassium (K); Quantitative (24-hr)

Normal Values
25–125 mEq/24 hr or 25–125 mmol/24 hr
Varies with diet.

Explanation of Test
This test provides some insight into the electrolyte balance of the body by measuring the amount of potassium excreted in 24 hours. This measurement is useful in the study of renal and adrenal disorders and of water and acid–base imbalances. When a patient gives an obscure history in the presence of a known potassium deficit, evaluation of urinary potassium can be helpful in determining the origin of the deficit.

Potassium acts as a part of the body's buffer system; therefore, potassium balance serves a vital function in the body's overall electrolyte balance. Because the kidneys cannot conserve potassium, this balance is regulated by the kidneys' excretion of potassium through the urine.

Procedure
1. A 24-hour urine container is labeled with the name of the patient, test, and date.
2. Urine must be refrigerated or collected in an iced container.
3. General instructions for 24-hour urine collection are followed.
4. Exact start and ending of the collection are recorded on the specimen container and the patient's record.
5. Send the specimen to the laboratory refrigerator when the test is completed.

Clinical Implications
A. *Elevated levels*
   1. Found in:
      (a) Chronic renal failure
      (b) Diabetic and renal tubular acidosis
      (c) Dehydration
      (d) Starvation
      (e) Primary aldosteronism
      (f) Cushing's disease
      (g) Salicylate toxicity
      (h) Mercurial chlorothiazide, ammonium chloride, and Diamox diuretics
B. *Decreased levels*
   1. Associated with
      (a) Malabsorption syndrome
      (b) Diarrhea
      (c) Acute renal failure
      (d) Adrenocortical insufficiency (can be normal or decreased)
      (e) Excessive mineralocorticoid activity (aldosterone)
         Because licorice contains a mineralocorticoid compound, people who consume large amounts of licorice may have lowered urinary potassium levels.
   2. In patients with potassium deficiency, regardless of the cause, the urine pH tends to fall. This fall occurs because hydrogen ions are secreted in exchange for sodium ions, inasmuch as both potassium and hydrogen are excreted by the same mechanism.
C. *Cautionary findings*
   1. In excessive vomiting or stomach suctioning, the accompanying alkalosis maintains urinary potassium excretion at levels inappropriately high for the degree of actual potassium depletion.
   2. In diabetes insipidus, urinary potassium is normal.

Interfering Factors
Factors vary with dietary intake.

Patient Preparation

1. Instruct the patient about the purpose of the test, collection and refrigeration of 24-hour urine specimen. Give a written reminder.
2. Food and fluids are permitted and encouraged.

Clinical Alert

1. Because electrolyte and water balance are so closely associated, determine the patient's state of hydration by checking daily weight, accurate intake and output, and by observing and recording skin turgor and appearance of the tongue and urine.
2. Observe for signs of muscle weakness, tremors, and changes in electrocardiograms. The level of potassium increase or decrease at which these symptoms become apparent varies from patient to patient.

Uric Acid; Quantitative (24-hr)

Normal Values

250–750 mg/24 hr on normal diet or 1.48–4.43 mmol/day
120 mg/24 hr on a purine-free diet or 2.48 mmol/day
1000 mg/24 hr on a high-purine diet or 5.90 mmol/day

Explanation of Test

Uric acid formation occurs as a result of the metabolic breakdown of nucleic acids; purines are the principal source of this breakdown. The test is indicated in the investigation of metabolic disturbances to identify gout and diagnose kidney disease. It will also reflect the effect of uricosuric agents when these drugs are used, by indicating the total amount of uric acid excreted.

Procedure

1. A 24-hour urine container with preservative added is labeled with the name of the patient, test, and date.
2. General instructions for 24-hour urine collection are followed.
3. Exact start and ending of the collection are recorded on the specimen container and the patient's record.
4. Send the specimen to the laboratory when the test is completed.

Clinical Implications
A. *Increased levels* (uricosuria)
1. Found in
(a) Gout
(b) Chronic myelogenous leukemia
(c) Polycythemia vera
(d) Liver disease
(e) Febrile illness
(f) Toxemias of pregnancy
(g) Fanconi's syndrome
2. Cytotoxic drugs to treat lymphoma and leukemia often cause greatly increased urinary uric acid levels.
3. High uric acid concentration plus low urine pH may lead to uric acid stones in the urinary tract.
B. *Decreased levels*
Found in kidney disease (chronic glomerulonephritis) because impaired renal function depresses uric acid excretion.

Interfering Factors
1. Many drugs, such as
(a) Salicylates
(b) Thiazide diuretics
(c) Chronic alcohol ingestion
2. Radiograph contrast media can markedly increase uric acid levels.

Patient Preparation
1. Instruct the patient about the purpose of the test, collection, and refrigeration of 24-hour urine specimen. Give a written reminder.
2. Food and fluids are permitted and encouraged. In some diagnostic situations, a diet high or low in purines may be ordered during the test period.

Calcium; Quantitative (24-hr) Sulkowitch

Normal Values
24-hour levels
100–300 mg/average diet or 2.50–7.50 mmol/day
50–150 mg/low-calcium diet or 1.25–3.75 mmol/day

Explanation of Test
The bulk of the calcium discharged by the body is excreted in the stool. However, there is a small quantity of calcium that is normally excreted in the urine, the amount increasing or decreasing as a result of changes in the quantity of dietary calcium ingested.

The 24-hour test is most often ordered to determine the function of the parathyroid gland, which maintains a balance between calcium and phosphorus by means of parathyroid hormone. Hyperparathyroidism is a generalized disorder of calcium, phosphate, and bone metabolism that results from an increased secretion of parathyroid hormones and an increased excretion of urinary calcium. In hypoparathyroidism, the urinary calcium is decreased.

Procedure
1. A 24-hour urine container is labeled with the name of the patient, test, and date.
2. An acid-washed bottle is required if not ordered with any other tests. See chart on page 146 regarding 24-hour urine collection data.
3. General instructions for 24-hour urine collection are followed.
4. Exact start and ending of the collection are recorded on the specimen container and the patient's record.
5. Send the specimen to the laboratory when the test is completed.

Clinical Implications
A. *Increased levels*
  1. Caused by
      (a) Hyperparathyroidism (results in constant 3+ to 4+ Sulkowitch tests)
      (b) Sarcoidosis
      (c) Primary cancers of breast and lung
      (d) Metastatic malignancies
      (e) Myeloma with bone metastasis
      (f) Wilson's disease
      (g) Renal tubular acidosis
      (h) Glucocorticoid excess
      (i) Fanconi syndrome
      (j) Vitamin D intoxication
  2. Increased urinary calcium almost always accompanies elevated blood calcium levels.
  3. Calcium excretion greater than intake is always excessive, and excretion above 400 to 500 mg/24 hours is reliably abnormal.
  4. Increased excretion of calcium occurs whenever calcium is mobilized from the bone, as in metastatic cancer and prolonged skeletal immobilization.
  5. When calcium is excreted in increasing amounts, a potential for nephrolithiasis or nephrocalcinosis is created.
B. *Decreased levels*
  1. Caused by
      (a) Hypoparathyroidism (hypocalcemia caused by hypoparathyroidism is usually associated with a negative reaction)

    (b) Vitamin D deficiency (vitamin D is necessary for absorption of calcium)

    (c) Malabsorption syndrome

Interfering Factors

A. *False elevated levels* are due to

  1. High sodium and magnesium intake

  2. Very high milk intake

  3. Some drugs

  4. Level higher immediately after meals

B. *False-negative levels* are due to

  1. Increased dietary phosphates

  2. Alkaline urine

  3. Some drugs

Patient Preparation

1. Instruct the patient about the purpose of the test, collection of 24-hour urine specimen. Give a written reminder.
2. Food and fluids are permitted and encouraged.
3. If the urine calcium test is done because of a metabolic disorder, the patient should eat a low-calcium diet and be on calcium medication restrictions for a 1- to 3-day period prior to collection of the specimen.
4. If the patient has a history of renal stone formation, a general diet will be prescribed.

Clinical Alert

1. Observe patients with very low urine calcium levels for signs and symptoms of tetany.
2. The first sign of calcium imbalance may be the occurrence of pathologic fracture that can be related to calcium excess.
3. The Sulkowitch test can be used in an emergency, especially when hypercalcemia is suspected, because hypercalcemia is life-threatening. A fasting, first morning specimen is examined for turbidity. Normal is 8 to 12 mg/dl; increased is greater than 12 mg/dl.

Magnesium; Quantitative (24-hr)

Normal Values

6.0–10.0 mEq/24-hr or 3.00–5.00 mmol/24-hr

Explanation of Test

A 24-hour urine test is useful in the evaluation of renal disease and magnesium deficiency. In magnesium deficiency, urine magnesium decreases before serum magnesium.

Procedure

1. A 24-hour urine specimen is obtained in a metal-free container with no preservative.
2. Exact starting and ending times should be recorded.

Clinical Implications

1. *Increased excretion* is associated with
    (a) Drugs such as thiazide, diuretics, ethacrynic acid, alcohol, corticosteroids, platinum therapy, and aldosterone.
    (b) Bartter's syndrome.
2. *Decreased excretion* is associated with
    (a) Renal disease
    (b) Magnesium deficiency

Oxalate; Quantitative (24-hr)

Normal Values

Urine: 8–40 mg/24 hr or 91–456 μmol/24 hr

Explanation of Test

This test is of value in diagnosing systemic poisoning due to ethylene glycol poisoning, kidney stones, and primary hyperoxalurea, a genetic disorder.

Procedure

A 24-hour urine specimen is collected using hydrochloric acid as a preservative. See page 146 for specifics.

Interfering Factors

Foods such as rhubarb, strawberries, beans, beets, spinach, and tomatoes, gelatin, chocolate, cocoa, and tea, as well as calcium and ascorbic acid and some drugs increase excretion.

Clinical Implications

1. *Increased values* are associated with
    (a) Ethylene glycol poisoning
        (>150 mg/day or >1710 μmol/day)
    (b) Primary hyperoxaluria
        (100–600 mg/day or 1140–6840 μmol/day
        [nephrocalcinosis])

(c) Diabetes
(d) Cirrhosis
(e) B$_6$ deficiency
(f) Sarcoidosis
(g) Steatorrhea due to pancreatic insufficiency
(h) Celiac disease
(i) Bacterial overgrowth
(j) Ileal resection
(k) Jejuno-ileal shunt
(l) Biliary tract disease
(m) Small bowel disease

2. *Decreased values* are associated with renal failure.

Patient Preparation
Explain the purpose and procedure of the test. No foods that increase excretion are to be eaten.

Follicle-Stimulating Hormone (FSH); Luteinizing Hormone (LH)

Normal Values
FSH
Men: 1–20 IU/24 hr
Women: 5–20 IU/24 hr
Postmenopausal: 30–440 IU/24 hr
Midcycle peak: 15–30 IU/24 hr

LH
Men: 5–20 IU/24 hr
Women: 5–15 IU/24 hr follicular phase
Postmenopausal: 50–100 IU/24 hr
Midcycle peak: 30–95 IU/24 hr
See your laboratory for values in infants and children.

Explanation of Test
This 24-hour urine test measures the gonadotropic hormones FSH and LH and may be helpful in determining whether a gonadal insufficiency is primary or due to insufficient stimulation by the pituitary hormones. Production of these gonadotropins is believed to be under control of the pituitary gland. In women, FSH promotes maturation of the ovarian follicle, and the maturing follicle produces estrogens. As the levels of estrogen rise, luteinizing hormones are produced. Together, FSH and LH induce ovulation. In men, FSH produces spermatogenesis, and LH stimulates the secretion of androgens and increased synthesis of testosterone. In women, LH acts on the interstitial cells, resulting in synthesis of androgens, estrogens, and progesterone.

Follicle-stimulating hormone is an aid in studying various causes of hypothyroidism in women as well as endocrine dysfunction in men. In primary ovarian failure or testicular failure, FSH is increased. Measuring urine FSH and LH are of value for children with endocrine problems related to precocious puberty. Urine assays are also used to monitor ovulatory cycles of *in vitro* fertilization patients.

Procedure
1. A 24-hour urine container is labeled with the name of the patient, test, and date. The 24-hour urine collection minimizes the problems with episodic secretion spikes that occur with blood serum specimens.
2. Urine is collected either with a preservative or refrigerated only.
3. A blood sample of at least 3 ml can also be obtained. Sometimes multiple blood specimens are necessary because of episodic release of FSH from the pituitary gland. An isolated sample may be at the peak or valley of secretion.
4. In anovulatory fertility problems, the presence or absence of a midcycle peak can be established by a series of daily blood specimens.
5. When all the urine is collected, the specimen is sent to the laboratory refrigerator.

Clinical Implications
A. *Decreased FSH levels* occur in
   1. Feminizing and masculinizing ovarian tumors when production is inhibited as a result of increased estrogen
   2. Failure of pituitary or hypothalamus
   3. Anorexia nervosa
   4. Neoplasm of testes or adrenal glands that secrete estrogens or androgens
B. *Increased FSH levels* occur in
   1. Turner's syndrome (ovarian dysgenesis). Approximately 50% of patients with primary amenorrhea have Turner's syndrome.
   2. Hypogonadism and primary gonadal failure
   3. Complete testicular feminization syndrome
   4. Precocious puberty, either idiopathic or secondary to a central nervous system lesion
   5. Klinefelter's syndrome
C. *Both FSH and LH are increased* in
   (a) Primary gonadal failure
   (b) Complete testicular feminization syndrome
   (c) Precocious puberty
D. *Decreased FSH and LH* occur in
   Failure of pituitary or hypothalamus

Patient Preparation
Instruct the patient about the purpose of the test and collection of 24-hour urine specimen. Give a written reminder.

Pregnanediol

Normal Values
This test is difficult to standardize; it varies with age, sex, and weeks of pregnancy.

Men: 0–1 mg/24 hr
Women: Pregnancy: 6–100 mg/24 hr
         Postmenopausal—0.2–1 mg/24 hr

Explanation of Test
This test is a measurement of ovarian and placental function. It is indicated when a deficiency of progesterone is suspected. Combined deficiency of estrogen and progesterone is evidenced by menstrual irregularities and difficulty in conceiving and maintaining a pregnancy. Specifically, it measures the hormone progesterone and its principal excreted metabolite, pregnanediol. Progesterone has its main effect in the endometrium by causing the endometrium to enter the secretory phase and become ready for implantation of the blastocyte if fertilization has occurred.

Pregnanediol excretion is high in pregnancy and low in luteal deficiency or placental failure.

Procedure
1. A 24-hour urine container is labeled with the name of the patient, test, and date.
2. Refrigeration of the specimen may be required or a boric acid preservative added. Check your laboratory policy.
3. General instructions for 24-hour urine collection are followed.
4. Exact start and ending of the collection are recorded on the specimen container and the patient's record.
5. When all urine is collected, the specimen is sent to the laboratory refrigerator.

Clinical Implications
A. *Increased levels* are associated with
   1. Luteal cysts of ovary
   2. Arrhenoblastoma of the ovary
   3. Hyperadrenocorticism
B. *Decreased levels* are associated with
   1. Amenorrhea
   2. Threatened abortion (sometimes)
   3. Fetal death
   4. Toxemia

Patient Preparation
1. Instruct the patient about the purpose of the test and collection of 24-hour urine specimen. Give a written reminder.
2. Food and fluids are permitted.

Pregnanetriol

Normal Values
Adults: up to 2 mg/24 hr or <5.04 µmol/day
Children: up to 1.5 mg/24 hr or <4.46 µmol/day
Infants: up to 0.2 mg/24 hr or up to 0.59 µmol/day

Explanation of Test
Pregnanetriol is a compound substance reflecting one segment of adrenocortical activity. Pregnanetriol should not be confused with pregnanediol, despite the similarity of name. Pregnanetriol is a precursor in adrenocorticoid synthesis and arises from 17-hydroxyprogesterone, not from progesterone.

This 24-hour urine test is done to diagnose adrenocortical dysfunction, adrenogenital syndrome, a defect in 21-hydroxylation. The diagnosis of adrenogenital syndrome is considered in the following instances:

1. Adult women who show signs and symptoms of excessive androgen production with or without hypertension
2. Craving for salt
3. Sexual precocity in boys
4. Infants who exhibit signs of failure to thrive
5. External genitalia in women (pseudohermaphroditism)

In boys, differentiation must be made between a virilizing tumor of the adrenal gland, neurogenic and constitutional types of sexual precocity, and interstitial cell tumor of the testes.

Procedure
1. A 24-hour urine container is labeled with the name of the patient, test, and date.
2. Refrigeration of the specimen may be required; some laboratories may require boric acid preservative.
3. General instructions for 24-hour urine collection are followed.
4. Exact start and ending of the collection are recorded on the specimen container and the patient's record.
5. When all urine is collected, the specimen is sent to the laboratory.

Clinical Implications
Elevated pregnanetriol levels occur in

1. Congenital adrenocortical hyperplasia
2. Stein–Leventhal syndrome

Patient Preparation
1. Instruct the patient about the purpose of the test and collection of 24-hour urine specimen. Give a written reminder.
2. Food and fluids are permitted.

5-Hydroxyindoleacetic Acid (5-HIAA)
(5-Hydroxy 3, Serotonin, Indoleacetic Acid)

Normal Values
Qualitative: negative
Quantitative: 2–8 mg/24 hr or 10.4–41.6 μmol/24 hr

Explanation of Test
The qualitative random sample test may be done for screening purposes, followed by a quantitative 24-hour test if need be, or the 24-hour test may be done initially.

The urine test is conducted to diagnose a functioning carcinoid tumor, which is indicated by significant elevation of 5-hydroxyindoleacetic acid (5-HIAA), a denatured product of serotonin. Serotonin is a vasoconstricting hormone normally produced by the argentaffin cells of the gastrointestinal tract. The principal function of the cells is to regulate smooth muscle contraction and peristalsis.

Procedure
1. No bananas, pineapple, tomatoes, eggplants, or avocados are to be eaten during the 24-hour test because they contain serotonin (5-hydroxyindoleacetic acid is a metabolic product of serotonin).
2. A 24-hour urine container with preservative is labeled with the name of the patient, test, and date.
3. General instructions for 24-hour urine collection are followed.
4. Exact start and ending of the collection are recorded on the specimen container and the patient's record.
5. Send the specimen to the laboratory refrigerator when the test is completed.

Clinical Implications
1. Levels over 100 mg/24 hr are indicative of large carcinoid tumor, especially when metastatic. However, this increase occurs in only 5% to 7% of patients with carcinoid tumor.

2. *Levels greater than* 10 mg but less than 100 mg are found in
   (a) Hemorrhage
   (b) Thrombosis
   (c) Nontropical sprue
   (d) Severe pain of sciatica or skeletal and smooth muscle spasm
   (e) Oat cell cancer of bronchus
   (f) Bronchial adenoma of carcinoid type
3. *Decreased levels* are found in
   (a) Depressive illness
   (b) Small intestinal resection
   (c) Mastocytosis
   (d) Phenylketonuria (PKU)
   (e) Hartnup's disease

Interfering Factors

A. *False positives*
   1. Bananas, pineapples, plums, walnuts, eggplants, tomatoes, and avocados may increase the 5-HIAA level, for these foods contain serotonin.
   2. A number of drugs may cause false positives.
B. *False negatives*
   Specific drugs may cause false negatives (depressing 5-HIAA).

Patient Preparation

1. Instruct the patient about the purpose of the test and collection of the 24-hour urine specimen. Give a written reminder.
2. Food and water are permitted and encouraged. Foods high in serotonin content are not to be eaten during the test.

Clinical Alert

The patient should take no drugs for 72 hours before the test, if at all possible.

Vanillylmandelic Acid (VMA) (Catecholamines, 3-Methoxy-4-Hydroxymandelic Acid)

Normal Values

Vanillylmandelic acid up to 7 μg/mg/24 hr or up to 35.4 μmol/24 hr
Catecholamines
Epinephrine: 0–15 μg/24 hr or 0.0–81.9 nmol/24 hr
Norepinephrine: 0–100 μg/24 hr or 0–591 nmol/24 hr
Metanephrine: 0.25–0.8 mg/24 hr or 1.27–4.06 μmol/day
Dopamine: 65–400 μg/24 hr or 424–2612 nmol/24 hr

Explanation of Test
This 24-hour urine test of adrenomedullar function is primarily done when a person with hypertension is suspected of having pheochromocytoma, a tumor of the chromaffin cells of the adrenal medulla. (Less than 1% of hypertensive patients have pheochromocytoma.) The principal substances formed by the adrenal medulla and excreted in the urine include VMA, epinephrine, norepinephrine, metanephrine, and normetanephrine. These compounds contain a catechol nucleus and an amine group and are thus referred to as *catecholamines.* The major portion of the hormones are changed into metabolites, the principal one being 3-methoxy-4-hydroxymandelic acid, or VMA.

Vanillylmandelic acid is the main urinary metabolite of the catecholamine group, having a urine concentration much greater than the other amines (10 to 100 times). It is also easier to detect owing to simpler laboratory methods than the methods that must be used for catecholamine determination. Testing for VMA is important in pheochromocytoma because these tumors secrete excessive amounts of catecholamine, resulting in high urine levels of VMA.

Procedure
1. A 24-hour urine container with preservative is labeled with the name of the patient, test, and date.
2. General instructions for 24-hour urine collection are followed.
3. Exact start and ending of the collection are recorded on the specimen container and the patient's record.
4. When all the urine is collected, the specimen is sent to the laboratory refrigerator.

Clinical Implications
A. *Elevated levels of VMA*
   1. High levels found in pheochromocytoma
   2. Slight to moderate elevations in
      (a) Neuroblastomas
      (b) Ganglioneuromas
      (c) Ganglioblastomas
B. *Elevated catecholamines*
   Found in
   (1) Pheochromocytoma
   (2) Neuroblastomas
   (3) Ganglioneuromas
   (4) Ganglioblastomas
   (5) Progressive muscular dystrophy
   (6) Myasthenia gravis

Interfering Factors
A. *Increased levels of VMA* are caused by
   1. Starvation. (For this reason, the test should *not* be scheduled while the patient is NPO.)

2. Many foods such as the following:
   (a) Tea
   (b) Coffee
   (c) Cocoa
   (d) Vanilla
   (e) Fruit, especially ba-
       nanas
   (f) Fruit juice
   (g) Chocolate
   (h) Cheese
   (i) Cider vinegar
   (j) Gelatin foods
   (k) Salad dressing
   (l) Carbonated drinks, ex-
       cept gingerale
   (m)Jelly and jam
   (n) Candy and mints
   (o) Cough drops
   (p) Chewing gum
   (q) Foods containing artifi-
       cial flavoring or coloring
   (r) Foods containing licorice
3. Many drugs will cause increased VMA levels.
B. *False decreased levels* of VMA are caused by
   1. Alkaline urine
   2. Uremia (causes toxicity and impaired excretion of VMA)
   3. Radiographic iodine contrast agents (For this reason, an intra-
      venous pyelogram should not be scheduled prior to a VMA test.)
   4. Specific drugs
C. *Interfering factors in determining catecholamine levels*
   1. Vigorous exercise may cause increase.
   2. Certain drugs may cause increase.

Patient Preparation
1. Instruct the patient about the purpose of the test and collection of
   the 24-hour urine specimen. Give a written reminder.
2. Explain diet and drug restrictions.
3. Diet restrictions will vary among laboratory policies, but coffee,
   tea, bananas, cocoa products, vanilla products, and aspirin are always excluded for 3 days (2 days prior to testing and day of the test).
4. Many laboratories require that all drugs be discontinued for 3 to 7
   days before testing.
5. Rest and adequate food and fluids are encouraged, and stress is to
   be avoided during the test.

Patient Aftercare
Restricted foods, drugs, and activity are permitted as soon as the test is
completed.

17-Ketosteroids (17-KS);
17-Hydroxycorticosteroids (17-OHCS)

Normal Values
17-Ketosteroids (17-KS)
Men: 8–20 mg/24 hr

Women: 6–15 mg/24 hr
Children: 0–2 mg/24 hr

17-Hydroxycorticosteroids (17-OHCS)
Men: 3–10 mg/24 hr
Women: 2–6 mg/24 hr

Explanation of Test

These 24-hour tests of adrenal function measure the excretion of urinary steroids and are indicated in the investigation of endocrine disturbances of the adrenals and testes.

Urinary steroids can be divided into three main groups:

17-ketosteroids (17-KS)—adrenal hormones and metabolites of testicular androgens. In men, the adrenals produce two thirds of 17-KS, whereas the testes produce the remainder. In women the adrenals produce all of these hormones. In both sexes, 17-KS decline with age.

17-ketogenic steroids (17-KGS)—adrenal cortex activity

17-hydroxycorticosteroids (17-OHCS)—Porter–Silber chromogens

Procedure

1. A 24-hour urine container with preservative is labeled with the name of the patient, test, and date.
2. General instructions for 24-hour urine collection are followed.
3. Exact start and ending of the collection are recorded on the specimen container and the patient's record.
4. Send the specimen to the laboratory when the test is completed.

Interfering Factors

1. Severe stress and obesity will cause increased levels of ketosteroids and hydroxycorticosteroids.
2. Ketosteroid levels are often increased in the third trimester of pregnancy.
3. Many drugs affect test outcomes.

The 17-ketosteroids are excreted in the urine as the sulfates and glucuronides of androsterone.

Dehydroepiandrosterone (DHEA)
Etiocholanalase
11-beta hydroxyandrosterone
11-beta hydroxyetiocholanolone
11-ketoandrosterone
and
11-ketoetiocholanolone

Increased 17-KS
1. Adrenal carcinomas
2. Pregnancy
3. Premature infants
4. ACTH administration
5. Testicular interstitial cell tumors
6. Cushing's syndrome
7. Nonmalignant virilizing adrenal tumors
8. Androgenic arrhenoblastoma
9. Luteal cell ovarian tumors
10. Female pseudohermaphroditism
11. Adrenogenital syndrome associated with adrenal hyperplasia

Decreased 17-KS
1. Addison's disease
2. Panhypopituitarism
3. Myxedema
4. Nephrosis
5. Castration or eunuchoidism in man
6. Gout
7. Chronic illness
8. Thyrotoxicosis

Increased 17-OHCS
1. Any acute illness
2. Cushing's disease
3. Adrenal adenoma
4. Carcinoma
5. Ectopic ACTH syndrome
6. Severe hypertension
7. Acromegaly
8. Thyrotoxicosis

Decreased 17-OHCS
1. Addison's disease
2. Congenital adrenal hyperplasia
3. Hypopituitarism
4. Hypothyroidism

Patient Preparation
1. Instruct the patient about the purpose of the test and collection of 24-hour urine specimen. Give a written reminder.
2. Food and fluids are permitted and encouraged.

Porphyrins and Porphobilinogens

Normal Values
Porphobilinogens: 0–2 mg/24 hr or negative or 0–8.8 μmol/24 hr
Children: <1 μg/24 hr
Uroporphyrins: >60 μg/24 hr
DAL or ALA: 1.5–7.5 mg/24 hr
Coproporphyrin: <180 μg/24 hr

Explanation of Test

Porphyrins are cyclic compounds formed from delta-aminolevulinic acid (DAL or ALA), which is important in the formation of hemoglobin and other hemoproteins that function as carriers of oxygen in the blood and tissues. In health, insignificant amounts of porphyrin are excreted in the urine. However, in certain conditions, such as porphyria (disturbance in metabolism of porphyrin), liver disease, lead poisoning, and pellagra, there is an increased level of porphyrins, as well as DAL and ALA in the urine. Disorders in porphyrin metabolism also result in porphobilinogen.

In acute attacks of porphyria, the patient may suffer skin lesions, abdominal pain, neuropathy, and mental disturbances. The urine of patients with this disease usually has a pinkish to reddish black tinge and will become darker upon standing.

In the laboratory, the urine is tested for the presence of porphyrins, porphobilinogen, and DAL or ALA. It is also given the black light screening test (porphyrins are fluorescent when exposed to black or ultraviolet light). See Chapter 2 for other tests for porphyria.

Procedure

1. A 24-hour clean-catch urine container is labeled with the name of the patient, test, and date.
2. Refrigeration is usually required. The specimen is kept protected from exposure to light.
3. General instructions for 24-hour urine collection are followed.
4. Exact start and ending of the collection are recorded on the specimen container and the patient's record.
5. Send the specimen to the laboratory when the test is completed. Preservative is usually added in the laboratory.
6. Porphobilinogens are always done with the porphyrin test. Should a single, freshly voided specimen be ordered, only a porphobilinogen will be done. Protect specimen from light. Take specimen to laboratory immediately. The test must be performed within 60 minutes of voiding for test to be valid. If possible, obtain specimen between 10:00 AM and 2:00 PM
7. Observe and record the color of urine. If porphyrins are present, the urine may have a grossly recognizable amber red or burgundy color. It may vary from pale pink to almost black. Some patients will excrete a urine of normal color that turns dark after standing in the light.

Clinical Implications

A. *Porphyria*
   1. In the porphyrias, the urine contains increased amounts of porphyrins and porphobilinogens and may not contain increased quantities of DAL or ALA.

   2. Excretion of ALA and DAL is elevated in acute intermittent porphyria, an hepatic porphyria that is aggravated by alcohol, barbiturates, and other drugs affecting the liver.

B. *Lead poisoning*
1. ALA or DAL will be present in the urine.
2. Porphyrins may or may not be present in the urine.

C. *Other conditions with increased levels of porphyrins*

1. Cirrhosis	6. Heavy metal poisoning
2. Infectious hepatitis	7. Carbon tetrachloride or
3. Hodgkin's disease	benzine toxicity
4. Some cancers	8. Vitamin deficiency
5. Central nervous system disorders	

D. A number of drugs may cause false-positive tests.

Patient Preparation

1. Instruct the patient about the purpose and collection of a 24-hour urine specimen. Give a written reminder.
2. Food and fluids are permitted; alcohol and excessive fluid intake during collection should be avoided.

Clinical Alert

This test should not be ordered for patients receiving Donnatal and other barbiturate preparations. However, if intermittent porphyria is the reason for testing, the test should be done with the patient receiving these medications because these drugs may provoke an attack of porphyria.

Formiminoglutamic (FIGLU) Acid Excretion Test

Normal Values
Less than 35 mg/day or less than 201 μmol/day

Explanation of Test
This 24-hour test is ordered in the evaluation of folic acid deficiency. It is an indirect test for folate; when histidine is administered to a person with a folic acid deficiency, FIGLU acid will increase. The test is not useful in pregnant women.

Procedure
1. The 24-hour urine collection begins after dose(s) of histidine.
2. A container containing 12 ml of glucose acetic acid is required. Refrigeration is also required.

3. Label the container with the name of the patient, test, and date.
4. Follow general instructions for 24-hour urine collection.
5. Record exact start and ending of the collection on both the specimen container and the patient's record.
6. Send the specimen to the laboratory when the test is completed.

Clinical Implications
1. Increased values (>35 mg/dl) are associated with
   (a) Folate deficiency
   (b) Primary vitamin B_{12} deficiency
   (c) Protein malnutrition
   (d) Megaloblastic anemia
   (e) Hereditary spherocytosis
   (f) Alcoholics with and without liver disease

Interfering Factors
1. Drugs that decrease values include those that cause megaloblastic anemia.
2. Decreases occur in persons with low histidine intake and normal persons.
3. Increased levels are associated with pregnancy (especially older women), parity, and toxemia.

Patient Preparation
1. Instruct the patient about the purpose of the test and collection of the 24-hour urine specimen using a preservative. Give a written reminder.
2. Food and fluids are permitted. Check with laboratory for any dietary guidelines regarding histidine intake.

Amylase Excretion/Clearance

Normal Values
0–275 U/L or 14 units/hr
1500–6000 Somogyi units/24 hr or 277–1110 U/24 hr

Background
Amylase is an enzyme that changes starch to sugar. It is produced in the salivary glands, pancreas, liver, and fallopian tubes and normally is excreted in small amounts in the urine. If there is an inflammation of the pancreas or salivary glands, much more of the enzyme enters the blood and more amylase is excreted in the urine.

Explanation of Test

This test of blood and urine is an indication of pancreatic function and is done to differentiate acute pancreatitis from peptic ulcer and other disorders in which amylase is increased. The timed urine and amylase test (2 hours or 24 hours) is ordered to detect inflammation of the salivary glands or pancreas, to monitor treatment of acute pancreatitis, and to recognize recurrent attacks of acute pancreatitis in persons who exhibit severe abdominal pain.

The 2-hour amylase excretion in the urine is a more sensitive test than either the serum amylase or lipase test. In patients with acute pancreatitis, the urine often shows a prolonged elevation of amylase as compared to the short-lived peak in the blood. However, urine amylase may be elevated when blood amylase is within normal range, and, conversely, the blood amylase may be elevated when urine amylase is within normal range. The 24-hour level may be normal even when some of the 1- or 2-hour specimens show increased values.

Procedure

A venous blood sample of 4 ml may be collected at the same time a random urine specimen is obtained.

1. A 1-hour, 2-hour, or 24-hour timed specimen will be ordered. A 2-hour specimen is usually collected.
2. No preservative or refrigeration is required.
3. General instructions for a timed or 24-hour urine collection are followed.
4. Exact start and ending of the collection are recorded on the specimen container and on the patient's record.
5. Send the specimen to the laboratory refrigerator when the test is completed.

Clinical Implications

1. Elevated levels of urine amylase are associated with acute pancreatitis, choledocholithiasis, and peptic ulcer.
2. Patients with acute pancreatitis have values about 900 units/hour during the first 2 days of the attack; it increases sooner than blood amylase. Urine amylase also stays elevated longer in acute pancreatitis.
3. Values will increase about five per unit in pancreatitis; in other disorders associated with hyperamylase, the level is less than 5%.

Patient Preparation

1. Instruct the patient about the purpose of the test and collection of the urine specimen. Give a written reminder for 2-hour or 24-hour test.
2. Encourage fluids during test if fluids are not restricted for other medical reasons.

Phenylketonuria (PKU) **in Blood and Urine**

Normal Values
Blood <4 mg/100 ml
Urine: Negative dipstick; no observed color change

Explanation of Test
Routine blood and urine tests are done on newborns to detect PKU, a genetic disease that can lead to mental retardation and brain damage if untreated. This disease is characterized by a lack of the enzyme that converts phenylalanine, an amino acid, to tyrosine, which is necessary for normal metabolic function. If tyrosine accumulates in the tissues, phenylpyruvic acid, a metabolite of phenylalanine, will be produced, resulting in brain damage. Phenylalanine can be detected in the blood of an abnormal child in 4 days. Phenylpyruvic acid appears in the urine of an abnormal child about 2 to 8 weeks after birth. Current practice is to test for PKU either with a blood phenylalanine test or with a phenylpyruvic acid urine test.

Procedure (Collecting Blood Sample)
1. After the skin is cleansed with an antiseptic, the infant's heel is punctured with a sterile disposable lancet.
2. If bleeding is slow, it is helpful to hold the leg dependent for a short time before spotting the blood on the filter paper.
3. The circles on the filter paper must be filled completely. This can best be done by placing one side of the filter paper against the infant's heel and watching for the blood to appear on the front side of the paper and completely fill the circle.

Procedure (Collecting Urine Sample in Nursery or at Home)
1. The reagent strip is either dipped into a fresh sample of urine or pressed against a wet diaper.
2. After exactly 30 seconds, the strip is compared to a color chart scaled at concentrations of 0, 15, 40, and 100 mg phenylpyruvic acid.

Clinical Implications
1. In a positive test for PKU, the blood phenylalanine is greater than 15 mg/100 ml. Blood tyrosine is less than 5 mg/100 ml. It is never increased in PKU.
2. The urine test is positive in PKU.

Interfering Factors
1. Premature infants, infants weighing less than 11 kg (5 lb) may have elevated phenylalanine and tyrosine levels without having the genetic disease. This is probably a result of delayed development of appropriate enzyme activity in the liver.

2. Large amounts of ketones in urine will produce an atypical color reaction.

Instructions to Mothers

1. Inform the mother about the purpose of the test and the method of collecting the specimens.
2. Most parents would be interested in knowing that PKU (a genetic disease in which a defective gene is passed on from each parent) was first recognized about 40 years ago by a young mother of two mentally retarded children. She was aware that the urine of these children had a peculiar odor, and on the basis of this was able to have a biochemist study the urine and identify phenylpyruvic acid. About 20 years ago, the first successful dietary treatment (restriction of phenylalanine as in milk) of newborn babies identified as having PKU was started, resulting in normal mental development.

Clinical Alert

1. The blood test must be performed at least 3 days after birth or after the child has had a chance to ingest protein (milk) for a period of 24 hours.
2. Urine testing is usually done at the 4- or 6-week checkup if a blood sample was not obtained.
3. PKU studies should be done on all infants 5 lb or more before they leave the hospital.

Tubular Reabsorption Phosphate (TRP)

Normal Values
82%–95% on normal diet or 0.82–0.95

Explanation of Test
This test is done to detect hyperparathyroidism. A fasting blood and a 24-hour or a 4-hour urine sample is obtained to determine the levels of phosphorus and creatinine. The results of the test are based on the ratio of creatinine clearance to phosphate clearance. The TRP is a rough estimation of the level of parathyroid hormone in the blood. The test is based on the fact that excessive parathyroid hormone increases renal tubular reabsorption of phosphate. However, the test has a limited value, and a determination of increased calcium in the blood is still essential for the exact diagnosis of hyperparathyroidism.

Procedure

1. An overnight fast from food is usually necessary. Water is permitted.
2. A venous blood sample will be obtained the morning of the day the test is completed.
3. A 24-hour urine container (also used for 4-hour test) with preservatives is labeled with the name of the patient, test, and date.
4. General instructions for 24-hour or 4-hour urine collection are followed.
5. A good time to do this test is from noon to noon, although it is not necessary.

   Exact start and ending of the collection are recorded on the specimen container and the patient's record.

   Send the specimen to the laboratory refrigerator when the test is completed.

Clinical Implications

1. In hyperparathyroidism, the reabsorption of phosphate is increased.
2. The TRP is decreased in hypoparathyroidism.

Interfering Factors

False-positive results may occur in the presence of uremia, renal tubular disease, osteomalacia, and sarcoidosis.

Patient Preparation

1. Instruct the patient about the purpose of the test, collection of 24-hour or 4-hour urine specimen, overnight fast if ordered, and blood sample. A normal or phosphate diet will be ordered. Give a written reminder.
2. If fasting is ordered, encourage the patient to drink water.

D-**Xylose Absorption**

Normal Values

Urine: Adult—>4 g/after 5 hr
Blood: Adult—>25 mg/dl
Blood: Child—>30 mg/dl after 1 hr
Urine: Child—>16% ingested dose

Explanation of Test

This test is an indirect measure of intestinal absorption and is used in the differential diagnosis of steatorrhea. The usual problem is the differentiation of pancreatic from enterogenous steatorrhea. When D-xylose (which is not metabolized by the body) is administered orally, blood and urine levels are checked for absorption rates. Absorption is normal in pancreatic steatorrhea but will be impaired in enterogenous steatorrhea.

Procedure
1. No food or liquids by mouth after midnight on the day of the test.
2. Have the patient void between 8:00 and 9:00 AM. Discard urine.
3. Then give dose of D-xylose orally. Dissolve in water. Follow immediately with additional water. Note time and record on the patient's record. No further fluids or food until the test is completed.
4. Exactly 2 hours later, a venous blood sample of 3 ml is obtained.
5. The patient must remain stationary until test is completed.
6. Save all urine voided during the test. Five hours after the test is started, have the patient void. Add this urine to collected urine, if any. Send the urine specimen to the laboratory.

Clinical Implications
Decreased levels in

Enterogenous steatorrhea
Malabsorption

Patient Preparation
Explain the purpose and procedure of the test and collection of the urine specimen.

Patient Aftercare
Provide food and fluids, and allow patient to be ambulatory.

> **Clinical Alert**
>
> Nausea, vomiting, and diarrhea may occur as side effects of D-xylose, especially if more than 5 g of drug are given.

Creatinine/Creatinine Clearance

Normal Values
Urine creatinine
>Men: <150 mg/24 hr
>Women: <250 mg/24 hr
Creatinine clearance: 70–130 ml/min

Explanation of Test

This blood and urine test is a specific measurement ordered to determine kidney function, primarily glomerular filtration. It measures the rate at which creatinine is cleared from the blood by the kidney. Clearance of a substance may be defined as the imaginary volume (ml/min) of plasma from which the substance would have to be completely extracted in order for the kidney to excrete that amount in 1 minute. (See Chapter 6 for blood creatinine.)

Creatinine is a substance that, in health, is easily excreted by the kidney. Creatinine is the byproduct of muscle energy metabolism and is produced at a constant rate depending on the muscle mass of the individual. Endogenous production of creatinine is constant as long as muscle mass remains constant. Because all the creatinine that is filtered in a given time interval appears in the urine, the creatinine is equivalent to the glomerular filtration rate (GFR). A disorder of kidney function prevents excretion of creatinine. More than 50 of the total kidney nephrons have to be altered to reflect change in the normal value. Creatinine is co-ordered with virtually every quantitative urine test. Creatinine is measured along with other urinary constituents to assess the accuracy of the collection and to interpret the excretion rate of specific urinary constituents.

Procedure

1. A 12-hour or 24-hour urine container is labeled with the name of the patient, test, and date.
2. Refrigeration may be necessary or keep the specimen on ice. Check laboratory policy.
3. General instructions for 24-hour urine collection are followed.
4. Exact start and ending of the collection are recorded on the specimen container and the patient's record.
5. Send the specimen to the laboratory refrigerator when the test is completed.
6. A venous blood sample of 7 ml for serum creatinine is obtained the morning of the day that the 12-hour or 24-hour collection will be completed.

Clinical Implications

1. A normal clearance cannot be used as a standard for a patient who is known to have existing renal disease.
2. A decreased clearance gives a reliable indication of impaired kidney function.
3. However, a normal blood creatinine does not always indicate unimpaired renal function.

Interfering Factors

Phenacetin will cause creatinine clearance to be decreased.

> **Clinical Alert**
>
> A 24-hour urine test for cyclic adenosine monophosphate (cAMP) is a second-order test in difficult-to-diagnose cases of primary hyperparathyroidism. Urine excretion of cAMP is compound with a measurement of glomerular filtration.

Patient Preparation

1. Instruct the patient about the purpose of the test and collection of the urine specimen. Give a written reminder.
2. Food and fluids are permitted. Encourage fluids so that voiding is easier, because a large urine flow is best for greatest accuracy of the test. Avoid coffee, tea, and vigorous exercise during the test.

Cystine

Normal Values

Qualitative: Negative
Quantitative: Children under 8—2–13 mg/24 hr
                 Children over 8 and adults—10–100 mg/24 hr

Explanation of Test

These tests of urine are useful in the differential diagnosis of cystinuria, an inherited disease characterized by bladder calculi (cystine has a low solubility). In cystinosis, cystine is deposited in lung tissues. A positive test is confirmed in a 24-hour collection.

Procedure

1. A random urine specimen of 20 ml is obtained for a quantitative screen.
2. If a 24-hour urine specimen is ordered, it is collected in a container with a preservative. Follow general procedures for collection of a 24-hour specimen.
3. Schedule before an intravenous pyelogram.
4. Notify the laboratory if the patient is taking penicillamine.

Clinical Implications

Values are increased in

1. Cystinuria (up to 20 times normal) in which there is excess urinary excretion of lysine, ornithine, arginine, and cystine
2. Cystinosis (no excess of lysine, ornithine, or arginine)

> **Clinical Alert**
>
> Persons with cystinuria can be put on a special diet that minimizes formation of kidney stones.

Hydroxyproline

Normal Values
Total: 0–6 mg/24 hr
Free: 0–2 mg/24 hr

Explanation of Test
This study is an indication of bone reabsorption in various disorders, as well as an indication of the degree of destruction from primary or secondary bone tumors. It is an important measurement as a determinant of the severity of Paget's disease and the response to treatment. Hydroxyproline is an amino acid that is increased during periods of rapid growth, bone diseases, and some endocrine disorders. Less than 10% is normally free; almost all is peptide bound. In adults, hydroxyproline excretion reflects bone resorption, whereas alkaline phosphatase reflects bone formation.

Procedure
1. A 2-hour specimen is usually obtained after an overnight fast.
2. Notify the laboratory of the patient's age and sex.
3. A 24-hour urine specimen may also be collected. No preservative is required.
4. Follow the general 24-hour collection procedure. The laboratory will record the total 24-hour volume.
5. A blood sample is the preferred method of testing in the first few months of life.

Clinical Implications
1. *Free hydroxyproline is increased* in
   (a) Hydroxyprolinemia, a hereditary autosomal recessive condition
   (b) Familial iminoglycinuria, also inherited
2. *Total hydroxyproline levels are increased* in
   (a) Hyperparathyroidism   (e) Osteoporosis
   (b) Paget's disease   (f) Bone tumors
   (c) Marfan syndrome   (g) Myeloma
   (d) Klinefelter's syndrome

Lysozyme

Normal Values
Blood plasma: 2.8–15.8 μg/ml
Urine: 1.3–3.6 mg/24 hr

Background
Lysozyme (muramidase) in blood or urine comes from degradation of granulocytes and monocytes.

Explanation of Test
This test of blood and urine is used in the investigation of leukemia, chronic infections, and renal graft rejection.

Procedure
1. A venous blood sample of 10 ml or a urine specimen is collected.
2. Follow general instructions for random collection or 24-hour urine collections.

Clinical Implications
1. *Levels are elevated* in
    (a) Acute myelomonocytic leukemia
    (b) Chronic granulocytic leukemia
2. *Levels may be elevated* in
    (a) Renal disorders
    (b) Regional enteritis
    (c) Chronic infections
    (d) Renal homograft rejection (especially urine)

Myoglobin

Normal Values
Urine: <20 ng/dl

Increases slightly with age.

Background
Myoglobin is the oxygen-binding protein of striated muscle. It resembles hemoglobin, but it is unable to release oxygen except at extremely low tension. Injury to skeletal or cardiac muscle will result in release of myoglobin. It is rapidly excreted from the blood into the urine; there is no threshold level.

Explanation of Test
Urine myoglobin tests are helpful in evaluating a variety of conditions, including some metabolic diseases. See Chapter 2 for myoglobin in blood.

Procedure
1. A urine sample of at least 1 ml is collected.
2. The urine must test positive for hemoglobin before proceeding with the test.

Clinical Implications
A. *Increased values* are associated with
1. Myocardial infarction
2. Other muscle injury, sports, and car accidents
3. Polymyositis
4. Hereditary myoglobinuria
5. Phosphorylase deficiency
6. Unknown metabolic defects
7. Crushing injuries
8. Progressive muscle disease
9. Hyperthermia and malignant hypertension
10. Electric shock
11. Some viral illnesses

Clinical Alert

If large amounts of myoglobin are presented to the kidney, anuria may result from renal damage.

Pregnancy Tests

Normal Values
Negative in blood and urine.

Background
From the earliest stage of development (9 days old), the placenta produces hormones, either on its own or in conjunction with the fetus. The very young placental trophoblast produces appreciable amounts of a hormone, human chorionic gonadotropin (HCG), that is excreted in the urine. Human chorionic gonadotropin is not found in the urine of normal, young, nonpregnant women.

Explanation of Test
Increased urinary levels of HCG form the basis of most tests for pregnancy and for trophoblastic tumors in men. All pregnancy tests are designed to detect HCG. Human chorionic gonadotropin is present in blood and urine whenever there is living chorionic/placental tissue. Human chorionic gonadotropin can be further identified as alpha or beta HCG. Human chorionic gonadotropin can be detected in the urine of pregnant women 26 to 36 days after the first day of the last men-

strual period, or 8 to 10 days after conception. Pregnancy tests should be negative 3 to 4 days after delivery.

The tests using female rats or male frogs have been supplanted by immunologic tests that are more accurate, easier to perform, and do not require a laboratory to maintain animal facilities. New urine tests are just as sensitive as the serum tests. Quantitative analysis of HCG aids in making a differential diagnosis of a viable pregnancy versus a nonviable pregnancy, twins or multiple gestations, or developing hydatidiform mole.

Procedure (for Urine Test)

1. An early morning urine specimen is collected. The first morning specimen generally contains the greatest concentration of HCG. However, specimens collected at any time may be used, but the specific gravity must be at least 1.005.
2. A 24-hour specimen is collected for quantitative studies. Then the general procedure for collection of 24-hour urine specimens is followed.
3. Grossly bloody specimens are not acceptable; in this instance, a catheterized specimen should be obtained.

Clinical Implications

1. A positive result usually indicates pregnancy. Only two thirds of women with ectopic pregnancies will have positive pregnancy tests.
2. Positive results also occur in
   (a) Choriocarcinoma
   (b) Hydatidiform mole
   (c) Testicular tumors
   (d) Chorioepithelioma
   (e) Chorioadenoma destruens
   (f) Conditions with a high erythrocyte sedimentation rate such as acute salpingitis
   (g) Cancer of lung, stomach, colon, pancreas, and breast

Interfering Factors

1. *False-negative tests* and falsely low levels of HCG may be due to a dilute urine (low specific gravity) or a specimen obtained too early in pregnancy.
2. *False-positive tests* are associated with
   (a) Proteinuria
   (b) Hematuria
   (c) Presence of excess pituitary gonadotropin (HLH) as in menopausal women
   (d) Drugs
      1. Anticonvulsants
      2. Antiparkinsons
      3. Hypnotics
      4. Tranquilizers

Clinical Alert

The presence of HCG in urine should be interpreted in conjunction with other clinical and laboratory data available to the clinician.

Estrogen Fractions/Urine and Serum

Normal Values
Vary widely between women and men, pregnancy, menopausal state, and follicular, ovulatory, and luteal stage of menstrual cycle

Explanation of Test
These measurements are useful along with gonadotropins in evaluating menstrual and fertility problems, feminization in men, estrogen-producing tumors and pregnancy. Estradiol (E_2) is the most active of endogenous estrogens. Estriol (E_3) levels in both plasma and urine rise as pregnancy advances, with significant amounts being produced in the third trimester.

Procedure
1. A venous blood sample can be obtained.
2. A 24-hour urine can be collected using a preservative. Refrigerate.
3. General collection procedures for 24-hour specimen are followed.

Clinical Alert

1. If estriol levels are higher than expected, one of the following may be indicated
   (a) Gestation more advanced than expected
   (b) More than one fetus
   (c) Laboratory error

Clinical Implications
1. *Estrogen values are increased* in
   (a) Ovarian tumors producing estrogen
   (b) Testicular tumors
   (c) Tumors or hyperplasia of the adrenal cortex
   (d) True precocious puberty
   (e) Corpus luteum cyst
   (f) Liver cirrhosis
   (g) Stein–Leventhal syndrome

2. *Estrogen values are decreased* in
   (a) Hypofunction or dysfunction of pituitary and adrenal glands
   (b) Primary ovarian malfunction
   (c) Menopause
   (d) Anovulatory bleeding
   (e) Inadequate luteal phase
3. *Estriol values are decreased* in
   (a) Placental insufficiency
   (b) Fetal distress—an abrupt drop of 40% or more on two consecutive days
   (c) Fetal outcome is considered favorable if the movement is upward
   (d) Other causes of decreased estriol levels include
       (1) Anemia
       (2) Malnutrition
       (3) Pyelonephritis
       (4) Intestinal disease
       (5) Hemoglobinopathies

Patient Preparation
1. Explain the purpose and procedure of the test.
2. Address the issue of compliance. The patient must be able to adjust daily activities to accommodate to the urine collection.

Amino Acids (Total/Fractions)

Normal Values
Urine and blood
Age-dependent

Explanation of Test
This test is used as the initial screen for inborn errors of metabolism and transport when genetic abnormalities are suspected, such as mental retardation, reduced growth rates, or various other unexplained symptoms. More than 50 aminoacidopathies are now recognized.

Procedure
1. A fasting blood specimen may be obtained.
2. Urine specimens, random or 24-hour collection, preserved with boric acid are collected for the initial screening procedure.

Clinical Implications
1. *Total serum amino acids are increased* in
   (a) Diabetes with ketosis
   (b) Malabsorption
   (c) Hereditary fructose intolerance

(d) Conditions with severe brain damage

(e) Reye's syndrome

(f) Acute and chronic renal failure

(g) Eclampsia

(h) Specific amino acidopathies

2. *Total serum amino acids are decreased* in

(a) Adrenocortical hyperfunction

(b) Huntington's chorea

(c) Phlebotomus fever

(d) Nephritic syndrome

(e) Rheumatoid arthritis

(f) Hartnup disease

(g) Fever

(h) Malnutrition

3. *Total urine amino acids are increased* in

(a) Viral hepatitis

(b) Multiple myeloma

(c) Hyperparathyroidism

(d) Rickets (vitamin D)

(e) Osteomalacia

(f) Hereditary fructose intolerance

(g) Galactosemia

(h) Cystinosis

(i) Wilson's disease

(j) Hartnup disease

4. *Fractions of total amino acids include*

Alanine
Alpha-amino-N-butyric acid
Alpha-aminoodysic acid
Anserine
Arginine
Argininosuccinic acid
Asparagine
Aspartic acid
Beta-alanine
Beta-aminoisobutyric acid

Carnosine
Citrulline
Cystine
Ethanolamine
Glutamic acid
Glutamine
Glycine
Histidine
Hydroxyproline
Isoleucine
Leucine
Lupine
Methionine

1-Methylhistidine
3-Methylhistidine
Ornithine
Phenylalanine
Phosphaethanolamine
Proline
Sarcosine
Serine
Taurine
Threonine
Tryptophan
Valine

BIBLIOGRAPHY

Ames Company: Factors Affecting Urine Chemistry Tests. Elkhart, IN, Ames Company, 1982

Baselt RC: Analytical Procedures for Therapeutic Drug Monitoring and Emerging Toxicology, 2nd ed. Littletown, MA, PSG Publishing, 1987

Blair ER et al (eds): Damon Clinical Laboratories Handbook. Stow, OH, Lexi-Comp, Inc, 1989

Boehringer Mannheim Diagnostics: Urinalysis Today. Indianapolis, IN, 1986

Brady S: Urodynamics: An overview. Urological Nursing 9(1):837–841, January/March 1990

Cella JH, Watson J: Nurses' Manual of Laboratory Tests. Philadelphia, FA Davis, 1989

Collins WG: Drug Abuse Testing in the Workplace. MLO 19(2), February 1987

Graff L: A Handbook of Routine Urinalysis. Philadelphia, JB Lippincott, 1983

Gray M et al: Urodynamics in the computer age. Urological Nursing 9(2):16–17, October/December 1988

Hawkes RL, Clancy CN: Urine Testing for Drugs of Abuse. NIDA Research Monograph B, DHHS Pub. No. (ADM) 87–1481, 1986

Henry JB (ed): Todd–Sanford–Davisohn Clinical Diagnosis and Management by Laboratory Methods, 18th ed. Philadelphia, WB Saunders, 1990

Jolleff CR: Albumin. Beckman Monograph. Brea, CA, Beckman Instruments, 1989

Klaassen CD et al: Casorett and Doull's Toxicology: The Basic Science of Poisons, 3rd ed. New York, Macmillan, 1986

Leavelle DE (ed): Mayo Medical Laboratories: Interpretive Handbook. Rochester, MN, Mayo Medical Laboratories, 1990

Lipo RF: Crises: Substance Abuse in the Workplace: Solutions for Business and Industry. Oak Creek, WI, Chem-Bio Corp, 1986

Maternal substance use and neonatal drug withdrawal (Protocol). J Perinat Med 8(4):387–392, Fall 1988

Morris A et al: Current issues in the laboratory diagnosis of urinary tract infections. NZ J Med Lab Technol 44(3):67–70, August 1990

Pappas AA, Fody EP, Cannon D: Clinical toxicology. Paper presented at meeting of American Society of Clinical Pathologists. Excerpted from Laboratory Management, November, 1987

Sacher RA, McPherson RA: Widmann's Clinical Interpretation of Laboratory Tests, 10th ed. Philadelphia, FA Davis, 1991

Smith Kline Bio-Science Laboratories: The Smith Kline Bio-Science Laboratories Handbook, 14th ed. Van Nuys, CA, Smith Kline Bio-Science Laboratories, 1987

Steele S: Phenylketonuria: Counseling and teaching functions of the nurse on the interdisciplinary team. Issues Compr Pediatr Nurs 12(5): 395–409, September/October 1989

Strasinger SK: Urinalysis and Body Fluids. Philadelphia, FA Davis, 1985

Tietz NW (ed): Clinical Guide to Laboratory Tests, 2nd ed. Philadelphia, WB Saunders, 1990

Whittier FC: Proteinuria: Incidental finding or tip of the iceberg? Consultant 22(2): 151–156, 1982

FECAL STUDIES

Introduction: Formation and Composition of Feces

The elimination from the body of waste products of digestion is essential to health. These excreted waste products are known as *stool* or *feces*. Stool examination is often done in the evaluation of gastrointestinal disorders, and results are helpful in detecting gastrointestinal bleeding and obstruction, obstructive jaundice, parasitic disease, dysentery, ulcerative colitis, and increased fat excretion.

An adult excretes 100 to 300 g of fecal matter a day, and of this as much as 70% may be water. The feces are what remains of the 8 to 10 L of fluid that enter the intestinal tract each day. Food and fluid taken orally, saliva, gastric secretions, pancreatic juice, and bile contribute to the formation of feces.

Feces are composed of

1. Waste residue of indigestible material such as cellulose in food eaten over the previous 4 days
2. Bile (pigments and salts); color is normally due to bile pigments that have been altered somewhat by bacterial action
3. Intestinal secretions, including mucus
4. Leukocytes that migrate from the bloodstream
5. Shed epithelial cells
6. Large numbers of bacteria that make up to one third of total solids
7. Inorganic material (10%–20%) that is chiefly calcium and phosphates
8. Undigested or unabsorbed food (present in very small quantities)

The output of feces depends on a complex series of absorptive, secretory, and fermentative processes. Normal function of the colon involves three physiologic processes: (1) absorption of fluid and electrolytes, (2) contractions that churn the contents, expose contents to the mucosa, and transport the contents to the rectum, and (3) defecation.

The small intestine is approximately 23 feet long, and the large intestine is 4 to 5 feet long. The small intestine degrades ingested fats, proteins, and carbohydrates to absorbable units and absorbs them. Pancreatic, gastric, and biliary secretions operate in the luminal contents to prepare them for active mucosal transport. Other active substances absorbed in the small intestine include fat-soluble vitamins, iron, and calcium. Vitamin B_{12}, after combining with intrinsic factors, is absorbed in the ileum. The small intestine also absorbs as much as 9.5 L of water and electrolytes for return to the bloodstream. Small intestine contents (chyme) begin to enter the rectum as soon as 2 to 3 hours after a meal, but the process is not complete until 6 to 9 hours after eating.

The large intestine performs less complex functions than the small intestine. The proximal or right colon absorbs most of the remaining water. Colonic absorption of water, sodium, and chloride is a passive process. Daily water excretion in the feces is only about 100 ml. The motility of the colon consists mainly of moving the luminal contents to and fro by seemingly random contractions of circular smooth muscle. More propulsive activity (peristalsis) occurs after eating. These peristaltic waves are caused by the gastrocolic and duodenocolic reflexes, which are initiated after meals and which are caused by the filling of the duodenum by food from the stomach. The muscles of the colon are innervated by the autonomic nervous system. The parasympathetic nervous system stimulates movement and the sympathetic system inhibits movement. Massive peristalsis usually occurs several times a day. Resultant distention of the rectum initiates the urge to defecate. In persons with normal motility and with a mixed dietary intake, transit time in the colon is 24 to 48 hours.

Normally evacuated feces reflect the shape and caliber of the colonic lumen. The normal consistency is somewhat plastic, neither fluid, mushy, nor hard; the usual brown color results from bacterial degradation of bile pigments; the odor is produced by indole, skatole, and butyric acid. Degradation of undigested protein produces a foul odor, as does excessive carbohydrate ingestion.

Appearance

Stool examination should include size, shape, consistency, color, odor, and presence or absence of blood, mucus, pus, tissue fragments, food residues, bacteria, or parasites. (See Chap. 7 for a discussion of microbiologic analysis of feces.) The gross appearance of feces should be assessed before administration of barium, laxatives, or enemas.

Patients and health personnel may dislike examining, collecting, and delivering feces for examination. However, this natural aversion must be overcome when considering the value of a feces examination in diagnosing many clinical conditions and diseases of the gastrointestinal tract and in providing information relating to the liver and pancreas.

Random Collection of Stool Specimens

Stool specimens are sometimes analyzed for diagnostic purposes. Some of the more frequently ordered tests on feces are tests for blood, bile, parasites, and parasite eggs (ova). Stool is also examined in the laboratory by *chromatographic* analysis for the presence of gallstones. The recovery of a gallstone from feces provides the only proof that a common duct stone has been dislodged and excreted. A lipid profile of gallstones will reveal the cholesterol content of stones.

Feces should be collected in a dry, clean, urine-free container. The entire stool should be collected and transferred to a container, using tongue blades. For best results, stool specimens should be covered and delivered to the laboratory immediately after collection. When possible, the specimen should be uncontaminated with urine or other body secretions. Depending on the examination to be performed, the specimen either should be refrigerated or kept warm. Generally, the laboratory will furnish detailed instructions as to the preserving of the feces specimen.

Ova and Parasites
Warm stools are best for detecting ova and parasites. Do *not* refrigerate specimens for ova and parasites. They will not live much below body temperature. Urine also will destroy parasites.

Culture for Enteric Pathogens
1. Some coliform bacilli produce antibiotic substances that destroy enteric pathogens. Refrigerate immediately.
2. A diarrheal stool will usually give good results.
3. A freshly passed stool is the choice specimen.
4. Stool specimens preferably should be collected before antibiotic therapy is initiated and as early in the course of disease as possible.
5. It is recommended that the entire passed stool be sent for examination. If mucus or blood is present, it definitely should be included with the specimen because parasites are more likely to be found in these substances. If for some reason only a small amount of stool can be used for a specimen, this amount should be suitable for examination; a stool the size of a walnut is usually adequate.
6. Do not use a stool that has been passed into the toilet bowl or that has been contaminated with barium, other radiographic media, or urine.
7. Accurately label all stool specimens with the patient's name, date, and reason for testing. Care should be taken that the outside of the container remain uncontaminated.

Interfering Factors
1. Red meat interferes with some tests and usually should be omitted from the diet for 3 days before a test for blood.
2. Stool specimens from patients receiving barium, bismuth, oil, or antibiotics are not satisfactory.
3. Bismuth from paper towels and toilet tissue interferes with tests.

Patient Preparation
1. Explain the purpose and procedure of the test.
2. Instruct the patient to defecate in a clean bedpan or large-mouthed container.

3. Instruct the patient *not to urinate* into the bedpan or collecting container.
4. Remind him that no toilet paper should be placed in the bedpan or container because it interferes with testing.
5. If the patient has diarrhea, newspaper (not paper towels, which contain bismuth) can be deposited into the toilet bowl and the diarrheal stool obtained above the water level of the toilet bowl.

> **Note:** This method may be used if the patient collects the stool specimen at home. Another method uses a large plastic bag attached by adhesive tape to the toilet seat. After collection, the bag can be placed in the gallon container.

Clinical Alert

Often the physician will order both ova and parasite testing and culture. In this case, the specimen should be divided in half—one portion refrigerated (for culture testing) and one portion kept at room temperature (for ova and parasite testing). There are commercial collection kits that require the stool to be divided and placed into separate vials for better recovery of ova and parasites and enteric pathogens.

Consistency, Shape, Form, and Amount

Normal Values
100–200 g/day

Plastic, soft, formed; soft and bulky on a high vegetable diet; small and dry on a high meat diet; seeds and vegetable skins present (Table 4–1).

Explanation of Test
Normally evacuated feces reflect the shape and caliber of the colonic lumen as well as the colonic motility. The bowel habits of healthy persons vary widely. For this reason, the words *diarrhea* and *constipation* have little meaning except when viewed as a change from the customary individual pattern. Detailed information is important in evaluating either abnormality.

Procedure
See "Random Collection of Stool Specimens," page 227.

TABLE 4–1.
Normal Values in Stool Analysis

Macroscopic Examination	Normal
Amount	*0–200 g/day*
Color	Brown
Odor	Varies with *p*H of stool and depends on bacterial fermentation and putrefaction
Consistency	Plastic; not unusual to see suds and vegetable skins; soft and bulky in a high vegetable diet; small and dry in a high meat diet.
Size, shape	Formed
Gross blood	None
Mucus	None
Pus	None
Parasites	None

Microscopic Examination	Normal
Fat	Colorless, neutral fat (18%) and fatty acid crystals and soaps
Undigested food, meat fibers, starch, trypsin	None to small amount
Eggs and segments of parasites	None
Yeasts	None
Leukocytes	None

Chemical Examination	Normal
*p*H	Neutral or weakly alkaline
Occult blood	Negative
Urobilinogen	40–280 mg/24 hr
Porphyrins	$\left\{\begin{array}{l}\text{coproporphyrins: 200 g/24 hr}\\ \text{protoporphyrins: 1500 g/24 hr}\\ \text{uroporphyrins: 1000 g/24 hr}\end{array}\right.$
Nitrogen	1–2 g/24 hr
Bile	Negative in adults, positive in children
Trypsin	Positive in small amounts in adults; present in greater amounts in normal children
Osmolality, used with serum osmolality to calculate osmotic gap	No established normal. Useful formula is $2\times$ (serum Na + serum K) = stool osmolality $\pm$ 30 mOsm.

Clinical Implications
1. The consistency of feces may change in various disease states.
   (a) Diarrhea mixed with mucus and red blood cells is associated with
(1) Typhus	(4) Amebiasis
(2) Typhoid	(5) Large bowel cancer
(3) Cholera	
   (b) Diarrhea mixed with mucus and white blood cells is associated with
(1) Ulcerative colitis	(4) Salmonellosis
(2) Regional enteritis	(5) Intestinal tuberculosis
(3) Shigellosis	
   (c) "Pasty" stool is associated with a high fat content.
       (1) A significant increase of fat is usually detected grossly.
       (2) In obstruction of the common bile duct, the fat gives a putty-like appearance to the stool.
       (3) In sprue and celiac disease, the appearance of the stool often resembles aluminum paint due to fatty acid.
       (4) In cystic fibrosis, the increase of neutral fat gives a greasy, "butter stool" appearance.
   (d) A bulky, frothy stool is associated with sprue and celiac disease.
2. Alterations in size or shape indicate altered motility or abnormalities in the colonic wall.
   (a) A narrow, ribbon-like stool suggests the possibility of spastic bowel, rectal narrowing or stricture, decreased elasticity, or a partial obstruction.
   (b) Excessively hard stools are usually due to increased absorption of fluid as a result of prolonged contact of luminal contents with the mucosa of the colon because of delayed transit time.
   (c) A very large caliber stool indicates dilatation of the viscus.
   (d) Small, round, hard stools (scybala) accompany habitual, moderate constipation.
   (e) Severe fecal retention can produce huge impacted masses with a small amount of pasty stool as overflow.

Assessment of Diarrhea and Constipation
1. When patients complain of diarrhea and constipation, it is important to obtain and record
   (a) An estimate of volume and frequency of fecal output
   (b) Consistency, blood, pus, mucus, oiliness, and bad odor (obtain through direct examination)
   (c) Reduction or increase in frequency of defecation
   (d) Sensations of rectal fullness with incomplete evacuation of stools
   (e) Painful defecation due to hard stools

2. Assess the patient's emotional status. In many instances, psychological stress is the major reason for altered bowel habits.

Odor and pH

Normal Values
Characteristic odor varies with the pH of stool; normal pH is neutral or weakly alkaline.

Explanation of Test
Substances called indole and skatole, formed by intestinal putrefaction and fermentation by bacteria, are primarily responsible for the odor of normal stools. An observation should be made about the odor of feces. The pH is dependent on bacterial fermentation and putrefaction in the bowel.

Interfering Factors
1. Carbohydrate fermentation changes the pH to acid.
2. Protein breakdown changes the pH to alkaline.

Color

Normal Values
Brown

Explanation of Test
The color of the feces should be noted, because it can provide information on pathologic conditions, organic dysfunction, bleeding, diet, and intake of drugs. An abnormality in color may aid the clinician in selecting appropriate diagnostic chemical and microbiologic tests of stool.

The brown color of normal feces is probably due to stercobilin (urobilin), a bile pigment derivative, which results from the action of reducing bacteria in bilirubin and undetermined factors.

Procedure
See "Random Collection of Stool Specimens," page 227.

Clinical Implications
1. The color of feces changes in disease states.
    (a) Yellow to yellow green—severe diarrhea
    (b) Green—severe diarrhea
    (c) Black—usually the result of bleeding into the upper gastrointestinal tract

(d) Tan or clay colored—associated with blockage of the common bile duct as well as pancreatic insufficiency, which produces a pale, greasy, acholic stool. In these instances, reduced quantities of bile pigments enter the intestine because of intrinsic hepatobiliary disease or obstruction.

(e) Red—possible result of bleeding from the lower gastrointestinal tract

2. Grossly visible blood always indicates an abnormal state.

(a) Blood streaked on the outer surface usually indicates hemorrhoids or anal abnormalities

(b) Blood present in stool can also arise from abnormalities higher in the colon. If transit time is sufficiently rapid, blood from the stomach or duodenum can appear as bright or dark red in stool.

Interfering Factors

1. Stool darkens on standing.
2. Color is influenced by diet, food dyes, certain foods, and drugs.

(a) Yellow to yellow green color occurs in the stool of breast-fed infants who lack normal intestinal flora. It also occurs in sterilization of bowel by antibiotics.

(b) Green color occurs in diets high in chlorophyll-rich vegetables such as spinach, with the use of the drug calomel, and in antibiotic therapy.

(c) Black or very dark brown color may be due to drugs such as iron, charcoal, and bismuth, to foods such as cherries, or to an unusually high proportion of meat in the diet.

(d) Light-colored stool with little odor may be due to diets high in milk and low in meat.

(e) Clay-like color may be due to a diet with excessive fat intake, bile duct obstruction, or barium used in radiograph examinations.

(f) Red color may be due to a diet high in beets or use of drugs such as Bromsulphalein (sodium sulfobromophthalein) and laxatives of vegetable origin.

(g) Certain color changes may result from drugs.

(1) Black—iron salts, bismuth salts, charcoal
(2) Green—mercurous chloride, indomethacin, calomel
(3) Green to blue—dithiazanine
(4) Brown staining—anthraquinones
(5) Red—phenolphthalein, pyrvinium pamoate, tetracyclines in syrup, Bromsulphalein
(6) Yellow—santonin
(7) Yellow to brown—senna
(8) Light—barium
(9) Whitish discoloration—antacids

(10) Orange red—phenazopyridine
(11) Pink to red to black—anticoagulants (excessive dose), or salicylates causing internal bleeding

Clinical Alert

A complete dietary and drug history will help to differentiate significant abnormalities from interfering factors.

Blood in Stool

Normal Values
Negative.

Explanation of Test
The normal person passes 2.0 to 2.5 ml of blood into the gastrointestinal tract daily. Passage of more than 2.8 ml of blood in 24 hours is an important sign of gastrointestinal disease. Blood is most commonly seen when hemorrhoids and anal fissures are present. Detection of occult (hidden) blood in the stool is very useful in detecting or localizing disease of the gastrointestinal tract. This test will demonstrate the presence of blood in upper gastrointestinal bleeding, as in the presence of gastric ulcer. The real benefit is screening for colonic carcinoma and other sources of occult bleeding.

Procedure
Chemical Tests for Occult Blood in Stool
Tests for detecting blood in feces use substances that depend on peroxidase content as an indication of hemoglobin content to cause a color change in the stool specimen being tested. The reagent substances used differ in sensitivity. All the commercial tests have sensitivities intended to be consistent in the uses for which they are designed. The sensitivities are adjusted to detect blood loss greater than 5 to 10 ml/day. Hematest is more sensitive and also has more false positives. Hemocult (guaiac) is less sensitive and has fewer false positives.

Clinical Implications
1. A dark red to black tarry appearance of the stool is indicative of a loss of 0.50 ml to 0.75 ml of blood from the upper gastrointestinal tract. Smaller quantities of blood in the gastrointestinal tract can produce similar stools or appear as bright red blood.
2. A stool should be considered grossly bloody only after chemical

testing to prevent confusing bloody stool with coloring from diet or drugs (see section on color).

3. Blood in the stool is abnormal and should be reported and recorded.
4. Gross or occult blood in the stool may indicate chronic nonspecific ulcerative colitis, or carcinoma of the colon.
5. Stool specimens may be positive for blood in diaphragmatic hernia.
6. Occult blood may appear in the stool in diverticulitis, gastric carcinoma, and gastritis.
7. To be completely valid, the test employed must be repeated three to six times on different samples. The patient's diet should be free of meats, fish, and vegetable sources of peroxidase activity. Only after following this regimen can a positive series of tests be considered an indication for further evaluation of the patient.

Interfering Factors

Drugs such as salicylates, steroids, indomethacin, colchicine, iron (when used in massive therapy), and rauwolfia derivatives are associated with increased gastrointestinal blood loss in normal persons and with even more pronounced bleeding when disease is present. Gastrointestinal bleeding can also follow parenteral administration of these drugs.

1. Foods
   (a) Meat in the diet contains hemoglobin and myoglobin and enzymes that can give false-positive tests for up to 4 days after eating.
   (b) Vegetables with peroxidase activity (*e.g.*, turnips, horseradish).
2. Vitamin C (ascorbic acid) taken in quantities greater than 500 mg/ day may cause a false-negative test for occult blood in the stool.
3. Drugs that may cause a false-positive test for occult blood include
   (a) Boric acid   (d) Iodine
   (b) Bromides   (e) Inorganic iron
   (c) Colchicine   (f) Oxidizing agents
4. The testing method must be followed exactly or the results are not reliable.
   (a) Use an aliquot from the center of the formed stool.
   (b) Time the reaction exactly.
   (c) Liquid stools may cause false negatives with filter paper methods.
5. Other factors that affect the test
   (a) Medications: For 2 days before and during the test, do not ingest alcohol, aspirin, or vitamin C.
   (b) Bleeding hemorrhoids
   (c) Collection of specimen during menstrual period

(d) Other diseases of the gastrointestinal tract (*e.g.*, colitis, gastritis, ulcers)

Patient Preparation

It is recommended that the patient be placed on a high-residue diet starting 2 days before and continuing through the test period. Diet may include

1. Meats: only small amounts of chicken, turkey, and tuna
2. Vegetables: generous amounts of both raw and cooked vegetables, including lettuce, corn, spinach, carrots, and celery. Avoid those with high peroxidase activity.
3. Fruits: plenty of fruits, especially prunes and apples
4. Cereals: bran and bran-containing cereals
5. Moderate amounts of peanuts and popcorn daily. If any of the above foods are known to cause discomfort, the patient is instructed to inform his physician.

The following foods should be avoided:

1. Meat: Diet should not include any red or rare meat.
2. Fruits and vegetables containing high peroxidase activity, such as turnip, cauliflower, broccoli, cantaloupe, horseradish, and parsnip

Mucus in Stool

Normal Values
Negative.

Explanation of Test
The mucosa of the colon secretes mucus in response to parasympathetic stimulation. Mucus in the stool appears in conditions of parasympathetic excitability.

Procedure
See "Random Collection of Stool Specimens," page 227.

Clinical Implications
1. Presence of recognizable mucus in a stool specimen is abnormal and should be reported and recorded.
2. Translucent gelatinous mucus clinging to the surface of formed stool occurs in
   (a) Spastic constipation   (c) Emotionally disturbed patients
   (b) Mucous colitis   (d) Excessive straining at stool
3. Bloody mucus clinging to the feces is suggestive of neoplasm or inflammation of the rectal canal.

4. In villous adenoma of the colon, copious quantities of mucus may be passed (up to 3–4 L in 24 hours).
5. Mucus with pus and blood is associated with
   (a) Ulcerative colitis
   (b) Bacillary dysentery
   (c) Ulcerating cancer of colon
   (d) Acute diverticulitis
   (e) Intestinal tuberculosis
   } rarely

Collection of 24-, 48- and 72-Hour Stool Specimens

This test is used with testing for fat and urobilinogen.

Special Instructions for Submitting Individual Specimens
1. Collect all stool specimens for 1 to 3 days. The entire stool should be collected.
2. Label specimens as to *Day 1, Day 2, Day 3*, time of day, patient's name, and purpose of examination.
3. Submit individual specimens to the laboratory as soon as they are collected.

Special Instructions for Submitting Total Specimens
1. Obtain a 1 gallon container from the laboratory (paint cans are often supplied).
2. Save all stool and place in the container. Keep refrigerated or in a container with canned ice. Replace ice daily.
3. At the end of the collection period, return the properly labelled container to the laboratory.

Fat in Stool

Normal Values
In a normal diet, fat in stool will be up to 20% of total solids
Lipids measured as fatty acids: <7 g/24 hr

Explanation of Test
This test is helpful in diagnosing malabsorption syndromes such as pancreatic insufficiency and Whipple's disease in which steatorrhea is a prominent feature.

Procedure
1. Collect a random stool specimen or a 72-hour specimen. If a 72-hour specimen is required, each individual stool specimen is collected and identified with the name of the patient, time, and date and sent

immediately to the laboratory. Indicate the length of the collection period.
2. Follow the procedure for the collection of random or 72-hour specimens.
3. A diet of more than 60 g of fat for 6 days prior to sampling is recommended.

Clinical Implications
1. Increases in fecal fat and fatty acids are associated with
   (a) Enteritis and pancreatic diseases when there is a lack of lipase
   (b) Surgical removal of a section of the intestine
   (c) Malabsorption syndromes
2. A stool specimen high in fat content will have a pasty appearance and can be detected by gross examination.
3. A high fat value is indicative of steatorrhea and excessive fat loss in the stool.
4. In chronic pancreatic disease, fat is more than 10 g in 24 hours. Excessive fecal nitrogen is also found as the pancreas is destroyed.

Interfering Factors
1. Increased neutral fat may occur under the following conditions:
   (a) With the use of rectal suppositories and oily creams applied to the perineum
   (b) With the ingestion of castor oil, mineral oil, and Metamucil
   (c) With the ingestion of dietetic low-calorie mayonnaise
2. Barium and bismuth interfere with test results.

Clinical Alert

Record the appearance and odor of all stools in persons suspected of having steatorrhea. The typical stool is foamy, greasy, soft, and foul smelling.

Patient Preparation
1. Explain the purpose of the test, interfering factors, and the procedure for the collection of specimens.
2. For a 72-hour stool collection, a diet containing 60 to 100 g of fat, 100 g of protein, and 180 g of carbohydrate is ordered for 6 days before and during the test. Follow the procedure for the collection of 72-hour stool specimens.

An additional fecal test that can be used in the evaluation of malabsorption syndrome, pancreatic dysfunction, and gastrocolic fistula is a determination for meat fibers. There are no meat fibers in the normal stool.

Procedure for Meat Fibers

1. The patient must eat an adequate amount of red meat for 24 to 72 hours before testing.
2. Specimens obtained with a warm saline enema or Fleet Phospho-Soda are acceptable. Specimens obtained with mineral oil, bismuth, or magnesium compounds cannot be used.
3. Examination for meat fibers yields correlate with amount of fat excretion.

Urobilinogen in Stool

Normal Values

30–200 mg/100 g of feces
125–250 Erlich units/24 hr

Explanation of Test

This test is done to determine excess production of urobilinogen in the investigation of hemolytic diseases. Determination of this substance is an estimate of the total excretion of bile pigments, which are the breakdown products of hemoglobin. Increased destruction of red blood cells as in hemolytic anemia increases the amount of urobilinogen excreted. Normally, 80% to 90% of excreted bile pigment measured as fecal urobilinogen is derived from old erythrocytes that have lived 100 to 120 days.

Liver disease in general reduces the flow of bilirubin to the intestine and thereby decreases the fecal excretion of urobilinogen. In addition, complete obstruction of the bile duct reduces urobilinogen to very low levels.

Procedure

See "Random Collection of Stool Specimens," page 227. Send the specimen to the laboratory at once.

Clinical Implications

1. *Increased values* are associated with hemolytic anemias.
2. *Decreased values* are associated with
   (a) Complete biliary obstruction
   (b) Severe liver disease
   (c) Oral antibiotic therapy that alters intestinal bacterial flora
   (d) Decreased hemoglobin turnover as in aplastic anemia

Bile in Stool

Normal Values
Adults: negative
Children: positive

Explanation of Test
A test for bile in the stool is helpful in determining the presence and degree of biliary tract obstruction in jaundiced patients

Procedure
A random stool specimen is obtained.

Clinical Implications
1. Normally, unaltered bile is never found in feces.
2. In diarrheal stools, bile may be present.
3. Increased levels occur in hemolytic jaundice.
4. Implications closely follow urobilinogen in the stool.

Trypsin in Stool

Normal Values
Positive in small amounts in 95% of normal persons. Present in greater amounts in the stools of normal children. Trypsin is destroyed by bacteria in the gastrointestinal tract in older children and adults.

Explanation of Test
This test is helpful in indicating pancreatic function and to rule in or rule out inability to split carbohydrates, protein, and fats by this pancreatic enzyme.

Procedure
1. Collect a first morning specimen and send it to the laboratory. Three separate fresh stools are usually collected.
2. In older children, a cathartic is ordered prior to obtaining a specimen.

Interfering Factors
No trypsin activity is detectable in constipated stools owing to the prolonged exposure to intestinal bacteria.

Clinical Implications
Absence of trypsin is presumptive evidence of pancreatic deficiency and is usually accompanied by the absence of lipase and amylase.

Clinical Alert

Positive results for trypsin should be checked again in a week to rule out the possibility that the positive reaction might be due to the action of proteolytic bacteria of the intestines.

Leukocytes in Stool

Normal Values
Negative.

Explanation of Test
Microscopic examination of the feces for white blood cells is often helpful in differentiating between bacterial dysentery or ulcerative colitis when there are increased leukocytes and the diarrhea caused by a virus or toxin such as viral gastroenteritis when white blood cells are absent. Persons with localizing abscesses and fistulas communicating with the bowel lumen will also have increased leukocytes and pus in the feces. Recognizable pus is seldom seen in stools unless there is a draining rectal infection or ulcerating or fungating process.

Clinical Implications
1. Large amounts of pus accompany
   - (a) Chronic ulcerative colitis
   - (b) Chronic bacillary dysentery
   - (c) Localized abscesses
   - (d) Fistulas to sigmoid rectum or anus
2. Primary mononuclear leukocytes appear in typhoid.
3. Primary polymorphonuclear leukocytes appear in
   - (a) Shigellosis
   - (b) Salmonellosis
   - (c) Invasive *Escherichia coli* diarrhea
   - (d) Ulcerative colitis
4. Absence of leukocytes is associated with
   - (a) Cholera
   - (b) Nonspecific diarrhea
   - (c) Viral diarrhea
   - (d) Amebic colitis
   - (e) Noninvasive *E. coli* diarrhea
   - (f) Toxigenic bacteria—staphylococcus, *Clostridium* cholera
   - (g) Parasites—*Giardia, Entamoeba*

Procedure
See "Random Collection of Stool Specimens," page 227.

Clinical Alert
Pus in the stool is abnormal and should be reported.

Nitrogen in Stool

Normal Values
1 g–2 g/24 hr

Explanation of Test
This test is used along with the measurement of fecal fat in the evaluation of chronic progressive pancreatitis. In the course of this disease, as the pancreas is destroyed, amylase and lipase will revert to normal. However, very high levels of fecal fat and nitrogen will continue to be found.

Procedure
See the procedure for 48- to 72-hour stool collection (p. 237).

Clinical Implications
Increased levels (more than 2.5 g/day) are associated with chronic progressive pancreatitis.

Porphyrins in Stool

Normal Values
Coproporphyrin: <200 μg/24 hr
Uroporphyrin: <1000 μg/24 hr
Protoporphyrin: <1500 μg/24 hr

Explanation of Test
Analysis of fecal porphyrins is especially helpful in the differential diagnoses of coproporphyrin, porphyria variegata, or protoporphyria. The pattern of excretion in feces and urine and accumulation within the red blood cells provide the basis for detecting and differentiating the porphyrias (see "Porphyrins and Porphobilinogens," p. 206, and red cells, pp 61 and 63).

Procedure
Collect a 24-hour stool specimen. See your laboratory for specific protocols. Fecal porphyrins can be qualitatively estimated by acid extraction and ultraviolet light; in erythropoietic protoporphyria, the fecal specimen may fluoresce due to high protoporphyrin levels.

Clinical Implications
1. *Increased fecal coproporphyrin* is associated with
   (a) Coproporphyria, persistently high (hereditary)
   (b) Porphyria variegata
   (c) Protoporphyria
   (d) Hemolytic anemia
2. *Increased fecal protoporphyrin* is associated with
   (a) Porphyria variegata
   (b) Protoporphyria
   (c) Acquired liver disease

BIBLIOGRAPHY

Bai JC et al: Fecal fat concentration in the differential diagnosis of steatorrhea. Am J Gastroenterol 84(1):27–36, 1984.

Bauer JD: Clinical Laboratory Methods, 9th ed. St. Louis, CV Mosby, 1982

Berkam R (ed): Merck Manual of Diagnosis and Theory, 15th ed. Rahway, NJ, Merck & Co., 1987

Blair ER et al (eds): Damon Clinical Laboratories Handbook. Stow, Ohio, Lexi-Comp, 1989

Bradley GM: Fecal analysis: Much more than an unpleasant necessity. Diagn Med 3(2):64–67, 1980

Braunwald E, Isselbacher KJ, Petersdorf RG et al (eds): Harrison's Principles of Internal Medicine, 11th ed. New York, McGraw–Hill, 1987

Cneasy TS et al: Floating faeces in steatorrhea—A new sign. Clin Radiol 39(6):692, 1988

Helena Laboratories: Colorscreen Self-Test: A Technical Overview. Beaumont, TX, Helena Laboratories, 1989

Henry JB: Todd–Sanford–Davidsohn Clinical Diagnosis and Management by Laboratory Methods, 18th ed. Philadelphia, WB Saunders, 1990

Krom FA et al: Clinitesting neonatal stools. Neonatal Netw 8(2):37–40, October 1989

Lawson JM et al: Collagenous colitis: An association with fecal leukocytes. Clin Gastroenterol 10(6):672–675, 1988

Newcomb PA et al: Efficacy of fetal occult blood screening. Prev Med 18:780, 1989

Ravel R: Clinical Laboratory Medicine, 5th ed. Chicago, Year Book Medical Pub, 1989

Sacker RA, McPherson RA: Widmann's Clinical Interpretation of Laboratory Tests, 10th ed. Philadelphia, FA Davis, 1991

Sheller MG: Stool specimens: Key to detecting intestinal invaders. RN 43(10):50–53, 1980

Sleisinger MH, Fordtran JS (eds): Gastrointestinal Disease, 4th ed. Philadelphia, WB Saunders, 1989

Sonnenwirth AC, Jarett L: Gradwohl's Clinical Laboratory Methods and Diagnosis, 8th ed. St. Louis, CV Mosby, 1980

Tressler KM: Clinical Laboratory and Diagnostic Tests. Significance and Nursing Implications, 2nd ed. Norwalk, CT, 1988.

Venina P et al: Fecal fat concentration in the differential diagnosis of steatorrhea. Am J Gastroenterol 84(10):27–36, 1984

CEREBROSPINAL FLUID STUDIES

Description, Formation, and Composition of Cerebrospinal Fluid

Background

Cerebrospinal fluid (CSF) is a clear, colorless liquid formed within the cavities or ventricles of the brain by the choroid plexus and diffused blood plasma. Approximately 500 ml of the fluid are formed per day, although there are only 120 ml to 150 ml in the system at any one time. CSF is completely replaced about three times a day.

Circulating slowly from the ventricular system into the spaces surrounding the brain and spinal cord, CSF serves as an hydraulic shock absorber, diffusing the force from a hard blow to the skull that might otherwise cause severe injury. CSF also helps to regulate intracranial pressure, which may change according to blood flow, and to transport nutrients and waste products. This fluid is believed to influence other control mechanisms such as glucose levels on the hypothalamus and hunger sensations and eating behaviors.

Most constituents of CSF are present in the same or lower concentrations as in the blood plasma, except for chloride concentrations, which are usually higher. Thus, like blood plasma, CSF contains few cells and little protein. Disease, however, can cause elements ordinarily restrained by the blood–brain barrier to enter the spinal fluid. Erythrocytes and leukocytes can enter the CSF from the rupture of blood vessels or from meningeal reaction to irritation. Bilirubin, normally not present, can be found in the spinal fluid after intracranial hemorrhage. In such cases, the arachnoid granulations and the nerve root sheaths will reabsorb the bloody fluid. Normal CSF pressure will consequently be maintained by the absorption of CSF in amounts equal to production. Blockage will cause an increase in the amount of CSF, resulting in hydrocephalus in infants or increased pressure in adults. The normal pressure of CSF is approximately 100 ml to 200 ml of water in the lateral decubitus position. Of the many factors that regulate the level of CSF pressure, venous pressure is the most important, because the reabsorbed fluid ultimately drains into the venous system.

Despite the continuous production (about 0.3 ml minute) and reabsorption of CSF and the exchange of substances between the CSF and the blood plasma, considerable pooling occurs in the lumbar sac. The lumbar sac at L4 to L5 is the usual site for puncture because damage to the nervous system is unlikely to occur in this area. In infants, the spinal cord is situated more caudally than in adults (L3–L4 until 9 months, when the cord ascends to L1–L2), and a low lumbar puncture should be made. The removal of CSF can give rise to a headache. This is because when fluid is withdrawn from the ventricle or subarachnoid spaces, free nerve endings along the major vessels of the inner dura are stretched as a result of the partially collapsed brain tugging on the meninges.

General Observations: Explanation of Test

Cerebrospinal fluid is usually obtained by lumbar puncture. A lumbar puncture is done for the following reasons:

1. To examine the spinal fluid, as in cases of suspected meningitis and intracranial hemorrhage

TABLE 5–1.
Normal CSF Values in Adults

Volume	90–150 ml; child: 60–100 ml
Clarity	Crystal clear, colorless
Pressure	50–180 m H_2O
Total cell count	0–5 WBC/μl
	(All cells are lymphocytes; PMNs and RBCs absent)
Specific gravity	1.006–1.008
Osmolality	280–290mOsm/kg
Clinical Tests	
Glucose	40–70 mg/dl
Protein	15–45 mg/dl (lumbar)
	15–25 mg/dl (cisternal)
	5–15 mg/dl (ventricular)
Lactic acid	24 mg/dl
Glutamine	6–15 mg/dl
A/G ratio (albumin to globulin)	8:1
Chloride	118–132 mEq/L
Urea nitrogen	6–16 mg/dl
Creatinine	0.5–1.2 mg/dl
Cholesterol	0.2–0.6 mg/dl
Uric acid	0.5–4.5 mg/dl
Bilirubin	0 (none)
LDH	1/10 that of serum
Electrolytes and pH	
pH	7.30–7.40
Chloride	118–132 mEq/L
Sodium	144–154 mEq/L
Potassium	2.0–3.5 mEq/L
CO_2 content	25–30 mEq/L (mmol)
P_{CO_2}	42–53 mm Hg
P_{O_2}	40–44 mm Hg
Calcium	2.1–2.7 mEq/L
Magnesium	2.4–mEq/L
Syphilis	
VDRL	Negative

2. To determine level of CSF pressure to document impairment of CSF flow or to lower the pressure by removal of a volume of fluid. (Fluid removal can be dangerous; the brain stem could be dislocated.)
3. To introduce anesthetics, drugs, and radiographic contrast media

Examination of CSF
Certain observations are made every time lumbar puncture is performed (Table 5–1):

1. General appearance, consistency, and tendency to clot are noted.
2. Pressure is measured.
3. Cell count is performed in laboratory to distinguish types of cells present; this must be done within 2 hours.
4. Protein, chloride, and sugar concentrations are determined.
5. Other clinical serologic and bacteriologic tests are done when the patient's condition warrants them (e.g., tests for aerobes and anaerobes, tuberculosis.)
6. There are tumor markers in CSF that are useful as supplements to CSF cystology analysis. (Table 5–2).

Note: Blood levels should always be measured simultaneously with CSF.

TABLE 5–2.
Tumor Markers in CSF

Determination	Used in Diagnosis of	Normal Value
Alpha-fetaprotein (AFP)	CNS dysgerminomas and meningeal carcinomatosis	<1.5 mg/ml
Beta-glucuronidase	Possible meningeal carcinomatosis	<49 mU/L Indeterminate 49–70 mU/L Suspicious >70 mU/L
Carcinoembryonic antigen (CEA)	Meningeal carcinomatosis: intradural or extradural, or brain parenchymal metastasis from adenocarcinoma. Although the assay appears to be specific for adenocarcinoma and squamous cell carcinoma, increased CEA values in CSF are not seen in all such tumors of the brain.	<0.6 mg/ml
Human chorionic gonadotropin (HCG)	Adjunct in determining CNS dysgerminomas and meningeal carcinomatosis	<0.21 U/L

Procedure for Sterile Lumbar Puncture (Spinal Tap)

1. The patient is usually placed in a side-lying position with head flexed onto the chest and knees drawn up to but not compressing the abdomen to bow the back. This position helps to increase the space between the lower lumbar vertebrae so that the spinal needle can be inserted with ease between the spinal processes. However, a sitting position (patient straddles a straight-backed chair) with head flexed to chest can be used. The patient is helped to relax with soothing words and instructed to breathe slowly and deeply with mouth open.

2. The puncture site is selected, usually between L4 and L5 or lower. There is a little bone at the L5-S interspace ("surgeon's delight") that facilitates puncture. The site is thoroughly cleansed with an antiseptic solution, and the surrounding area is draped with sterile towels. However, care should be taken so that drapes do not obscure important landmarks.

3. A local anesthetic is injected slowly into the dermis.

4. A spinal needle with stylet is inserted into the midline between the spines of the lumbar space. The needle is to enter the subarachnoid space. The patient may feel the entry ("pop") of the needle through the dura mater. Patient should then be helped to straighten the legs slowly to relieve abdominal compression.

5. The stylet is removed and a manometer is attached to the needle to record the opening CSF pressure.

   Note: If the initial pressure is normal, the Queckenstedt's test may be done. This test is not done if a central nervous system (CNS) tumor is suspected. In this test, pressure is placed on both jugular veins to occlude them temporarily and to produce an acute rise in CSF fluid. Normally, pressure rapidly returns to average levels. Total or partial spinal block is diagnosed if the lumbar pressure fails to rise when both jugular veins are compressed or if the pressure requires more than 20 seconds to fall after compression is released. Pressure reading is height-dependent, and sitting equals pressure in the midventricular system.

6. A specimen of CSF is removed and is usually collected in three tubes. Tubes are labeled, 1, 2, and 3 in correct order of collection. A closing pressure reading may be done, and the needle is withdrawn. In cases of increased intracranial pressure, very little fluid is withdrawn.

7. A small sterile dressing is applied to the puncture site.

8. Tubes should be correctly labeled with the proper number (1, 2, or 3), the patient's name, and date. Specimens of CSF must be deliv-

ered immediately to laboratory personnel. The spinal fluid should never be placed in the refrigerator provided for other specimens. Refrigeration will alter test results if bacteriologic and fungal studies are done. Analysis should be started immediately. If viral studies are to be done, the specimen should be frozen.

9. Record the completion time of the procedure, the condition and reaction of the patient, the appearance of the CSF, and the pressure readings. Time specimens are sent to the laboratory.

Patient Preparation
1. Explain the purpose of the test; give a step-by-step description of the procedure.
2. Help the patient to be as relaxed as possible. Breathing slowly and deeply may help the patient to relax. Tell the patient to refrain from breath holding, straining, and talking during the procedure.

Patient Aftercare
1. The patient should lie prone (flat or horizontal) usually for 4 to 8 hours. Alternatively, the patient may lie on the abdomen to help prevent headache. Turning from side to side is permitted.
2. Women will have difficulty voiding in this position. The use of a "fracture bedpan" may help to alleviate voiding problems.
3. Fluids are encouraged to help in the prevention and relief of possible headache.
4. Observe the patient for important changes in his neurologic state, such as a change in his conscious state and in his pupils. Elevated temperature, increased blood pressure, irritability, as well as numbness and tingling sensations in the lower extremities should also be assessed.
5. If headache should occur, administer ordered analgesics and encourage a longer period of bed rest.
6. Check the puncture site for leakage.

Clinical Alert

1. Extreme caution should be used in lumbar puncture when intracranial pressure is elevated, especially when papilledema or split cranial sutures are present. However, in some cases of increased intracranial pressure, such as with a comatose patient, intracranial bleeding, or suspected meningitis, the need to establish a diagnosis is absolutely essential and outweighs the danger of the procedure.
2. Other contraindications to lumbar puncture are
   (a) Suspected epidural infection

> (b) Infection or severe dermatologic disease in the lumbar area, which may result in spinal fluid infiltration and infectious complications
> (c) Severe psychiatric problems or chronic back pain in neurotics
> 3. If there is a sign of leakage at the puncture site, notify the physician immediately.

Pressure of CSF

Normal Values
50–180 mm H_2O lateral decubitus
To midventricular position when sitting
This value is height-dependent and will change if patient is in a horizontal or sitting posture.

Background
The pressure should be measured before any fluid is withdrawn. CSF pressure is directly related to pressure in the jugular and vertebral veins that connect with the intracranial dural sinuses and the spinal dura. In conditions such as congestive heart failure and obstruction of the superior vena cava, CSF pressure is increased, but in circulatory collapse, it is decreased.

Clinical Implications
1. *Increases* in pressure can be a significant finding in
   (a) Intracranial tumors or abscess
   (b) Purulent or tuberculous meningitis
   (c) Inflammatory processes of meninges
   (d) Hypo-osmolality due to hemodialysis
   (e) Congestive heart failure
   (f) Acute observation of superior vena cava
   (g) Subarachnoid hemorrhage
   (h) Cerebral edema
2. *Decreases* in pressure can be a significant finding in
   (a) Circulatory collapse
   (b) Severe dehydration
   (c) Hyperosmolality
   (d) Leakage of spinal fluid
   (e) Complete subarchnoid block
3. *Significant variations* between opening and closing CSF pressures can be found in
   (a) Tumors or spinal blockage when there is a large pressure drop indicative of a small CSF pool

(b) Hydrocephalus when there is a small pressure drop that is indicative of a large CSF pool

Clinical Alert

If initial pressure is near 200 mm, only 1 to 2 ml of fluid should be removed. Spinal cord compression or cerebellar herniation could result. See **Note** in procedure for spinal tap for Queckenstedt's test.

Interfering Factors
1. Slight elevations of pressure may occur in an anxious patient who holds his or her breath or tenses muscles.
2. If a patient's knees are flexed too firmly against the abdomen, venous compressions will cause an elevation in pressure. This can occur in patients of normal weight and in the obese.

Color, Turbidity of CSF

Normal Value
Crystal clear and colorless, like water

Background
A slight color change may be difficult to detect, and CSF should be compared with a test tube of distilled water held against a white background. If there is no turbidity, a newspaper can be read through the tube. Inflammatory diseases, hemorrhage, tumors, and trauma bring about an elevated cell count and a corresponding change in appearance.

Clinical Implications
1. Abnormal colors (see Table 5–3)—their causes and indications:
   (a) Blood (the blood is evenly mixed in all three tubes in subarachnoid and cerebral hemorrhage). The supernate is also xanthochromic after centrifugation—at least 400 cells/μl must be present before turbidity is detected. Clear CSF fluid does not rule out intracranial hemorrhage.
   (b) Turbid fluid usually indicates increased white blood cells, (WBCs), red blood cells, (RBCs), or microorganisms such as yeast and bacteria.
   (c) Xanthochromia (pale to dark yellow)
       (1) Bilirubin, as in bilirubinemia (conjugated in adults; unconjugated in infants)

TABLE 5-3.
Color Changes in CSF Suggestive of Disease States*

Appearance	Condition
Opalescent, slightly yellow with delicate clot	Tuberculous meningitis
Opalescent to purulent, slightly yellow with coarse clot	Acute pyogenic meningitis
Slightly yellow; may be clear or opalescent with delicate clot	Acute anterior poliomyelitis
Bloody; purulent; may be turbid	Primary amebic meningoencephalitis
Generally clear, but may be xanthochromic	Tumor of brain or cord
Xanthochromic	Toxoplasmosis

* *Color and clot changes are only very general indications of disease states. They must not be thought of as specific indicators.*

(2) Yellow pigments usually signify previous bleeding, as in subarachnoid hemorrhage, from lipid RBCs, severe jaundice, or high protein level. The xanthochromia grading range is 1+ to 4+.

(3) Methoglobin

(4) If the CSF protein is more than 150 mg/dl, the fluid will be slightly yellow.

(5) Bleeding into CSF is associated with a corresponding increase in protein, about 1 mg/dl/700 RBC/μl. Clots will form in CSF with high protein levels (fibrinogen).

(6) Carotene, as in systemic carotenemia

(7) Melanin, from meningeal melanosarcoma

Interfering Factors

1. If the blood in the specimen is due to trauma during lumbar puncture, the fluid in the third tube is usually lighter in color than tube number one and tube number two.

2. Contamination of the specimen with a skin disinfectant will cause an abnormal color.

Microscopic Examination of Cells; Total Cell Count; Differential Cell Count of CSF

Normal Values

0–5 WBC/μl or 0–5 10^6 WBC/L (mononuclear cells; lymphocytes and monocytes)

Background
CSF is essentially free of cells. When the cells are counted, they are identified by cell type, and the percentage of cell type is compared to the total number of white cells present. In general, inflammatory disease, hemorrhage, neoplasms, and trauma will cause an elevated cell count.

Clinical Implications
A. *White cell counts*
   1. An increase in the number of WBCs in CSF is termed *pleocytosis.* Disease processes may lead to abrupt increases or decreases (shift to the right or left); usually there are no WBCs in CSF.
   2. White cell counts above 500 usually arise from a purulent infection and are predominantly granulocytes (neutrophils).
      (a) Increases in neutrophils are associated with
      (1) Bacterial meningitis
      (2) Early viral meningitis
      (3) Early tuberculosis
      (4) Mycotic meningitis
      (5) Amebic encephalomyelitis
      (6) Early stages of meningovascular syphilis
      (7) Aseptic meningitis
      (8) Septic emboli due to bacterial endocarditis
      (9) Osteomyelitis of skull or spine
      (10) Subdural empyema
      (11) Cerebral abscess
      (12) Phlebitis of dural sinuses or cortical veins
      (b) Noninfectious causes of neutrophilia are
      (1) Reaction to central nervous system hemorrhage
      (2) Reaction to repeated lumbar puncture
      (3) Injection of foreign materials into subarachnoid space such as a contrast medium or anticancer drugs
      (4) Pneumoencephalogram
      (5) Chronic granulocytic leukemia involving the central nervous system
      (6) Lumbar puncture with needle contaminated by detergent
      (7) Metastatic tumor
      (8) Infarct

Clinical Alert

Neutrophilic reaction classically suggests meningitis due to pyogenic organism.

   3. White counts of 300 to 500 with predominately mononuclear cells are indicative of

(a) Viral infections such as poliomyelitis and aseptic meningitis
(b) Syphilis of CNS
(c) Tuberculous meningitis
(d) Tumor or abscess (WBCs may also be normal in these conditions)
(e) Partially treated bacterial meningitis
(f) Multiple sclerosis (50% of cases)
(g) Encephalopathy due to drug abuse
(h) Guillain–Barré syndrome
(i) Acute disseminated encephalomyelitis
(j) Sarcoidosis of meninges
(k) Polyneuritis
(l) Periarteritis of central nervous system

4. White cell counts with 40% or more monocytes are seen after subarachnoid hemorrhage.

B. *Other Cells*

1. Malignant cells (lymphocytes or histiocytes) may be present with primary and metastatic brain tumors, especially with meningeal extension.
2. Increased numbers of plasma cells may occur in association with lymphocytic reactions.

(a) Subacute and chronic inflammatory processes
(b) Multiple sclerosis
(c) Leukoencephalitis
(d) Delayed hypersensitivity responses
(e) Subacute viral encephalitis
(f) Meningitis (tuberculous or fungal)
(g) Some brain tumors

These cells are responsible for an increase in IgG and for altered patterns in immunoelectrophoresis.

3. Macrophages are present in traumatic and ischemic cranial infarcts, tuberculous or mycotic meningitis, reaction to erythrocytes, foreign substances, or lipids in the CSF.
4. Glial, ependymal, and plexus cells may be present after surgical procedures or trauma to the central nervous system.
5. Leukemic cells appear in CSF after several remissions have been achieved by chemotherapy. Leukemic cells may appear in CSF during apparent remission and after chemotherapy has been discontinued.

Chloride in CSF

Normal Values
Adult: 118–132 mEq/L
Child: 111–130 mEq/L

Background
Any condition that alters the blood plasma chloride level will also affect the CSF level. Chlorides in CSF are higher (1.2–1) than in blood plasma. The measurement of CSF chloride is most useful in the diagnosis of tuberculous meningitis.

Clinical Implications
Decreased levels are associated with

1. Tuberculous meningitis
2. Bacterial meningitis

Interfering Factors
1. Concurrent intravenous administration of chloride will invalidate test results.
2. Test values are invalidated if blood, as in a traumatic tap, is mixed with the specimen.

Glucose in CSF

Normal Values
Adult: 40–70 mg/dl
Child: 60–80 mg/dl

Background
The CSF glucose level varies with the blood glucose levels. CSF is usually 60% to 70% of blood glucose. A blood glucose specimen should be obtained at least 30 to 60 minutes before lumbar puncture for comparisons. Any changes in blood sugar are reflected in the CSF after 1 to 3 hours.

Explanation of Test
This measurement is helpful in determining impaired transport of glucose from plasma to CSF and increased use of glucose by the central nervous system, leukocytes, and microorganisms. As evidenced by decreased CSF glucose, accurate evaluations of CSF glucose require a relatively constant level of plasma glucose.

Clinical Implications
1. *Decreased levels* are associated with
    (a) Pyogenic, tuberculous, and fungal infections
    (b) Lymphomas with meningeal spread
    (c) Leukemia with meningeal spread
    (d) Mumps meningoencephalitis (usually normal in viral meningoencephalitis)
    (e) Hypoglycemia

Note: *All types* of organisms consume glucose, and decreased glucose reflects bacterial activity.

2. Increased levels are associated with diabetes.
3. CSF glucose levels are usually normal in some viral infections of the brain and meninges and in aseptic meningitis.

Clinical Alert

1. Glucose oxidase test strips are of no clinical value for distinguishing CSF leakage from nasal or ear secretions. Diagnosis of CSF rhinorrhea and otorrhea must be made by other means such as cotton pledgets examined for radioactivity after administration of technetium-99m.
2. Panic value is less than 20 mg/dl.

Glutamine in CSF

Normal Values
6–20 mg/dl
Reference values vary.

Background
Glutamine is synthesized in brain tissue from ammoniaic and glutamic acid. Production of glutamine provides a mechanism for removing ammonia from the central nervous system.

Explanation of Test
This measurement is used as a determination of hepatic encephalopathy and cerebrospinal fluid acidosis.

Procedure
In the laboratory, glutamine levels can be measured by a simple method that releases ammonia and is measured by a colorimetric reaction.

Clinical Implications
Increased levels are associated with

1. Hepatic encephalopathies
2. Reye's syndrome
3. Hepatic coma
4. Cirrhosis
5. Hypercapnia

Lactic Acid in CSF

Normal Values
24 mg/dl (reported reference intervals vary)

Background
The source of lactic acid in the cerebrospinal fluid is probably central nervous system anaerobic metabolism (see Chapter 14). Lactic acid in CSF may vary independently of the level in the blood. It appears that diffusion of lactic acid across the blood–CSF barrier is very slow.

Explanation of Test
Measurement of CSF lactate may be useful as a screening test to detect central nervous system disease and may be an aid in the differential diagnosis of bacterial meningitis versus viral meningitis if other conditions can be excluded.

Clinical Implications
Increased levels are associated with

1. Bacterial meningitis
2. Hypocapnia
3. Hydrocephalus
4. Brain abscess
5. Cerebral ischemia
6. Traumatic brain injury
7. Idiopathic seizures
8. Respiratory alkalosis
9. Low blood pressure
10. Low arterial Po_2
11. Cerebral infarct
12. Less than 50% of multiple sclerosis
13. Cancer of central nervous system

Lactate Dehydrogenase (LD/LDH) in CSF

Normal Values
One-tenth that of serum

Background
Although many different enzymes have been measured in CSF, only lactate dehydrogenase (LDH) appears useful clinically. Sources of LDH in normal CSF include diffusion across the blood–CSF barrier, diffusion across the brain–CSF barrier, and LDH activity in cellular elements of CSF such as leukocytes, bacteria, and tumor cells. Because the brain tissue is rich in LDH, damaged central nervous system tissue can cause increased levels of LDH in the cerebrospinal fluid.

Explanation of Test

Measurement of LDH in the CSF has been used for differential diagnosis of bacteria versus viral meningitis. High levels of LDH occur in about 90% of bacterial meningitis cases and in only 10% of viral meningitis cases. When high levels of LDH do occur in viral meningitis, the condition is usually associated with encephalitis and a poor prognosis. Tests of LDH isoenzymes have been used to improve the specificity of LDH measurements (see Chap. 6 for a complete description of isoenzymes).

Clinical Implications

1. Increased LDH levels are associated with
   (a) Bacterial meningitis
   (b) Viral meningitis (10% of cases)
   (c) Subarachnoid hemorrhage
   (d) Leukemia
   (e) Lymphoma
   (f) Metastatic carcinoma of the central nervous system
2. In viral meningitis, the presence of LDH 1, 2, 3 reflects a combined central nervous system lymphocytic reaction.
3. In bacterial meningitis, the LDH isoenzyme pattern reflects a granulocytic reaction with LDH 4 and 5 present.
4. High levels of LDH 1 and 2 in either viral or bacterial meningitis suggest extensive central nervous system damage and a poor prognosis.

Total Protein in CSF

Normal Values

15–45 mg/dl (lumbar)
15–25 mg/dl (cisternal)
 5–15 mg/dl (ventricular)

These values are age-dependent; for example, a lumbar protein may be 65 in a 65-year-old patient.

Background

CSF normally contains very little protein because the protein in blood serum is in the form of large molecules that do not cross the blood–brain barrier. However, the proportion of albumin to globulin is higher in CSF than in the blood plasma, because the albumin molecule is significantly smaller and can more easily cross the blood–brain barrier. Increased permeability of the blood–brain barrier to protein occurs in infections.

Clinical Implications

1. Moderate to marked increases in total protein levels and alterations in the ratio of albumin to globulin (A/G ratio) are caused by increased permeability of the blood–CSF barrier, obstructions in circulation of CSF, increased synthesis of protein within the central nervous system, or tissue degeneration as in Guillain–Barré syndrome and brain tumors. Increases may also be seen in

   (a) Purulent meningitis
   (b) Froin's syndrome
   (c) Tuberculous meningitis
   (d) Aseptic meningitis
   (e) Syphilis, neurosyphilis
   (f) Brain abscesses
   (g) Subarachnoid hemorrhage
   (h) Poliomyelitis
   (i) Collagen disease
   (j) Guillain–Barré syndrome

2. In most diseases, any changes in CSF cell count and protein are parallel. For example, as the CSF cell count rises, the CSF protein level also rises.

3. There is often some increase of protein level in multiple sclerosis.

4. A traumatic tap with a mixture of peripheral blood in the CSF may cause an increase in protein.

5. Decreased concentration of protein in CSF is caused by

   (a) Leakage of CSF
   (b) Removal of large volume of CSF
   (c) Increased intracranial pressure
   (d) Hyperthyroidism

Interfering Factors

Drugs may cause increased or decreased levels.

Syphilis Serology

Normal values negative (nonreactive). Neurosyphilis is characterized by an increase in protein, an increase in number of lymphocytes, and a positive test for syphilis (see Chap. 8).

Protein Electrophoresis of CSF; Albumin and Immunoglobulin G (IgG); Multiple Sclerosis Panel

Normal Values
Albumin: 11–48 mg/dl
Oligoclonal banding: none present
IgG: 0–4.5 mg/dl
IgG/albumin: 0.15–3.8
Pre-albumin: 2%–7%
Albumin: 52%–72%

Alpha$_1$: 1%–7%
Alpha$_2$: 3%–12%
Beta: 7%–23%
Gamma: 3%–13%

Explanation of Test

This measurement of albumin and IgG using immunoelectrophoresis is becoming accepted as a method of evaluating the integrity and permeability of the blood–CSF barrier and of the synthesis of IgG within the central nervous system. The most important clinical application of CSF protein fractionation is detection and diagnosis of multiple sclerosis. Abnormalities in CSF in multiple sclerosis include an increase in total protein primarily due to IgG. The IgG protein in multiple sclerosis and other neuropathies migrate as discrete populations rather than as a homogeneous band, and these have been called *oligoclonal bands*.

Clinical Implications

1. *Increases* in IgG or IgG/albumin index occur in
   (a) Infectious disease
   (b) Subacute sclerosing leukoencephalitis
   (c) Multiple sclerosis
   (d) Neurosyphilis
   (e) Chronic phases of central nervous system infections
   (f) Some patients with meningitis, Guillain–Barré syndrome, lupus erythematosus involving central nervous system, and other neurologic conditions
2. IgM is normally absent; it may be abnormally present in
   (a) Tumors of brain and meninges
   (b) Meningitis
   (c) Multiple sclerosis
3. Increased levels of albumin are associated with
   (a) Lesions of choroid plexus
   (b) Blockage of flow of CSF
   (c) Damage to blood and central nervous system
4. Increased levels of gamma globulins in the presence of normal albumin level are associated with
   (a) Multiple sclerosis
   (b) Neurosyphilis
   (c) Subacute sclerosing panencephalitis
   (d) Chronic phase of central nervous system infections
5. Oligoclonal bands are found in
   (a) Multiple sclerosis
   (b) Cryptococcal meningitis
   (c) Idiopathic polyneuritis
   (d) Neurosyphilis
   (e) Chronic rubella panencephalitis
   (f) Subacute sclerosing panencephalitis

Note: In order for this test to be valid, corresponding bands must not be present in the serum.

BIBLIOGRAPHY

Glasser L: Body fluids III: Tapping the wealth of information in CSF. Diagn Med 4(1):23–33, 1981

Henry JB (ed): Todd, Sanford, Davidsohn: Clinical Diagnosis and Management by Laboratory Methods, 18th ed. Philadelphia, WB Saunders, 1990

Kaplan A, Szabo L: Clinical Chemistry: Interpretation and Techniques, 3rd ed. Philadelphia, Lea & Febiger, 1988

Leavelle, DE (ed): Interpretive Handbook: Interpretive Data for Diagnostic Laboratory Tests. Rochester, MN, Mayo Medical Laboratories, 1990

Lipman T: Cerebrospinal fluids (unpublished thesis), Medical College of Wisconsin, 1984

McManus C, Hallsman KA: Cerebrospinal fluid analysis. Nursing 23(8): 43–47, 1982

Merritt HH: Textbook of Neurology, 8th ed. Philadelphia, Lea & Febiger, 1989

Ravel R: Clinical Laboratory Medicine, 5th ed. Chicago, Year Book Medical Pub, 1989

Sacher RA, McPherson RA: Widmann's Clinical Interpretation of Laboratory Tests, 10th ed. Philadelphia, FA Davis, 1991

Sonnenwirth AC, Jarett L (eds): Gradwohl's Clinical Laboratory Methods and Diagnosis, 8th ed. St. Louis, CV Mosby, 1980

Tietz NB (ed): Clinical Guide to Laboratory Tests, 2nd ed. Philadelphia, WB Saunders, 1990

Wolf JK: Practical Clinical Neurology. New York, Medical Examination Publishing, 1980

Wyngaarden JB, Smith LH (eds): Cecil's Textbook of Medicine, 8th ed. Philadelphia, WB Saunders, 1988

CHEMISTRY STUDIES

Introduction

Blood chemistry is a means of identifying many of the body's chemical constituents found in the blood. Although the relation of the abnormal levels of these constituents to disease can be evaluated, unfortunately, very few diseases show a single abnormality in body chemistry. Thus, it is often necessary to measure several body chemicals to establish a pattern of abnormalities characteristic of a particular disease. The quantity of blood that is drawn for samples will vary, depending on the method used in testing and the available equipment.

A wide range of tests falls into the category of blood chemistry. Some can be grouped under the broad headings of enzymes, electrolytes, blood sugar, protein or protein by-products, lipids, hormones, vitamins, minerals, and drug investigation. Others have no such common denominator. See Appendix for vitamins and minerals.

From the numerous tests included here, selected tests serve as screening devices in general patient care and help to identify target organ damage. Most of these tests constitute the patient profile that is obtained from the autoanalyzer printout shown in Fig. 6-1 (A–F).

General Biochemical Profiles

Profiles are a group of various tests that screen for certain conditions. Some of the more commonly offered profiles or panels are listed in Table 6-1.

(*text continues on page 271*)

TABLE 6–1.
Common Biochemical Profiles

Disorder	Tests Suggested
Cardiac enzymes	CPK, AST, LDH
Kidney functions and disease	UA, BUN, phosphorus, LDH, creatinine, creatinine clearance, uric acid, total protein, A/G ratio, albumin, globulins, calcium, glucose, cholesterol
Lipids	Cholesterol, triglycerides, lipoprotein electrophoresis (LDL, VLDL, HDL)
Liver function/disease	Total bilirubin, alkaline phosphatase, cholesterol, GGT, total protein, A/G ratio, albumin, globulins, AST, LDH, Australian antigen (hepatitis panel) prothombin time
Thyroid function	T_3, T_4, T_7, free thyroxine, TSH

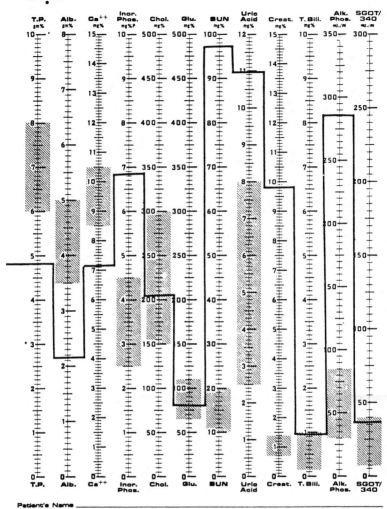

FIGURE 6–1A.

Chronic glomerulonephritis.   Alkaline phosphatase: high   Creatinine: high
Calcium: low   BUN: high   Total protein: low
Inorganic phosphorus: high   Uric acid: high   Albumin: low

FIGURE 6–1A-F.

Results of a multiparameter test provided by the Technicon SMA 12/60 System,
a multichannel system that can perform 12 blood chemistry analyses simultaneously. Certain patterns of increases and decreases in blood constituents are
associated with particular disease entities. The normal range for each constituent tested is indicated by a vertical shaded strip. (Used with permission of
Technicon Instruments Corporation, Tarrytown, NY)

FIGURE 6–1B.

Metastatic carcinoma of bone.
Calcium: high
Osteoblasts: proliferate
Alkaline phosphatase: dramatically increased

(**Note:** The shaded areas represent the normal values for a given analyte.)

S M A 12/60

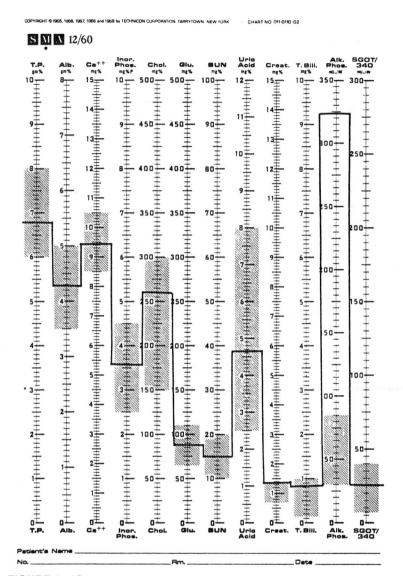

Patient's Name _____

No. _____ Rm. _____ Date _____

FIGURE 6–1C.
Metastatic carcinoma of liver.
Isolated elevation of alkaline phosphatase.

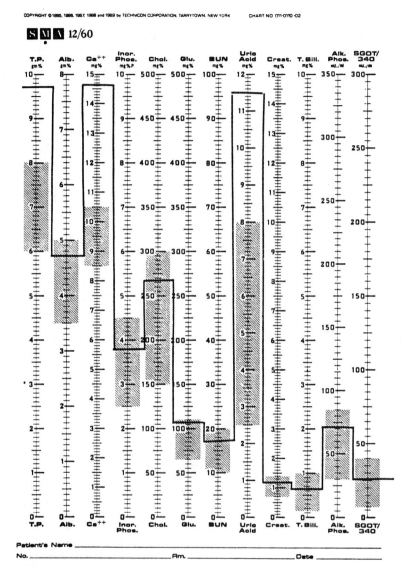

FIGURE 6–1D.
Multiple myeloma.
Calcium: elevated
Alkaline phosphatase: normal
Uric acid: elevated
Total protein: markedly elevated

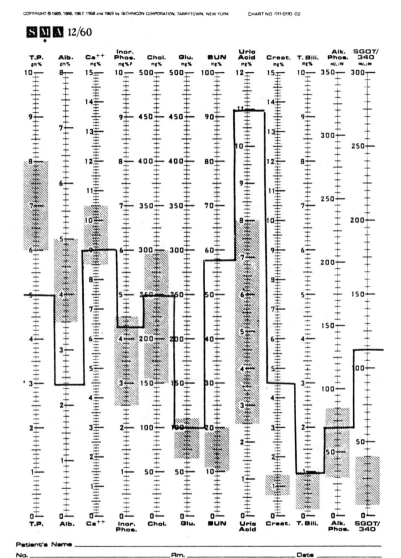

FIGURE 6–1E.
Acute eclampsia.
BUN: elevated
Uric acid: elevated
Creatinine: elevated
AST: elevated
Albumin: decreased
Total protein: decreased

FIGURE 6–1F.
Primary hyperparathyroidism.
Calcium: elevated
Alkaline phosphatase: elevated
Inorganic phosphorus: decreased

Use of the Autoanalyzer

The use of instrumentation in a laboratory setting has made it possible to conduct a wide variety of chemical tests on a single sample of blood. Autoanalyzers such as the Ektachem 700 by Kodak; the Automated Clinical Analyzer (ACA) by Dupont; Astra by Berkman; the Sequential Multiple Analyzer by Technicon (SMAC) (see Fig. 6-1, A–F) and the Multiple Sequential Screening Panel (MSSP) by Technicon can be used to process an individual specimen rapidly through a number of basic chemical analyses. The results of these tests are also recorded automatically and displayed for ease of interpretation; if an interface is available, the results can be transmitted directly to the hospital or clinic computer.

Because of the speed of the autoanalyzer and the number of tests it can process in a short period of time, it has become a major means of screening patients. Not only does it provide a baseline for future comparisons, it also has uncovered unsuspected diseases and allowed for early diagnosis of diseases whose symptoms are either vague or absent.

Note: Normal or reference values for any chemistry determination will vary with the method or assay employed. For example, differences in substrates or temperature at which the assay is run will alter the "normal" range. It may be somewhat misleading to give normal ranges, for they will vary from laboratory to laboratory. (See Chap. 1, p. 6 regarding normals.)

The blood chemistries usually recorded include

Albumin	Glucose
Alkaline phosphatase	Inorganic phosphorus
Aspartate transaminase (AST)	Total bilirubin
Blood urea nitrogen (BUN)	Total protein (TP)
Calcium (Ca^{2+})	Triglycerides
Cholesterol	Uric acid
Creatinine	

Various combinations of these chemical values provide insight into liver function, kidney disease, cardiovascular and pulmonary disorders, hematologic and reticuloendothelial dysfunction, and possible cancerous conditions.

Use of Multiple Laboratories

It is important to realize that, for economic reasons, it is not possible to do all the tests listed in this book in one hospital or clinic laboratory. In many cases, a number of tests are sent out to reference or commercial laboratories. A certain percentage of these tests will fall into the category of being too sophisticated or of too low a volume to obtain reliable results. This is one of the reasons why test results are not immediately available for interpretation.

ELECTROLYTE TESTS

Calcium (Ca^{2+})

Normal Values

Total: 8.8–10.0 mg/dl
        2.20–2.55 mmol/L
Children: (4–20)
          9.2–11.0 mg/dl
          2.3–2.75 mmol/L

Ionized: 1.09–1.33 mmol/L
         4.4–5.4 mg/dl
         2.1–2.6 mEq/L
Children: 1.10–1.50 mmol/L
          4.40–6.00 mg/dl

Background

The bulk of body calcium (98%–99%) is stored in the skeleton and teeth, which act as huge reservoirs for maintaining the blood levels of calcium. About 50% of the blood calcium is ionized; the rest is protein-bound. However, only ionized calcium can be used by the body in such vital processes as muscular contraction, cardiac function, transmission of nerve impulses, and blood clotting. Yet the ionized calcium cannot be measured independently of the total calcium levels. Therefore, the 50% ratio is only estimated and can fluctuate depending on general acid–base balance. In acidosis, the ionized calcium will be higher than 50%; in alkalosis, it will be lower.

The amount of protein in the blood will also affect calcium levels, because 50% of the blood calcium is protein-bound. Thus, a decrease in serum albumin would result in a profound decrease in total serum calcium. However, the decrease does not alter the concentration of the ionized form.

A patient suffering from a deficiency of ionized calcium will show signs of tetany accompanied by muscular twitching and eventual convulsions (a neuromuscular response to the decreased calcium at the nerve junctions).

Factors Influencing Calcium Levels

A. *Parathyroid hormone*
   1. Blood calcium is regulated by parathyroid hormone, which exerts a direct effect on bone to release calcium into the blood.
   2. Parathyroid hormone also acts on both the intestines, increasing absorption of calcium, and the kidneys, causing calcium to be reabsorbed by the proximal tubules.

B. *Calcitonin*
   This hormone lowers blood calcium levels by increasing calcium clearance by the kidneys.

C. *Vitamin D*
   It stimulates calcium absorption by the intestines.
D. *Estrogens and androgens*
   1. Estrogens increase calcium deposits in the bones. (Osteoporosis, following menopause, may respond to estrogen therapy.)
   2. Androgens. Hyperfunction of the adrenal cortex or thyroid may result in hypocalcemia and bone decalcification.
E. *Carbohydrates and lactose*
   1. Carbohydrates increase intestinal absorption of calcium.
   2. Addition of lactose to the diet increases the absorption and retention of calcium.

Explanation of Test

This test measures the concentration of total calcium in the blood and is used as a measure of parathyroid function, calcium metabolism, and in the evaluation of malignancies.

Hyperparathyroidism and cancer are the most common causes of hypercalcemia, and hypoalbuminemia is the most common cause of reduced total calcium. A test for the ionized fraction of calcium will reflect the functional states of calcium metabolism better than the total calcium.

Procedure

A venous blood sample of 5 ml is obtained.

Clinical Implications

A. *Normal levels of total calcium* combined with other findings
   1. Normal calcium levels with overall normal findings in other tests indicate that there are no problems with calcium metabolism.
   2. Normal calcium and abnormal phophorus indicate impaired calcium absorption due to alteration of parathyroid hormone activity or secretion. In rickets, the calcium level may be normal or slightly lowered and the phosphorus level is depressed.
   3. Normal calcium and elevated blood urea nitrogen (BUN) indicate
      (a) Possible secondary hyperparathyroidism. Initially, a lowered serum calcium results from uremia and acidosis. The lower calcium level stimulates the parathyroid to release parathyroid hormone, which acts on bone to release more calcium.
      (b) Possible primary hyperparathyroidism. Excessive amounts of parathyroid hormone cause elevation in calcium levels, but secondary kidney disease would cause retention of phosphate and concomitant lower calcium.

4. Normal calcium and decreased serum albumin
This is indicative of hypercalcemia, because there should be a decrease in calcium when there is a decrease in albumin because 50% of serum calcium is protein-bound.

B. *Hypercalcemia* (increased total calcium levels)
Hypercalcemia is associated with many disorders, but its greatest clinical importance rests in its association with *cancer*, including multiple myeloma, parathyroid tumors, nonendocrine tumors producing a parathyroidlike substance, and cancers metastasizing to the bone. Increased calcium levels are caused by or associated with

1. Hyperparathyroidism due to
   (a) Parathyroid adenoma
   (b) Hyperplasia of parathyroid glands } Associated with hypophosphatemia
2. Cancer
   (a) Metastatic cancers involving bone. Cancers of lung, breast, thyroid, kidney, and testes may metastasize to bone.
   (b) Hodgkin's disease and other lymphomas
   (c) Multiple myeloma in which there is extensive bone destruction
   (d) Lung and renal cancers may produce parathyroid hormone, resulting in symptoms of hypercalcemia.
   (e) Sarcoidosis due to increased IgG or IgA
   (f) Leukemia
3. Addison's disease
4. Hyperthyroidism
5. Paget's disease of bone (also accompanied by high levels of alkaline phosphatase)
6. Prolonged immobilization
7. Bone fractures combined with bedrest
8. Excessive intake of vitamin D
9. Prolonged use of diuretics, thiazides
10. Respiratory acidosis
11. Milk–alkali syndrome (history of peptic ulcer could indicate excessive intake of milk and antacids)

C. *Hypocalcemia* (decreased total calcium levels)
Commonly caused by or associated with
1. Pseudohypocalcemia (hyperproteinemia), which is a reflection of reduced albumin (as revealed by a serum protein electrophoresis). It is the reduced protein that is responsible for the low calcium, because 50% of the calcium total is protein-bound.

Note: Excessive use of intravenous fluids will decrease albumin levels and thus decrease the amount of calcium.

2. Hypoparathyroidism (primary is very rare), which may be due to accidental removal of parathyroid glands during a thyroidectomy, irradiation, hypomagnesemia, gastrointestinal disorders, renal wasting
3. Hyperphosphatemia, which is due to renal failure, laxatives, cytotoxic drugs
4. Malabsorption, which is due to sprue, celiac disease, pancreatic dysfunction (fatty acids combine with calcium and are precipitated and excreted in the feces)
5. Acute pancreatitis
6. Alkalosis (calcium ions become bound to protein)
7. Osteomalacia
8. Diarrhea
9. Rickets

D. *Increased ionized calcium*
   1. Primary hyperparathyroidism
   2. Ectopic parathyroid hormone–producing tumors
   3. Excess intake of vitamin D
   4. Various malignancies

E. *Decreased ionized calcium*
   Primary hypoparathyroidism is associated with low ionized calcium level and low total calcium level.

Clinical Alert

Panic Levels
<7.0 mg/dl, associated with tetany
>11.0 mg/dl, suggestive of hyperparathyroidism
>13.5 mg/dl, associated with hypercalcemic coma and metastatic cancer

Rapid treatment of hypercalcemia with substance such as calcitonin solution is indicated.

Interfering Factors
1. Thiazide diuretics may lead to impairment of urinary calcium excretions and consequent hypercalcemia.
2. In patients with renal insufficiency who are undergoing dialysis, a calcium–ion exchange resin is sometimes used for hyperkalemia. The use of this resin may lead to increased calcium levels.
3. Increased intake of magnesium and phosphates and the excessive use of laxatives may lower the blood calcium level. This occurs

because of the increased intestinal loss of calcium these elements produce.

4. When decreased calcium levels are due to magnesium deficiency, as in poor absorption from the bowel, the administration of magnesium will correct the calcium deficiency.

5. If a patient is known to have or suspected of having a pH abnormality, a concurrent pH should be requested with ionized calcium.

6. Many drugs may cause increased or decreased levels of calcium. Calcium supplements taken shortly before specimen collection will cause a falsely high value.

Chloride (Cl^-)

Normal Values
Adult: 98–106 mmol/L or Newborn: 96–110 mmol/L

Chloride, a blood electrolyte, is an anion that exists predominantly in the extracellular spaces, and in a lesser preponderance in the intravascular spaces and in the cell itself. Chemically, it exists primarily in combinations as sodium chloride or hydrochloric acid.

Chloride maintains cellular integrity through its influence on osmotic pressure. It is also significant in monitoring acid–base balance and water balance.

Chloride has the reciprocal power of increasing or decreasing in concentration whenever changes occur in the concentration of other anions. In metabolic acidosis, there is a reciprocal rise in chloride concentration when the bicarbonate concentration drops. Similarly, when aldosterone directly causes an increase in the reabsorption of sodium (which is a positive ion), the indirect effect is an increase in the absorption of chloride (the negative ion).

Chlorides are excreted with cations (positive ions) during massive diuresis from any cause and are lost from the gastrointestinal tract as a result of vomiting, diarrhea, or intestinal fistulas.

Explanation of Test
Alteration of serium chloride is seldom a primary problem. Thus, the measurement of chlorides is usually done for its inferential value and is helpful in diagnosing disorders of acid–base and water balance. Because of the relatively high concentration of chloride in the gastric juices, prolonged vomiting may lead to considerable chloride loss and lowered serum level.

Chloride is the least important electrolyte to measure in an emergency, but it is especially important to measure in the correction of hypokalemic alkalosis. If potassium is supplied without chloride, hypokalemic alkalosis may persist.

Procedure

A venous blood sample of 5 ml is obtained.

Clinical Implications

1. Whenever the serum level is much lower than 100 mEq/L, the urinary excretion of chloride falls to a very low level.
2. The reason why decreased chloride levels often occur in acute infections is not clear.
3. Chloride measurements are of limited value in renal disease for the reason that plasma chloride can be maintained near normal limits even when a considerable degree of renal failure is present.
4. *Decreased chloride levels* occur in
   - (a) Severe vomiting
   - (b) Severe diarrhea
   - (c) Ulcerative colitis
   - (d) Pyloric obstruction
   - (e) Severe burns
   - (f) Heat exhaustion
   - (g) Diabetic acidosis
   - (h) Addison's disease
   - (i) Fever
   - (j) Acute infections such as pneumonia
   - (k) Use of drugs such as mercurial and chlorothiazide diuretics
5. *Increased chloride levels* occur in
   - (a) Dehydration
   - (b) Cushing's syndrome
   - (c) Hyperventilation
   - (d) Eclampsia
   - (e) Anemia
   - (f) Cardiac decompensation
   - (g) Some kidney disorders

Interfering Factors

1. The plasma chloride concentration of infants is usually higher than that of children and adults.
2. Many drugs may cause a change in chloride levels.

Clinical Alert

1. If an electrolyte disorder is suspected, daily weight and accurate fluid intake and output should be recorded.
2. Panic value for serum chloride is <70 or >120 mEq/L; <70 or >120 mmol/L.

Phosphate (P)/Inorganic Phosphorus (PO₄)

Normal Values

Adults: 2.7–4.5 mg/dl or 0.87–1.45 mmol/L
Children: 4.5–5.5 mg/dl   1.45–1.78 mmol/L

Explanation of Test

Approximately 85% of the body's total phosphorus content is combined with calcium in the bone. The remainder is located within the cells. Most of the phosphorus in the blood exists as phosphates or esters.

Phosphate is required for generation of bony tissue and functions in the metabolism of glucose and lipids, in the maintenance of acid–base balance, and in the storage and transfer of energy from one site in the body to another. Phosphorus enters the cell with glucose and is lowered after carbohydrate ingestion. For these reasons, blood phosphate levels must be controlled within reasonably constant limits.

Phosphate levels are always evaluated in relation to calcium levels because there is an inverse relationship between the two. When calcium levels are decreased, phosphorus levels increase. When phosphorus levels decrease, calcium levels increase. An excess in serum levels of one causes the kidneys to excrete the other. Many of the causes of elevated calcium are also causes of lower phosphorus levels. As with calcium, the controlling factor is parathyroid hormone.

Procedure

A venous blood sample of 5 ml is obtained.

Clinical Implications

A. *Hyperphosphatemia* (increased phosphorus levels)

The most common causes of elevated blood phosphate levels are found in association with kidney dysfunction and uremia. This is because phosphate is so closely regulated by the kidneys.

(a) Renal insufficiency and severe nephritis (accompanied by elevated BUN and creatine)

(b) Hypoparathyroidism (accompanied by elevated phosphorus, decreased calcium, and normal renal function)

(c) Hypocalcemia

(d) Excessive intake of alkali (possible history of peptic ulcer)

(e) Excessive intake of vitamin D

(f) Fractures in the healing stage

(g) Bone tumors

(h) Addison's disease

(i) Acromegaly

B. *Hypophosphatemia* (decreased phosphorus levels)

(a) Hyperparathyroidism (accompanied by elevated calcium; no renal disease)

(b) Rickets (childhood) or osteomalacia (adult)

(c) Diabetic coma because of increased carbohydrate metabolism

(d) Hyperinsulinism

(e) Continuous administration of intravenous glucose in a nondiabetic patient.

Interfering Factors
1. Normally high in children
2. Falsely increased by hemolysis of blood
3. Vitamin D can be the cause of elevation; drugs can also be the cause of decreases.
4. The use of laxatives or enemas containing large amounts of sodium phosphate will cause increased phosphorus levels. With the oral intake of the laxative, the blood level may increase as much as 5 mg/dl 2 to 3 hours after the dose. This increased level is only temporary (5–6 hours), but this factor should be considered when abnormal levels are seen that cannot otherwise be explained.

Clinical Alert

When phosphorus rises rapidly, calcium drops—watch for arrhythmias and muscle twitching.

Magnesium (Mg^{2+})

Normal Values
Adult: 1.3–2.1 mEq/L or 0.65–1.05 mmol/L
Newborn: 1.2–1.8 mEq/L or 0.6–0.9 mm/L

Background
Because all natural foods are rich in magnesium, magnesium deficiency is rare in a normal diet. Ingestion of magnesium increases not only the amount of magnesium absorbed but also the amount of calcium absorbed. On the other hand, a high phosphate diet suppresses both magnesium and calcium absorption.

Magnesium is required for the use of adenosine triphosphate (ADP) as a source of energy. It is therefore necessary for the action of numerous enzyme systems such as

1. Carbohydrate metabolism
2. Protein synthesis
3. Nucleic acid synthesis
4. Contraction of muscular tissue

Along with sodium, potassium, and calcium ions, magnesium also regulates neuromuscular irritability. In addition, it is needed in the clotting mechanism.

Magnesium and calcium are intimately tied together in their body functions, and deficiency of either one has a significant effect on the metabolism of the other. This is because of magnesium's importance in the absorption of calcium from the intestines and in calcium metabolism. A magnesium deficiency will result in the draft of calcium out of the bones, possibly resulting in abnormal calcification in the aorta and the kidney in the absence of a calcium pump mechanism. This condition responds to administration of magnesium salts.

Normally, 95% of the magnesium that is filtered through the glomerulus is reabsorbed in the tubule. When there is decreased kidney function, greater amounts of magnesium are retained, resulting in increased blood serum levels.

Explanation of Test

Measurement of magnesium levels is used as an index to metabolic activity in the body and to renal function.

The bulk of total magnesium in the body is concentrated in the bone, cartilage, and within the cell itself.

Procedure

A venous blood sample of 4 ml is obtained. Avoid hemolysis.

Clinical Implications

A. *Reduced magnesium levels* occur in

(a) Chronic diarrhea
(b) Hemodialysis
(c) Chronic renal disease
(d) Hepatic cirrhosis
(e) Chronic pancreatitis
(f) Use of diuretics
(g) Aldosteronism
(h) Ulcerative colitis
(i) Hyperaldosteronism
(j) Toxemia of pregnancy
(k) Hyperthyroidism and hypoparathyroidism
(l) Excessive lactation
(m) Malabsorption syndromes
(n) Chronic alcoholism
(o) Prolonged gastric drainage

In magnesium deficiency states, urinary magnesium decreases before the serum does.

B. *Increased magnesium levels* occur in

(a) Renal failure or reduced renal function
(b) Diabetic acidosis before treatment
(c) Hypothyroidism
(d) Addison's disease
(e) Adrenalectomy
(f) Controlled diabetes in older persons
(g) Use of antacids containing magnesium (*e.g.*, milk of magnesia)
(h) Dehydration
(i) Use of thiazides
(j) Use of ethacrynic acid

Interfering Factors

1. Prolonged salicylate therapy, lithium, and magnesium products (antacids, laxatives) will cause falsely increased magnesium levels, particularly if there is renal damage.

2. Calcium gluconate, as well as a number of other drugs, can inter-fere with testing methods and cause falsely decreased results.
3. Hemolysis will invalidate results because about three-fourths of the magnesium in the blood is found intracellularly in the red blood cells.

Clinical Alert

1. Treatment of diabetics in coma will often result in low plasma magnesium levels. This is because magnesium moves with potassium into the cells after insulin administration.
2. Magnesium deficiency may cause apparently unexplained hypocalcemia and hypokalemia. In these instances, patients may have neurologic and/or gastrointestinal symptoms.
3. Signs of too much magnesium (which acts as a sedative) include
   (a) Lethargy, flushing, nausea, vomiting, slurred speech
   (b) Weak or absent deep tendon reflexes
   (c) Electrocardiogram: prolonged PR and Q–T intervals, widened QRS; bradycardia
   (d) Hypotension, drowsiness, and respiratory depression

Treatment involves

   (a) Withholding source of magnesium excess
   (b) Promoting excretion
   (c) Giving calcium salts
   (d) Hemodialysis
4. Signs of insufficient magnesium include
   (a) Muscle tremors, twitching, tetany
   (b) Hypocalcemia
   (c) Hyperactive deep tendon reflexes
   (d) Electrocardiogram: prolonged P–R and Q–T intervals; broad, flat T waves; premature ventricular contractions; ventricular tachycardia; and fibrillation
   (e) Anorexia, nausea, and vomiting
   (f) Lethargy and insomnia

Treatment involves

   (a) Administering magnesium salts
   (b) Reducing auditory, mechanical, and visual stimuli
5. Panic levels for serum magnesium are <0.5 or >3.0 mEq/L; <0.5 or >3.0 mmol/L.

Potassium (K$^+$)

Normal Values
Adult: 3.5–5 mEq/L or 3.5–5.0 mmol/L
    A very narrow range of normal
Newborn: 3.7–5.9 mEq/L or 3.7–5.9 mmol/L
    Child: 3.4–4.7 mEq/L or 3.4–4.7 mmol/L

Background
Potassium is the principal electrolyte (cation) of intracellular fluid and the primary buffer within the cell itself. Ninety percent of potassium is concentrated within the cell; only small amounts are contained in bone and blood. A kilogram of tissue such as red blood cell or muscle contains about 90 mEq of potassium. Damaged cells release potassium into the blood.

The body is adapted to efficient potassium excretion. Normally, 80% to 90% of the cells' potassium is excreted in the urine by the glomeruli of the kidneys. The remainder is excreted in sweat and in the stool. Even when no potassium is taken into the body (as in a fasting state), 40 to 50 mEq are still excreted daily in the urine. The kidneys do not conserve potassium, and when an adequate amount of potassium is not ingested, a severe deficiency will occur. Potassium balance is maintained in adults on an average dietary intake of 80 to 200 mEq/day. The minimum daily need is about 30 mEq; the maximum daily tolerance to an acute load is 400 mEq. The normal intake, minimal needs, and maximum tolerance for potassium are almost the same as those for sodium.

Potassium plays an important role in nerve conduction and muscle function. Moreover, it helps maintain acid–base balance and osmotic pressure. Along with calcium and magnesium, potassium controls the rate and force of contraction of the heart and, thus, the cardiac output. Evidence of a potassium deficit can be noted on an electrocardiogram (ECG) by the presence of a U wave.

Potassium and sodium ions are particularly important in the renal regulation of acid–base balance because hydrogen ions are substituted for sodium and potassium ions in the renal tubule. Potassium is more important than sodium because potassium bicarbonate is the primary intracellular inorganic buffer. In potassium deficiency, there is a relative deficiency of intracellular potassium bicarbonate and the pH is relatively acid. The respiratory center responds to the intracellular acidosis by lower Pco$_2$, through the mechanism of hyperventilation.

Concentration of potassium is greatly affected by the adrenal hormones. A potassium deficiency will cause a significant reduction in protein synthesis.

Evaluation of Test

This test is used to evaluate changes in body potassium and is helpful in diagnosing disorders of acid–base and water balance in the body. It is not an absolute value and varies with the circulatory volume and other factors. Because a totally unsuspected potassium imbalance can suddenly prove lethal, its development must be anticipated. Thus, it is important to check this value in severe cases of Addison's disease, uremic coma, intestinal obstruction, acute renal failure, gastrointestinal loss in the administration of diuretics, steroid therapy, and cardiac patients on digitalis.

Procedure

1. A venous blood sample of 5 ml is obtained.
2. Hemolysis in obtaining the sample should be avoided; it will give falsely elevated results.
3. The sample must be delivered to the laboratory and spun at once to separate cells from serum. Potassium leaks out of the cell and will be falsely elevated after 4 hours.

Clinical Implications

A. *Hypokalemia*
 1. Values of 3.5 mEq/L are more commonly associated with deficiency, rather than normality.
 2. A falling trend (0.1–0.2 mEq/day) is indicative of a developing potassium deficiency.
  (a) Most frequent cause of potassium deficiency is gastrointestinal loss.
  (b) Most frequent cause of potassium depletion is intravenous (IV) fluid administration without adequate potassium supplements.
 3. *Decreased levels* (hypokalemia) are associated with
  (a) Diarrhea
  (b) Pyloric obstruction
  (c) Starvation
  (d) Malabsorption
  (e) Severe vomiting
  (f) Severe burns
  (g) Primary aldosteronism
  (h) Excessive ingestion of licorice
  (i) Renal tubular acidosis
  (j) Diuretic administration
  (k) Other drugs such as
   (1) Steroids
   (2) Estrogens
  (l) Familial periodic paralysis

(m)Liver disease with ascites
(n) Chronic stress
(o) Crash dieting without potassium
(p) Chronic fever
B. *Hyperkalemia* (increased levels of 5.5)
The most frequent causes of increased levels are
1. Renal failure
   (a) Oliguria
   (b) Anuria
2. Cell damage as in burns, accidents, surgery, chemotherapy, disseminated intravascular coagulation (damaged cells will release potassium into the blood)
3. Acidosis (drives potassium out of the cells)
4. Addison's disease
5. Selective hypoaldosteronism
6. Internal hemorrhage
7. Uncontrolled diabetes
8. Acidosis

Interfering Factors
1. Opening and closing the fist ten times with a tourniquet in place results in an increase of the potassium level by 10% to 20%. For this reason, it is recommended that the blood sample be obtained without a tourniquet, or that the tourniquet be released after the needle has entered the vein and 2 minutes are allowed to elapse before the sample is withdrawn.
2. Drug usage
   (a) The IV use of *potassium penicillin* may cause hyperkalemia; *penicillin sodium* may cause an increased excretion of potassium.
   (b) Glucose tolerance testing or the ingestion and administration of large amounts of glucose in patients with heart disease may cause a decrease of as much as 0.4 mEq/L in potassium blood levels.
   (c) A number of drugs interfere with potassium levels.

(*text continues on page 287*)

Clinical Alert

1. Serum potassium panic values are 2.5 mEq/L or less or 6.5 mEq/L or greater. These levels (<2.5 or >6.5 mmol/L) may cause heart problems leading to death.
2. The most common cause of hypokalemia in patients receiving IV fluids is water and sodium chloride administration with-

out adequate replacement for potassium lost in urine and drainage fluids. A patient receiving IV fluids needs potassium every day. The minimum daily dose should be 40 mEq, but the optimum daily dose ranges between 60 and 120 mEq. Potassium needs are greater in tissue injury, wound infection, gastric intestinal or biliary drainage. If adequate amounts of potassium are not given in IV solution (40 mEq/day), hypokalemia will develop eventually.

Patients receiving more than 10 mEq KCL in 100 cc of IV solution should be ECG-monitored for potential arrhythmias if the IV rate is 100 ml/hr or greater. Concentrated doses of IV potassium should always be administered via volume-controlled IV infusion devices. A burning sensation felt at the site of needle insertion may indicate that the concentration is toxic and the IV rate can be reduced. Some physicians will order a small dose of Xylocaine to be added to IV potassium to eliminate the "burning" sensation some patients experience. Always be sure to check for Xylocaine allergies prior to administration of this local anesthetic.

3. Patients taking digitalis and diuretics should be watched closely for hypokalemia because cardiac arrhythmias can occur. Hypokalemia enhances the effect of digitalis preparations, creating the possibility of digitalis intoxication from even an average maintenance dose. Digitalis, diuretics, and hypokalemia are a potentially lethal combination.

4. The potassium blood level rises 0.6 mEq/L for every 0.1 decrease in blood pH.

5. Hyperkalemia can be altered by the use of hypertonic ion exchange resins orally, or by an enema (Kayexalate) to remove excess potassium.

6. If there is a massive loss of extracellular potassium, the potassium within the cells may have to support potassium concentration in the blood. This process cannot be measured directly and can only be inferred from an understanding of clinical signs. Recognizing signs and symptoms of hypokalemia and hyperkalemia is very important, because many of them originate in the nervous and muscular systems and are usually nonspecific and similar.

7. *Evaluating Changes in Body Potassium*
How to recognize an excess K$^+$ or K$^+$ deficiency or depletion even when the blood level is normal

Hyperkalemia (Excess potassium)	Hypokalemic (deficiency of K^+)
1. Record fluid intake and output.	1. Record fluid intake and output.
2. Check blood volume and venous pressure, which will give a clue to dehydration or circulatory overload.	2. Check blood volume and venous pressure, which will give a clue to circulatory overload or dehydration.
3. Identify ECG changes. (a) Elevated T-wave heart block (b) Flattened P wave (c) Cardiac arrest may occur without any warning other than ECG changes.	3. Identify ECG changes. (a) Depressed T waves (b) Peaking of P waves
4. Observe for slow pulse and oliguria.	4. Observe for dehydration caused by severe vomiting, hyperventilation, sweating, diuresis, nasogastric tube with gastric suction. Accurately record state of hydration or dehydration.
5. Observe for neuromuscular changes, such as (a) Muscle weakness and impaired muscle function (b) Flaccid paralysis (c) Tremors, twitching preceding actual paralysis	5. Observe for neuromuscular changes, such as (a) Fatigue (b) Muscle weakness, muscle pain, flabby muscles (c) Paresthesia (d) Hypotension and rapid pulse (e) Respiratory muscle weakness leading to paralysis, cyanosis, and respiratory arrest (f) Anorexia, nausea, vomiting, paralytic ileus (g) Apathy, drowsiness, irritability, tetany, coma

Clinical Alert

Be on the alert for these arrhythmias that may occur with hyperkalemia.

1. Sinus bradycardia
2. Sinus arrest
3. First-degree atrioventricular block
4. Nodal rhythm

5. Idioventricular rhythm
6. Ventricular tachycardia
7. Ventricular fibrillation
8. Ventricular arrest

Be on the alert for the following arrhythmias, which may occur with hypokalemia.

1. Ventricular premature beats
2. Atrial tachycardia

3. Nodal tachycardia
4. Ventricular tachycardia
5. Ventricular fibrillation

Sodium (Na$^+$)

Normal Values

Adult: 135–148 mmol/L or 135–148 mEq/L
Newborn: 134–144 mmol/L or 134–144 mEq/L
Child: 138–144 mmol/L or 138–144 mEq/L

Sodium, a blood electrolyte, is the most abundant cation (90% of the electrolyte fluid) and the chief base of the blood. Its primary functions in the body are to chemically maintain osmotic pressure and acid–base balance and to transmit nerve impulses. The body has a strong tendency to maintain a total base content, and only slight changes are found even under pathologic conditions.

Sodium concentration is under the control of the kidneys and the central nervous system acting through the endocrine system. In health, the level of sodium is kept constant within narrow limits despite wide fluctuations in dietary intake. An average dietary intake of 90 to 250 mEq/day is enough to maintain sodium balance in adults. The minimum daily need is approximately 15 mEq.

Explanation of Test

Determinations of plasma sodium levels are useful in detecting gross changes in water and salt balance but are of little help in detecting early or subtle changes. Urinary sodium is a more sensitive indicator of altered sodium balance. Numerous factors, as listed below, determine the content and volume of urine excreted. These, in turn, determine the content and flow rate in the renal vein returning processed blood.

Mechanisms for maintaining a constant sodium level in the plasma and extracellular fluid include

1. *Renal blood flow*
    (a) Increased renal blood flow to the glomeruli will result in increased sodium and chloride excretions.
    (b) Decreased renal blood flow to the glomeruli will result in sodium and chloride retention and edema. This occurs in patients with reduced cardiac output.
2. *Carbonic anhydrase enzyme activity*
    (a) The level of activity of this system is an important factor in control of the rate of sodium excretion.
    (b) Inhibition of carbonic anhydrase enzyme activity results in increased sodium reabsorption in the tubules.
3. *Aldosterone*
    (a) Aldosterone acts on the distal tubules and also affects sodium reabsorption.
    (b) Regulation of aldosterone secretion is
        (1) Primarily by the renin–angiotensin system
        (2) Secondarily by ACTH, sodium, and potassium concentration
    (c) In primary hyperaldosteronism, sodium will be retained and hypertension will result. In exchange for sodium, potassium will often be excreted and decreased potassium may be found in this condition.
4. *Action of other steroids* whose plasma level is controlled by the anterior pituitary gland
    These steroids can cause salt and water retention. During the menstrual cycle, estrogen and progesterone cause salt and water retention before menstruation and diuresis if fertilization has not taken place.
5. *Renin enzyme secretion*
    Renin is a potent stimulus to aldosterone secretion. It regulates renal blood flow, the glomerular filtration rate, and salt and water excretion. In renal diseases, excessive amounts of renin secreted into the plasma result in salt and water retention and hypertension.
6. *Antidiuretic hormone (ADH), vasopressin secretion*
    (a) ADH controls the reabsorption of water at the distal tubules of the kidney.
    (b) Secretion of this hormone is responsive to changes in extracellular fluid volume.

Procedure
A venous blood sample of 5 ml is obtained.

Clinical Implications

A. *Hyponatremia* (decreased levels)

1. Hyponatremia usually reflects a relative excess of body water rather than a low total body sodium.

2. *Reduced* sodium levels (hyponatremia) are associated with
   (a) Severe burns
   (b) Severe diarrhea
   (c) Vomiting
   (d) Excessive IV induction of nonelectrolyte fluids
   (e) Addison's disease (lack of adrenal steroids impairs sodium reabsorption)
   (f) Severe nephritis
   (g) Pyloric obstruction
   (h) Malabsorption syndrome
   (i) Diabetic acidosis
   (j) Drugs
       (1) Mercurial diuretics
       (2) Chlorothiazide diuretics
   (k) Edema
   (l) Excessive sweating accompanied by large amounts of water by mouth
   (m)Stomach suction accompanied by water or ice chips *by mouth*

B. *Hypernatremia* (increased levels)

1. Increased sodium levels are uncommon, but when they do occur they are associated with
   (a) Dehydration and insufficient water intake
   (b) Conn's syndrome
   (c) Primary aldosteronism
   (d) Coma
   (e) Cushing's disease
   (f) Diabetes insipidus
   (g) Tracheobronchitis

Clinical Alert

1. IV therapy considerations are as follows:
   (a) Sodium balance is maintained in adults with an average dietary intake of 90 to 250 mEq/day. The maximum daily tolerance to an acute load is 400 mEq/day. If a patient is given 3 L of isotonic saline in 24 hours, he will receive 465 mEq of sodium. This amount exceeds the average, healthy adult's tolerance level. It will take a *healthy* person 24 to 48 hours to excrete the excess sodium.

(b) After surgery, trauma, or shock, there is a decrease of extracellular fluid volume. Replacement of extracellular fluid is essential if water and electrolyte balance is to be maintained. The ideal replacement IV solution should have a sodium concentration of 140 mEq/L.
2. Check patients for signs of edema or hypertension.
3. Panic values are <120 or ≥155 mEq/L or <120 or >155 mmol/L.

Interfering Factors
Many drugs may cause falsely increased or decreased levels of blood sodium.

Osmolality and Water-load Test

Normal Values
Serum
Adult: 275–295 m/Osmol/kg
Newborn: as low as 266 mOsmol/kg

Urine Osmolality
Random: 50–1200 m/Osmol/L
After 12-hr fluid restriction: >850 m/Osmol/L
Ratio of serum/urine Osmolality: 1.0–3.0

Background
In health, a change in osmolality produces a sequence of physiologic events that maintains homeostasis. Increased osmolality will stimulate secretion of ADH that acts on renal tubules. This results in reabsorption of water, more concentrated urine, and less concentrated serum. Low serum osmolality suppresses the release of ADH, water reabsorption is decreased, and large amounts of dilute urine are produced.

Explanation of Test
This test is used as an indication of fluid and electrolyte balance and to rule out the presence of organic acids, sugars, or ethanol. It is helpful in evaluating hydration status, seizures, liver disease, ADH function, liver disease, coma, and in toxicology work-up.

Serum osmolality increases with dehydration and decreases with overhydration. In general, the same conditions that reduce or increase serum sodium affect the osmolality.

Procedure
A venous blood sample of at least 6 ml is obtained. It is determined in the laboratory by the number (not the nature) of dissolved solute particles in solution.

Interfering Factors
1. Decreases are associated with attitude, diurnal variation with water retention at night, and some drugs.
2. Some drugs will cause increases.

Clinical Implications
1. *Increased values* (hyperosmolality) are associated with
   (a) Water restriction or loss
   (b) Brain trauma with impaired release of ADH
   (c) Hypercalcemia
   (d) Diabetes mellitus due to increased glucose
   (e) Diabetes insipidus
   (f) Cerebral lesions (often with tube feeding)
2. *Decreased values* (hypoosmolality) are associated with
   (a) Loss of sodium with diuretics and low salt diet
   (b) Addison's disease
   (c) Adrenogenital syndrome
   (d) Inappropriate secretions of ADH, as in trauma and cancer of lung
   (e) Excessive water replacement

Clinical Alert

1. Panic serum values are results that are less than 240 or greater than 321. A value of 385 relates to stupor in hyperglycemia. Values of 400 to 420 are associated with grand mal seizures; values greater than 420 are deadly.
2. The patient receiving intravenous fluids should have a normal osmolality. If the osmolality increases, the fluids contain relatively more electrolytes than water. If it falls, relatively more water than electrolytes is present.
3. If the ratio of serum sodium to serum osmolality falls below 0.43, the outlook is guarded. This ratio may be distorted in drug intoxication.

Water-load or dilution test may be done to investigate impaired renal excretion of water.

Procedure for Water-load Test

1. The ideal position during testing period is the recumbent position, because in an upright position the response to water loading is reduced.
2. One hour before testing, the patient is given 300 ml of water to replace fluid lost during the overnight fast. This water is not counted as part of the test load.
3. The patient drinks a test load of water (calculated as 20 ml/kg of body weight) within 30 minutes.
4. After water is consumed, all urine is collected for the next 4 to 5 hours, and each voiding is checked for its amount, osmolality, and specific gravity. When the test is completed, a blood sample is obtained for osmolality and the entire volume of urine obtained is checked for osmolality.

Patient Preparation

1. Explain the purpose and procedure. The test takes 5 to 6 hours to complete.
2. No food, alcohol, medications, or smoking for 8 to 10 hours before testing.
3. The patient may experience nausea, abdominal fullness, fatigue, and desire to defecate.

Clinical Alert

1. Observe for adverse reactions to water-load test such as extreme abdominal discomfort, shortness of breath, or chest pain.
2. If water clearance is impaired, the water load will not induce diureses and maximum urinary dilution will not occur.
3. Accurate results may not be obtained if nausea, vomiting, or diarrhea occur or if disturbance in bladder emptying is present.

BLOOD SUGARS AND RELATED TESTS

Cortisone Glucose Tolerance

Normal Values

At 1 hour: blood glucose 160 mg/dl
At 2 hour: blood glucose 140 mg/dl
(Add an additional 18 mg/dl at age 40 and for each decade over 40 years.)

Explanation of Test
This is a glucose tolerance test based on the fact that cortisone increases blood glucose. The test is also known as the "steroid challenge" test because cortisone acetate is given before the standard glucose tolerance test is begun.

Indications for Test
1. When the results of the standard glucose tolerance test are doubtful, and altered carbohydrate metabolism is strongly suspected
2. In patients with suggestive signs of vascular or neurologic disease
3. In persons with a strong family history of diabetes
4. In women whose pregnancies were complicated by glycosuria and delivery of large infants

Procedure
The procedure is the same as for the glucose tolerance test with the following exceptions:

1. An oral dose of cortisone acetate is given 8 hours before glucose ingestion and again 2 hours before glucose is given.
2. A venous blood sample is obtained after the second dose of cortisone.

Clinical Implications
If the 2-hour level is above 140 mg/dl, a person is considered to be prediabetic and should be followed closely for the development of diabetes.

Interfering Factors
See "Glucose Tolerance Test."

C-Peptide

Normal Values
0.78–1.89 ng/ml or 0.26–0.62 nmol/L

Background
C-peptide is formed during the conversion of proinsulin to insulin in the beta cells of the pancreas. It is secreted into the blood serum in almost equal concentration with insulin. Normally, a strong correlation exists between levels of insulin and C-peptide, except possibly in obese persons and in the presence of islet cell tumors.

Explanation of Test
The measurement of C-peptide levels provides a reliable indication of beta and secretory function and insulin secretions. This determination has its most useful application in the evaluation of endogenous secre-

tion of insulin when the presence of circulatory insulin antibodies interferes with the direct assay of insulin. This situation is most likely to occur in diabetics who have been treated with bovine or pork insulin. This test is also useful in evaluating hypoglycemic states, in identifying surreptitious injection of insulin, and in confirming of remission of diabetes mellitus. Furthermore, monitoring following pancreatectomy for removal of cancer can provide a means of detecting the presence of residual tissue.

Procedure
A fasting venous blood sample of 1 ml is obtained.

Clinical Implications
1. *Increased values* are associated with endogenous hyperinsulinism and insulin-dependent diabetic persons when a high level of insulin is also present.
2. *Decreased levels* are associated with persons who have been surreptitiously injecting insulin and who have both hypoglycemia and high insulin levels.
3. *Normal levels* are found in persons who have had a remission of diabetes mellitus.

Patient Preparation
1. Explain the purpose and procedure of the test.
2. Caution the patient to fast from food for 8 to 12 hours. Water is permitted.

Glucagon

Normal Values
50–200 pg/ml or ng/L plasma

Glucagon response in normal person after a standard test meal of carbohydrates, fat, and protein is a gradual increase from 92 plus or minus 12 pg/ml to a peak of 125 plus or minus 13 pg/ml.

In a glucose tolerance test, glucagon levels will significantly decline from fasting levels during the hyperglycemic first hour in normal persons.

Background
Glucagon is a peptide hormone that originates in the alpha cells of the islets of Langerhans. In the liver, this hormone promotes glucose production. This action of glucagon is opposed by that of insulin. The normal coordinated release patterns of this hormone provide a sensitive control mechanism for glucose production and storage. For example, low glucose levels result in release, whereas conditions of hyper-

glycemia reduce circulating glucagon levels to approximately 50% of the amount in the fasting state.

It is now believed that the kidneys play an important role in the metabolism of glucagon. Studies reveal that elevated fasting levels of glucagon in patients with renal failure return to normal following successful renal transplantation. On the other hand, renal rejection has resulted in a dramatic rise in glucagon levels several days before changes in creatinine levels.

Abnormally high levels of glucagon recede once insulin therapy begins to control diabetes, and levels slowly revert to normal in persons on maintenance doses of insulin. Also, in contrast to the normal person, glucagon secretion in diabetics does not decrease following ingestion of a carbohydrate meal. However, an arginine infusion causes greatly increased glucagon secretion in normal persons.

Explanation of Test

This measurement has clinical significance in two ways. Glucagon deficiency reflects a general loss of pancreatic tissue. Compelling evidence for glucagon deficiency is the failure of glucagon levels to rise during arginine infusion. Hyperglucagonemia (increased glucagon levels) occurs in diabetes, acute pancreatitis, and in situations in which catecholamine secretion is greatly augmented, as in pheochromocytoma and in the presence of infection.

Procedure

Five venous blood samples of 5 ml are obtained in heparinized or EDTA containers. Special handling is required because glucagon is highly susceptible to enzymatic degradation. Blood-drawing tubes must be iced and plasma frozen as soon as possible.

Clinical Implications

1. *Increased levels* are associated with
   (a) Acute pancreatitis, such as occurs when there is an alpha cell tumor of the pancreas
   (b) Diabetes mellitus. Persons with severe diabetic ketoacidosis are reported to have levels five times normal fasting levels despite marked hyperglycemia.
   (c) Glucagonoma
   (d) Uremia
2. *Reduced levels* are associated with
   (a) Inflammatory disease when there is a loss of pancreatic tissue
   (b) Neoplastic replacement of the pancreas
   (c) Surgical removal of the pancreas

Interfering Factors

Increased levels occur in vigorous exercise and in trauma. Recently administered radiopharmaceuticals will affect test outcome.

Patient Preparation

No preparation is necessary unless glucose tolerance testing is to be done or if arginine infusion is ordered. In this case, check with your testing laboratory for specific protocols.

Glucose; Fasting Blood Sugar (FBS)

Adult: Fasting serum—70–110 mg/dl or 3.89–6.11 mmol/L
      Fasting whole blood—60–100 mg/dl or 3.33–5.53 mmol/L
      Nonfasting—85–125 mg/dl >50 yr or 70–115 mg/dl <50 yr
Child: 60–100 mg/dl or 3.33–5.55 mmol/L

Explanation of Test

The purpose of this test is to detect any disorder of glucose metabolism, mainly diabetes, and it is used as an aid in diabetes management. Glucose is formed from the digestion of carbohydrates and the conversion of glycogen by the liver. Two hormones directly regulate blood glucose: glucagon and insulin. Glucagon accelerates the breakdown of glycogen in the liver, causing blood glucose to rise. Insulin increases the permeability of cellular membranes to glucose, transports glucose into cells for metabolism, and further stimulates formation of glucogen and reduces blood glucose levels. Getting insulin into the cells where metabolism takes place requires insulin and insulin receptors. Following a meal, insulin will be released by the pancreas to help the body use glucose, provided there are enough insulin receptors. Insulin binds to special receptors on the surface of target cells such as fat and muscle. This causes channels to open that allow glucose to pass into cells where it can be used to make energy. As glucose is metabolized by the cells, blood glucose falls and none passes into the urine. Other hormones that contribute to glucose metabolism are ACTH, adrenocorticosteroids, epinephrine, and thyroxine.

    The test for blood sugar is used to detect disorders of metabolism that may be the result of one of several causes.

1. Inability of the beta islet cells of the pancreas to produce insulin
2. Reduced number of insulin receptors
3. Inability of the intestines to absorb glucose
4. Inability of the liver to accumulate and break down glycogen
5. The presence of increased amounts of hormones (*i.e.*, ACTH)

In most cases, any degree of elevated blood sugar (hyperglycemia) indicates diabetes. At the same time, it is important to remember that in mild cases of diabetes, the blood sugar may be within normal ranges. Therefore, in any suspected cases of diabetes, a glucose tolerance test is in order (see p. 303).

Although diabetes is the most readily suspected disorder in the presence of hyperglycemia, other diseases may be responsible for the elevated blood sugar and therefore should not be dismissed.

Clinical Alert

1. If a known or suspected diabetic is experiencing dizziness, weakness, or fainting, a blood sugar test must be done before any insulin is given. The same symptoms may be present for both insulin reaction and high blood sugar. If there will be a delay in obtaining a blood glucose measurement, when in doubt about signs and symptoms the patient is presenting, *give glucose, (e.g., orange juice).*
2. Frequent determinations of blood glucose are, in many situations, more desirable than monitoring urine glucose. Hence, blood glucose monitoring facilitates regulation of diabetes and may increase the likelihood of achieving ideal control in type 1 diabetes that approximates euglycemia.

Procedure

1. A venous blood sample of 5 ml is drawn while the patient is in a fasting state. If the patient is a known diabetic, blood should be drawn before insulin or oral hypoglycemics are given.
2. Self-monitoring of blood glucose requires one large drop of fingertip blood and can be done using reagent strips, with or without a glucometer.

Clinical Implications

A. *Elevated blood sugar* (hyperglycemia)
   1. Diabetes
      Values over 120 mg/dl on several testings may indicate diabetes mellitus. Except for diabetes, the FBS rarely exceeds 120 mg/dl.
   2. Other possible conditions
      (a) Cushing's disease (increase in glucocorticoids causes increase in blood sugar)
      (b) Acute stress (such as in myocardial infarction or severe infections, such as meningitis or encephalitis)
      (c) Pheochromocytoma
      (d) Pituitary adenoma (growth hormone leads to elevated blood sugar)
      (e) Hyperthyroidism
      (f) Adenoma of pancreas (may result in production of glucagon, which counteracts insulin)
      (g) Pancreatitis

      (h) Brain trauma or brain damage
      (i) Chronic liver disease
      (j) Chronic illness
      (k) Prolonged physical inactivity
      (l) Chronic malnutrition (insufficient intake)
      (m)Potassium deficiency

B. *Lower glucose levels* (hypoglycemia)
1. Overdose of insulin (most frequent cause)
2. Addison's disease (hypoglycemia is accompanied by elevated potassium and decreased sodium and elevated BUN)
3. Bacterial sepsis
4. Islet cell carcinoma of pancreas (secretes excessive amount of insulin)
5. Hepatic necrosis
6. Hypothyroidism
7. Glycogen storage disease
8. Psychogenic causes

Interfering Factors
1. Steroids, diuretics, and many other drugs
2. Pregnancy (normally a slight elevation in glucose)
3. Anesthesia (sometimes in excess of 200 mg/dl)
4. Overweight
5. Infections of adrenals
6. Stress

Patient Preparation
1. Because FBS is being tested, the patient must fast for 12 hours.
2. Water is permitted.

Patient Aftercare
1. The patient may eat or drink as soon as the blood sample is drawn.
2. Persons with values of 200 mg/dl or greater should be placed on a strict I and O (intake and output).

Clinical Alert

1. A confirmed fasting level (two or more tests) above 140 mg/dl is diagnostic of diabetes mellitus. In this case, a glucose tolerance test should not be done.
2. When the value is greater than 300 mg/dl, there will be an increased urinary output with greater chance of dehydration.
3. When glucose is less than 30 mg/dl or 1 to 7 mmol/L, brain damage is possible.
4. When glucose is greater than 300 mg/dl or 16.7 mmol/L, coma is possible.

2-Hour Postprandial Blood Sugar (2-hr PPBS)

Normal Values
Less than 120 mg/dl or <6.7 mmol/L

Explanation of Test
A *postprandial* test, a test taken *after* a meal, is an excellent screening test for diabetes. Glucose concentration in a fasting blood specimen obtained 2 hours after a meal is rarely elevated in normal persons but is significantly increased in diabetic patients. It is also used to monitor insulin therapy and to confirm diabetes in a patient with a FBS less than 120 mg/dl.

Procedure
1. For best results, the patient should be on a high carbohydrate diet 2 to 3 days before testing.
2. After an overnight fast (water is permitted), the patient eats a high carbohydrate breakfast. The meal should include orange juice, cereal with sugar, toast, and milk.
3. Two hours after the patient finishes eating breakfast, a venous blood sample of 5 ml is obtained.
4. Record the time that breakfast is completed, and notify the laboratory.

Clinical Implications
Values above 140 mg/dl are abnormal. This figure applies only to adults under 50 years of age. The level should be raised to 160 mg/dl for those in their 60s and to as much as 180 mg/dl for people over 60.

A. *Increased levels* occur in many stressful or serious conditions, such as the following:
1. Malnutrition
2. Advanced cirrhosis of liver
3. Cushing's syndrome
4. Acromegaly
5. Hyperthyroidism
6. Pheochromocytoma
7. Lipoproteinemias
8. Myocardial or cerebral infarction
9. Some malignancies
10. Pregnancy
11. Anxiety states

B. *Decreased levels* occur in
1. Anterior pituitary insufficiency
2. Islet cell adenoma
3. Steatorrhea
4. Addison's disease

C. A 2-hour postprandial glucose greater than 200 ml/dl is consistent with a diagnosis of diabetes mellitus.

Interfering Factors
Smoking and/or coffee drinking may raise blood glucose level.

Patient Preparation
1. Instruct the patient about the purpose and procedure of the test. The patient must fast from food overnight, at least 12 hours, and can drink water but no other liquids.
2. The patient should remain at rest during the 2-hour interval.

Patient Aftercare
After the blood sample is drawn, the patient may eat and drink normally.

Clinical Alert

1. Values of 140 to 200 mg/dl indicate decreased tolerance and warrant the use of a glucose tolerance test.
2. Test results are reliable only if the patient is properly prepared.

Glycosylated Hemoglobin (HbA$_{1c}$); Glycohemoglobin (G-Hb); Diabetic Control Index

Normal Values
Results expressed as percent of total hemoglobin.
Normal (nondiabetic): 4.0%–7.0%
Diabetic: >7%

Background
Glycohemoglobin is one of the types of minor hemoglobins found in everyone. Hemoglobin A$_1$ undergoes change or glycosylation to hemoglobin A$_{1a}$, A$_{1b}$, and A$_{1c}$ by a slow, nonenzyme process within the red blood cells during their circulating life span of 120 days. Most simply put, glycohemoglobin is blood glucose bound to hemoglobin. The red cell, as it circulates, combines some of the glucose from the bloodstream with its own content of hemoglobin to form glycohemoglobin in a one-way reaction. The amount of glycosolated hemoglobin found and stored by the erythrocyte depends on the amount of glucose available to it over the 120-day life span of the red blood cell. In diabetes with hyperglycemia, the increase in glycohemoglobin is usually caused by an increase in HbA$_{1c}$. The glucose concentration will increase when hyperglycemia caused by insulin deficiency develops. This glycosylation is irreversible.

Explanation of Test

This test is an index of long-term glucose control. Glycosylated hemoglobin monitoring reflects the average blood sugar level for the 2- to 3-month period before the test. The more glucose the red blood cell is exposed to, the higher the percentage of glycosylated hemoglobin. The test provides information about the success of treatment of diabetes such as adequacy of dietary or insulin therapy, allows determination of duration of hyperglycemia in new cases of juvenile onset diabetes with acute ketoacidosis, provides a sensitive estimate of glucose imbalance in mild cases of diabetes, and is an evaluation of effectiveness of old and new forms of therapy such as oral hypoglycemic agents, single or multiple insulin injections, and B-cell transplantation. Test results are not affected by time of day, meal intake, exercise, just-administered diabetic drugs, emotional stress, or patient cooperation.

The measurement may be of particular value for specific groups of patients. These groups include diabetic children, diabetics in whom the renal threshold for glucose is abnormal, unstable insulin-dependent diabetics in whom blood sugars vary markedly from day to day, patients who do not test urine regularly for glucose, and persons who, before their scheduled appointments, will change their usual habits, dietary or otherwise, so that their metabolic control appears better than it actually is.

Procedure

A venous blood sample of at least 3 ml is obtained.

Clinical Implications

1. Values are increased in poorly controlled and newly diagnosed diabetes. In these instances, HbA$_{1c}$ levels comprise 8% to 12% of the total hemoglobin.
2. With optimal insulin control, the HbA$_{1c}$ levels return toward normal.
3. A diabetic patient who has only recently come under good control may still have a high concentration of glycosylated hemoglobin. This level will decline only gradually as newly formed red blood cells with nearly normal glycosylated hemoglobin replace older red blood cells with high concentrations of glycosylated hemoglobin.
4. Good control: <9.0%
   Fair control: 9.0%–12.0%
   Poor control: >12.0%

Interfering Factors

1. Spurious results should be expected in every case of hemoglobinopathy distinguishable from hemoglobin A by electrophoresis.
2. Decreased value in pregnancy and sickle cell anemia; increased value in thalassemia.

Clinical Alert

Confusion in interpretation of results may occur because there are two tests for determining glycosylated hemoglobin. The most specific test measures hemoglobin A_1, which includes hemoglobin A_{1a}, A_{1b}, and A_{1c}. There are different expected values for each test. Keep in mind that hemoglobin A_1 is always 2% to 4% higher than A_{1c}.

Insulin

Normal Values
Adult: 6–24 μU/ml by radioimmunoassay or 35–145 pmol/L
Newborn: 3–20 μ/U/ml

Background
Insulin, a hormone produced in the pancreas by the beta cells of the islets of Langerhans, regulates the metabolism of carbohydrates along with liver, adipose, muscle, and other target cells and is responsible for maintaining a constant level of blood glucose. The rate of insulin secretion is determined primarily by the level of blood glucose perfusing the pancreas and is also affected by hormonal status, the autonomic nervous system, and nutritional status.

Explanation of Test
This measurement of the insulin secretory response to glucose may be of value in establishing the diagnosis of insulinoma and in the evaluation of abnormal carbohydrate and lipid metabolism. Insulin levels are also helpful in supporting the diagnosis of diabetes in persons with borderline abnormalities of the glucose tolerance procedures. This determination is invaluable in the investigation of fasting hypoglycemic patients and may be useful in the differentiation of islet cell neoplasms.

The insulin study can be ordered in conjunction with the glucose tolerance test or in conjunction with a one-time fasting glucose.

Procedure
1. A fasting blood sample of 4 ml is obtained.
2. If ordered in conjunction with the glucose tolerance test, blood specimens should be obtained before ingesting 100 g of glucose and obtained again at 30, 60, and 120 minutes after glucose ingestion.

Clinical Implications
Increased values are associated with

A. Insulinoma. Diagnosis of insulinoma is based on
   1. Association of hyperinsulinemia with hypoglycemia
   2. Persistent hypoglycemia along with hyperinsulinemia between 2 and 3 hours after injection of tolbutamide
   3. Failure of C-peptide suppression when plasma glucose is 40 mg/dl or less. After 100 g of glucose, normal serum insulin will rise less than 2 μU/ml to 25 to 231 in one-half hour, 18 to 276 in 1 hour, 16 to 166 in 2 hours, and 4 to 38 in 3 hours. The results may be too variable to be of diagnostic usefulness.
B. Acromegaly
C. Cushing's syndrome

Interfering Factors
Falsely increased values are associated with food intake, obesity, and use of oral contraceptives.

Patient Preparation
1. Explain the purpose and procedure of the test.
2. The patient should be fasting overnight unless otherwise directed.
3. Water is permitted.

Standard Oral Glucose Tolerance Test (OGTT)

Normal Values
FBS: <115 mg/dl or <64 mmol/L
90 minutes: <200 mg/dl or <11.1 mmol/L
2 hours: <140 mg/dl or <7.8 mmol/L
3 hours: <125 mg/dl.

All three blood values must be met to be considered normal. All urines are negative for glucose.

Explanation of Test
This timed test of blood and urine is done to rule out diabetes (see box on p. 304) by determining the rate of removal of a concentrated dose of glucose from the bloodstream. In the healthy person, the insulin response to a large oral dose of glucose is almost immediate, peaking in 30 to 60 minutes and returning to normal within 3 hours. In this instance, it can be assumed that sufficient insulin is present to allow glucose to leave the blood and enter the cells of the body.

Testing is usually done in the morning after an overnight fast. The glucose tolerance test is indicated when there is sugar in the urine or when the fasting blood sugar or 2-hour postprandial blood sugar is more than slightly elevated. The glucose tolerance test is more definite than a 2-hour postprandial blood sugar test in diagnosing hypoglyce-

---

**Type 1: Insulin-Dependent
Diabetes Mellitus (IDDM)**

1. Persons who
   (a) Lack insulin
   (b) Have plentiful receptor sites
   (c) Require insulin injections
   (d) Are usually young

**Type 2: Noninsulin-Dependent
Diabetes Mellitus (NIDDM)**

1. Persons who
   (a) Have insulin but whose body cells cannot use it
   (b) Have reduced number of insulin-receptor sites
   (c) Are usually older, obese, and physically inactive
   (d) Require life-style change and possibly oral medication

---

mia and malabsorption syndrome. It is also ordered in a questionable diagnosis of Cushing's syndrome or acromegaly.

Indications for Test
The glucose tolerance test rather than the 2-hour postprandial blood sugar test should be done on certain patients, particularly those with

1. Family history of diabetes
2. Obesity
3. Unexplained episodes of hypoglycemia
4. History of recurrent infections such as boils and abscesses
5. (In women) a history of delivery of large infants, stillbirths, neonatal death, premature labor, and abortions
6. Transitory glycosuria or hyperglycemia in pregnancy, surgery, trauma, stress, myocardial infarction, ACTH administration

Tolerance tests can also be performed for pentose, lactose, galactose, and *D*-xylose (see p. 307).

Procedure
This is a timed test. A 2-hour test is ordered for diabetes detection in men and nonpregnant women; a 3-hour test for pregnant women; and a 5-hour test to evaluate possible hypoglycemia.

1. A diet containing at least 150 g of carbohydrates should be eaten for 3 days before the test.
2. Drugs that may influence the test should be discontinued for 3 days before the test.

(a) Hormones, including oral contraceptives
(b) Salicylates
(c) Diuretic agents
(d) Hypoglycemic agents
3. Insulin or oral hypoglycemics should not be given until after test is completed.
4. A sample of 5 ml of venous blood is drawn after an overnight fast. At least three other blood samples will be obtained (dependent on physician's order and laboratory practice).
5. The patient is given a drink of a very sweet commercial preparation liquid, containing 75 g of glucose. He is encouraged to drink it all quickly. All the solution must be taken.
6. Blood and urine samples are usually obtained at intervals of 30 minutes, 1, 2, and sometimes 3 hours after ingestion of glucose, and are tested for glucose.
7. Inclusion of the fifth hour specimens of both blood and urine is valuable in detecting hypoglycemia.

Clinical Implications
1. In type 2 onset diabetes, the secretion of insulin is delayed, followed by a slightly higher than normal glucose level at 2 hours. Blood glucose is elevated until the 2-hour point.
2. In overt diabetes, there is no secretion of insulin, resulting in above-normal glucose levels throughout the test.
3. In hypoglycemia, the blood glucose is below normal after the 2-hour point and low up to 4 to 5 hours because of high insulin levels.
4. Tolerance tests can also be performed for pentose, lactose, galactose, and D-xylose.
5. Diagnostic criteria of 1979 National Diabetes Data Group
   (a) *Diabetic glucose tolerance test*
       Fasting: <140 mg/dl
       2 hr: >200 mg/dl
       ½, 1, or 1½ hr: >200 mg/dl
   (b) *Gestational diabetes (two or more must be met and exceeded)*
       Fasting: >105 mg/dl
       1 hr: >190 mg/dl
       2 hr: >165 mg/dl
       3 hr: >145 mg/dl
   (c) *Impaired glucose tolerance (IGT) test (all three must be met)*
       Fasting: <140 mg/dl
       2 hr: 140–200 mg/dl
       ½, 1, or 1½ hr: >200 mg/dl
   (d) Glucose values above the normal value concentrations, but below the criteria for diabetes or IGT, should be considered nondiagnostic for these conditions.

Interfering Factors
1. Smoking will increase the glucose level.
2. Inadequate diet (such as weight reducing diet) before testing can diminish carbohydrate tolerance and suggest a false diabetes.
3. Levels tend to increase normally in older persons; the maximum can reach 200 mg/dl.
4. Prolonged administration of oral contraceptives will give significantly higher glucose levels in the second hour or in later blood specimens.
5. Bed rest over a lengthy period of time will influence glucose tolerance. For this reason, the test should be performed on ambulatory patients, not on patients whose condition requires bed rest.
6. Infectious diseases and surgery will affect tolerance. Two weeks of recovery should be allowed before the test.
7. Certain drugs will impair glucose tolerance.

   (a) Insulin   (g) Estrogens
   (b) Oral hypoglycemics   (h) Ferrous ascorbinate
   (c) Large doses of salicylates   (i) Nicotinic acid
   (d) Thiazide diuretics   (j) Phenothiazines
   (e) Oral contraceptives   (k) Lithium
   (f) Corticosteroids   (l) Metapyrone

   These drugs should be discontinued, if possible, for at least 3 days before the test.
8. If the patient vomits the glucose solution, the test is invalid and has to be repeated after 3 days.

Patient Preparation
1. Instruct the patient about the purpose and procedure of the test and leave him a written reminder.
   (a) Stress a normal diet with high carbohydrates (150 g) for 3 days preceding the test.
   (b) Fasting is required for at least 12 hours before the test and for not more than 16 hours.
   (c) Water is permitted and encouraged.
2. Determine the patient's weight and record it.
3. Collect urine and blood specimens and test for glucose, recording exact time of collection. Have the patient empty his or her bladder for each specimen.
   (a) No liquids can be taken other than water.
   (b) No food is to be eaten during the test periods.
   (c) No alcohol should be taken the previous evening.
   (d) Encourage the patient to stay in bed or rest quietly during the test period. Weakness or feeling faint may occur during the test, and exercise also changes glucose results.

(e) No smoking is allowed during the test.

(f) Coffee and unusual physical exercise should be avoided for at least 8 hours before the test.

Patient Aftercare

1. The patient may eat and drink normally as soon as the test is over.
2. Administer insulin or oral hypoglycemics to diabetics as soon as the test is completed.

Clinical Alert

1. This test is contraindicated in patients who have had a recent history of surgery, myocardial infarction, or labor and delivery, for these conditions can cause erroneous results (altered carbohydrate tolerance).
2. Record and report any reactions during the test. Weakness, faintness, and sweating may occur between the second and third hours. If this occurs, a blood sample for sugar is drawn immediately, and the test is discontinued.
3. The test should be postponed in the event of unexpected illness such as fever or gastritis or if there has been ingestion of food within 8 hours.
4. If the fasting blood sugar is over 200, the glucose tolerance test is usually not done. If it is done, the patient should be monitored very carefully for severe reaction or even coma.

Lactose Tolerance

Normal Values

A rise in glucose greater than 20-mg/dl and no abdominal symptoms such as pain or diarrhea

Explanation of Test

This is a glucose tolerance test to diagnose intestinal disaccharidase (lactase) deficiency.

Procedure

1. Follow instructions for the glucose tolerance test.
2. A fasting specimen is obtained and the patient is given 100 g of lactose in 200 ml of water.
3. Blood samples are drawn at 15, 30, 60, and 120 minutes for glucose.

Clinical Implications

A "flat" lactose tolerance finding is suspicious of a deficiency. However, this test should be followed by a monosaccharide tolerance test such as glucose galactose tolerance test.

END PRODUCTS OF METABOLISM AND OTHER TESTS
Ammonia

Normal Values

Adult: 15–45 μgN/dl or 11–32 μmol/L
Newborn: 90–150 μgN/dl or 64–107 μmol/L

There is a great deal of variation in reported values because of methods used.

Background

Ammonia, one of the end products of protein metabolism, is formed from the action of bacteria on proteins in the intestines and from hydrolysis of glutamine in the kidneys. The liver normally removes most of the ammonia from the portal vein blood flow and converts ammonia to urea. Because any appreciable level of ammonia in the blood would affect acid–base balance and brain function, an adequate mechanism for its removal is essential. The liver accomplishes this by synthesis of urea for excretion by the kidney.

Explanation of Test

Measurement of blood ammonia levels is used to evaluate metabolism as well as the progress of severe liver disease and response to treatment.

Procedure

1. A fasting venous blood sample of 3 ml is obtained.
2. The sample is placed in an iced container, and the test must be performed within 20 minutes.
3. The laboratory should be notified of all antibiotics the patient is receiving because of the possibility of these drugs lowering ammonia levels.

Clinical Implications

Increased ammonia levels occur in

1. Liver disease
2. Hepatic coma due to
   (a) Cirrhosis
   (b) Severe hepatitis
3. Severe heart failure
4. Azotemia
5. Cor pulmonale
6. Hemolytic disease of the newborn
7. Pulmonary emphysema

8. Acute bronchitis
9. Pericarditis

10. Myelocytic and lymphatic leukemia
11. Reye's syndrome

Patient Preparation
1. Instruct the patient to fast for 8 hours before the blood test.
2. Water is permitted.

Interfering Factors
1. Ammonia levels vary with protein intake.
2. Exercise may cause an increase in ammonia levels.
3. There are many drugs that may affect blood ammonia levels.

Clinical Alert

In patients with impaired liver function demonstrated by elevated ammonia levels, the blood level can be lowered by reduced protein intake and by use of antibiotics to reduce intestinal bacteria counts.

Bilirubin

Normal Values
Total bilirubin: 0.2–1.0 mg/dl or 3.4–17.1 μmol/L
Conjugated: 0.0–0.2 mg/dl or 0.0–3.4 μmol/L
Indirect unconjugated: 0.2–0.8 mg/dl or 3.4–13.68 μmol/L
Newborn: 1.5–12.0 mg/dl or 26–205 μmol/L

Background
Bilirubin, resulting from the breakdown of hemoglobin in the red blood cells, is a by-product of hemolyis (red blood cell destruction). It is produced by the reticuloendothelial system. Removed from the body by the liver, which excretes it into the bile, it gives the bile its major pigmentation.

Usually a small amount of bilirubin is found in the serum. A rise in serum levels will occur if there is an excessive destruction of red blood cells or if the liver is unable to excrete the normal amounts of bilirubin produced.

There are two forms of bilirubin in the body: (1) indirect or unconjugated bilirubin (which is protein bound), and (2) direct or conjugated bilirubin that circulates freely in the blood until it reaches the liver, where it is conjugated with glucuronide transferase and then excreted into the bile. An increase in protein-bound bilirubin (unconjugated bilirubin) is more frequently associated with increased destruction of red blood cells (hemolysis); an increase in free-flowing bilirubin is more likely seen in dysfunction or blockage of the liver.

A routine examination measures only the total bilirubin. A normal level of total bilirubin rules out any significant impairment of the excretory function of the liver or excessive hemolysis of red cells. Only when the levels are elevated will there be a call for differentiation of the bilirubin according to the conjugated and unconjugated levels.

Jaundice/Icterus

Excessive amounts of bilirubin eventually seep into the tissues, which then assume a yellow hue. The yellow color is a clinical sign of jaundice. In newborns, signs of jaundice may indicate hemolytic anemia or congenital icterus. If the bilirubin levels reach a critical point in the infant, damage to the central nervous system may occur in a condition known as *kernicterus*. Therefore, in these infants, it is the level of bilirubin that is the deciding factor in the decision to do an exchange transfusion.

Explanation of Test

The measurement of bilirubin is important in evaluating liver function, hemolytic anemias, and hyperbilirubinemia (in newborns).

Procedure

1. A venous sample of 5 ml is obtained before the patient eats breakfast.
2. The sample must be protected from ultraviolet light.
3. Air bubbles and unnecessary shaking of the sample are to be avoided while blood is collected.
4. If the specimen cannot be examined immediately, then it should be stored in a refrigerator and in darkness.
5. In infants, blood must be collected from a heel puncture. Two full micro blood sampling tubes are collected. (In newborns, the sample size is 0.3 ml.)

Clinical Implications

A. *Bilirubin elevations accompanied by jaundice* may be due to hepatic, obstructive, or hemolytic causes.
   1. *Hepatocellular jaundice* results from injury or disease of the parenchymal cells of the liver and can be caused by
      (a) Viral hepatitis
      (b) Cirrhosis
      (c) Infectious mononucleosis
      (d) Reactions of certain drugs such as chlorpromazine
   2. *Obstructive jaundice* is usually the result of obstruction of the common bile or hepatic ducts due to stones or neoplasms. The obstruction produces high conjugated bilirubin levels due to bile regurgitation.
   3. *Hemolytic jaundice* is due to overproduction of bilirubin result-

ing from hemolytic processes that produce high levels of unconjugated bilirubin. Hemolytic jaundice can be found in

    (a) Hemolytic disease of the newborn (erythroblastosis fetalis)

        (1) Rh incompatibility

        (2) **ABO** incompatibility (less severe hemolytic anemia)

    (b) Pernicious anemia

    (c) Sickle cell anemia

    (d) Transfusion reactions

    (e) Crigler–Najjar syndrome (a severe disease that results from a genetic deficiency of a hepatic enzyme needed for the conjugation of bilirubin)

B. *Elevated* **nonconjugate** *bilirubin levels* occur in

  1. Hemolytic anemias

  2. Trauma in the presence of a large hematoma

  3. Hemorrhagic pulmonary infarcts

  4. Crigler–Najjar syndrome (rare)

  5. Gilbert's disease (rare)

C. *Elevated* **conjugate** *bilirubin levels* occur in

  1. Cancer of the head of the pancreas

  2. Choledocholithiasis

  3. Dubin–Johnson syndrome

D. *Elevated* **conjugate and nonconjugate** *levels (with the conjugate levels more elevated)* occur in

  1. Hepatic metastasis   4. Cholestasis secondary to drugs

  2. Hepatitis   5. Cirrhosis

  3. Lymphoma

Interfering Factors

1. A 1-hour exposure of the specimen to sunlight or high-intensity artificial light at room temperature will decrease the bilirubin content.

2. Contrast media 24 hours before measurement may cause an altered reaction.

3. A high-fat meal may cause decreased bilirubin levels by interfering with the clinical reactions.

4. Air bubbles and shaking of the specimen may cause decreased levels.

5. Foods (carrots, yams) and drugs increase the yellow hue in the serum.

Clinical Alert

In newborns, if total bilirubin approaches 16 mg/dl, aggressive treatment has to be initiated immediately (exchange transfusion) or mental retardation will result.

Blood Urea Nitrogen (BUN)

Normal Values
Adult: 7–18 mg/dl or 2.5–6.4 mmol/L
Child: 5–18 mg/dl or 1.8–6.4 mmol/L

Explanation of Test
Urea is formed in the liver and constitutes the major nonprotein nitrogenous end product of protein catabolism. The urea is then carried to the kidneys by the blood to be excreted in the urine.

The test for BUN, measuring the nitrogen portion of urea, is used as a gross index of glomerular function and the production and excretion of urea. Rapid protein catabolism and impairment of kidney function will result in an elevated BUN. The rate at which the BUN rises is influenced by the degree of tissue necrosis, protein catabolism, and the rate at which the kidneys excrete the urea nitrogen.

The BUN is less sensitive than creatinine clearance tests and may not be abnormal until the creatinine clearance is moderately abnormal.

Procedure
A venous blood sample of at least 5 ml is obtained. The amount drawn depends on the method and type of equipment used.

Clinical Implications
A. *Increased BUN levels (azotemia)*
   1. The most common cause of increased BUN level is inadequate excretion due to kidney disease or urinary obstruction, frequently occurring in cases of prostate enlargement.
      (a) An increased BUN of 50 to 150 mg/100 ml indicates serious impairment of renal function.
      (b) An increased BUN of 150 to 250 mg/100 ml is definitive for severely impaired renal failure.
   2. *Increased BUN levels* are associated with
      (a) Impaired renal function
      (b) Shock
      (c) Dehydration
      (d) Gastrointestinal hemorrhage
      (e) Infection
      (f) Diabetes
      (g) Some malignancies
      (h) Acute myocardial infarction
      (i) Chronic gout
      (j) Excessive protein intake or protein catabolism

      Increases of 50 mg/100 ml/day in the BUN have occurred in previously healthy people who have undergone *severe crushing injuries* or are suffering from *overwhelming infection*.
B. *Decreased BUN levels* are associated with
      (a) Liver failure

(b) Negative nitrogen balance, as may occur in malnutrition, excessive use of intravenous fluids, and physiologic hydremia of pregnancy
(c) Impaired absorption as in celiac disease
(d) Nephrotic syndrome (occasionally)
(e) Overhydration (excessive intravenous fluids)
   A further decreased BUN of 6 to 10 mg/100 ml is possible in overhydration.
(f) Pregnancy

Interfering Factors
1. A combination of a low protein and a high carbohydrate diet can cause a decreased BUN level.
2. The BUN is normally lower in children and women because they have a smaller muscle mass than adult men.
3. Increased BUN values normally occur in late pregnancy and infancy because of increased use of protein.
4. Older persons may have an increased BUN when their kidneys are not able to concentrate urine adequately.
5. Decreased BUN values may occur normally earlier in pregnancy because of physiologic hydremia.
6. Many drugs may cause increased and decreased BUN levels.

Clinical Alert

1. If a patient is confused, disoriented, or has convulsions, the BUN should be checked. If the level is high, it may help to explain these signs and symptoms.
2. In patients with an elevated BUN, fluid and electrolyte regulation may be impaired.
3. Excessive intravenous fluids can result in lowered BUN levels.
4. Panic value of BUN is greater than 100 mg/dl.

Cholinesterase RBC (Pseudocholinesterase)

Normal Values
0.5–1.5 mg/dl
8–18 U/ml
8–18 kU/L

Values vary with substrate and method.

Explanation of Test
The primary use of the measurement of serum cholinesterase (CHS) is to monitor the effect of muscle relaxants such as succinylcholine that are used in surgery. Patients for whom suxamethonium anesthesia is planned should be tested for the presence of atypical cholinesterase variants, which are incapable of hydrolyzing this widely used muscle relaxant. It is also used when poisoning by pesticides such as parathion or malathion is suspected. Severe insecticide poisoning causes headaches, visual distortions, nausea, vomiting, pulmonary edema, confusion, convulsions, respiratory paralysis, and coma.

Clinical Implications
Patients who are homozygous for the atypical gene that controls serum cholinesterase activity have low levels of cholinesterase that are not inhibited by dibucaine. Those persons with normal serum cholinesterase activity show 70% to 90% inhibition by dibucaine.

1. Low or absent levels are associated with
   (a) Persons who will not be able to hydrolyze drugs such as muscle relaxants in surgery. These patients may have a prolonged period of apnea if they are given succinylcholine.
   (b) Poisoning from organic phosphate insecticides
   (c) Parenchymatous liver diseases
      (1) Hepatitis
      (2) Cirrhosis with jaundice
   (d) Conditions that may have decreased blood albumin, such as malnutrition, anemia, infections, skin diseases, and acute myocardial infarction.

Clinical Alert

In industrial exposure, workers should not return to work until values rise to 75% of normal. Red blood cell cholinesterase regenerates at the rate of 1% per day. Plasma cholinesterase regenerates at the rate of 25% in 7 to 10 days.

Creatinine

Normal Values
Adult: 0.6–1.2 mg/dl or 53–106 μmol/L
Child: 0.3–0.7 mg/dl or 27–62 μmol/L

Explanation of Test

Creatinine is a by-product in the breakdown of muscle creatine phosphate resulting from energy metabolism. It is produced at a constant rate depending on the muscle mass of the person and is removed from the body by the kidneys. Production of creatinine is constant as long as muscle mass remains constant. A disorder of kidney function reduces excretion of creatinine, resulting in increased levels of blood creatinine.

The test is used to diagnose impaired renal function. It is a more specific and sensitive indicator of kidney disease than BUN, although in chronic renal disease, BUN correlates more accurately with symptoms of uremia than does the blood creatinine.

Procedure

A venous blood sample of 5 ml is obtained.

Clinical Implications

A. *Increased creatinine levels* occur in

1. Impaired renal function
2. Chronic nephritis
3. Obstruction of the urinary tract
4. Muscle disease
   (a) Gigantism
   (b) Acromegaly
   (c) Myasthenia gravis
5. Muscular dystrophy
6. Poliomyelitis
7. Diabetic acidosis
8. Starvation
9. Hyperthyroidism

Interfering Factors

1. High levels of ascorbic acid can cause a falsely increased level.
2. Drugs that influence kidney function plus other medications can cause a change in the blood creatinine.
3. A diet high in meat will cause increased levels.

Clinical Alert

1. A normal blood serum creatinine does not always indicate unimpaired renal function. A normal value cannot be used as a standard for a patient who is known to have existing renal disease.
2. Panic value is 10 mg/dl in nondialysis patients.
3. Creatinine should always be checked before giving nephrotoxic chemotherapeutics such as
   (a) Methotrexate
   (b) Cisplatin
   (c) Cytoxan
   (d) Mithramycin
   (e) Semustine

Sweat Test

Normal Values
Sweat Sodium Normals
Normal: 10–40 mmol/L or mEq/L
Cystic fibrosis: >70 mmol/L or mEq/L
Sweat Chloride Normals
Normal: 0–35 mmol/L
Cystic fibrosis: 60–200 mmol/L

Explanation of Test
This test has become the cornerstone of diagnosis for cystic fibrosis when the outcome is taken in conjunction with clinical, radiological, and stool tests. It is known that persistent, abnormally high concentrations of sodium and chloride appear in the secretions of eccrine sweat glands in cystic fibrosis. The abnormality is present at birth and persists throughout life. This study is based on techniques inducing sweating that is stimulated by pilocarpine iontophoresis, followed by chemical analysis to determine sodium and chloride content.

Interfering Factors
1. The sweat test does not retain its value after puberty because levels may vary over a very wide range.
2. Dehydration and edema, particularly of areas where sweat is collected, may interfere with test results.

Procedure
1. The forearm is the preferred site for stimulation of sweating, but in thin or small babies the thigh or back may be a better area to use. It may be necessary to stimulate sweating in two places to obtain enough sweat, especially in young infants. At least 100 μL of sweat is necessary. In cold weather or if the room is cold, a warm covering should be placed over the arm or site of sweat collection.
2. Sweat is produced by transporting positive pilocarpine ions into the skin. This is commonly achieved by applying gauze pads or filter paper saturated with a measured amount of pilocarpine to the skin and attaching electrodes through which a current of 4 to 5 milliamperes is delivered at intervals for a total of 5 minutes.
3. The electrodes and pad are removed, and the area is thoroughly washed with distilled water and carefully dried.
4. Successful iontophoresis is indicated by a red area about an inch in diameter that appears where the electrode was placed.
5. The skin is scrubbed thoroughly with distilled water and dried carefully. The area for sweat collection must be completely dry, free from contamination by powder or antiseptic, and the skin must be free of any area that might ooze.

6. Collection of sweat can occur by applying preweighed filter or sweat collection cups that are taped securely over the red spot. The inside surfaces of the collecting device should never be touched.
7. The paper is left on for at least 1 hour before removal and is then placed on a preweighed flask to avoid evaporation. The flask is again weighed.
8. If the cup is used, it is left on for 1 hour and then carefully removed by scraping it across the iontophoresed area. This "puddles" the sweat in the cup to reduce evaporation and to redissolve any salts left by the evaporation. Suction capillary tubes are used to take sweat out of the collection cups.

Clinical Implications

1. Children with cystic fibrosis will have sodium and chloride values above 60 mEq/L (mmol/L).
2. Borderline or gray-zone cases are those with values between 40 and 60 mEq/L for both sodium and chloride and require retesting. Potassium values do not assist in differentiating these borderline cases.
3. In adolescence and adulthood, levels over 100 mEq/L usually indicate cystic fibrosis.
4. Elevated sweat electrolytes can be associated with
   (a) Addison's disease
   (b) Congenital adrenal hyperplasia
   (c) Ectodermal dysplasia with hypoparathyroidism with sensorineural deafness
   (d) Pitressin-resistant diabetes insipidus
   (e) Glucose-6-phosphatase deficiency
   (f) Fucosidosis
   (g) Nephrotic syndrome

Clinical Alert

1. The test should always be repeated if the result, the clinical features, and the stool microscopy do not fit together.
2. The test can be used to exclude the diagnosis of cystic fibrosis in siblings of diagnosed patients.
3. There have been reports of cystic fibrosis patients with normal sweat electrolyte levels.

Patient Preparation

1. Explain the purpose and procedure of the test.
2. Inform the patient that a slight stinging sensation is usually experienced, especially in fair-skinned persons.

Uric Acid

Normal Values
Men: 3.5–7.2 mg/dl or 0.21–0.42 mmol/L
Women: 2.6–6.0 mg/dl or 0.154–0.35 mmol/L
Children: 2.0–5.5 mg/dl or 0.12–0.32 mmol/L

Explanation of Test
Uric acid is formed from the breakdown of nucleonic acids and is an end product of purine metabolism. In humans, a lack of the enzyme uricase allows this poorly soluble substance to accumulate in body fluids. Two thirds of the uric acid produced daily is excreted by the kidneys, whereas the remaining one third exits by the stool. The basis for this test is that an overproduction of uric acids occurs in conditions in which there is excessive cell breakdown and catabolism of nucleonic acids (as in gout), excessive production and destruction of cells (as in leukemia), or an inability to excrete the substance produced (as in renal failure).

Measurement of uric acid is used most commonly in the evaluation of renal failure, gout, and leukemia. In hospitalized patients, renal failure is the most common cause of elevated uric acid levels, and gout is the least common cause. This test is also valuable in assessing the prognosis of eclampsia because of the uric acid level's ability to reflect the extent of liver damage in toxemia of pregnancy.

Procedure
A venous blood sample of 5 ml is obtained.

Clinical Implications
A. *Elevated levels* (hyperuricemia)
1. Increased levels of blood uric acid are associated with nitrogen retention and with increases in urea, creatinine, and other non-protein nitrogenous substances of the blood. These findings are usually interpreted as another indication of decreased *kidney function* (renal failure).
2. Increased levels are found in *gout,* but the increase may be slight in the early stages of the disease. The amount of increase is not directly related to the severity of the disease.
3. Other conditions associated with elevated uric acid levels
   (a) Leukemia
   (b) Acute stages of infectious diseases such as infectious mononucleosis
   (c) Lymphomas
   (d) Metastatic cancer
   (e) Severe eclampsia
   (f) Starvation
   (g) Shock
   (h) Alcoholism
   (i) Chemotherapy for cancer
   (j) Violent exercise
   (k) Multiple myeloma

(l) Metabolic acidosis
(m) Diabetic ketosis (ketoaci-
    dosis)

(n) Lead poisoning
(o) Polycythemia
(p) Hemaglobinopathies

B. *Decreased levels*
  1. Uric acid level should fall in patients who are treated with uri-
     cosuric drugs such as allopurinol, probenecid, and sulfinpyra-
     zone.
  2. Fanconi syndrome
  3. Nepolastic disease
  4. Wilson's disease

Interfering Factors
1. Stress will cause increased levels.
2. Some drugs may cause an increase or a decrease in uric acid blood
   levels.

HORMONE TESTS

Androstanedione

Normal Values
Premenopausal women: 0.6–3 μg/ml

Background
Androstanedione is one of the major androgens produced in women by
the ovaries, and to a lesser extent in the adrenals. This hormone is
converted to estrogens by hepatic enzymes.

Explanation of Test
This hormone measurement is helpful in the evaluation of conditions
characterized by hirsutism and possible excessive ovarian androgen
production.

Procedure
1. A venous blood sample of 5 ml is obtained in the morning.
2. This specimen should be collected 1 week before or after the menstrual period.
3. Record data of the last menstrual period on the laboratory form.

Clinical Implications
Increased values are associated with

1. Stein–Leventhal syndrome
2. Cushing's syndrome
3. Certain ovarian tumors
4. Ectopic ACTH-producing
   tumor

5. Late-onset congenitive adrenal hyperplasia
6. Ovarian stromal hyperplasia

Aldosterone

Normal Values
Plasma is taken with the patient in an upright position for 4 hours and
with unrestricted salt intake
Women: 5–30 ng/dl or 0.14–0.83 nmol/L
Men: 6–22 ng/dl or 0.17–0.61 nmol/L
Two to three times higher in pregnancy
Urine: >35–80 μg/day or > 97–222 mmol/day

Background
This hormone, which is derived from cholesterol, is the most potent of
the mineralocorticoids. Its foremost physiologic effect is that of regulating the transport of ions across cell membranes, particularly those of
the renal tubes. This hormone causes the retention of sodium and chloride and the elimination of potassium and hydrogen. The second major
effect is the maintenance of blood pressure and blood value. Minute
quantities will depress the urinary and salivary sodium-to-potassium
ratio primarily because of decreased sodium excretion.

The three main factors that apparently affect aldosterone levels
include the renin–angiotensin system, the plasma–potassium concentration, and adrenocorticotropic hormone. The renin–angiotensin system appears to be the major mechanism that controls extracellular
fluid by regulation of aldosterone secretion. Potassium loading results
in increased aldosterone levels, whereas a potassium-deficient diet in
the presence of aldosterone excess will result in a lowered aldosterone
level. Increased concentrations of potassium in the blood plasma directly stimulate adrenal production of the hormone. The ACTH may
affect aldosterone production in conditions of acute stress, burns, hemorrhage, and other pathologic conditions. Under physiologic conditions, ACTH seems to have little effect on aldosterone production.

Procedure
1. A venous blood specimen of 10 ml in heparin or EDTA is obtained.
   The cells must be separated from plasma immediately. The specimen should be obtained in the morning after the patient has been
   upright for at least 4 hours.
2. Specify and record the source of the specimen, such as from a peripheral vein, and so forth.
3. A 24-hour urine specimen is obtained.
4. It is recommended that urine be refrigerated during collection.

Explanation of Test
This test is useful in detecting primary or secondary aldosteronism.
Patients with primary aldosteronism characteristically have hyperten-

sion, muscular pains and cramps, weakness, tetany, paralysis, and polyuria.

Clinical Implications

1. *Elevated levels occur in primary aldosteronism,* as in
   - (a) Aldosterone-producing adenoma
   - (b) Adrenal cortical hyperplasia
   - (c) Indeterminate hyperaldosteronism
   - (d) Glucocorticoid remediable hyperaldosteronism
2. *Elevated levels also occur in secondary aldosteronism* when aldosterone output is elevated due to external stimuli or because of greater activity in the renin–angiotensin system, as in
   - (a) Salt depletion
   - (b) Potassium loading
   - (c) Large doses of ACTH
   - (d) Cardiac failure
   - (e) Cirrhosis of liver with ascites
   - (f) Nephrotic syndrome
   - (g) Bartter's syndrome
   - (h) Postsurgical syndrome
   - (i) Hypovolemia and hemorrhage

Interfering Factors

Values are increased in pregnancy and by posture.

Patient Preparation

1. Explain the purpose and procedure of the test.
2. Diuretic agents, progestational agents, estrogens, and licorice should be discontinued for 2 weeks before the test.
3. The patient's diet for 2 weeks before the test should be normal and include 3 g of sodium per day.
4. Check with your laboratory for special protocols.

Antidiuretic Hormone (ADH)

Normal Values

1–5 pg/ml or < 1.5 mg/L

Background

The ADH is excreted by the posterior pituitary gland. When ADH activity is present, small volumes of concentrated urine are excreted. When ADH is absent, large amounts of diluted urine are produced.

Explanation of Test

This measurement of the level of ADH is useful in the differential diagnosis of polyuric and hyponatremic states.

Inappropriate secretion of ADH is associated with a number of abnormal findings: decreased blood sodium and chloride associated with normal blood potassium, carbon dioxide, and urea nitrogen; decreased blood osmolality; increased urine osmolality; increased ratio of urine to blood osmolality; and increased urine sodium. It will respond to water restriction but not to administration of isotonic or hypertonic saline.

Procedure
Venous blood samples are drawn into three specimen tubes that are immediately chilled.

Clinical Implications
Increased secretion of ADH is associated with

1. Acute intermittent porphyria
2. Brain tumor
3. Pneumonia
4. Pulmonary tuberculosis
5. Systemic neoplasms

Chorionic Gonadotropin, Human Chorionic Gonadotropin (HCG)

Normal Values
Men and nonpregnant women: 3 IU/L or mU/ml

Explanation of Test
This test is used as a marker in the diagnosis of testicular and trophoblastic tumors. Serial monitoring is used to follow tumor response to surgery and chemotherapy. In this test, which uses antibodies specific to the beta subunit of HCG, luteinizing hormone (LH) can be differentiated from HCG.

Procedure
A venous blood sample of 5 ml is obtained.

Interfering Factors
1. Lipemia
2. Hemolysis

Clinical Implications
1. Values below normal will be seen in threatened abortion and ectopic pregnancy.
2. *Increased values* are associated with
   (a) Hydatidiform mole
   (b) Choriocarcinoma
   (c) Seminoma
   (d) Ovarian and testicular teratomas
   (e) Multiple pregnancy
   (f) Neoplasms of stomach, pancreas, lung, colon, and liver

Cortisol (Hydrocortisone)

Normal Values
8:00 AM: 5–23 μg/dl or 138–635 μmol/L
4:00 PM: 3–15 μg/dl or 83–414 μmol/L

Background
Cortisol, compound F, is a glucocorticosteroid of the adrenal cortex and affects metabolism of proteins, carbohydrates, and lipids. Cortisol (hydrocortisone) is the most potent of the glucocorticoids and inhibits the effect of insulin. Cortisol stimulates glucogenesis by the liver and decreases the rate of glucose use by the cells. In the healthy person, the secretion rate of cortisol is higher in the early morning (6–8 AM) and lower in the evening (4–6 PM). This variation is lost in patients with Cushing's syndrome and in persons under stress.

Explanation of Test
This is a test of adrenal hormone function. Cortisol is elevated in adrenal hyperfunction and decreased in adrenal hypofunction.

Procedure
Venous blood samples of 5 ml are obtained in the morning and evening.

Clinical Implications
Extreme elevation in the morning and no variation later in the day suggest carcinoma.

A. *Decreased levels* are expected in
   1. Liver disease
   2. Addison's disease
   3. Anterior pituitary hyposecretion
   4. Hypothyroidism
   5. Therapy with dexamethasone, prednisone, and prednisolone (steroids)
B. *Increased levels* are found in
   1. Hyperthyroidism
   2. Stress (trauma, surgery)
   3. Obesity
   4. Cushing's syndrome (high upon rising but no variation later in the day)

Interfering Factors
1. Pregnancy will cause an increased value.
2. There is no normal diurnal variation in patients under stress.
3. Drugs such as spironolactone and oral contraceptives will give falsely elevated values.

Cortisol Suppression
(Dexamethasone Suppression) (DST)

Normal Values
8:00 AM: 6–26μg/dl
4:00 PM: 2–18μg/dl
Morning following administration of dexamethasone: 5 μg/dl

Explanation of Test
This study is a screening test for Cushing's syndrome and to identify depressed persons who are likely to respond to antidepressants or electroshock therapy. It is based on the fact that ACTH production will be suppressed in normal persons after a low dose of dexamethasone, whereas it is not in Cushing's syndrome or in some depressed persons.

Procedure
1. Venous blood samples will be obtained the day following administration of dexamethasone.
2. Late in the afternoon or at bedtime, dexamethasone tablets are administered by mouth. The dosage varies according to weight.

Interfering Factors
False positive tests may occur in

1. Pregnancy
2. High doses of estrogens
3. Anorexia nervosa
4. Uncontrolled diabetes
5. Trauma
6. Fever
7. Dehydration
8. Acute withdrawal from alcohol

Clinical Implications
No diurnal variation or suppression will occur

1. In Cushing's syndrome
2. In conditions of high stress
3. In depressed persons who are most likely to respond to somatic intervention
4. In patients who fail to take dexamethasone
5. If Dilantin has been administered

Patient Preparation
1. Explain the purpose and procedure of the test.
2. All medications should be discontinued for 24 to 48 hours before the study. Especially important are aldactone, estrogens, birth control pills, cortisol, tetracyclines, stilbestrol, and Dilantin.
3. Weigh the patient and record his or her weight.

Cortisol Stimulation (Cortrosyn Stimulation)

Normal Values
Rise: >7 ng/dl
Peak: >20 ng/dl

Explanation of Test
This study is a good test to detect adrenal insufficiency. Cortrosyn is a synthetic subunit of ACTH that exhibits the full corticosteroid stimulating effect of ACTH in normal persons. Failure to respond is an indication of adrenal insufficiency.

Procedure
1. A fasting venous blood sample of 4 ml is obtained.
2. Cortrosyn is administered intramuscularly.
3. Additional blood specimens of 4 ml are obtained 30 and 60 minutes after administration of Cortrosyn.

Clinical Implications
Absent or blunted response occurs in

1. Adrenal insufficiency
2. Hypopituitarism
3. Prolonged steroid administration

Gastrin

Normal Values
Adult: <60 yr—<100 pg/ml or 100 ng/L
　　　≥60 yr—increases related to decline in production of acid
Child: 10–125 pg/ml or ng/L

Background
Gastrin is a hormone secreted by the mucosa of the pylorus of the stomach. The gastrin is absorbed into the blood and returned to the stomach, where it stimulates the secretion of gastric acid. Excessive production of gastrin, then, can result in hypersecretion of gastric acid. Hydrochloric acid, one of the gastric secretions, in turn inhibits the secretion of gastrin.

Explanation of Test
Although elevated levels of gastrin are found in disorders such as pernicious anemia, measurement of serum gastrin is generally used to diagnose a stomach disorder.

Procedure
A fasting venous blood sample of at least 5 ml is obtained.

Interfering Factors
Values will be falsely increased in nonfasting patients, diabetics taking insulin, and after gastroscopy.

Clinical Implications
Increased gastrin levels are found in

1. Stomach cancer because of significant reduction of gastric acid secretion
2. Gastric and duodenal ulcers
3. Zollinger–Ellison syndrome
4. Pernicious anemia (low secretion of hydrochloric acid results in elevated gastrin levels)
5. End-stage renal disease (gastrin is metabolized by the kidneys)
6. Elderly patients, because of reduced secretion of hydrochloric acid

Patient Preparation
1. The patient should be in a fasting state for 12 hours preceding the test.
2. Water is permitted.

Growth Hormone (hGH)

Normal Values
Men: <5 ng/ml or <5 µg/L
Women: <10 ng/ml or <10 µg/L
Children: 0–10 ng/ml or 0–10 µg/L
Newborn: 10–40 ng/ml or µg/L

Background
Growth hormone or somatotrophin is essential to the growth process and has an important role in the everyday metabolism of adults. It is released by the pituitary gland secondary to certain stimuli, exercise, deep sleep, hypoglycemia, and ingestion of protein. It also stimulates the production of RNA, mobilizes fatty acids from fat deposits, and is intimately connected with insulinism. If the pituitary gland secretes too little or too much in the growth phase of life, dwarfism or giantism will result. An excess of growth hormone during adulthood leads to acromegaly.

Explanation of Test
The test is used to confirm hypo- or hyperpituitarism so that therapy can be instituted as soon as possible. Challenge or stimulation tests are generally used to detect growth hormone deficiency.

Clinical Implication
1. Levels will rise 15 times normal by the second day of starvation. Levels will also rise after 2 hours of sleep.
2. Increased levels are associated with giantism and acromegaly.
3. Decreased levels are associated with dwarfism.
4. Following challenge testing to establish a pattern, the appropriate response is debatable. A response equal to or greater than 7 ng/ml is clearly normal. Also, the suppression of growth hormone levels of 0 to 3 ng/ml in 30 minutes to 2 hours following the ingestion of 100 g of glucose is considered a normal response in adults. In children, a rebound-stimulation effect may be seen from 2 to 5 hours following administration of glucose.

Interfering Factors
1. *Increased levels* are associated with the use of oral contraceptives and estrogens.
2. *Decreased levels* are associated with obesity and the use of corticosteroids.

Procedure
1. A fasting venous blood sample of at least 5 ml is obtained.
2. Check with your laboratory for specific challenge protocols for stimulation tests such as insulin-induced hypoglycemia, arginine transfusion, glucagon infusion, L-dopa, and propanolol with exercise.

Patient Preparation
1. Explain the purpose and procedure of the test.
2. Advise the patient to fast from food for 8 to 10 hours. For true baseline levels to be obtained, the patient should be free of stress and at complete rest in a quiet environment for at least 30 minutes before specimen collection. Water is permitted.

Prolactin (HPRL)

Normal Values
Nonpregnant women: 5–40 ng/ml or ug/L
Pregnant women: <400 ng/ml or ug/L by third trimester
Men: <20 ng/ml or ug/L

Background
Prolactin is a pituitary hormone essential for initiating and maintaining lactation. The sex difference in prolactin does not occur until puberty, when increased estrogen production results in higher prolactin levels in women. Circadian changes in prolactin concentration in

adults are marked by episodic fluctuation and a sleep-induced peak in the early morning hours.

Explanation of Test
This test may be helpful in the diagnosis, management, and follow-up of a prolactin-secreting tumor in persons who have secondary amenorrhea or galactorrhea with hyperprolactinemia and infertility. It is also useful in the management of hypothalamic disease and to monitor surgery, chemotherapy, and radiation treatment of prolactin-secreting tumors.

Procedure
A 12-hour fasting venous blood sample of at least 5 ml is obtained. Specimens should be drawn in the morning.

Clinical Implications
Increased values are associated with

1. Galactorrhea and/or amenorrhea
2. Diseases of the hypothalamus and pituitary stalk
3. Prolactin-secreting pituitary tumors
4. Acromegaly
5. Ectopic production of malignant tumors
6. Hypothyroidism
7. Renal failure
8. Anorexia nervosa

Interfering Factors
1. Increased values are associated with newborns, pregnancy, postpartum period, stress, exercise, sleep, nipple stimulation and lactation.
2. Drugs may increase values (estrogens, methyldopa, tricyclic antidepressants, phenothiazines, antihypertensives).
3. Other drugs may decrease values.

Clinical Alert

Dopaminergic drugs inhibit prolactin secretion. Administration of L-dopa can reduce prolactin levels back to normal in galactorrhea, hyperprolactinemia, and pituitary tumor.

Parathyroid Hormone Assay; Parathyrin; Parathormone (PTH-C Terminal)

Normal Values
N-terminal: 236–630 pg/ml as bovine PTH 230–630 ng/L
C-terminal: 410–1760 pg/ml as bovine PTH 410–1760 ng/L

Parathormone: 20–70 μl Eq/ml or 20–70 mEq/L
Varies greatly with method used.

Background
Parathormone (PTH) is a polypeptide hormone produced in the parathyroid gland, and it is one of the major factors in the regulation of calcium concentration in extracellular fluid. Three molecular forms of PTH exist: (1) intact, also called native or glandular hormone; (2) multiple N-terminal fragments; and (3) C-terminal fragments.

Explanation of Test
This test is used in studies of altered calcium metabolism and is helpful in establishing a diagnosis of hyperparathyroidism and in distinguishing nonparathyroid from parathyroid causes of hypercalcemia. A decrease in the level of ionized calcium is the primary stimulus for PTH secretions, whereas a rise in calcium inhibits secretions. This relationship is lost in hyperthyroidism, and PTH will be inappropriately high in relation to calcium.

The C assays tend to have higher values and are more widely accepted as better indications of hyperparathyroidism. Creatinine is usually determined with all PTH assays to determine kidney function.

Clinical Implications
1. *Increased PTH values* occur in
    (a) Chronic renal failure. This is a cause of secondary hyperparathyroidism.
    (b) Pseudohyperparathyroidism. There is a primary defect in renal tubular responsiveness to PTH (slight increase).
    (c) Vitamin D deficiency (moderate)
    (d) Malabsorption (moderate)
    (e) Rickets (moderate)
    (f) Osteomalacia (moderate)
2. *Decreased PTH values* occur in nonparathyroid hypercalcemia, as in
    (a) Use of thiazide diuretics
    (b) Mild alkali syndrome
    (c) Vitamin A and D intoxication
    (d) Hematologic malignancies (some)
    (e) Sarcoidosis
    (f) Graves' disease
    (g) Permanent postoperative hypoparathyroidism
3. *Increased PTH-N values* occur in
    (a) Pseudohypoparathyroidism
    (b) Secondary hyperparathyroidism
    (c) Primary hyperparathyroidism
4. *Decreased PTH-N values* occur in
    (a) Hypoparathyroidism
    (b) Neoplasms
    (c) Nonparathyroid hypercalcemia

5. *Increased PTH-C values* occur in
   (a) Pseudohypoparathyroidism
   (b) Secondary hyperparathy-
      roidism
   (c) Primary hyperparathy-
      roidism
   (d) Neoplasms
6. *Decreased PTH-C values* occur in
   (a) Hypoparathyroidism
   (b) Nonparathyroid hyper-
      calcemia

Interfering Factors
1. Elevated blood lipids interfere with results.
2. Milk ingestion may falsely lower PTH levels.

Procedure
1. A 10-hour fasting venous blood sample of at least 6 ml is obtained
   (3 ml in two separate vials).
2. The specimen is obtained in the early morning.
3. If the patient cannot fast, notify the laboratory.

Progesterone

Normal Serum Values
Follicular phase: 0.02–0.9 ng/ml or 0.06–2.86 nmol/L
Luteal phase: 6–30 ng/ml or 19.08–95.40 nmol/L
Rises 16–24 hours before ovulation, reaches maximum 6–10 days after
   urinary total estrogen peak.

Explanation of Test
This test is done as part of a fertility study to confirm ovulation and in
the evaluation of the function of the corpus luteum. Several samples
during the cycle are necessary. Ovarian production of progesterone is
low during the follicular (first) phase of the menstrual cycle. After ovulation, progesterone levels rise for 4 to 5 days and then fall. During
pregnancy, there is a gradual increase from the 9th to 32nd week, often
to 100 times the level in the nonpregnant woman. Levels of progesterone in twin pregnancy will be higher than in a single pregnancy.

Procedure
1. A venous blood sample is obtained. The test request should include
   sex, day of last menstrual period, and trimester of pregnancy.
2. Urine tests can also be done.

Clinical Implications
1. *Increased levels* are associated with
   (a) Congenital adrenal hyper-
      plasia
   (b) Lipid ovarian tumor
   (c) Molar pregnancy
   (d) Chorionepithelioma of
      ovary

2. *Decreased levels* are associated with
   (a) Threatened abortion   (b) Galactorrhea–amenorrhea
                                                syndrome

Somatomedin-C, Insulin-like Growth Hormone

Normal Values

Men
    0–8 years: 4–87 ng/ml
    9–10 years: 26–98 ng/ml
    11–13 years: 44–207 ng/ml
    14–16 years: 48–255 ng/ml
    Adults: 42–110 ng/ml

Women
    0–8 years: 7–110 ng/ml
    9–10 years: 39–186 ng/ml
    11–13 years: 66–215 ng/ml
    14–16 years: 96–256 ng/ml
    Adults: 42–110 ng/ml

Explanation of Test

This test is used to monitor the growth of children as well as in the diagnosis of acromegaly and hypopituitarism. Normal somatomedin results are evidence against a deficiency of growth hormone.

Procedure

Fasting (preferred) venous blood sample is obtained.

Clinical Implications

1. *Increased levels* are associated with acromegaly.
2. *Decreased levels* are associated with
   (a) Dwarfism   (d) Kwashiorkor
   (b) Hypopituitarism   (e) Laron dwarfism
   (c) Hypothyroidism   (f) Cirrhosis of liver

Testosterone

Normal Values

Men: 500–860 ng/dl or 500–860 mmol/L
Women: 26–54 ng/dl or 26–54 nmol/L

Background

Testosterone is a hormone responsible for the development of male secondary sexual characteristics. This substance is synthesized mainly in the Leydig cells of the testes. It is secreted by the adrenal glands and testes in men and by the adrenal glands and ovaries in women. Excessive production induces premature puberty in men and masculinity in women. A small portion of total testosterone exists in the free or unbound state and is available for entry into cells of the target organs.

Explanation of Test

Routine testosterone measurements in men have been found useful in the assessment of hypogonadism, pituitary gonadotropin function, impotency, and cryptorchidism; these measurements are also useful in the detection of ovarian and adrenal tumors in women.

Procedure

1. Three venous blood samples of 10 ml may be obtained from men.
2. Five venous blood samples of 10 ml may be obtained from women. (The quantity will vary according to laboratory procedure.)
3. Indicate sex and age on the laboratory form.

Clinical Implications

1. *Decreased total testosterone levels in men* are associated with
   (a) Hypogonadism
   (b) Klinefelter's syndrome
   (c) Hypopituitarism
   (d) Orchidectomy
   (e) Estrogen therapy
2. *Increased total testosterone levels in women* are associated with
   (a) Adrenal neoplasms
   (b) Ovarian tumors, benign or malignant
   (c) Polycystic ovaries
3. *Increased free testosterone levels* are associated with
   (a) Female hirsutism
   (b) Polycystic ovaries
   (c) Virilization
4. *Decreased free testosterone levels* are associated with hypogonadism.

Interfering Factors

In adult men, an inverse correlation of free testosterone with age occurs. The upper limit of normal range generally decreases from the age of 20 to 60 years. The lower range of free normal does not change significantly with age.

ENZYME TESTS

Acid Phosphatase

Normal Values

Men: 0.15–0.65 BLB (Bersey, Lowry, and Brock) units at 37°C or 2.5–11.7 U/L

Women: 0.02–0.55 BLB units at 37°C or 0.3–9.2 U/L

Explanation of Test

Acid phosphatases are enzymes that are widely distributed in tissue, including the bone, liver, spleen, kidney, red blood cells, and platelets. However, their greatest importance is found in the prostate gland, where acid phosphatase activity is 100 times higher than in other tissue.

For this reason, the test of acid phosphatase levels is used to diagnose metastatic cancer of the prostate and to follow the effectiveness of treatment. It is known that elevated levels of acid phosphatase are seen in patients with prostate cancer that has metastasized beyond the capsule to other parts of the body, especially the bone. It is believed that once the carcinoma has spread, the prostate starts to release acid phosphatase, resulting in an increase in blood level. The prostatic fraction procedure specifically measures the concentration of prostatic acid phosphatase secreted by cells of the prostate gland in contrast to the total enzyme activity, which is an indirect measurement.

Acid phosphatase is also present in high concentration in seminal fluid. Tests for this enzyme may be used to investigate rape.

Procedure
A venous blood sample of 10 ml is obtained.

Clinical Implications
1. A significantly elevated value nearly always is indicative of metastatic cancer of the prostate. If the tumor is successfully treated, this enzyme level will drop within 3 to 4 days after surgery or 3 to 4 weeks after estrogen administration.
2. Moderately elevated values also occur in the absence of prostate disease in
   (a) Paget's disease
   (b) Gaucher's disease
   (c) Hyperparathyroidism
   (d) Multiple myeloma
   (e) Any cancer that has metastasized to the bone
   (f) Hepatitis
   (g) Obstructive jaundice
   (h) Acute renal impairment
   (i) Sickle cell crisis
   (j) Excessive destruction of platelets
3. Levels are reported to be elevated in the bone marrow of patients with prostatic cancer metastatic to the bone.

Interfering Factors
Drugs may cause *increased* and *decreased* levels.

Prostate-Specific Antigen (PSA)

Normal Values
Men under 40: 0–2.7 ng/ml
Men over 40: 0–4.0 ng/ml

Explanation of Test
This enzyme test is done to detect the presence of prostate-specific antigen. It is included in this chapter because in clinical practice paral-

lel testing for both PSA and prostate acid phosphatase (PAP) increases detection of early stage prostate cancer. This test is done to determine the effectiveness of therapy for prostate cancer and is used as an early indicator of prostate cancer recurrence. Its greatest value is as a marker in the follow-up of patients at high risk for disease progression (Tietz, 1990).

Procedure
A venous blood sample of 2 ml is obtained. Inform the laboratory of patient's age. Collect specimen prior to palpation of the prostate.

Clinical Implications
1. Increases occur in prostate cancer (80% of patients). A lesser increase is seen in benign prostate hypertrophy.
2. Increases above 4.0 ng/ml have been reported in about 8% of patients with no prostatic malignancies and benign diseases (Mayo, 1990).
3. If a prostate tumor is completely removed, the antigen will not be detected.

Interfering Factors
Transient increases occur followng prostate palpation.

Alanine Aminotransferase (ALT); Serum Glutamic-Pyruvic Transaminase (SGPT)

Normal Values
Women: 7–17 U/L at 30°C
Men: 7–24 U/L at 30°C
Children: 5–28 U/L at 30°C

Explanation of Test
This test of enzyme levels is done primarily to diagnose liver disease. High concentratons of this enzyme occur in the liver, and relatively low concentrations are found in the heart, muscle, and kidney. These enzymes are also used to monitor the course of treatment for hepatitis, active postnecrotic cirrhosis, or the effects of drug treatment that might be toxic to the liver. This test is also used to differentiate between hemolytic jaundice and jaundice due to liver disease. In comparison to aspertate amino transferase (AST), the ALT test is more specific for liver malfunction. In addition, this enzyme is elevated in myocardial infarction.

Procedure
1. A 5-ml sample of venous blood is obtained.
2. Hemolysis should be avoided during collection of the specimen.

Clinical Implications
A. *Increased levels* are found in
   1. Hepatocellular disease (moderate to high increase)
   2. Active cirrhosis (mild increase)
   3. Metastatic liver tumor (mild increase)
   4. Obstructive jaundice/biliary obstruction (mild to moderate increase)
   5. Infection or toxic hepatitis
   6. Infectious mononucleosis
   7. Pancreatitis (mild increase)
   8. Myocardial infarction
   9. Delerium tremens
   10. Severe burns
   11. Trauma
   12. Shock
B. AST/ALT *comparison*
   1. Although the AST level is always increased in acute myocardial infarction, the ALT level does not always increase proportionately.
   2. The ALT is usually increased more than the AST in acute extrahepatic biliary obstruction.
   3. ALT is less sensitive than AST to alcoholic liver disease.

Interfering Factors
1. Many drugs may cause falsely increased levels.
2. Salicylates may cause decreased or increased levels.

Clinical Alert

There is a correlation between the presence of elevated serum ALT and antibodies to the hepatitis B virus core antigen in a blood donor with the risk of non-A non-B hepatitis developing in the blood recipient. Therefore, persons with elevated ALT levels should *not* donate blood.

Alkaline Phosphatase (ALP)

Normal Values
Adult: 20–70 U/L
Child: 20–150 U/L

Explanation of Test

Alkaline phosphatase is an enzyme originating mainly in the bone, liver, and placenta, with some activity in the kidney and intestines. It is called *alkaline* because it functions best at a *p*H of 9.

This enzyme test is used as a tumor marker and an index of liver and bone disease when correlated with other clinical findings. In bone disease, the enzyme rises in proportion to new bone cell production resulting from osteoblastic activity and the deposit of calcium in the bones. In liver disease, the blood level rises when excretion of this enzyme is impaired as a result of obstruction in the biliary tract.

Procedure

A venous blood sample of 10 ml is obtained.

Clinical Implications

A. *Elevated levels*
   1. Liver disease (correlates with abnormal liver function tests)
     An elevation of ALP is often associated with elevated AST and elevated bilirubin.
     (a) Marked increases
        (1) Obstructive jaundice (gallstones obstructing major biliary ducts; accompanying elevated bilirubin)
        (2) Space-occupying lesions of the liver such as cancer and abscesses
        (3) Hepatocellular cirrhosis
        (4) Biliary cirrhosis
        (5) Liver metastasis
     (b) Moderate increases
        (1) Hepatitis
        (2) Pregnancy
        (3) Pancreatitis
   2. Bone disease
     (a) Marked increases
        (1) Paget's disease   (3) Osteitis deformans
        (2) Metastatic bone disease   (4) Osteogenic sarcoma
     (b) Moderate increases
        (1) Osteomalacia (elevated levels help differentiate between osteomalacia and osteoporosis, in which there is no elevation)
        (2) Rickets
   3. Other diseases
     (a) Hyperparathyroidism (accompanied by hypercalcemia)
     (b) Infectious mononucleosis
     (c) Leukemia
B. *Reduced levels*
   1. Hypophosphatasia (markedly reduced)

2. Malnutrition
3. Hypothyroidism
4. Pernicious anemia
5. Scurvy
6. Milk–alkali syndrome
7. Placental insufficiency
8. Dwarfism

Interfering Factors
1. A variety of drugs produces mild to moderate elevations or decreased levels of ALP.
2. Young children, those experiencing rapid growth, pregnant women, and all post-menopausal women have physiologically high levels of ALP.
3. The level is slightly increased in older persons.
4. After IV administration of albumin, there is sometimes a marked increase for several days.

Alkaline Phosphatase Isoenzymes

Normal Values
AP-1, Alpha 2: Values are reported as weak, moderate, or strong
AP-2, Beta 1: Values are reported as weak, moderate, or strong
AP-3, Beta 2: Values are reported as weak, moderate, or strong

Background
The isoenzymes of ALP are produced by various tissues. AP-1, Alpha 2 is heat labile and is produced in the liver and by proliferating blood vessels. AP-2, Beta 1 is heat stable and is produced by bone and placental tissue. The intestinal isoenzyme AP-3, Beta 2 is present in small quantities in Group O and B individuals. AP-1 and 2 can be partially distinguished in the laboratory by heating and urea testing. Placental ALP is still more stable to heat than urea.

Explanation of Test
This is done when the total ALP is abnormal and it is used primarily to distinguish between bone and liver origin of ALP.

Procedure
A venous blood sample of 5 ml is obtained.

Clinical Implications
1. Osteoblastic bone tumors increase the bone ALP in the blood serum; less than 25% is thermostabile in bone disease.
2. Liver diseases such as cancer and biliary obstruction increase the liver isoenzyme; more than 25% is thermostabile in hepatic disease.

3. The intestinal isoenzyme may be increased in patients with cirrhosis.
4. The placental isoenzyme is increased in some patients with cancer (carcinoplacental antigen) and normally in pregnancy.
5. *Normal values* are observed in

   (a) Poliomyelitis
   (b) Myasthenia gravis
   (c) Multiple sclerosis
   (d) Neurogenic muscle atrophy

Aldolase (ALS)

Normal Values
1.5–12.0 μ/L at 37°C

Background
Aldolase is a glycolytic enzyme that catalyzes the breakdown of fructose 1,6-diphosphate into the triase phosphates. This is one of the important reactions in the intermediary glycolytic breakdown of glucose. This enzyme has a widespread distribution throughout most tissues of the body.

Explanation of Test
This test is helpful in diagnostic situations where cell destruction and necrosis or increased membrane permeability may have occurred, as in acute hepatitis, progressive muscular atrophy, myocardial infarction, and malignancy.

Procedure
A fasting venous blood sample of 5 ml is usually obtained.

Clinical Implications
1. The *highest levels* are found in muscular dystrophy.
2. The *lesser elevations* are found in

   (a) Dermatomyositis
   (b) Polymyositis
   (c) Limb-girdle muscular dystrophy
3. *Normal or moderately elevated values* are found in

   (a) Chronic hepatitis
   (b) Portal cirrhosis
   (c) Obstructive jaundice
4. *Increased levels* are also associated with

   (a) Gangrene
   (b) Prostate tumors
   (c) Trichinosis
   (d) Some carcinomas metastatic to the liver
   (e) Some blood dyscrasias
   (f) Delirium tremens
   (g) Burns
   (h) 20% of cancer patients (more frequent with liver involvement)

Patient Preparation

Explain the purpose and procedure of the test. Advise the patient to fast from food from midnight before the specimen is obtained. Water is permitted.

Serum Angiotensin-Converting Enzyme (SACE)

Normal Values

6.1–21.1 U/L for patients >20 yr of age

Background

Angiotensin I is produced by the action of resin on angiotensinogen. Angiotensin I-converting enzyme (CE) catalyzes the conversion of angiotensin I to the vasoactive peptide, angiotensin II. Angiotensin I is concentrated in the proximal tubules.

Explanation of Test

This test is primarily used in the study of persons with sarcoidosis to evaluate the severity and activity of the disease. Serum angiotensin-converting enzyme (SACE) levels are significantly higher in 79% of patients with active sarcoidosis. However, about 5% of the normal adult population have elevated levels.

Procedure

A venous blood sample of at least 5 ml is obtained.

Clinical Implications

1. *Increased levels* are associated with
   (a) Sarcoidosis: SACE levels reflect the severity of the disease, with 68% positivity in stage 1 disease, 86% in stage 2, and 92% in stage 3.
   (b) Gaucher's disease
   (c) Leprosy
2. *Decreased levels* occur in many persons with the disease who are treated with prednisone.

Interfering Factors

The test should not be done on persons under age 20 because they normally have a very high level of SACE.

Amylase

Normal Values

50–150 μ/L
25–130 IU/L by enzymatic method

Background

Amylase is an enzyme that changes starch to sugar. It is produced in the salivary glands, pancreas, liver, and fallopian tubes. If there is an inflammation of the pancreas or salivary glands, much more of the enzyme enters the blood. Amylase levels in the urine reflect blood changes by a time-lag of 6 to 10 hours (see *"Amylase Excretion/Clearance,"* Chap. 3).

Explanation of Test

This test is used to diagnose and monitor treatment of acute pancreatitis and to detect inflammation of salivary glands.

Procedure

A venous blood sample of 10 ml is obtained.

Clinical Implications

A. *Increased levels*
1. Greatly increased in acute nonhemorrhagic pancreatitis early in the course of the disease. The increase begins in 3 to 6 hours after the onset of pain.
2. Increases also occur in
   (a) Acute exacerbation of chronic pancreatitis
   (b) Partial gastrectomy
   (c) Obstruction of pancreatic duct
   (d) Perforated peptic ulcer
   (e) Alcohol poisoning
   (f) Mumps
   (g) Obstruction or inflammation of salivary duct or gland
   (h) Acute cholecystitis
   (i) Intestinal obstruction with strangulation
   (j) Ruptured tubal pregnancy
   (k) Ruptured aortic aneurysm
B. *Decreased levels* occur in
1. Acute pancreatitis subsidence
2. Hepatitis
3. Cirrhosis of liver
4. Toxemia of pregnancy
5. Severe burns
6. Severe thyrotoxicosis

Clinical Alert

1. The amylase/creatinine clearance can be used to differentiate cause if etiology is a problem.
2. Serum panic level is greater than 600 IU/liter.

Aspartate Amino Transferase (AST) or Serum Glutamic-Oxaloacetic Transaminase (SGOT)

Normal Values
Men: 8–20 μ/L at 30°C
Women: 6–18 μ/L at 30°C
Children: 25–75 μ/L

Explanation of Test
AST is an enzyme present in tissues of high metabolic activity. It occurs in decreasing concentration in the heart, liver, skeletal muscle, kidney, brain, pancreas, spleen, and lungs. The enzyme is released into the circulation following the injury or death of cells. Any disease that causes change in these highly metabolic tissues will result in a rise in AST. The amount of AST in the blood is directly related to the number of damaged cells and the amount of time that passes between injury to the tissue and the test. Following severe cell damage, the blood AST level will rise in 12 hours and remain elevated for about 5 days.

Procedure
A venous sample of 5 ml is obtained. Hemolysis during the procedure should be avoided.

Clinical Implications
A. *Increased levels* occur in
   1. Myocardial infarction (MI)
      (a) In MI, the AST level may be increased 4 to 10 times the normal values.
      (b) The AST level reaches a peak in 24 hours and returns to normal by the third or fourth day. Secondary rises in AST levels suggest extension or recurrence of MI.
      (c) The AST curve in MI parallels that of creatine phosphokinase, (see p. 342).
      (d) Elevated levels do not always indicate MI in suspected patients. Severe arrhythmias and severe angina can also cause elevation.
   2. Liver disease
      (a) Level is always elevated in cirrhosis of the liver.
      (b) In liver disease, the level may be 10 to 100 times the normal.
      (c) Liver diseases associated with elevated AST levels
         (1) Acute hepatitis
         (2) Active cirrhosis
         (3) Infectious mononucleosis with hepatitis
         (4) Hepatic necrosis
         (5) Primary or metastatic carcinoma

3. Other diseases associated with elevated AST levels
   (a) Acute pancreatitis
   (b) Trauma and irradiation of skeletal muscle
   (c) Acute hemolytic anemia
   (d) Acute renal disease
   (e) Severe burns
   (f) Cardiac catheterization and angiography
   (g) Recent brain trauma with brain necrosis
   (h) Crushing injuries
   (i) Progressive muscular dystrophy
   (j) Pulmonary emboli
   (k) Gangrene
   (l) Malignant hyperthermia

B. *Decreased levels* occur in
   1. Beriberi
   2. Uncontrolled diabetes mellitus with acidosis
   3. Liver disease occasionally may cause a decrease instead of the expected increase.

Interfering Factors
1. Slight decreases occur during pregnancy when there is abnormal metabolism of pyridoxine.
2. Many drugs can cause elevated levels.
3. Salicylates may cause falsely decreased or increased AST levels.
4. Alcohol ingestion

Clinical Alert

For diagnosis of MI, the AST levels should be done on three consecutive days because the peak is reached in 24 hours and levels are back to normal in 3 to 4 days.

Creatine Phosphokinase (CPK); Creatine Kinase (CK) and Isoenzymes

Normal Values

Men		*Isoenzymes*
6–11 years	56–185 U/L	MM: 100%
12–18 years	35–185 U/L	MB: 0%
≥19 years	38–174 U/L	BB: 0%

Women	
6–7 years	50–145 U/L
8–14 years	35–145 U/L
15–18 years	20–100 U/L
≥19 years	96–140 U/L
Newborn	68–580 U/L

Explanation of Test

Creatine kinase (CK) is an enzyme found in high concentrations in the heart and skeletal muscles and in much smaller concentrations in the brain tissue. Because CK exists in relatively few organs, this test is used as a specific index of injury to myocardium and muscle. Thus, it is important in the diagnosis of myocardial infarction and as a reliable measure of skeletal muscle diseases such as muscular dystrophy. In fact, CK levels can prove helpful in recognizing muscular dystrophy before clinical signs appear. This test is also of value in following the course of inflammatory muscle disease. Creatine kinase levels may rise significantly with central nervous system disorders such as Reye's syndrome. The determination of CK isoenzymes may be helpful in a differential diagnosis.

CPK/CK Isoenzymes

CPK can be divided into three isoenzymes: MM or CK_3, BB or CK_1, and MB or CK_2. CK-MM is the isoenzyme that makes up almost all the circulatory enzymes in healthy persons. Skeletal muscle contains primarily MM; cardiac muscle, MM and MB; and brain tissue, gastrointestinal and genitourinary tracts, BB. Normal CK levels are virtually 100% MM isoenzyme. A slight increase in total CPK is reflected from elevated BB from central nervous system injury. The isoenzyme studies help distinguish whether the CPK originated from the heart (MB) or the skeletal muscle (MM). Thus, elevation of MM levels is an indication of skeletal muscle injury. Elevation of MB, the cardiac enzyme, provides a more definitive indication of myocardial cell damage or death than total CK alone.

CK-BB may be a useful marker for monitoring therapy in cancer of the lung, breast, and prostate.

Procedure

A blood sample of at least 5 ml is obtained by venipuncture. If a patient has been receiving multiple injections intramuscularly, this fact should be noted on the laboratory requisition.

Clinical Implications of Total CK Levels

A. Myocardial infarction (MI)
1. Rise starts soon after an attack (about 4–6 hours) and reaches a peak of at least several times normal within 30 hours.
2. CK rises before and falls earlier than AST.
3. Level returns to normal 2 to 3 days after infarction. Thus, if patient is seen within this period following an infarction, the CK levels can help determine that an infarction did occur.
4. If the CPK rise is extensive, some clinicians believe the infarcted area is extensive and the prognosis is thus unfavorable. Others believe that subendocardial infarction causes greater increases in CPK because of easy diffusion of CPK from cell to blood.

B. Other diseases and procedures that cause increased CK levels
   1. Acute cerebrovascular disease
   2. Progressive muscular dystrophy (levels may reach 300–400 times normal)
   3. Dermatomyositis (involves muscle inflammation and neurons) and polymyositis
   4. Delirium tremens and chronic alcoholism (an episode of acute intoxication may be accompanied by CK levels comparable to those found in MI)
   5. Electric shock
   6. Myxedema
   7. Cardiac surgery
   8. Cardiac defibrillation
   9. Electromyography
   10. Convulsions, cerebral infarction, ischemia, or subarachnoid hemorrhage
   11. Hypokalemia
   12. Hypothyroidism
   13. Acute psychosis
   14. Central nervous system trauma
   15. Pulmonary infarction or edema (rise in CK levels is unexplainable)
C. Normal values are found in myasthenia gravis and multiple sclerosis.

Clinical Implications of CK Isoenzymes

A. Elevated MM isoenzyme levels occur in
   1. Muscle trauma
   2. Following intramuscular injections
   3. Shock
   4. Postoperatively in major surgical procedures
   5. MI (may remain elevated 4 or 5 days following MI)
B. Elevated MB isoenzyme levels occur in
   1. Myocardial infarct (rises in 4–6 hours after MI; not demonstrable after 24–36 hours) (>5 in MI)
   2. Myocardial ischemia
   3. Duchenne's muscular dystrophy
   4. Polymyositis
   5. Significant myoglobinuria
   6. Reye's syndrome
C. BB (CK_1) elevations are seen in
   1. Biliary atresia
   2. Some breast, small cell, lung, and prostate cancers
   3. Severe shock syndrome (some)
   4. Brain injury

D. After an MI, MB appears in the serum between 6 and 12 hours and remains for about 18 to 32 hours. The finding of MB in a patient with chest pain is diagnostic of MI. In addition, if there is a negative CK-MB for 48 hours or more following a clearly defined episode under question, it is clear that the patient has not had an MI.

E. MB may also be present in the serum of some patients with some forms of muscular dystrophy. This is significant because, normally, only MM is present in serum.

Interfering Factors
1. Strenuous exercise (up to three times normal) and surgical procedures that damage skeletal muscle may cause increased levels.
2. High doses of salicylates may cause increased levels.
3. Athletes have a higher value because of greater muscle mass.
4. Multiple intramuscular injections may cause increased levels.
5. Drugs may cause increased levels.
6. Childbirth
7. Hypothermia

Galactose-1-Phosphate Uridyl Transferase, Galactokinase

Normal Values
Galactose-1-phosphate uridyl transferase: 18.5–28.5 U/g of hemoglobin
Galactokinase: 12.1–39.7 μ/g of hemoglobin

Background
The enzyme galactose-1-phosphate uridyl transferase is needed in the use of galactose-1-phosphate so that it does not accumulate in the body.

Explanation of Test
This measurement is used to identify a defect in the use of galactose, which can result in widespread tissue damage and abnormalities such as cataracts, liver disease, and renal disease. This effect usually occurs in infants and children.

Procedure
A venous blood sample of at least 1 ml is obtained.

Clinical Implications
Decreased values are associated with galactosemia, a rare genetic disorder transmitted as an autosomal recessive gene.

Clinical Alert

Parents of infants and children with positive test results should be instructed that the disease can be treated by removing galactose-containing foods, especially milk, from the diet.

Hexosaminidase; Total and A

Normal Values
Total: 10.4–23.8 U/L
A: 56%–80% of total

Background
Hexosaminidase A is a lysosomal isoenzyme, a deficiency of which characterizes patients with Tay–Sachs disease. In the brains of affected children, there is a 100 times increase of ganglioside due to a deficiency of this enzyme.

Explanation of Test
This determination is a diagnostic test for Tay–Sachs disease and can be of help in identifying carriers among persons with no family history of Tay–Sachs. This condition is due to an autosomal recessive trait found predominantly, but not exclusively, in Ashkenazic Jews and is characterized by the appearance during infancy of psychomotor deterioration, blindness, cherry red spot on the macula, and an exaggerated extension response to sound.

Procedure
A fasting venous blood sample of at least 1 ml is obtained.

Clinical Implications
1. The total value may be normal or decreased in this disease, but an almost total deficiency of the A component is diagnostic of Tay–Sachs disease or G_{M2} gangliosidosis.
2. In a variant of Tay–Sachs disease, Sandhoff's disease, both A and B are defective, causing an absence of this enzyme.

Interfering Factors
Total values are increased in pregnancy owing to the appearance of a third heat-stable enzyme.

Lactic Acid Dehydrogenase (LD, LDH)

Normal Values
Values for the normal range of LD activity in serum vary considerably, depending on the direction of the enzyme reaction, the type of method used, and the experimental parameters. For the pyruvate → lactate reaction at 30°C and at a pH of 7.4, a range of 95 to 200 U/L represents the experience of most workers.

Background
Lactic acid dehydrogenase is an intracellular enzyme that is widely distributed in the tissues of the body, particularly in the kidney, heart, skeletal muscle, brain, liver, and lungs. Increases in the reported value usually indicate cellular death and leakage of the enzyme from the cell.

Explanation of Test
Although elevated levels of LDH are nonspecific, this test is useful in confirming myocardial or pulmonary infarction when viewed in relation to other test findings. For example, LD remains elevated longer than CK in myocardial infarction (MI). It is also helpful in the differential diagnosis of muscular dystrophy and pernicious anemia. More specific findings may be found by breaking down the LDH into its five isoenzymes. (When LD values are reported or quoted, *total* LDH is meant.) LDH is also valuable as a tumor marker in seminoma or germ cell testis tumor, especially when AFP and HCG are not produced in the tumor.

Procedure
1. A venous blood sample of 5 ml is obtained.
2. Avoid hemolysis in obtaining blood sample.

Clinical Implications
A. Myocardial infarction

   The elevation of LDH that follows an MI is characterized by
   1. High levels (2–10 times normal) within 12 to 24 hours of infarction (18 hours).
   2. Elevations that may continue for 6 to 10 days (longer than SGOT or CK). For this reason, LDH determinations may be useful in the late diagnosis of MI. Elevations usually return to normal in 8 to 14 days.

B. Pulmonary infarction

   In pulmonary infarction, there is usually an increased LDH within 24 hours of the onset of pain. The pattern of normal SGOT and elevated LDH that levels off 1 to 2 days after an episode of chest pain provides evidence for pulmonary infarction.

C. Conditions in general and according to degree of increase in levels

1. *Elevated levels* of LDH are observed in a variety of conditions, such as

   (a) Acute MI
   (b) Acute leukemia
   (c) Hemolytic anemias
   (d) Hepatic disease
   (e) Skeletal muscle necrosis
   (f) Sprue
   (g) Acute pulmonary infarction
   (h) Malignant neoplasms, extensive cancer
   (i) Acute renal infarctions and chronic renal disease
   (j) Shock with necrosis of minor organs
   (k) Myxedema

2. The *greatest increase* (2–40 times) of LDH is seen in

   (a) Megaloblastic anemias
   (b) Extensive cancer
   (c) Shock and anoxia

3. *Moderate increase* (2–4 times) of LDH is seen in

   (a) Myocardial infarction
   (b) Pulmonary infarction
   (c) Granulocytic or acute leukemia
   (d) Hemolytic anemia
   (e) Infectious mononucleosis
   (f) Progressive muscular dystrophy

4. *Slight increases* occur in

   (a) Delirium tremens
   (b) Hepatitis
   (c) Obstructive jaundice
   (d) Cirrhosis
   (e) Mononucleosis
   (f) Hemolysis (prosthetic heart valve)
   (g) Shock and anoxia

D. Angina and pericarditis do *not* produce LDH elevations.

E. *Decreased LD levels* are associated with a good response to cancer therapy.

F. *Elevated urine LD levels* occur in

1. Cancer of kidney or bladder
2. Glomerulonephritis
3. Malignant hypertension
4. Lupus nephritis
5. Acute tubular necrosis
6. Renal transplantation and hemograft rejection
7. Pyelonephritis (sometimes)

Interfering Factors

1. Strenuous exercise and the muscular exertion involved in childbirth will cause increased levels.
2. Skin diseases can cause falsely increased levels.
3. Hemolysis of red blood cells due to freezing, heating, or shaking the blood sample will cause falsely increased levels.
4. Some drugs may cause increased and decreased levels.

Electrophoresis of LDH (LD) Isoenzymes

Normal Values

Isoenzyme Normals	*Percents of Total*
LD_1	14–26
LD_2	29–39
LD_3	20–26
LD_4	8–16
LD_5	6–16

Explanation of Test

Electrophoresis or separation of LDH identifies the five isoenzymes or fractions of LDH, each with its own physical characteristics and electrophoretical properties. Fractionating the LDH activity sharpens its diagnostic value, because LDH is found in many organs. The LD isoenzymes are released into the bloodstream when tissue necrosis occurs. However, a complete knowledge of the clinical history is necessary to interpret properly the resulting patterns. The isoenzymes are elevated in terms of patterns established, not on the basis of the value of a single isoenzyme.

The five isoenzyme fractions of LDH show different patterns in various disorders. Abnormalities in the pattern suggest which tissues have been damaged and help to diagnose MI, pulmonary infarction, and liver disease. (This test is sensitive enough to detect increased hepatic fraction in infectious hepatitis before clinical jaundice appears.) It is in confirming the diagnosis of suspected MI that the separation of LD finds its most frequent application, especially when a second infarct occurs shortly after the first. In these cases, the ECG is already abnormal, but the isoenzyme pattern will show increased LD_1, indicating the release of more of the cardiac isoenzyme.

Procedure

A venous blood sample of 5 ml is obtained. Avoid hemolysis.

Clinical Implications

Abnormal patterns reflect damaged tissue.

1. LD_1 and LD_2 are increased in MI and in some hemolytic anemias.
2. The LD pattern will be essentially the same in MI, pernicious anemia, and renal infarction. This is because red blood cells and the kidney have an isoenzyme pattern similar to that of heart muscle.
3. LD_3 is increased in pulmonary infarction and extensive pneumonia.
4. LDH_5 is increased in various malignancies and liver disease but has had limited clinical use. An increase in LD_2, LD_3, and LD_4 is common in malignant disease.

5. In most cancers, one to three of the bands (LD_2, LD_3, and LD_4) are frequently increased. A notable exception is in seminomas and dysgerminomas when LD_1 and LD_2 are increased. Frequently, an increase in LD_3 may be the first indication of the presence of cancer.

Clinical Alert

Because erythrocytes and kidney cells contain the same isoenzymes as heart muscle, patients with pernicious anemia or renal infarction may have the same serum isoenzyme patterns as those with MIs.

Lipase

Normal Values
Vary with methodology used
Using the Shihalsi/Bishop assay, the normals are 4–24 U/L

Explanation of Test
Lipase functions in the body to change fats to fatty acid and glycerol. The major source of this enzyme is the pancreas. Therefore, lipase appears in the bloodstream following damage to the pancreas.

The test is used to diagnose pancreatitis and to differentiate pancreatitis from an acute surgical abdominal emergency. When secretions of the pancreas are blocked, the blood serum lipase levels rise.

Procedure
A venous blood sample of 5 ml is obtained.

Clinical Implications
A. *Elevated levels in pancreatic disorders*
    1. Elevation of lipase may not occur until 24 to 36 hours after onset of illness.
    2. Elevation occurs later than amylase and persists longer than changes in blood amylase, which is also related to pancreatic disorders (up to 14 days).
    3. Lipase level may be high when amylase levels are normal.
    4. Thus, the lipase test is useful in late diagnosis of acute pancreatitis.
B. *Increased lipase values* are associated with
    1. Pancreatitis
    2. Obstruction of the pancreatic duct
    3. Pancreatic carcinoma

4. Acute cholecystitis
5. Cirrhosis
6. Severe renal disease
7. High intestinal obstruction
C. Usually normal in mumps

Interfering Factors
Some drugs may increase or decrease the level.

5'-Nucleotidase

Normal Values
10.6–17.5 U/L

Background
5'-nucleotidase is an enzyme that has a wide distribution throughout the body and blood. It is known to appear in the serum in diseases of the liver.

Explanation of Test
This measurement provides supportive evidence in the diagnosis of liver disease and helps to differentiate skeletal disorders along with the investigation of alkaline phosphatase. The two tests combined may provide definitive diagnoses of Paget's disease or rickets, in which high levels of alkaline phosphatase accompany normal or marginally increased 5'-nucleotidase activity.

Procedure
A venous blood sample of 5 ml is obtained.

Clinical Implications
1. *Increases* are associated with diseases of liver such as
   (a) Extrahepatic obstruction
   (b) Cholecystosis caused by chlorpromazine
   (c) Hepatic carcinoma
   (d) Biliary cirrhosis
2. Usually does not increase in skeletal disease.

Renin

Normal Values
Ages 20–39: Normal sodium diet: 0.6–4.3 ng/ml/hr or μg/L/hr
Restricted sodium diet: 2.9–24.0 ng/ml/hr or μg/L/hr
Ages ≥40: Normal sodium diet: 0.6–3.0 ng/ml/hr
Restricted sodium diet: 2.9–10.8 ng/ml/hr

Background
Renin is an enzyme that converts angiotensinogen to angiotensin I. Derived from the liver, angiotensinogen is an alpha-2 globulin in the serum. Angiotensin I is then converted in the lung to angiotensin II. Angiotensin II is a potent vasopressor agent responsible for hypertension of renal origin, as well as a powerful releaser of aldosterone from the adrenal cortex. Both angiotensin II and aldosterone increase blood pressure. It is known that renin levels increase when there is decreased renal perfusion pressure and when there is decreased delivery of sodium and water to the vascular pole of the glomerulus.

Relationship of Plasma Renin to Hyperaldosteronism
Increased aldosterone production associated with decreased renin and normal 17-OH corticosteroids is practically diagnostic of primary hyperaldosteronism, whether hypokalemia is present or not.

Explanation of Test
This test of renin activity is most useful in the differential diagnosis of hypertension, either essential, renal, or renovascular. In primary hyperaldosteronism, the findings will demonstrate that aldosterone secretion is exaggerated and secretion of renin is suppressed. This test is of considerable importance because the number of patients suffering from this disorder can be very substantial.

Procedure
1. A fasting venous blood sample of 10 ml is obtained. It is important to use EDTA as the anticoagulant because it aids in preservation of any angiotensin formed before examination.
2. A second, nonfasting specimen may be ordered with exercise.

Clinical Implications
1. *Increased levels* are associated with
   - (a) Hypertension of renal origin
   - (b) Addison's disease
   - (c) Salt-losing nephropathy
   - (d) Hemorrhage
2. *Decreased levels* are associated with
   - (a) Salt-retaining steroid therapy
   - (b) Antidiuretic hormone therapy

Patient Preparation
1. Explain the purpose and procedure of the test.
2. A regular diet that contains 180 mEq of sodium and 100 mEq of potassium must be maintained for 3 days before the specimen is obtained.
3. Instruct the patient that it is necessary to be in a supine position for at least 1 hour before obtaining the specimen.

4. Drugs that interfere with testing, along with licorice, should be terminated at least 2 weeks before testing. Check with your laboratory and pharmacy.

Interfering Factors
1. Levels may vary in normal persons and will rise under influences that tend to shrink the intravascular fluid volume.
2. Values will be higher when the patient is in an upright position early in the day, in low salt diets, during pregnancy, and with drugs such as diuretics, antihypertensives, estrogen, and oral contraceptives.

Challenge Test
A challenge test has been recommended to distinguish primary from secondary hyperaldosteronism on the basis of renin levels, with the patient in both the recumbent and upright positions and after the patient has been maintained on a low salt diet. In normal persons and in those with essential hypertension, renin concentration will be increased by the reduction in volume due to sodium restriction and the upright position. In primary aldosteronism, volume depletion does not occur and renin concentration remains low.

General Procedure for Renin Stimulation Test
1. The patient should be admitted to the hospital for this test. On admission, weight is obtained and recorded.
2. A diet containing reduced sodium content supplemented with potassium is given for 3 days, along with diuretics (such as furosemide or chlorothiazide) as ordered.
3. Weigh again on the third day, record, and see that the patient remains upright for 4 hours doing normal activities.
4. A venous heparinized blood sample for renin is obtained at 11 AM or when renin activity is usually at its maximum. Place it in ice and send it immediately to the laboratory.

Interpretation of Renin Stimulation Test
In normal persons and most hypertensive patients, the stimulation of a low salt diet, a diuretic, and upright posture will raise renin activity to very high levels and result in weight loss. However, in primary aldosteronism, the plasma level is expanded and remains so. In these patients, there is little if any weight loss and the renin level is very low or undetectable. It is important to keep in mind that a response within the normal range can occur in the presence of aldosterone.

Patient Preparation
1. Explain the purpose and procedure of the test.
2. Check with the individual laboratory for specific practices. The purpose of the preparation is to deplete the patient of sodium.

Uroporphyrinogen-1-Synthase (U1S)

Normal Values
Women: 8–16.8 nmol/L/sec
Men: 7.9–14.7 nmol/L/sec

Background
This enzyme in the red blood cells is needed to convert porphobilinogen to uroporphyrinogen. This enzyme will be diminished in any person with acute intermittent porphyria.

Explanation of Test
This measurement can be used in the detection of acute intermittent porphyria in the latent stage as well as in the confirmation of a diagnosis during an acute episode. It can most significantly be used to detect affected persons before occurrence of a first acute episode. Persons with latent acute intermittent porphyria can be identified. This is important because acute episodes of this disorder can be fatal.

Procedure
1. A fasting venous blood sample of at least 10 ml is obtained. The specimen must be placed in wet ice at once.
2. Include the patient's hematocrit on the laboratory request.

Clinical Implications
Decreased values are associated with

1. Acute intermittent porphyria (50% below that of normal individuals)
2. Values between 6 nmol/L/sec and 8 nmol/L/sec are suggestive but indeterminate.

Patient Preparation
Advise the patient about fasting. Water is permitted.

Gamma-Glutamyl Transferase (GGT); Gamma-Glutamyl Transpeptidase (γGT); Gamma-Glutamyl Transferase (γGT)

Normal Values
Men: 6–28 U/L at 25°C
Women: 4–18 U/L at 25°C

Background
The enzyme γ-glutamyl transpeptidase is present mainly in the liver, kidney, prostate, and spleen. The liver is considered the source of normal serum activity, despite the fact that the kidney has the highest

level of the enzyme. This enzyme is believed to function in the transport of amino acids and peptides into cells across the cell membranes and to be involved in glutathione metabolism. Men will have higher normal levels because of the large amounts found in the prostate.

Explanation of Test
This test is used to determine liver cell dysfunction and to detect alcohol-induced liver disease. It is also an efficient way to screen for the consequences of chronic alcoholism. The GGT is very sensitive to the amount of alcohol consumed by chronic drinkers. It can be used to monitor the cessation or reduction of alcohol consumption. γGT activity is elevated in all forms of liver disease. This test is much more sensitive than either the alkaline phosphatase test or the transaminase test in detecting obstructive jaundice, cholangitis, and cholecystitis.

Procedure
A venous blood sample of 5 ml is obtained.

Clinical Implications
1. Increased γGT levels are associated with
   - (a) Cholecystitis
   - (b) Cholelithiasis
   - (c) Cancer metastatic to the liver
   - (d) Cirrhosis of the liver
   - (e) Acute pancreatitis
   - (f) Cancer of the bile duct
   - (g) Alcoholism (occult)
   - (h) Barbiturate use
   - (i) Lipoid nephrosis
   - (j) Obstruction to biliary tract
   - (k) Hepatotoxic drugs for treatment of cancer increase levels more than the cancer itself
2. In MI, γGT is usually normal. However, if there is an increase, it occurs about the fourth day after an MI and probably implies liver damage secondary to cardiac insufficiency.
3. Values are not elevated in
   - (a) Bone disorders
   - (b) Pregnancy
   - (c) Skeletal muscle disease
   - (d) Neonatal hepatitis
   - (e) Renal failure

DRUG MONITORING

Explanation of Test
Therapeutic drug monitoring is widely accepted as a reliable and practical approach to managing individual patient drug therapy. Determination of drug levels is especially important when the potential for drug toxicity is significant or when inadequate or undesirable response follows the use of a standard dose. It provides an easier and more rapid estimation of dosage requirements than does observation of the drug effects themselves. For some drugs, it is routinely useful (digoxin); for others, it can be helpful in certain situations (antibiotics).

(*text continues on page 359*)

TABLE 6–2.
Blood Plasma Concentration of Commonly Monitored Drugs

Drug	Therapeutic* Maintenance	Toxic† (Panic or Critical)
Acetaminophen (Tylenol)	1–30 µg/ml or 66–199 µmol/L	>200 µg/ml or >1324 µmol/L
Alcohol (Ethanol)	Driving while intoxicated: 100 mg/dl or 10.9–21.7 mmol/L	>400 mg/dl >86.8 mmol/L
Amitriptyline (Elavil)	120–250 mg/ml or 433–903 nmol/L	>500 mg/ml or >1805 nmol/L
Bromide	750–1500 µg/ml or 9.4–18.7 nmol/L	>1250 µg/ml or >15.6 nmol/L
Carbamazepine (Tegretol)	8–12 µg/ml or 34–51 µmol/L	>15 µg/ml or >63 mol/L
Chlordiazepoxide (Librium)	700–1000 ng/ml or 2.34–3.34 µmol/L	>5000 ng/ml or >16.70 µmol/L
Desopyramide (Norpace)	Variable	>7 µg/ml or >20.7 µmol/L
Diazepam (Valium)	100–1000 ng/ml or 0.35–3.51 µmol/L	>5000 ng/ml or >17.55 µmol/L
Digitoxin	20–35 ng/ml or 26–46 nmol/L	>45 ng/ml or >59 nmol/L
Digoxin	CHF: 0.8–1.5 ng/ml or 1.0–1.9 nmol/L Arrhythmias: 1.5–2.0 ng/ml 1.9–2.6 nmol/L	>25 ng/ml or >3.2 nmol/L
Doxepin	30–150 ng/ml or 107–537 nmol/L	>500 ng/ml or >1790 nmol/L
Ethchlorvynol (Placidyl)	2–8 µg/ml or 14–55 µmol/L	>20 µg/ml or >138 µmol/L
Glutethimide (Doriden)	2–6 µg/ml or 9–28 µmol/L	>5 µg/ml or >23 µmol/L

Drug	Therapeutic Value*	Toxic Value†
Imipramine (Tofranil)	125–250 ng/ml or 446–893 nmol/L	>500 ng/ml or >1785 nmol/L
Lithium	0.6–1.2 mEq/L or 0.6–1.2 mmol/L	>2 mEq/L or >2 mmol/L
Lidocaine (Xylocaine)	1.5–6.0 µg/ml or 6.4–25.6 µmol/L	6–8 µg/ml or 25.6–34.2 µmol/L
Methotrexate	Variable	48 hrs after high dose: 454 mg/ml or 1000 mmol/L
Methyprylon (Noludar)	8–10 µg/ml or 45–55 µmol/L	>50 µg/ml or >275 µmol/L
Phenobarbital	15–40 g/ml or 65–172 mol/L	Varies 35–80 g/ml or 151–345 mol/L
Phenytoin (Dilantin)	10–20 g/ml or 40–79 mol/L	Varies with symptoms
Procainamide (Promestyl)	4–10 g/ml or 17–42 mol/L	10–12 g/ml or 42–51 mol/L
Primidone (Mysoline)	5–12 g/ml or 23–35 mol/L	15 g/ml or 69 mol/L
Propranolol (Inderal)	50–100 mg/ml or 193–386 nmol/L	Not defined
Quinidine	Varies considerably	Quite variable
Salicylate	<100 µg/ml or <724 µmol/L	begins at 100 µg/ml or begins at 724 µmol/L
Theophylline	Bronchodilator: 8–20 µg/ml or 44–111 µmol/L; Premature apnea: 6–13 µg/ml or 33–72 µmol/L	>20 µg/ml or >111 µmol/L
Valproic Acid (Depakene)	50–100 g/ml or 347–693 µmol/L	100 g/ml or 693 µmol/L

* Therapeutic value refers to expected drug concentration associated with desirable clinical effects in majority of the patient population treated.
† Toxic values refer to the drug concentration associated with undesirable effects or, in certain cases, death.

TABLE 6–3.
Blood Plasma Concentration of Commonly Monitored Antibiotics

Antibiotic	Peak*		Trough†	
Amikacin	Therapeutic:	25–35 μg/ml or 43–60 μml/L	Less severe infections: 1–4 μg/ml	
	Toxic:	>35–40 μg/ml or >60–80 μmol/L	Therapeutic: Toxic:	1.71–6.84 μmol/L >10–15 μg/ml or >17–26 μmol/L
Ethosuximide			Therapeutic: Toxic:	40–100 μg/ml or 283–708 μmol/L >150 μg/ml or >1062 μmol/L
Gentamicin	Less severe infection: Therapeutic:	5–8 μg/ml	Less severe: Therapeutic:	<1 μg/ml or <2.09 μ/mol/L
	Toxic:	>10–12 μg/ml or 21–25 μmol/L	Toxic:	>2–4 μg/mL or >4–8 μmol/L
Kanamycin	Therapeutic:	25–35 μg/ml or 52–72 μmol/L	Less severe: Therapeutic:	1–4 μg/mL or 2–8 μmol/L
	Toxic:	>35–40 μg/mL or 72–82 μmol/L	Toxic:	>10–15 μg/ml >21–31 μmol/L
Tobramycin	Less severe: Therapeutic:	5–8 μg/mL or 11–17 μmol/L	Less severe: Therapeutic:	<1 μg/ml or <2 μmol/L
	Toxic:	<10–12 μg/mL or 21–26 μmol/L	Toxic:	>2–4 μg/mL or >4–9 μmol/L

* Peak drug level refers to maximum drug concentration achieved following administration of a single dose. For a specific drug, both the concentration achieved and time interval between dosing and peak drug level required may vary considerably from patient to patient.
† Trough drug level refers to minimum drug concentration following administration of a single dose.

Drugs that can be monitored by serum levels include analgesics, tranquilizers, hypoglycemics, sedatives, antidepressants, antibiotics, anticonvulsants, antineoplastics, bronchodilators, cardiac drugs (Tables 6-2 and 6-3), and drugs of abuse. (Urine drug testing is explained in Chap. 3, *Urine Studies.*)

Indications for Testing

1. The drug source, dose, or regimen is changed.
2. Noncompliance (nonadherence) is suspected, and patient motivation to maintain medication is poor.
3. Physiologic status is altered by factors such as weight, menstrual cycle, body water, stress, age, and thyroid function.
4. Coadministered (multiple) drugs cause synergistic or antagonistic drug reaction.
5. Pathology that influences drug absorption and elimination, such as
   (a) Cardiovascular dysfunction
   (b) Liver clearance
   (c) Renal clearance (urinary output and *p*H)
   (d) Gastrointestinal/poor absorption
   (e) Altered plasma protein binding (or change in blood proteins that carry drug)
6. Some drugs have a very small safety range (therapeutic window).

Clinical Alert

1. Reliable clinical assessment of changes in patient's condition, and knowledge of drug interaction must be used to aid in the interpretation of test results.
2. The importance of sampling time in obtaining value therapeutic drug monitoring data cannot be understated. Whatever sampling procedure is used, such as *peak* or *maximum* concentration or *trough* or *minimum drug* concentration, it is important that the same time interval between sampling and dose administration be used consistently when comparing results from serial samples on the same patient.
3. *Elimination half-life* refers to time required to eliminate pain from the body and reduce by one-half the drug concentration in the body after the initial distribution phase is complete. Under certain conditions, elimination half-life dates are useful in estimating how long one should wait following initiation of therapy before sampling.
4. Factors influencing drug and chemical concentrations in living patients are frequently altered significantly after death.

Ethanol (Ethyl Alcohol)

Normal Values
None detected

Explanation of Test
The test, done to detect the presence of alcohol, is an indication of overdose and alcohol-impaired driving.

Procedure
1. A venous blood sample of 5 ml is obtained from the arm in living persons. From dead persons, take samples from the aorta.
2. A 20-ml sample of urine or gastric contents can be used.
3. Breath analyzer measures ethanol content at the end of expiration, following a deep inspiration.

Clinical Implications
1. At levels of 50 to 100 mg/dl, certain signs and symptoms are reported:
   (a) Flushing
   (b) Slowing of reflexes
   (c) Impaired visual acuity
2. At levels higher than 100 mg/dl, central nervous system depression is reported.
3. At levels higher than 400 mg/dl, death is reported.

Interfering Factors
Increased blood ketones, as in diabetic ketoacidosis, can falsely elevate blood or breath test results.

Clinical Alert

1. A value of greater than 300 mg/dl is a critical or panic value. Report and initiate overdose treatment at once.
2. Proper collection, handling, and storage of the blood alcohol specimen is essential when the question of sobriety is raised.

PROTEIN TESTS

Ceruloplasmin

Normal Values
Adults: 17–34 mg/dl or 229–431 mg/L
Neonate: slightly lower

Background
Ceruloplasmin is a protein that transports copper. About 95% of the copper in blood serum is normally in ceruloplasmin.

Explanation of Test
This measurement is a direct determination of copper in the blood serum. It should be determined in any person under age 30 with hepatitis, cirrhosis, hemolysis, or neurologic symptoms to attain early diagnosis and treatment of Wilson's disease.

Procedure
A venous blood sample of at least 5 ml is obtained. Place the specimen on ice or freeze.

Interfering Factors
1. Values are increased in the first trimester of pregnancy and in consumption of estrogen or birth control pills.
2. Values are decreased in newborns.

Clinical Implications
1. *Increased values* are associated with
   (a) Rheumatoid arthritis (will even give the blood greenish cast)
   (b) Biliary cirrhosis
   (c) Some infectious diseases
   (d) Thyrotoxicosis
   (e) Cancer
2. *Decreased levels* are associated with
   (a) Wilson's disease (in most cases). Decreased ceruloplasmin with increased copper occurs only in Wilson's disease in normal infants less than 6 months of age.
   (b) Menkes' steely-hair disease
   (c) Severe copper deficiency that accompanies long-term hyperalimentation and parenteral nutrition
   (d) Transient deficiencies in nephrosis, sprue, and kwashiorkor

---

Mucoproteins (Seromucoid)

Normal Values
83–203 mg/L
Average: 135 mg/L

Background
Mucoproteins are amino compounds whose action in the body is undetermined. It is known that in diseases such as cancer, infections, and inflammations, there is an increase of mucoproteins in the blood. In cancer, the more widespread the condition, the greater the increase in mucoproteins.

Explanation of Test

This test has its greatest value as a guide to the successful treatment of cancer, indicated by a decrease in mucoproteins and in the differential diagnosis of liver diseases.

Procedure

A venous blood sample of 10 ml is obtained.

Clinical Implications

A. *Increased levels* are found in
   1. Cancer
   2. Rheumatoid arthritis
   3. Infections
   4. Ankylosing spondylitis
B. *Decreased levels* are found in
   1. Infectious hepatitis
   2. Infectious cirrhosis

Proteins: Albumin and Globulin; A/G Ratio

Normal Values

Total protein: 6–8 g/dl or 60–80 g/L
Albumin: 3.8–5.0 g/dl or 38–50 g/L
Globulin: 2.3–3.5 g/dl or 23–35 g/L
Albumin–globulin ratio: greater than 1
Albumin–binding capacity: 91%–127%

Explanation of Test

Proteins and nucleic acids, the structural components of a cell, serve as biocatalysts (enzymes), regulators of metabolism (hormones), and preservers of genetic makeup (chromosomes). Amino acids are the building blocks of protein.

Much clinical information is obtained by examining and measuring proteins because of the involvement of proteins in so many functions. The three major catagories of protein are tissue or organ proteins, plasma proteins, and hemoglobin. Because of its large size, muscle mass provides the greatest amount of protein in conditions of deprivation. Tissue protein in muscle mass has the largest buffering capacity of the protein sites.

Plasma proteins serve as a source of nutrition for the body tissues and function in body buffering ability by combining with hemoglobin to exert an effect comparable to that of bicarbonate and other inorganic blood buffer systems.

Albumin and Albumin/Globulin Ratio

Albumin is a protein that is formed in the liver and that helps to maintain normal distribution of water in the body (colloidal osmotic pressure). It also helps in the transport of blood constituents such as ions, pigments, bilirubin, hormones, fatty acids, enzymes, and certain drugs. Approximately 52% to 60% of total protein is albumin; the rest is globulin, which functions in antibody formation, and other plasma protein (fibrinogen and prothrombin) functioning in coagulation.

Although the serum globulins function mainly as immunologic agents, they also play a part in maintaining the osmotic pressure of the blood; they are less effective than the serum albumin in this role because the globulin molecule is so much larger than the albumin molecule. Normally, the capillary walls are impermeable to the plasma protein, but in certain diseases the albumin will "seep through." The larger globulins, however, remain within the bloodstream and assume the major function in maintaining osmotic pressure. Because of the globulin's inability to function as effectively as the albumin, the osmotic pressure may be below normal, even though the total protein is retained at normal levels. Thus, the ratio of albumin to globulin becomes an important indicator of certain disease states, although a high ratio is usually clinically insignificant.

Albumin-Binding Capacity

The albumin-binding capacity (ABC) indicates the number of available bilirubin binding sites on albumin. The unconjugated bilirubin is carried in serum attached to albumin. Infants with elevated unconjugated bilirubin and a low ABC are more likely to develop kernicterus.

Procedure

A venous blood sample of at least 0.5 ml is obtained.

Clinical Implications

A. *Decreased albumin levels*
   1. Severe hypoalbuminemia is often associated with edema and decreased transport function such as hypocalcemia.
   2. Decreased albumin levels are caused by many different conditions
      (a) Inadequate iron intake
      (b) Severe liver diseases
      (c) Malabsorption
      (d) Diarrhea
      (e) Eclampsia
      (f) Nephrosis
      (g) Exfoliative dermatitis
      (h) Third-degree burns

(i) Starvation

(j) Excessive administration of IV glucose in water

B. *Increased albumin levels* are generally not observed.

C. *Increase in total protein* (hyperproteinemia)

1. Increase in total protein may be due to hemoconcentration as a result of dehydration from loss of body fluid and may occur in vomiting, diarrhea, wound drainage, or poor kidney function.

   (a) Both albumin and globulins increase in the same proportions so that the albumin/globulin ratio is unchanged.

   (b) This is the only instance in which an increase in albumin is found.

2. When the total protein increases and the albumin is unchanged or slightly decreased while globulins increase, the albumin/globulin ratio falls markedly.

   Caused by

   (a) Lupus erythematosus

   (b) Rheumatoid arthritis and other collagen diseases

   (c) Chronic infections

   (d) Liver disease

   (e) Multiple myeloma, sarcoidosis, and other malignant tumors

   (f) Bacterial pneumonia

   (g) Chronic alcoholism

   (h) Leukemia

   (i) Rheumatic fever

   (j) Shock

   (k) Tropical disease

   (l) Tuberculosis

D. *Decrease in total protein* (hypoproteinemia)

1. Associated with low albumin and small change in globulin, resulting in low albumin/globulin ratio.

2. Due to

   (a) Increased loss of albumin in urine

   (b) Decreased formation in liver

   (c) Insufficient protein intake

   (d) Severe hemorrhage when the plasma volume is replaced more rapidly than the protein level

3. Associated conditions

   (a) Severe liver disease

   (b) Malabsorption

   (c) Nephrotic syndrome

   (d) Diarrhea

   (e) Exfoliative dermatitis

   (f) Severe burns

   (g) Dilution of excessive IV administration of glucose in water

> **Note:** The liver is so crucial to protein metabolism that liver disease is frequently associated with alterations in proteins and disturbances of protein metabolism. For example, in undernutrition and liver disease, the albumin level may be decreased by inadequate synthesis.

E. *Decreased ABC*
   Infants below 50% should be considered for possible exchange transfusion.

Interfering Factors
1. Low levels of albumin occur normally in all trimesters of pregnancy.
2. Bromsulphalein may cause a false elevation. Therefore, a serum protein test should not be done within 48 hours following a Bromsulphalein test.
3. Drugs interfere with total protein levels.

Clinical Alert

Observe, report, and record signs and symptoms of possible accompanying edema or hypocalcemia (see tests for calcium, p. 272).

LIPOPROTEIN TESTS

The lipids are fat substances and consist mainly of cholesterol, cholesterol esters, triglycerides, nonesterified fatty acids, and phospholipids. Elevations of levels are due to excess intake and production or decreased catabolism. Lipoproteins are macromolecular complexes of unique plasma proteins, known as *apoproteins*, and lipids that serve in the plasma to transport otherwise insoluble lipids. The lipoproteins can be divided into groups based on density, flotation characteristics, and electrophoretic mobility. These groups are chylomicrons; beta lipoproteins (low-density lipoproteins [LDL]); prebeta lipoproteins (very-low-density lipoproteins [VLDL]); and alpha lipoproteins (very-high-density lipoproteins [HDL]). Body lipids provide energy for metabolism and serve as precursors of steroid hormones (adrenals, ovaries, and testes) and bile acids. They also play an important role in the making of cell membranes. A lipod profile will include cholesterol, triglycerides, LDL, and HDL.

Lipoprotein fractionation is the single most useful combination of procedures used to detect genetically determined disorders of lipid metabolism and to assess the risk of coronary artery disease.

Lipoprotein measurement is important in both hyper- and hypo-lipidemia. The different types of hyperlipidemia are classified as I, IIa, IIb, III, IV and V. In coronary heart disease and other cardiovascular disorders, two types are most important and most noted: type II with cholesterol elevated, triglycerides slightly elevated; and type IV with cholesterol normal, triglycerides elevated. Types of hypolipidemia are types I, II, and III, which are initially detected by low levels of cholesterol.

Clinical Alert

1. The LDLs and HDLs have a combined function. Low-density lipoproteins carry most of the cholesterol in the body from the liver to other parts of the body, whereas HDLs carry excess cholesterol back to the liver for removal from the body. Levels of LDL and HDL are influenced by numerous apolypoproteins, which are involved in transfer reactions. High levels of LDL are atherogenic, whereas high levels of HDL are protective.
2. Therapy for hyperlipidemia should always begin with diet, and whenever possible, dieticians should supervise the patient's diet. The American Heart Association has an excellent resource that explains the diet.

Cholesterol

Normal Values
Normal values vary with age, diet, and from country to country. An upper limit of 200 mg/dl is desirable; as the blood level rises, the risk of atherosclerosis and heart disease increases.

Desirable range: 140–220 mg/dl or 3.63–5.70 mmol/L
Child: 70–175 mg/dl or 1.81–4.53 mmol/L

Background
Cholesterol, existing in muscles, red blood cells, and cell membranes, is used by the body to form steroid hormones, bile acids, and most cell membranes. Chemically, cholesterol exists in both a free and esterized form (60%–75%) in the body. Much of the cholesterol ingested is esterized in the intestines, but because it is also synthesized in the liver, cholesterol is transported in the blood by the LDLs (60%–75%) and HDLs (15%–35%).

High levels of cholesterol are associated with atherosclerosis and increased risk of coronary artery disease. There is evidence that populations consuming a smaller amount of fats in their caloric intake (by eating vegetables rather than animal fats) have a lower cholesterol level and a lower incidence of atherosclerosis and coronary disease.

Explanation of Test
The main use of cholesterol testing is to detect disorders of blood lipids and to evaluate the risk potential for atherosclerosis related to coronary artery disease. Cholesterol will be elevated in the hereditary hyperlipoproteinemias. This test is also used as a secondary aid in the study of thyroid and liver functions.

Procedure
A fasting venous blood sample of 5 ml is obtained.

Clinical Implications
1. The total blood cholesterol level is the basis for initial patient classification for risk of coronary heart disease (CHD).
    (a) All blood cholesterol levels above 200 mg/dl should be confirmed by repeat measurements, with the *average* used to guide clinical decisions.
    (b) Other CHD risk factors should be taken into account in selecting appropriate follow-up measures for patients with borderline-high cholesterol levels.
    (c) All patients with a level of 240 mg/dl or above, which is classified as high blood cholesterol, should receive a lipoprotein analysis. Patients with borderline-high blood cholesterol levels (200–239 mg/dl), who in addition have definite CHD or two other CHD risk factors, should also have a lipoprotein analysis performed. (Lipoprotein analysis = cholesterol, triglycerides, HDL + LDL.)
    (d) CHD risk factors include
    (1) Male sex
    (2) Family history of premature CHD (definite myocardial infarction or sudden death before age 55 in a parent or sibling)
    (3) Cigarette smoking (currently smokes more than 10 cigarettes/day)
    (4) Hypertension
    (5) Low HDL-cholesterol concentration (below 35 mg/dl confirmed by repeat measurement)
    (6) Diabetes mellitus
    (7) History of definite cerebrovascular or occlusive peripheral vascular disease
    (8) Severe obesity ($\geq$30% overweight)
    (e) In public screening programs, all patients with a level above 200 mg/dl should be referred to their physician for remeasurement and evaluation.

2. Conditions related to elevated cholesterol
   (a) Cardiovascular disease and atherosclerosis
   (b) Type II, familial hypercholesterolemia
   (c) Obstructive jaundice (also an increase in bilirubin)
   (d) Hypothyroidism (decreased in hyperthyroidism)
   (e) Nephrosis
   (f) Xanthomatosis
   (g) Uncontrolled diabetes
   (h) Nephrotic syndrome
   (i) Obesity
3. *Decreased levels* of cholesterol
   (a) Instances when cholesterol is not absorbed from the GI tract
(1) Malabsorption	(5) Sepsis
(2) Liver disease	(6) Stress
(3) Hyperthyroidism	(7) Drug therapy such as
(4) Anemia	antibiotics

   (b) Other conditions related to decreased cholesterol levels
(1) Pernicious anemia	(5) Terminal stages of de-
(2) Hemolytic jaundice	bilitating diseases such
(3) Hyperthyroidism	as cancer
(4) Severe infections	(6) Hypolipoproteinemias

   (c) Esterol fraction decreases in liver diseases, liver cell injury, malabsorption syndrome, and malnutrition.

Clinical Alert

The higher the cholesterol/HDL ratio, the greater the possible risk of developing atherosclerosis.

Cholesterol/HDL-C Ratio

Risk Level	Men	Women
1/2 average	3.43	3.27
Average	4.97	4.44
2 × average	9.55	7.05
3 × average	23.99	11.04

LDL CHOL/HDL-C Ratio

Risk Level	Men	Women
1/2 average	1.00	1.47
Average	3.55	3.22
2 × average	6.25	5.03
3 × average	7.99	6.14

Interfering Factors

1. Cholesterol is normally slightly elevated in pregnancy.
2. Estrogen decreases plasma cholesterol and oophorectomy increases it.
3. Many drugs may cause a change in the blood cholesterol levels.

Patient Preparation

1. Instruct the patient about fasting overnight for 12 hours before the test.
2. Water is permitted.
3. Before fasting, the patient should be on a normal diet for 7 days before testing.
4. No alcohol should be consumed for 24 hours before testing.
5. Lipid-lowering drugs such as estrogen, oral contraceptives, and salicylates should be withheld.

Clinical Alert

1. If the patient breaks the fast or is unable to fast, notify the laboratory.
2. Once hyperlipidemia has been definitely identified, the diet should include a decreased amount of animal fats and replacement of saturated fats with polyunsaturated fats.
3. Elevated levels should be confirmed by a repeat test.
4. At least 6 months of dietary therapy should be carried out before initiating drug therapy.

High-Density Alpha-1-Fraction Lipoprotein (HDL) Cholesterol

Normal Values

Men: 35–70 mg/dl or 30–70 g/L or 0.91–1.81 mmol/L
Women: 35–85 mg/dl or 30–80 g/L or 0.91–2.20 mmol/L
Children: 30–65 mg/dl or 0.78–1.68 mmol/L

Background

High-density lipoprotein is the cholesterol carried by the alpha lipoproteins. A high level of alpha-1-HDL is an indication of a healthy metabolic system in a person free of liver disease or intoxication of any form. It is believed that the HDLs serve as carriers that remove cholesterol from the peripheral tissues and transport it back to the liver for catabolism and excretion. HDL probably also inhibits cellular uptake of LDLs. These two mechanisms help to explain how the HDLs produce a protection in relation to the risk of CHD.

Explanation of Test

This measurement is used to assess the risk of coronary artery disease and to monitor persons with known low levels of HDLs. It is known that low levels of HDL cholesterol are associated with increased risk for atherosclerotic disease of the coronary arteries of men and women of age 50 and older. It is also recognized that the level of HDL cholesterol can be raised in some people by increasing physical activity. Among healthy persons, those who are more physically active tend to have higher alpha-1-HDL cholesterol levels.

Procedure

A fasting venous blood sample of 5 ml is obtained.

Clinical Implications

1. *Increased values*
    (a) Levels higher than 100 mg are associated with a chronic liver disorder or some form of chronic intoxication
    (b) Increased HDL with long-term aerobic exercise (*e.g.*, long-distance runners have higher levels of HDL)
2. *Decreased values* are associated with
    (a) Increased risk for CHD when HDL cholesterol is less than 35 mg/dl
    (b) Familial high alphalipoproteinemia
    (c) Hyperthyroidism
    (d) End-stage liver disease
    (e) Diabetes
    (f) Obesity
    (g) Chronic inactivity
    (h) Various drugs (birth control pills)
    (i) Cigarette smoking
    (j) Hypertriglyceridemia
3. Levels can be either high or low in primary biliary cirrhosis, chronic hepatitis, or alcoholism.

Interfering Factors

1. Decreased HDL is associated with smokers.
2. Increased HDL is associated with the moderate intake of alcohol.
3. Iodine contrast substances interfere with test results.
4. Recent weight gains or losses can interfere with test results.

Patient Preparation

1. Advise the patient about the purpose of testing and that overnight (12 hours) fasting is required. Water is permitted.
2. If possible, all medication should be withheld for 24 to 48 hours before testing. Confer with the attending physician.

3. Ask the patient if there has been any drastic change in weight in the last few weeks before testing.

Patient Aftercare

Persons with decreased HDL can be counseled to take measures to increase levels by losing weight, cutting down on calorie consumption, eating less red meat, and taking lecithin supplements. Moderate alcohol consumption is believed by some to be a factor in increased HDL.

Very-Low-Density Lipoproteins (VLDL)
and Low-Density Lipoproteins (LDL)

Desirable Values

LDL concentration (mg/dl)	Classification for Age 20 + Years
<130	Desirable LDL cholesterol
130–159	Borderline-high risk LDL
160 and above	High-risk LDL cholesterol

Normal Values
VLDL cholesterol: 25%–50% or 0.25–0.50

Background
VLDL is a major carrier of triglyceride (60%–70% triglyceride, 10%–15% cholesterol). Degradation of VLDL leads to a major source of LDL. Circulating fatty acids are vitalized by the liver to form triglycerides that are packaged with apoprotein and cholesterol and exported into the blood as VLDLs.

The LDLs are the cholesterol-rich remnants of the lipid transport vehicle VLDL. Because LDL has a longer half-life (3–4 days) than its precursor, VLDL, LDL is more prevalent in the blood. It is finally catabolized in the liver and possibly in nonhepatic cells as well.

Explanation of Test
This test is specifically done to determine the risk of CHD. The LDLs are closely correlated with an increased incidence of atherosclerosis and CHD. On the other hand, a decreased incidence of CDH is seen in persons with high levels of HDL. The VLDL cholesterol concentration is expressed as a percent of total cholesterol.

Procedure
The LDL cholesterol level is calculated by using the following formula (Friedwald formula):

LDL cholesterol =
total cholesterol − HDL cholesterol − (triglyceride/5)

Clinical Implications
Increased LDL levels are caused by

1. Familial type II hyperlipidemia
2. The secondary causes are as follows:
   (a) Diet high in cholesterol and saturated fat
   (b) Hypothyroidism
   (c) Nephrotic syndrome
   (d) Multiple myoloma
   (e) Hepatic disease
   (f) Pregnancy
   (g) Porphyria
   (h) Diabetes
   (i) Various drugs

Increased VLDL levels are caused by

1. Familial type IV hyperlipidemia
2. The secondary causes are as follows:
   (a) Alcoholism
   (b) Obesity
   (c) Diabetes mellitus
   (d) Chronic renal disease
   (e) Pancreatitis
   (f) Pregnancy
   (g) Various drugs (estrogens-progestins, birth control pills)

Triglycerides

Normal Values
Men: desirable level is 40–160 mg/dl or 0.45–1.81 mmol/L
Women: 35–135 mg/dl or 0.40–1.53 mmol/L
Children: 30–138 mg/dl or 0.34–1.56 mmol/L

Values are age- and diet-related. Values in the first two decades of life are slightly lower than those in subsequent years. Values in women are about 10 mg/dl lower than in men.

Background
Triglycerides account for more than 90% of dietary intake and comprise 95% of the fat stored in tissues. Because they are insoluble in water, they are the main plasma glycerol ester. They are stored in adipose tissue as glycerol, fatty acids, and monoglyceroids. The liver reconverts them to triglycerides.

Explanation of Test
This test is used to evaluate patients with suspected atherosclerosis and is used as an indication of the body's ability to metabolize fat. Elevated triglycerides along with elevated cholesterol are risk factors in atherosclerotic disease. Because cholesterol and triglycerides can

vary independently, measurement of both values is more meaningful than the measurement of either substance alone.

Procedure

A venous blood sample of at least 5 ml is obtained. Notify the laboratory of the patient's age and sex.

Clinical Implications

1. *Increased triglyceride levels* are believed to be a factor in increased risk for atherosclerosis.
   (a) Increased levels occur in
      (1) Types I, IIb, III, IV, and V hyperlipoproteinemias
      (2) Liver disease
      (3) Nephrotic syndrome
      (4) Hypothyroidism
      (5) Poorly controlled diabetes
      (6) Pancreatitis
      (7) Glycogen storage disease
      (8) Myocardial infarction (increases may last 1 year)
      (9) Metabolic disorders related to endocrinopathies
   (b) Many of the clinical conditions that cause an increase in cholesterol levels also cause an increase in triglycerides.
      (1) Nephrotic syndrome   (3) Toxemia
      (2) Pancreatic dysfunction   (4) Hypothyroidism
2. *Decreased levels* occur in malnutrition and congenital alpha–beta lipoproteinemia.
   (a) Chronic obstructive pul-   (c) Hyperthyroidism
       monary disease   (d) Malnutrition
   (b) Brain infarction   (e) Malabsorption syndrome

Patient Preparation

1. Instruct the patient about fasting overnight for 12 hours before the test.
2. Water is permitted.
3. Before fasting, the patient should be on a normal diet.
4. No alcohol should be consumed for 24 hours before testing.

Interfering Factors

1. A transient increase will occur following a heavy meal or alcohol ingestion.
2. Increased values are also associated with pregnancy and oral contraceptives.

Patient Aftercare

A person with high triglyceride levels should be counseled that weight reduction, low fat diet, and an exercise program can be factors that will reduce levels.

Lipoprotein Electrophoresis

Normal Values
On 12–14 hour fasting specimen

Chylomicrons: 0

Beta or LDL: 28%–53% or 0.28–0.53   Mass fraction of total lipoprotein

Pre-beta or VLDL: 3%–32% or 0.03–0.32   Mass fraction of total lipoprotein

Alpha or HDL: 24%–40% or 0.24–0.40   Mass fraction of total lipoprotein

Plasma appearance: Clear

Note: Chylomicrons are proteins that are derived from dietary sources and can extend into the pre-beta area when significantly increased. The term was first applied in 1920 to the description of particles visible in lymph and plasma after the eating of fats. In hyperchylomicronemia, chylomicrons are present and represent dietary fat in transport. The standing plasma contains a cream layer over a clear layer in type I hyperlipidemia, where chylomicrons are elevated, but not in type IV, where both chylomicrons and triglycerides are elevated, causing turbidity of infranate.

Free Fatty Acids

Normal Values
Adult: 239–843 μEq/L or 8–25 mg/dl or 0.30–0.90 mmol/L
Child: <31 mg/dl or <1.10 mmol/L

Background
Free fatty acids are formed by the breakdown of lipoproteins and triglycerides. High levels of free fatty acids are usually cleaned from the blood by the liver and then converted into lipoproteins. All but 2% to 5% of blood serum fatty acids are esterified. The nonesterified or free fatty acids are protein-bound. The amount of free fatty acids and triglycerides in the blood is derived from dietary sources, fat deposits, or synthesized by the body. Carbohydrates can be converted to fatty acids and then stored in fat cells as triglycerides.

Explanation of Test
This measurement of a lipid fraction is helpful in determining the metabolism of fats and carbohydrates. The ratio of fatty acid and car-

bohydrate use is altered in situations associated with fat breakdown such as fasting. Unusually high levels will be found in untreated diabetics. It has been shown that the response of free fatty acids to treatment occurs more rapidly than the responses of blood sugar, plasma carbon dioxide, or excretion of ketones in the urine. The test is also used in the diagnosis of secondary hypoproteinemia. Disorders identified with excess fatty acids are usually associated with high levels of VLDLs.

Procedure
A fasting blood sample of 5 ml is obtained. Serum should be separated from cells within 45 minutes of drawing and frozen at once.

Clinical Implications
Increased values are associated with

1. Uncontrolled diabetes mellitus
2. Excessive release of a lipoactive hormone such as epinephrine, norepinephrine, glucagon, thyrotropin, and adrenocorticotropin.
3. Prolonged fasting or starvation (as much as three times normal).

Interfering Factors
1. Values are increased by exercise, anxiety, lowered body temperature, and a number of drugs.
2. Values are decreased by food intake and a number of drugs.

Fatty Acid Profile of Serum Lipids

Normal Values
Linoleate: >25% of fatty acid in serum lipids
Arachidonate: >6% of fatty acids in serum lipids
Phytanate (phytanic acid): no more than 0.3% of fatty acids in serum lipids
Palmitate: 18%–26% of fatty acids in serum lipids

Explanation of Test
Measurement of these specific fatty acids can be useful in monitoring nutritional status in cases of malabsorption, starvation, and long-term intravenous feedings. It is also indicated in the differential diagnosis of polyneuropathy when Refsum's disease is suspected. The enzyme that degrades phytanic acid is lacking in the rare, inherited Refsum's disease.

Procedure
A venous blood sample of at least 5 ml of serum is obtained.

Clinical Implications

Decreased values are associated with

1. Zinc deficiency disease (lineolate and arachidonate)
2. Refsum's disease with polyneuropathy (phytanate). A level of 0.8% strongly suggests Refsum's disease, but the test should be repeated for confirmation.
3. Malabsorption
4. Starvation
5. Long-term intravenous therapy

THYROID FUNCTION TESTS

Laboratory determinations of thyroid function are useful in distinguishing patients with euthyroidism from those with hyperthyroidism or hypothyroidism (see Table 6–4, "Tests of Thyroid Function" on p. 377). In general, the most useful laboratory tests to confirm or exclude hyperthyroidism are total thyroxine (T_4), the free thyroxine index, and total triiodothyronine (T_3). The most useful tests to detect hypothyroidism are total T_4, the free thyroxine index, and thyroid-stimulating hormone (TSH). A thyrotropin-releasing hormone (TRH) stimulation test can be valuable in establishing the thyroid status in some patients with equivocal signs of thyroid dysfunction and borderline laboratory values. It should be kept in mind that values obtained for the assessment of thyroid function can be influenced by factors other than disease such as age, current illness, binding capacity of serum proteins, and some drugs.

To understand the thyroid function tests, it is necessary to understand these basic concepts.

1. The function of the thyroid gland is to take iodine from the circulating blood, combine it with the amino acid tyrosine, and convert it to the thyroid hormones T_4 and T_3. Iodine comprises about two thirds of the weight of the thyroid hormones.
2. Another function of the thyroid gland is to store T_3 and T_4 until they are released into the bloodstream under the influence of TSH from the pituitary gland.
3. Only a small amount of the hormones is not bound to protein. However, it is the free portion of the thyroid hormones that is the true determinant of the thyroid status of the patient.

TABLE 6–4.
Tests of Thyroid Function

These findings are intended only as an aid in evaluating thyroid function. In most instances, these procedures are used to confirm clinical impressions gained from history and physical examination.

Condition	T_4	T_3	FT_4	TBG	T_3UR	TSH	TRH Stimulation TSH	TRH Stimulation T_3/T_4	Antibodies
Hypothyroidism									
Primary	L	L,N	L	N	L	H	+	0	0,+
Primary with T_3Rx (euthyroid)	L	N	L	N	L,N	N(L)			0
Primary with T_3Rx (euthyroid)	N,H	N	N,H	N	N,H	N(L)			0
Secondary (pituitary)	L	L,N	L	N	L	N(L)	0	0	
Tertiary (hypothalamic)	L	L,N	L	N	L	N(L)	+	+	
Hyperthyroidism									
Graves' disease	H	H	H	N	H	N(I)	0	0	+
T_3 toxicosis	N	H	N	N	N	N	0	0	
Thyrotoxicosis factitia									
Due to T_3	L	H	L	N	L,N	N(L)	0	0	0
Due to T_4	H	N	H	N	N,H	N(L)	0	0	0
Hashimoto's thyroiditis	V	V	V	N	V	V	V	0	+++
Pregnancy, estrogens									
Excess TBG (euthyroid) hereditary	H	H	N	H	L	N			0
Androgens, steroids (high doses)									
Low TBG (euthyroid) hereditary	L	L	N	L	H	N			0
Nephrosis, cirrhosis	L	L	N	L	H	N	+	+	0
Diphenylhydantoin, salicylates (large doses)	L	L	N	N	H	N	+	+	0
X-ray contrast media	N	N	N	N	N	N	+	+	0

H, high; N, normal; L, may be low; +, responds or present; 0, no response or absent; V, variable.
(Adopted from Bio-Science Handbook, 12th ed. Van Nuys, CA, Bio-Science Laboratories, 1979, p. 52)

Calcitonin

Normal Values
Basal
Men: ≤19 pg/ml or ng/L
Women: ≤14 pg/ml or ng/L

Calcium infusion (2.4 mg of calcium/kg)
Men: ≤190 pg/ml or ng/L
Women: ≤130 pg/ml or ng/L

Pentagastrin injection (0.5 μg/kg)
Men: ≤110 pg/ml or ng/L
Women: ≤35 pg/ml or ng/L

Background
Calcitonin is a hormone secreted by the C cells or parafollicular cells of the thyroid gland. The main action of this hormone is to inhibit bone resorption by regulating the number and activity of osteoblasts. Calcitonin is secreted in direct response to high blood calcium levels and may prevent abrupt changes in calcium levels and the excessive loss of calcium.

Explanation of Test
This test is used in the differential diagnosis of cancer of the thyroid. Levels will be increased in medullary carcinoma (malignant C cell tumors), occasionally in patients with other tumors, and in some instances of renal failure.

Procedure
Two fasting specimens of 10 ml of venous blood are obtained.

Clinical Implications
1. *Increased levels* are associated with
   (a) Medullary thyroid cancers
   (b) C cell hyperplasia
   (c) Chronic renal failure
   (d) Pernicious anemia
   (e) Zollinger–Ellison syndrome
   (f) Cancer of lung, breast, and pancreas
2. In a small proportion of patients who do have medullary cancer, the fasting level of calcitonin is normal. In these instances, a provocative test using calcium or pentagastrin should be followed by an abnormally large increase in calcitonin levels.

Procedure
1. A pentagastrin injection is administered. Blood samples are drawn before the injection and 1.5 and 5 minutes after the injection.
2. Another method is to infuse calcium (2.4 mg/kg) over a 4-hour period and collect blood samples before infusion and again at 3 to 4 hours.

Interfering Factors
Levels are normally *increased* in

1. Pregnancy at term
2. Newborns

Clinical Alert

1. Screening of families of patients with proven medullary cancer of the thyroid is recommended because the tumor has both sporadic and familial incidence.
2. Also, if the stimulus test is normal in family members, it is advisable to repeat the calcium provocative test periodically.

Patient Preparation
1. Explain the purpose and procedure of the test.
2. Advise the patient to fast from food overnight. Water is permitted.

Free Thyroxine T$_4$ (FT$_4$)

Normal Values
0.8–2.4 ng/dl or 10.3–31.0 pmol/L
For patients on Synthyroid, up to 5.0 ng/dl

Background
Free thyroxine T$_4$ comprises a small fraction of the total thyroxine. The free T$_4$ is available to the tissues and is the metabolically active form of this hormone.

Explanation of Test
This is a measurement of that fraction (about 5%) of the circulatory thyroxine T$_4$ that exists in a free state, unbound to protein. It is commonly done to determine thyroid status, to rule out hypo- and hyperthyroidism, and to evaluate thyroid replacement therapy. This test has diagnostic value in situations in which total hormone levels do not correlate with the thyrometabolic state, and there is no reason to suspect an abnormality in binding protein levels. However, it is also a useful test when there are definite or probable abnormalities in binding levels. Demonstration of the free T$_4$ provides a more accurate picture of the thyroid status in persons with abnormal thyroxine binding globulin levels in pregnancy and in those who are receiving estrogens, hydrogens, phenytoin, and salicylates.

Procedure
A venous blood sample of at least 5 ml is obtained. Accurate results can be obtained in as little as 0.5 ml for pediatric cases.

Interfering Factors
1. Values are increased in infants at birth. This value rises even higher after 2 to 3 days of life.
2. Free T_4 levels are decreased in adolescents as compared to adults.
3. Heparin will cause falsely elevated values.

Clinical Implications
1. *Increased levels* are associated with
    (a) Graves' disease
    (b) Thyrotoxicosis due to T_4
2. *Decreased levels* are associated with
    (a) Primary hypothyroidism
    (b) Secondary hypothyroidism (pituitary)
    (c) Tertiary hypothyroidism (hypothalamic)
    (d) Thyrotoxicosis due to T_3
3. *Levels can be slightly elevated* in
    (a) Severe illness in nonthyroid disease
    (b) Cirrhosis of liver
4. *Values will be normal* in
    (a) T_3 toxicosis
    (b) Pregnancy
    (c) Nephrosis
    (d) Cirrhosis
    (e) Use of preceding radiographic contrast media
    (f) Use of drugs such as androgens, steroids (high doses), diphenylhydantoin, and salicylates (high doses), and estrogens

---

Free Triiodothyronine T_3 (FT$_3$)

Normal Values
Adult: 230–660 pg/dl or 3.54–10.16 pmol/L
Newborn: 390–430 pg/dl

Background
Free hormones are the best indicators of thyroid function. However, experts disagree on the selection of free T_3 versus the use of free T_4.

Explanation of Test
This is one of the determinations used in the evaluation of thyroid function and is a measure of that fraction of the circulatory T_3 that exists in the free state in the blood, unbound to protein. It is done to rule out T_3 toxicosis, hypothyroidism, and hyperthyroidism; to determine thyroid status; and to evaluate thyroid replacement therapy.

Procedure
A venous blood sample of at least 5 ml is obtained.

Interfering Factors

Significant quantities of radioactivity in the blood of the patient can result in serious errors. For this reason, the laboratory should be informed if the patient has recently received radioactive material.

Clinical Implications

1. *Increased values* are associated with hyperthyroidism and T$_3$ toxicosis.
2. *Decreased values* are associated with
   (a) Hypothyroidism (primary and secondary)
   (b) Nephrosis

Free Thyroxine Index (FTI) (T$_7$ Calculation)

Normal Values

Adult: 5.0–12.0 (these are arbitrary units)
Child: 5.5–10.0

Explanation of Test

This index is a simple mathematical calculation used to correct the estimated total thyroxine (T$_4$) for the amount of thyroxine binding globulin (TBG) present. To perform this calculation, two results are needed: the T$_4$ value and the T$_3$ uptake ratio. The product of these two members is the free thyroxine index (FTI). The FTI is useful in the diagnosis of hyper- and hypothyroidism, especially in patients with known or suspected abnormalities in thyroxine binding protein levels. In such cases, blood levels and clinical signs may seem contradictory unless both T$_4$ and TBG are considered as interrelated parameters of thyroid status. Measurement of the free T$_4$ also gives a more accurate picture of the thyroid status when the TBG is abnormal in pregnant women or those persons who are being treated with estrogen, androgens, phenytoin, or salicylates.

Procedure

Mathematical computation of T$_3$ uptake $\times$ T$_4$ = FTI.

Clinical Implications

Application of the equation of the FTI includes the following:

Status	TBG	T$_3$ Uptake	$\times$	T$_4$	=	FTI
Euthyroid	Normal	1.0		9.0		9.0
Euthyroid	Low	1.5		4.0		6.0
Euthyroid	High	0.6		16.0		9.6
Hypothyroid	High	0.7		4.0		2.8
Hyperthyroid	Low	1.3		13.0		16.9

Neonatal Thyrotropin-Releasing Hormone (TRH)

Normal Values
Normal adult: 5–60 pg/ml
Newborn: 30 minutes after delivery—78 pg/ml, dropping to normal by
  24 hours

Background
Neonatal primary hypothyroidism is characterized not only by low T_4
levels in blood serum but also by elevated thyrotropin-releasing hormone (TRH) levels (so as to differentiate from TSH test).

Explanation of Test
This measurement is best used as a confirmatory test for infants with
positive T_4 screens or low blood serum T_4 levels. Although TRH measurement has been suggested as the primary screening test for neonatal
hypothyroidism, infants with secondary (hypothalamic or hypopitui-
tary) hypothyroidism, which constitutes about 10% of all neonatal hypothyroid cases, would be missed in such a screening system.

Procedure
1. The skin is cleansed with an antiseptic, and the infant's heel is
   punctured with a sterile disposable lancet.
2. If bleeding is slow, it is helpful to hold the leg dependent for a short
   time before spotting the blood on the filter paper.
3. The circles on the filter paper must be completely filled. This can
   best be done by placing one side of the filter paper against the
   infant's heel and watching for the blood to appear on the front side
   of the paper and completely fill the circle.
4. Air dry for 1 hour, fill in all requested information, and send to the
   laboratory immediately.

Instruction to Mother
Inform the mother about the purpose of the test and the method of
collecting the specimens.

Clinical Implications
A positive test is associated with neonatal hypothyroidism.

Neonatal Thyroxine (T_4); Neonatal
Screen for Hypothyroidism

Alert Limits
1–5 days: ≤4.9 μg/dl equivalent
6–8 days: ≤4 μg/dl equivalent

9–11 days: ≤3.5 μg/dl equivalent
12–120 days: ≤3 μg/dl equivalent

Alert limits are defined as T_4 values that suggest hypothyroidism. A follow-up TSH paper test is advised in these cases.

Background
Normal brain growth and development cannot take place without adequate thyroid hormone. Congenital hypothyroidism (cretinism) is characterized by low levels of T_4 and elevated levels of TSH.

Explanation of Test
This is a screening test of thyroxine (T_4) activity to detect neonatal hypothyroidism. It can be used in infants aged 1 to 120 days. However, specimens should be obtained after the first 24 hours of life, preferably within the first week. Thyroxine is obtained from whole blood spotted on paper using a radioimmune assay technique.

Procedure
1. The skin is cleansed with an antiseptic, and the infant's heel is punctured with a sterile disposable lancet.
2. If bleeding is slow, it is helpful to hold the leg dependent for a short time before spotting the blood on the filter paper.
3. The circles on the filter paper must be completely filled. This can best be done by placing one side of the filter paper against the infant's heel and watching for the blood to appear on the front side of the paper and completely fill the circle.
4. Air dry for 1 hour, fill in all requested information, and send to the laboratory immediately.

Instructions to Mother
Inform the mother about the purpose of the test and the method of collecting the specimens.

Clinical Implications
A positive test is associated with hypothyroidism.

Clinical Alert
1. Do not interpret this test in terms of the blood serum T_4 values. This is an entirely different procedure using a different type of specimen.
2. Notify the attending physician and the mother of positive results within 24 hours.

Thyroglobulin (Tg)

Normal Values
<50 ng/ml

Background
Tg is present in normal blood and is composed of glycoprotein and the iodinated secretions of epithelial cells of the thyroid. These iodinated secretions contain both the precursors of T_4 and T_3 and these hormones themselves.

Explanation of Test
This test is helpful in the diagnosis of differentiated cancer of thyroid and hyperthyroidism. It is used to follow the course of patients with known differentiated or metastatic thyroid cancer. Levels will decrease following initial treatment, and in recurrence of metastasis, the level will again rise.

Procedure
A venous blood sample of 5 ml is obtained.

Clinical Implications
1. *Increased levels* are associated with
   (a) Untreated and metastatic differentiated thyroid cancers (elevated Tg in pleural effusions has been used as an indication of metastasis to the lungs)
   (b) Hyperthyroidism
   (c) Subacute thyroiditis (some cases)
   (d) Benign adenoma (some cases)
2. A correlation between elevated Tg levels and goiter size has been reported in nontoxic nodular growths.

Thyroid-Stimulating Hormone (TSH)

Normal Values
Adult: 0.5–6 milliIU/L
Neonate: 3–20 μIU/L by day 3 of life for both serum and spot test

Background
The thyroid is unique among the endocrine glands because it has a large store of hormone and a slow rate of normal turnover. Stimulation of the thyroid gland by the TSH, which is produced by the anterior pituitary gland, will cause the release and distribution of stored thyroid hormones. The TSH is also influenced by the parathyroid, which produces TRH. When T_4 and T_3 are too high, TSH secretion decreases.

When T_4 and T_3 are too low, TSH secretion increases. In primary hypothyroidism, TSH levels rise because of the low levels of thyroid hormone. If the pituitary fails in its function, TSH is not secreted, blood levels fall, and the thyroid becomes quiescent.

Explanation of Test
This measurement is used in the diagnosis of primary hypothyroidism when there is thyroid gland failure due to intrinsic disease, and it is used to differentiate primary from secondary hypothyroidism by determining the actual circulatory level of TSH. In principle, it is the same as the neonatal T_4 test. It is not the same measurement as the TSH stimulation test, in which the thyroid uptake of radioiodine is measured before and after the injection of TSH.

Procedure
A venous sample of at least 1 ml is obtained and measured by the radioimmune assay method.

Clinical Implications
1. *Increased levels* are seen in adults and neonates with primary hypothyroidism.
2. *Decreased levels* are associated with
   (a) Hyperthyroidism
   (b) Secondary and tertiary hypothyroidism

Interfering Factors
1. Values are normally high in neonatal cord blood. There is hypersecretion of TSH in newborns up to two to three times normal. The TSH level returns to normal by 14 days of life.
2. Values are suppressed during treatment with T_3, aspirin, corticosteroids, and heparin.
3. Values are abnormally increased during drug therapy with lithium, potassium iodide, and TSH injection.

Thyrotropin-Releasing Hormone (TRH) Stimulation Test

Normal Values
TSH should increase approximately two times baseline and is usually greater in women than in men.

Thirty Minutes After Stimulation
Child: 11–35 pIU/ml
Adult man: 15–30 pIU/ml
Adult woman: 20–40 pIU/ml

Background

The hypothalamus produces TRH, and the pituitary gland secretes TSH in response. Hypothalamic failure with lack of TRH leads to reduced thyroid function.

Explanation of Test

This test is done to assess the responsiveness of the anterior pituitary gland and to differentiate between the three types of hypothyroidism: primary, secondary, and tertiary. When TRH is injected, a rise in TSH indicates that the pituitary gland is functioning.

Procedure

1. A 400- to 500-μg bolus of TRH is given intravenously
   (a) Adult dose: 400–500 μg
   (b) Child dose: 7 μg/kg
2. Blood samples are obtained at intervals, and the TSH level is measured. The maximum response usually occurs in 20 minutes.
3. Check with your laboratory for specific procedures.

Clinical Implications

1. The TSH level shows a very slight increase or no response in hyperthyroidism.
2. In hypothyroidism, differing responses will be seen in the types of hypothyroidism.
   (a) In primary (thyroid gland failure), there is an increase of two or more times the normal response.
   (b) In secondary (anterior pituitary failure), there is no response.
   (c) In tertiary (hypothalamic failure), the TSH rises after a delay. Multiple injections of TRH may be necessary to induce the appropriate TSH response.

Thyroxine-Binding Globulin (TBG)

Normal Values

10–25 μg/dl or 100–250 μg/L as T_3 binding capacity
Total adult: 1.5–3.4 mg/dl or 15–34 mg/L
Child: 2.9–5.4 mg/dl or 29–54 mg/L

Background

Almost all of the thyroid hormones in the blood are bound to protein. These thyroxine-binding proteins play an important role in regulating the free FT_4. TBG is by far the most important determinant of the overall binding of T_4. For this reason, a measure of TBG is a good approximation of the thyroxine-binding function of the blood.

Explanation of Test

This measurement is useful in determining congenital excess or deficit of TBG and in confirming abnormalities of thyroxine-binding proteins suggested by the results of the T_3 uptake ratio. This measurement is the old T_3 test. When the TBG and T_4 are performed on the same blood sample, an accurate assessment of the state of thyroid function can be ascertained.

Procedure

A 2-ml specimen of venous blood is obtained.

Clinical Implications

1. *The TBG level is increased* in
   (a) Hypothyroidism
   (b) Pregnancy (in some sponta-neous aborters, the TBG level is not elevated)
   (c) Estrogen therapy
   (d) Oral contraceptives
   (e) Genetic and idiopathic hepatic disease
   (f) Prolonged perphenazine therapy
   (g) Acute intermittent por-phyria
2. *The TBG level is decreased* in
   (a) Nephrotic syndromes
   (b) Marked hypoproteinemia
   (c) Genetic and idiopathic liver disease
   (d) Uncompensated acidosis
   (e) Acromegaly
3. *The thyroxine prealbumin (TBPA) level is decreased* in
   (a) Thyrotoxicosis
   (b) Severe illness or trauma
   (c) Surgery
   (d) Parturition

Interfering Factors

Drugs may cause both increased and decreased levels.

Thyroid-Stimulating Immunoglobulins (TSI)

Normal Values

Present in only 5% of healthy people; 0–10 U/L; positive: >15 U/L

Background

Long-acting thyroid stimulator (LATS) is classified as a heterogeneous group of immunoglobulins and does not appear to have its origin in the pituitary gland. This factor has a longer-acting effect than the TSH and is found in the blood of some hyperthyroid patients. Renamed *thyroid-stimulating immunoglobulins* (TSI), these proteins can be now chemi-cally quantitated.

Explanation of Test

This test is very important in the evaluation of any person with thyroid disease, especially in identifying persons with malignant exophthalmos and Graves' disease.

Procedure

A venous blood sample of 5 ml is obtained. Notify the laboratory if iodine-131 has been administered within the past 48 hours. Serum must be frozen.

Clinical Implications

Increased levels are associated with

(a) Graves' disease, primary hyperthyroidism
(b) Persons prone to relapse of hyperthyroidism (used to follow treatment of Graves' disease)

Thyroxine; Total T_4

Normal Values

Adult: 5–12.5 μg/dl or 65–155 nmol/L
Child: 7.3–15 μg/dl or 94–194 nmol/L

Background

Thyroxine is the thyroid hormone that contains four atoms of iodine. Approximately 95% of thyroxine is bound to TBG as well as prealbumin and albumin. About 5% of the circulating T_4 is in the free or unbound portion.

Explanation of Test

Thyroxine is one of the thyroid panel tests used in the evaluation of thyroid function. It is a direct measurement of the concentration of T_4 in the blood serum. The measurement of total T_4 level is a good index of thyroid function when the TBG is normal. The increase in TBG levels normally seen in pregnancy and with estrogen therapy will increase the total T_4 levels. The decrease of TBG levels in persons receiving anabolic steroids, in chronic liver disease, and in nephroses will decrease the total T_4 value. This test is done commonly to rule out hyperthyroidism and hypothyroidism. The T_4 test also can be used as a guide in establishing and following maintenance doses of thyroid in the treatment of hypothyroidism. In addition, it also can be used in hyperthyroidism to follow the results of antithyroid drugs.

Procedure

A venous blood sample of at least 5 ml is obtained. If the patient is already receiving thyroid treatment, it must be stopped 1 month before the test to obtain a true picture of T_4. If a radioimmunoassay procedure is used in the laboratory, it is reported as T_4-RIA.

Interfering Factors

1. Total thyroxine levels increase during the second or third month of pregnancy as a result of increased estrogen production.
2. Values also are increased with the use of drugs such as estrogens and antiovulants.

Clinical Implications

1. *Values can be increased* in
   (a) Hyperthyroidism
   (b) Acute thyroiditis
   (c) Subacute thyroiditis
   (d) Hepatitis, early in disease (normal by 4 weeks)
2. *Values can be decreased* in
   (a) Cretinism
   (b) Myxedema
   (c) Hypothyroidism
   (d) Chronic thyroiditis (usually)
   (e) Subacute thyroiditis
   (f) Simmonds' disease
   (g) Nephrosis
   (h) Cirrhosis
   (i) Hypoproteinemia
   (j) Malnutrition

   The magnitude of decrease in values parallels the decrease in thyroid function. Therefore, lower values will occur in cretinism and myxedema than in mild hypothyroidism.
3. There is no typical androgen cancer of thyroid.
4. Values are usually normal in T_3 toxicosis.

Note: A thyroid panel usually consists of

1. T_3V
2. T_3-RIA
3. Free T_4 test
4. T_4-RIA (total T_4)
5. FTI

Triiodothyronine (T₃) by Radioimmunoassay (T₃-RIA)

Normal Values

Adult: 120–195 ng/dl or 1.86–3.00 nmol/L
Child: 90–240 ng/dl or 1.39–3.70 nmol/L

Background

T_3 has three atoms of iodine as compared with four atoms in T_4. T_3 is more active metabolically than T_4, but its effect is shorter. There is much less T_3 than T_4 in the serum, and it is bound less firmly to thyroid-binding globulin.

Explanation of Test

The measurement of T_3 is a quantitative determination of the total T_3 concentration in the blood and is the test of choice in the diagnosis of T_3 thyrotoxicosis. It is not the same as the T_3 uptake test that measures the unsaturated TBC in serum. It can also be very useful in the diagnosis of hyperthyroidism. T_3 thyrotoxicosis refers to a variant of hyperthyroidism in which a thyrotoxic patient will have elevated T_3 values and normal T_4 values. It is of limited value in diagnosing hypothyroidism.

Procedure

A venous blood sample of at least 5 ml is obtained.

Clinical Implications

1. *Increased values* are associated with
   (a) Hyperthyroidism
   (b) T_3 thyrotoxicosis
   (c) Daily dosage of 25 μg or more of T_3
   (d) Acute thyroiditis
   (e) Idiopathic TBG elevation
   (f) Daily dosage of 300 μg or more of T_4
2. *Decreased values* are associated with
   (a) Hypothyroidism (however, some clinically hypothyroid patients will have normal levels)
   (b) Starvation
   (c) Idiopathic TBG decrease
   (d) Acute illness

Interfering Factors

1. Values are increased in pregnancy and with the use of drugs such as estrogens and antiovulatory compounds.
2. Values are decreased in the use of drugs such as anabolic steroids, androgens, large doses of salicylates, and phenytoin.

Triiodothyronine Uptake Ratio (T_3UR, T_3UP)

Normal Values

0.8–1.30, which is a ratio between patient specimen and the standard control.

25%–35% uptake

Explanation of Test

This test is an indirect measurement of the unsaturated thyroxine-binding globulin (UTBG) in the blood. This determination is expressed in arbitrary terms and is inversely proportional to the TBG. For this reason, low T_3UR levels are indicative of situations that result in elevated levels of UTBG. For example, in hypothyroidism, when insufficient T_4 is available to produce saturation of TBG, UTBG is elevated and the T_3UR values are low. Similarly, in pregnant patients or those receiving estrogen, TBG levels are increased proportionately more than are T_4 levels, resulting in high levels of UTBG, which are reflected in low T_3UR results.

Clinical Implications
1. *Increased levels* are associated with
   (a) Hyperthyroidism
   (b) Nephrosis
   (c) Severe liver disease
   (d) Metastatic malignancy
   (e) Pulmonary insufficiency
   (f) Thyroxine and desiccated thyroid therapy
2. *Decreased levels* are associated with
   (a) Hypothyroidism
   (b) Normal pregnancy
   (c) Hyperestrogenic status
   (d) Triiodothyronine treatment for hypothyroidism
   (e) Propylthiouracil treatment for hyperthyroidism

Procedure
A venous blood sample of at least 2 ml is obtained.

Interfering Factors
1. *Decreased levels* occur in normal pregnancy and when estrogens and antiovulatory drugs are used.
2. *Increased levels* occur with drugs such as dicumarol, heparin, androgens, anabolic steroids, phenytoin, and large doses of salicylates.

> **Clinical Alert**
>
> This test has nothing to do with the actual T_3 blood level in spite of its name, which is sometimes confusingly abbreviated to the T_3 test. It is emphasized that the T_3 UR and the true T_3 (T_3 by RIA) are entirely different tests. The T_3 UR gives only an indirect measurement of overall binding.

BIBLIOGRAPHY

American Diabetes Association: The Physician's Guide to Type II Diabetes (NIDDM): Diagnosis and Treatment. New York, American Diabetes Association, 1984

Baines AD: Hormones and hypertension: Update in laboratory medicine. Ann Roy Coll Physicians Surgeons Can 21:95, 1988

Bauer D, Ditto W: Interpretation in Therapeutic Drug Monitoring. Chicago, American Society of Pathologists, 1981

Bauer JD: Clinical Laboratory Methods, 9th ed. St. Louis, CV Mosby, 1982

Berkow R (ed): Merck Manual of Diagnosis and Therapy, 14th ed. Rahway, NJ, Merck Sharp & Dohme, 1982

Blair ER et al (eds): Damon Clinical Laboratories Handbook. Stow, OH, Damon Corp., Lexi-Comp., 1989

Cello JP: Diagnostic approaches to jaundice. Hosp Pract 17(2):49–60, 1982

Cohen JA, Pantaleo N, Shell W: A message from the heart: What isoenzymes can tell you about your cardiac patient. Nursing 12(4):46–49, 1982

Damon Corp.: Clinical Laboratories Handbook. Stow, OH, Damon Corp., Damon Corp., Lexi-Comp, 1989

Goedeke Norris MK: Lab test tips—Assessing elevated potassium values. Nursing 91 21(1):31, Jan 1991

Grundy IM: The place of HDL in cholesterol management. Arch Intern Med 149:505–510, Mar, 1989

Hahn K: Clinical do's and don'ts: Testing blood glucose levels. Nursing 1989 19(12):66, Dec 1989

Hamilton AD et al: The introduction of a quality assessment schema for extra laboratory blood glucose analyses. Diabetic Med 6(5):444–447, Jul 1989

Heller JE: Prostatic acid phosphatase: Its current clinical status. J Urol 137:1091, 1987

Henry JB (ed): Todd, Sanford, Davidsohn: Clinical Diagnoses and Management by Laboratory Methods, 18th ed. Philadelphia, WB Saunders, 1990

Jacobs, DS et al: Laboratory Test Handbook. St. Louis, CV Mosby and Lexi-Comp., 1984

Kaplan MM: Clinical and laboratory assessment of thyroid abnormalities. Med Clin North Am 69:863, 1985

Kaye S: The collection and handling of the blood alcohol specimen. Am J Clin Pathol 74:743–746, 1980

Larson N: Manual of Endocrinology and Metabolism. Boston, Little, Brown & Co., 1986

Leavelle DE (ed): Mayo Medical Laboratories Interpretive Handbook. Rochester, MN, Mayo Medical Laboratories, 1990

MacMillan KM et al: Implementation of a successful bedside capillary blood glucose monitoring program by registered nurses in an acute care facility. Diabetes Ed 14(4):308–312, Jul/Aug 1988

Marchand A et al: The lab's role in cholesterol management. MLO 21(3):37–39, 42–45, Mar 1989

Moss DW: Diagnostic aspects of alkaline phosphatase and its isoenzymes. Clin Biochem 20:225, 1987

Munn NE: When the bile duct is blocked. RN 52(1):50–56, January 1989

National Cholesterol Education Program Report: NIH Publication No. 88–2920. U.S. Department of Health and Human Services, 1988

Ravel R: Clinical Laboratory Medicine: Clinical Application of Laboratory Data, 5th ed. Chicago, Year Book Medical Pub, 1989

Sacher RA, McPherson RA (eds): Widmann's Clinical Interpretation of Laboratory Tests, 10th ed. Philadelphia, FA Davis, 1991

Sunshine I: Preliminary tests for drugs of abuse. Clin Chem 34:331, 1988

Tabakoff B et al: Differences in platelet enzyme activity between alcoholics and non-alcoholics. N Engl J Med 318(3): 134, 1988

Tietz NW (ed): Clinical Guide to Laboratory Tests, 2nd ed. Philadelphia, WB Saunders, 1990

Tressler KM: Clinical Laboratory and Diagnostic Tests. Significance and Nursing Implications, 2nd ed. Norwalk, CT, Appleton and Lange, 1988

Wallach J: Interpretation of Diagnostic Tests, 4th ed. Boston, Little Brown & Co, 1986

MICROBIOLOGIC STUDIES

Introduction

Diagnostic Testing and Microbial Flora

Microorganisms in diagnostic testing are known as *pathogens*. The word *pathogenic* is usually defined as "causing infectious disease"; however, organisms that are pathogenic at certain times may reside in or on the human body at other times without causing disease. When these organisms are indeed present without causing harm to the host, they are considered *commensals*. But once they begin to multiply excessively and cause tissue damage, they are regarded as pathogens, for they will then have the potential for increasing pathogenicity (Table 7-1).

TABLE 7–1.

Pathogens Detectable in Body Tissue and Fluid by Diagnostic Methods

Nasopharynx	Sputum	Feces
Beta-hemolytic streptococci	*Blastomyces dermatitidis*	*Candida albicans*
Bordetella pertussis	*Bordetella pertussis*	*Campylobacter fetus*
Candida albicans	*Candida albicans*	*Clostridium botulinum*
Corynebacterium diphtheriae	*Coccidioides immitis*	*Entamoeba histolytica*
Hemophilus influenzae (large counts)	Hemolytic streptococci	*Escherichia coli* (in infants)
Meningococci	*Hemophilus influenzae*	*Mycobacterium tuberculosis*
Pneumococci (large counts)	*Histoplasma capsulatum*	*Proteus*
Staphylococcus aureus	*Klebsiella* species	*Pseudomonas* (large counts)
	Mycobacterium tuberculosis	*Salmonella*
	Yersinia pestis	*Shigella*
	Francisella tularensis	*Staphylococci*
	Pneumococci	*Vibrio cholerae*
	Staphylococcus aureus	*Vibrio comma*
	Mycoplasma species	*Vibrio parahaemolyticus*
	Eikenella corrodens	*Yersinia enterocolitica*
		Clostridium difficile

Urine	Skin	Ear
Beta-hemolytic streptococci, groups B & D	*Bacteroides* species	*Aspergillus fumigatus*
Coliform bacilli (100,000 count or more) including *Escherichia coli*, *Klebsiella*, *Enterobacter-Serratieae*	*Clostridium*	*Candida albicans* and other fungi
	Coliform bacilli	Coliform bacilli
	Fungi	Hemolytic streptococci
	Proteus	*Proteus* species
	Pseudomonas	Pneumococci (*Streptococcus pneumoniae*)
	Staphylococcus aureus	
	Streptococcus pyogenes	

(continued)

TABLE 7–1.
(Continued)

Urine	Skin	Ear

Enterococci
  *Streptococcus
  faecalis)*
Gonococci *(Neisseria
  gonorrhoeae)*
Klebsiella, positive and
  negative indole
*Mycobacterium
  tuberculosis*
Proteus species
*Pseudomonas
  aeruginosa*
Staphylococci, positive
  and negative
  coagulase
Staphylococcus aureus
*Staphylococcus sapro-
  phyticus*
Salmonella and *Shigella*
  species
Trichomonas vaginalis
*Candida albicans and
  other yeasts*
		*Pseudomonas
		  aeruginosa
		Staphylococcus aureus*

Cerebrospinal Fluid	Vaginal Discharge	Urethral Discharge

*Acinetobacter
  calcoaceticus
Bacteroides* species
*Brucella abortus
Coliform bacilli
Cryptococcus neoformans
Hemophilus influenzae
Leptospira* species
*Mycobacterium
  tuberculosis
Neisseria meningitidis*
Pneumococci,
  streptococcus
  pneumonia
*Pseudomonas
Staphylococci
Streptococci
Toxoplasma gondii
Viruses and fungi
Listeria monocytogenes*
	*Beta-hemolytic
	  streptococci
	Candida albicans
	Coliform bacilli
	Enterococci
	Gardnerella vaginalis
	Listeria monocytogenes
	Mycoplasma hominis
	Neisseria gonorrhoeae
	Treponema pallidum
	Hemophilus ducreyi
	Chlamydia trachomatis
	Herpes simplex virus
	Trichomonas vaginalis
	Ureaplasma urealyticum*
		*Acinetobacter
		  calcoaceticus
		Chlamydia trachomatis
		Coliform bacilli
		Cytomegalovirus
		Hemophilus ducreyi
		Herpes simplex virus
		Neisseria gonorrhoeae
		Treponema pallidum
		Trichomonas vaginalis*

Host Factors
Certain important factors, such as the following, influence the development of an infectious disease:

General health of the patient
Patient's defense mechanisms
Previous contact with the particular organism
Development of immune substances, or antibodies
Past clinical history
Type of tissue involved in the infection
Stress to the body, not necessarily of microbial origin
Age of patient
Exposure to antibiotics

Collection of Specimens

General Principles
The health care professional is responsible for the collection of specimens used for diagnostic examinations. Because procedures vary among the testing laboratories, it is recommended that you check with your laboratory for the preferred method of obtaining the specimen, delivering the specimen to the laboratory, preserving it when necessary, and reporting the results.

Precautions
Certain routine precautions must be taken in the collection and handling of specimens. Without these precautions, the patient's condition may be incorrectly diagnosed, much laboratory time wasted, and the pathogenic organisms transmitted to health care workers and to other patients.

Sources of Specimens
Microbiologic specimens may be collected from many sources: blood, pus or wound exudates, urine, sputum, feces, the genital tract, cerebrospinal fluid, an eye, or an ear. During collection, these general procedures should be followed:

1. Labeling of specimens
   Specimens should be labeled with
   (a) Patient's name, age, sex, address (or hospital number or physician's name and address)
   (b) Site of specimen (*e.g.*, throat, conjunctiva)
   (c) Time of collection
   (d) Nature of studies desired
   (e) Clinical diagnosis; microorganisms suspected

(f) Duration of illness

(g) Patient's immune state

(h) Previous infection

(i) Nature of any antibiotic therapy

(j) If in isolation, state type

(k) Any other information the laboratory requires

2. Avoiding contamination

   Collection should be as aseptic as possible. Observe the following:

   (a) Special kits may be required, such as

       (1) For anaerobes, syringe aspiration of pus or body fluid

       (2) Use of carbon dioxide–containing transport media for tissue specimens (rather than collection of specimens on swabs).

   (b) Use only sterile specimen containers.

   (c) Do not spill any material on the outside of the container.

   (d) Use only standard plugs to stopper tubes and bottles.

   (e) Discard plugs and caps that have come in contact with non-sterile surfaces.

3. Preserving specimens

   Prompt delivery to the laboratory is desirable; however, many specimens may be refrigerated (not frozen) for a few hours without any adverse effects. Note the following:

   (a) Urine cultures must be *refrigerated* if results of diagnostic tests are to be of value.

   (b) Cerebrospinal fluid specimens should be transported quickly to the laboratory. If this is impossible, the culture should be *incubated*, for the suspected meningococcus will not withstand refrigeration.

4. Transport of specimens

   Care and speed of transport of specimens to the laboratory is urged. The material should be transported quickly to prevent drying out of the specimen and consequent death of the microorganisms.

   (a) With anaerobic cultures, no more than 10 minutes should elapse between collection and culture.

   (b) Urine should be *refrigerated* during transport to the laboratory.

   (c) Specimens suspected of containing anaerobic bacteria should be injected into a butyl rubber-stoppered gassed-out glass tube.

   (d) Feces suspected of having *Salmonella* or *Shigella* organisms should be placed in a special transport medium such as buffered glycerol–saline if culturing will be delayed.

5. Quantity of specimens

   The quantity of specimens should be as large as possible. When only a small quantity is available, swabs should be moistened with sterile saline. This procedure is especially important in nasopharyngeal cultures.

6. Collection of specimens
   (a) Whenever possible, specimens should be collected before an antibiotic regimen is instituted.
   (b) Collection must be geared to the rise in symptoms. (The practitioner should be familiar with the clinical course of the suspected disease.)

Diagnosis of Bacterial Disease: General Observations

Bacteriologic studies are done to try to determine the specific organism that is causing an infection (Table 7-2). This organism may be specific for one disease, such as *Mycobacterium tuberculosis*, the causative agent of tuberculosis, or it may be organisms such as the *Staphylococcus* species that can cause a variety of infections. Antibiotic susceptibility or sensitivity tests are also done to determine the reactions of a specific organism to antibiotics.

The questions asked in searching for bacteria as the cause of a disease process are as follows: (1) Are bacteria responsible for this disease? (2) Is antimicrobial therapy indicated? Most bacterial diseases follow a febrile course. From a practical standpoint, relatively soon in the evaluation of a patient with fever a diagnosis must be reached and a decision made concerning antimicrobial therapy.

Disease due to anaerobic bacteria is commonly associated with localized necrotic abscesses, each of which may yield 2 to 13 different strains of bacteria. Because of the multiple species that can be isolated, the term *polymicrobic disease* is sometimes used to refer to anaerobic bacterial diseases. Diseases caused by anaerobic bacteria are in sharp contrast to the "one organism–one disease" concept that characterizes infections such as typhoid fever, cholera, and diphtheria. The isolation and identification of different strains of anaerobic bacteria are desirable so that appropriate therapy may be given. For instance, it is important when planning therapy for patients with anaerobic disease to know that certain drugs are not an effective or appropriate treatment.

Sensitivity (Susceptibility) of Bacteria to Antimicrobial Agents

A sensitivity (susceptibility) test detects the amount of antibiotic or chemotherapeutic agent required to inhibit the growth of bacteria. Often, a sensitivity test is ordered with a culture procedure. It is used

(*text continues on page 402*)

TABLE 7-2.
Bacterial Diseases and Their Laboratory Diagnosis

Disease	Causative Organism	Source of Specimen	Diagnostic Tests
Anthrax	*Bacillus anthracis*	Blood, sputum, sore, stool	Blood, sputum, and skin smear and culture; specific serologic test; biopsy
Brucellosis (undulant fever)	*Brucella melitensis, Br. abortus, Br. suis*	Blood, bone marrow	Blood and bone marrow culture; skin test; specific serologic test
Bubonic plague	*Yersinia pestis*	Buboes (enlarged and inflamed lymph nodes), blood, sputum	Skin, blood, and sputum smear; culture; agglutination test
Chancre	*Hemophilus ducreyi*	Penis	Penis smear culture; biopsy; serologic test
Cholera	*Vibrio cholerae*	Feces	Stool smear and culture; skin biopsy
Chlamydia, once considered virus because of small size	*Chlamydia psittaci (Psittacosis)* *Chlamydia trachomatis*	Blood, sputum, lung Vagina, urethra	Culture, smears
Diphtheria	*Corynebacterium diphtheriae*	Pharynx	Pharyngeal smear and culture
Dysentery	*Shigella dysenteriae*	Feces	Stool culture
Endocarditis	*Staphylococcus aureus*	Petechiae	Culture
Erysipeloid	*Erysipelothrix rhusio pathiae*	Lesion, blood	Culture
Glander's disease	*Pseudomonas mallei*	Skin sore, blood, sputum	Skin smear and culture; serologic test
Gonorrhea	*Neisseria gonorrhoeae*	Vagina, urethra, CSF, blood, joint fluid	Smear, culture, and serologic tests
Granuloma inguinale	*Calymmatobacterium granulomatis*	Penis, groin lesion	Smears and culture from penis and groin
Leprosy (Hansen's) disease	*Mycobacterium leprae*	Skin scrapings	Skin smear, biopsy, histamine lepromin, serologic test

Disease	Causative Organism	Specimen	Procedures
Listeriosis	*Listeria monocytogenes*	Pharynx, blood, CSF	Pharyngeal, blood, and CSF smears and culture; serologic test
Meningitis	*Neisseria meningitidis* *Angiostrongylus cantonensis*	Pharynx, CSF, blood	Pharyngeal, CSF, and blood smears and cultures
Pertussis (whooping cough)	*Bordetella pertussis*	Trachea, bronchi, nasopharynx	Cultures of swabs of trachea and nasopharynx and bronchi; serologic test
Pharyngitis	*Streptococcus pyogenes*	Pharyngeal swab, sputum	Smear of sputum and pharyngeal swab culture; antistreptolysin O (ASO) test; C-reactive protein (CRP) test; serologic test
Pneumonia	*Hemophilus influenzae,* *Klebsiella pneumoniae,* *Staphylococcus aureus,* *Streptococcus pneumoniae*	Pharyngeal swab, CSF, sputum, blood exudates, effusions	Smear and culture of sputum, blood, CSF, nasopharyngeal specimens, and exudates and effusions
Strep throat, scarlet fever, impetigo	*Streptococcus pyogenes*	Throat, lesion	Culture, serology
Tetanus	*Clostridium tetani*	Wound	Wound smear and culture
Toxic shock syndrome	*Staphylococcus aureus*	Tissue	Culture
Tuberculosis	*Mycobacterium tuberculosis*	Sputum, gastric washings, urine, CSF	Smear and culture of sputum; gastric washings, urine and CSF; skin biopsy; skin test
Tularemia	*Francisella tularensis*	Skin, lymph node, pharynx	Foshay skin test; serologic test
Typhoid	*Salmonella typhi*	Blood (after first week of infection); feces (after second week of infection)	Culture and serologic test
Whooping cough	*Bordetella pertussis*	Nasopharyngeal swab	Culture, fluorescent antibody

(Adapted from Collins RD: Illustrated Manual of Laboratory Diagnosis, 2nd ed. Philadelphia, JB Lippincott, 1975)

before selection of appropriate drugs or for the alteration of an already imposed regimen of treatment.

The most common and most useful test for antibiotic sensitivity is the disc method. A basic set of antibiotic-impregnated discs is available for routine testing against the commonly isolated microorganisms. Specific amounts of an antibiotic are inoculated with a culture of the specific bacteria to be tested. After a suitable period of incubation, sensitivity of the organisms is determined by microscopic observation of the presence or absence of growth in the antimicrobial agent and by measurement of disc zones. The diameters in millimeters are compared against standards to determine if the organism is truly sensitive or of intermediate category. The sensitive drug is preferred over the intermediate drug.

Clinical Implications
1. The term *sensitive* or *susceptible* implies that an infection caused by the strain tested, such as streptococcus, may be expected to respond favorably to the indicated antimicrobial, such as penicillin, for that type of infection and pathogen.
2. The term *intermediate* or *partially resistant* or *moderately susceptible* means that the strain tested is not inhibited completely by therapeutic concentrations of a specific drug.
3. *Indeterminant* means that the organism may be susceptible or resistant to this method of testing. Usually these organisms will be susceptible to high blood levels of antibiotics.
4. The organism is not inhibited.
5. Many physicians rely more on published reports of the antibiotics usually effective against the organism isolated than on the sensitivity report, for sensitivity is an *in vitro* (in glass) test, and the antibiotic will be working *in vivo* (in the body).

Diagnosis of Mycobacterial Infections

Mycobacteria contain several species pathogenic to humans (Table 7–3). *Mycobacterium* tuberculosis is spread from person to person by inhalation of air-borne respiratory secretions containing infectious mycobacteria expelled during coughing, sneezing, or talking. In homosexual patients with acquired immunodeficiency syndrome (AIDS), *Mycobacterium avium-intracellulare* (MAI) is acquired through the gastrointestinal tract, often by sexual transmission via infected semen.

Collection of Specimens
1. Sputum and bronchial aspirates and lavages are best for diagnosis of pulmonary infection. Purulent sputum from the first productive

TABLE 7–3.
Mycobacterial Infections and Their Laboratory Diagnosis

Causative Organism	Source of Specimen	Diagnostic Tests
Mycobacterium tuberculosis	Sputum, urine, CSF, tissue	Culture and smear; skin test
Mycobacterium avium-intracellulare	Sputum, stool, CSF, tissue, blood, semen, lymph nodes	Culture and smear
Mycobacterium kansasii	Skin, joint, lymph nodes, sputum, tissue	Culture and smear
Mycobacterium leprae	Cerebrospinal fluid, skin, bone marrow, lymph nodes	Histopathologic exam of lesion
Mycobacterium marinum	Joint, lesion	Culture and smear
Mycobacterium xenopi	Sputum	Culture and smear
Mycobacterium fortuitum	Surgical wound, bone, joint, tissue, sputum	Culture and smear
Mycobacterium chelonei	Surgical wound, sputum, tissue	Culture and smear

cough of the morning should be expelled into a sterile container. Approximately 5 to 10 ml should be collected. If the specimen is not processed immediately after collection, it should be refrigerated. Pooled specimens collected over several hours are not acceptable. For best results, three to five specmens collected over several days are recommended.

2. If unable to produce sputum, an early morning gastric aspirate can be cultured. The specimen must be hand delivered to the laboratory to be processed or neutralized immediately.

3. Urine from suspected renal disease patients should be an early morning specimen collected 3 days in a row. Pooled 24-hour urine collections are not recommended. If not processed immediately, the specimen should be refrigerated.

4. If tuberculosis meningitis is suspected, at least 10 ml of cerebrospinal fluid (CSF) is needed. Blood can be inoculated into biphasic blood culture media.

5. Sterile body fluids of all types, tissue biopsies, and aspirated material from skin lesions are acceptable for culture of mycobacteria. The least desirable specimen is a swab.

6. Feces are commonly the first specimen to be positive for MAI. An acid-fast stain is usually performed on a thin smear of feces. Culture is performed only if the smear is positive.

Diagnosis of Rickettsial Disease:
General Observations

Rickettsiae are small, gram-negative coccobacilli that structurally resemble bacteria, but on average are only one tenth to one half as large. Polychromatic stains (Giemsa stain) are better than simple stains or the gram stain for demonstrating rickettsiae in cells.

Rickettsiosis is the general name given to any disease caused by rickettsiae (Table 7-4). The organisms are considered to be *obligate intracellular parasites;* that is, they cannot exist anywhere except inside the bodies of living organisms. Diseases caused by rickettsiae are transmitted by *anthropod vectors* such as lice, fleas, ticks, or mites (see Table 7-5). Generally, these disease entities are divided into the following groups:

1. Typhus-like fevers
2. Spotted fever
3. Scrub typhus
4. Q fever
5. Other miscellaneous groups

Q fever, caused by *Coxiella burnetii,* is characterized by an acute febrile illness, severe headache, rigors, and possibly pneumonia or hepatitis. It may be a cause of encephalitis in children and has been isolated in breast milk and the placenta of infected mothers, making it possible for a fetus to be infected in utero. Both complement fixation and fluorescent antibody tests are available to detect antibody to the organism. *Coxiella burnetii* displays an antigenic variation during an infection. Phase I antibodies predominate during the chronic phase, whereas phase II antibodies predominate during the acute phase. A diagnosis is made when a phase I titer in a convalescent serum specimen is four times greater than that in an acute serum specimen.

Signs and Symptoms

1. Fever	5. Stupor and coma
2. Skin rashes	6. Headache
3. Parasitism of blood vessels	7. Ringing in the ears
4. Prostration	8. Dizziness

Note: Rickettsial diseases are often characterized by an incubation period of 10 to 14 days, with an abrupt onset of the preceding signs and symptoms following a history of arthropod bites.

TABLE 7-4.
Rickettsial Diseases and Their Laboratory Diagnosis

| Disease | | | Natural Cycle | | | Serologic Diagnosis | |
Group and Type	Agent	Geographical Distribution	Antropod	Mammal	Transmission to Man	Well-Felix Reaction	Complement Fixation
Typhus							
Epidemic	Rickettsia prowazekii	Worldwide	Body louse	Man	Infected louse feces into broken skin	Positive OX-19	
Brill's disease	R. prowazekii	North America, Europe	Recurrence years after original attack of epidemic typhus			Usually negative	Positive group- and type-specific
Endemic	R. typhi	Worldwide	Flea	Rodents	Infected flea feces into broken skin	Positive OX-19	
Spotted fever							
Rocky Mountain spotted fever	R. rickettsii	Western Hemisphere	Ticks	Wild rodents, dogs	Tick bite	Positive OX-19 OX-2	
North Asian tick-borne rickettsiosis	R. sibirica	Siberia, Mongolia	Ticks	Wild rodents	Tick bite	Positive OX-19 OX-2	
Boutonneuse fever	R. conorii	Africa, Europe, Middle East, India	Ticks	Wild rodents, dogs	Tick bite	Positive OX-19 OX-2	Positive group- and type-specific
Queensland tick typhus	R. australis	Australia	Ticks	Marsupials, wild rodents	Tick bite	Positive OX-19 OX-2	
Rickettsialpox	R. akari	North America, Europe	Blood-sucking mite	House mouse and other rodents	Mite bite	Negative	
Scrub typhus	R. tsutsugamushi	Asia, Australia, Pacific Islands	Tromiculid mite	Wild rodents	Mite bite	Positive OX-K	Positive in about 50% of patients
Q fever	Coxiella burnetti	Worldwide	Ticks	Small mammals, cattle, sheep and goats	Inhalation of dried, infected material	Negative	Positive
Trench fever	Rochalimaea quintana	Europe, Africa, North America	Body louse	Man	Infected louse feces into broken skin	Negative	Low titer

(Adapted from Davis BD et al: Microbiology, 4th ed. Philadelphia, JB Lippincott, 1990)

405

TABLE 7–5.
Modes of Transmission of the Major Rickettsial Diseases

Disease in Man	Etiologic Agent	Chain of Transmission
Epidemic typhus Endemic typhus	R. prowazekii R. typhi	. . Man→Louse→Man→Louse . . Rat→Rat flea→Rat→Rat flea→Rat . . . ↓ Man
Rocky Mountain spotted fever (boutonneuse fever, other spotted fevers	R. rickettsii	. . Tick→Tick→Tick→Tick . . . . ↓ Dog Man ↓ Tick→Man
Scrub typhus (tsutsugamushi fever)	R. tsutsugamushi	. . Mite→Field mouse→Mite→Field mouse . . . ↓ Man
Rickettsialpox	R. akari	. . Mite→House mouse→Mite→House mouse . . . ↓ Man
Q fever	Coxiella burnetii	. . Tick→Small mammal→Tick→Cattle . . . (airborne) (airborne) ↓ Man

(Adapted from Davis BD et al: Microbiology, 4th ed. Philadelphia, JB Lippincott, 1990)

Diagnosis of Parasitic Disease:
General Observations

Many parasitic infections are asymptomatic or produce only mild symptoms. Routine blood and stool examinations will uncover many unsuspected infections (Table 7-6).

Approximately 70 species of animal parasites commonly infect the body. More than half can be detected by examination of stool specimens, because the parasites inhabit the gastrointestinal tract and its environs. Of the parasites that can be diagnosed by stool examinations, one third are single-celled protozoa and two thirds are multicellular worms. Only six or seven of the intestinal protozoa are important clinically, but almost all of the worms are potentially pathogenic.

The diagnosis for parasites begins with the ova and parasite examination. Other options for intestinal disease include the examination of sigmoidoscopy smears, biopsy, radiologic studies using barium, and organism detection by serologic tests. For ova and parasite examination, three specimens should be collected every other day or within no more than a 10-day time frame.

For detection of *Giardia*, other diagnostic tests may be necessary. These include the Entero-test capsule (string test) and duodenal aspiration or biopsy.

Cryptosporidium parvum has been recognized as an animal parasite for years and is now infecting humans, especially compromised patients. Organisms have been recovered from the gallbladder and lung, in addition to stool specimen.

A tissue protozoa infecting humans is *Pneumocystis carinii*. This organism causes pneumonia in the compromised patient. An open lung biopsy or bronchoalveolar lavage (BAL) are the specimens of choice. For extraintestinal diagnosis of amebiasis, additional tests include hepatic scans, ultrasound, and needle aspiration.

Collection of Specimens

1. In general, it is not possible to identify accurately a parasite from one submitted specimen.
2. Most parasites in humans are identified from blood or feces, but organisms may also be obtained from urine, sputum, tissue fluid, and biopsies.

Clinical Alert

The number of worms harbored is the most important factor in the diagnosis of parasitic worms.

(*text continues on page 410*)

TABLE 7–6.
Parasitic Diseases and Their Laboratory Diagnosis

Disease	Causative Organism	Source of Specimen	Diagnostic Tests
Amebiasis	*Entamoeba histolytica*	Stool	Stool smear, rectal biopsy, and serologic test
Ascariasis	*Ascaris lumbricoides*	Stool, sputum	Stool and sputum smear
Cestodiasis of intestine (tapeworm disease)	*Taenia saginata* *Taenia solium* *Diphyllobothrium latum*	Stool	Stool smear and Scotch tape test
Chagas disease	*Trypanosoma cruzi*	Blood Spinal fluid	Blood and spinal fluid smear; animal inoculation
Cryptosporidiosis	*Cryptosporidium parvum*	Stool, lung, gallbladder	Stool, lung, and gallbladder smear
Cysticercosis	*Taenia solium larvae*		Muscle and brain cyst biopsy
Echinococcosis	*Echinococcus granulosus*	Sputum Urine	Sputum and urine smear; serologic test; Casoni skin test; liver and bone biopsy
Enterobiasis (pinworm disease)	*Enterobius vermicularis*	Stool	Scotch tape smear
Filariasis	*Wuchereria bancrofti*	Blood	Blood smear; lymph node biopsy
Giardiasis	*Giardia lamblia*	Stool, duodenal aspirate or biopsy	Stool smear, Enterotest
Hookworm disease	*Ancylostoma duodenale* *Necator americanus*	Stool	Stool smear
Isospora	*Isospora belli*	Stool	Stool smear
Kala-azar	Leishman's anemia	Liver Bone marrow	Liver, bone marrow, and blood smear and culture; animal inoculation; lymph node and spleen biopsy
Malaria	*Plasmodium falciparum*	Blood Bone marrow	Blood and bone marrow smear; serologic test; Wasserman test

Disease	Organism	Specimen	Method
	Plasmodium malariae		
	Plasmodium vivax		
	Plasmodium ovale		
Pneumocystis	Pneumocystis carinii	Lung biopsy, bronchoalveolar lavage	Smear
Onchocerciasis	Onchocerca volvulus		Skin biopsy
Paragonimiasis	Paragonimus westermani	Sputum Stool	Sputum and stool smear; serologic test; skin test
Scabies	Sarcoptes scabiei	Skin	Skin smear; serologic test; skin test
Schistosomiasis of intestine and bladder	Schistosoma mansoni Schistosoma japonicum Schistosoma haematobium	Stool Urine	Urine and stool smear; serologic test; skin test; rectal, bladder, and liver biopsy
Strongyloidiasis	Strongyloides stercoralis	Stool Duodenal aspirate	Stool and gastric smear
Toxoplasmosis	Toxoplasma gondii		Animal inoculation; serologic test; skin test
Trichinosis	Trichinella spiralis		Serologic test; skin test; muscle biopsy
Trichomoniasis	Trichomonas vaginalis	Vagina Bladder Urethra	Vaginal and urethral smear and culture
Trichuriasis	Trichuris trichiura	Stool	Stool smear
Trypanosomiasis	Trypanosoma rhodesiense Trypanosoma gambiense	Blood Spinal fluid Lymph node	Blood, spinal fluid, and lymph node smear; animal inoculation; serologic test
Visceral larva migrans	Toxocara canis Toxocara cati		Serologic test; skin test; liver biopsy

(Adapted from Collins RD: Illustrated Manual of Laboratory Diagnosis, 2nd ed. Philadelphia, JB Lippincott, 1975)

Clinical Considerations

A. General
   1. *Eosinophilia* is regarded as a definite indication of a parasitic infection. Infections with parasitic worms and protozoa may have associated eosinophilia, which varies considerably depending on the reaction of the patient.
   2. Protozoa and helminths, particularly larvae, may be found in various organs and tissues of the body, as well as in the blood.
B. According to specimen
   1. *Hepatic puncture* is useful in the diagnosis of visceral leishmaniasis. Liver biopsy may reveal toxocaral larvae and schistosomal worms and eggs.
   2. *Bone marrow* may be examined in trypanosomiasis and malaria when the blood is negative. Specimens are obtained by puncturing the sternum, crest of the ilium, vertebral processes, trochanter, or tibia.
   3. *Lymph nodes* may be examined for the diagnosis of trypanosomiasis, leishmaniasis, toxoplasmosis, and filariasis either by puncture or biopsy.
   4. Material from *mucous membranes* and *skin* may be obtained for examination by scraping, aspirating, or biopsy. Material may be obtained from the ulcer or nodule of the sore by puncturing the indurated margin of the lesion with a sterile hypodermic needle and aspirating gently.
   5. The *cerebrospinal fluid* may be examined for trypanosomes and toxoplasma.
   6. *Sputum* may be examined for presence of eggs of *Paragonimus westermani* (the lung fluke). Occasionally, the larvae and the hookworm of *Strongyloides stercoralis* and *Ascaris lumbricoides* may be coughed up during their pulmonary migration. In pulmonary echinococcosis (hydatid disease), the contents of the hydatid cyst may be evacuated in the sputum.

Diagnosis of Fungal Disease: General Observations

Fungal diseases, the mycoses, are now believed to be more common than in the past because of the widespread rise of the use of antibacterial agents and immunosuppressive drugs (Table 7-7). Fungi prefer the debilitated host, the individual with impaired immunity, chronic disease, or antibiotic therapy.

Of more than 50,000 species of fungi, approximately 50 are generally recognized as being pathogenic for humans. Fungi are organisms that live in a soil enriched by decaying nitrogenous matter and are capable of maintaining a separate existence by a parasitic cycle in humans or animals. The systemic mycoses are not communicable in the usual sense of human-to-human or animal-to-animal transfer. Humans become accidental hosts by the inhalation of spores or by their introduction into the tissues through trauma. Altered susceptibility may result in fungus lesions, as in patients having debilitating disease, diabetes, or impaired immunologic mechanisms resulting from steroid or antimetabolite therapy. Prolonged administration of antibiotics can result in a superinfection by a fungus.

Fungal diseases can be classified according to the type of tissues involved.

1. *Dermatophytoses* includes the superficial and cutaneous mycoses such as athlete's foot, ringworm, and "jock itch." Species of microsporum, epidermophyton, and trichophyton are the causative organisms of the dermatophytoses.
2. *Subcutaneous mycoses* involve the subcutaneous tissues and muscles.
3. *Systemic mycoses* involve the deep tissues and organs and are the most serious of all three groups.

Collection of Hair and Skin Specimens
1. Cleanse the area of suspected infection with 70% alcohol to remove bacteria.
2. Scrape the area with a sterile scalpel or wooden spatula, and place the specimen in a small sterile container with a lid.
3. Hair of the infected scalp or beard should be clipped and placed in a covered sterile container.
4. Hair stubs should be plucked out with a tweezer because the fungus is usually found at the base of the hair shaft. Using a Wood's light in a darkened room will help to identify the infected hairs.

Common Diagnostic Methods
1. Direct microscopic examination of material on a slide to determine whether a fungus is actually present
2. Use of a Wood's light to determine presence of a fungus. A Wood's light is a lamp using 3,660 Angstrom units of ultraviolet rays. When used in a darkened room, infected hairs will fluoresce a bright yellow-green color.
3. The potassium hydroxide (KOH) test to determine the presence of mycelial fragments, arthrospores, spherules, and budding yeast cells involves mixing the specimen in KOH on a glass slide, covering the slip, and applying gentle heat. The slide is examined microscopically for the above fungal elements.

(*text continues on page 414*)

TABLE 7-7.
Fungal Diseases and Their Laboratory Diagnosis

Disease	Causative Organism	Source of Specimen	Diagnostic Tests
Actinomycosis	*Actinomyces israelii*	Skin, subcutaneous tissue, sputum	Skin, subcutaneous tissue, and sputum culture and smear; biopsy
Aspergillosis	*Aspergillus fumigatus*	Sputum, tissue, ear	Culture, smear
Blastomycosis	*Blastomyces dermatitidis*	Skin, sputum	Skin and sputum smear and culture; serologic test; skin test
Candidiasis	*Candida albicans*	Mucous membrane, sputum	Mucous membrane and sputum smear and culture
Coccidioidomycosis	*Coccidioides immitis*	Sputum	Sputum smear, culture, animal inoculation, serologic test, skin test, biopsy
Cryptococcosis	*Cryptococcus neoformans*	CSF, Sputum, Urine	Serology, culture, smear
Histoplasmosis	*Histoplasma capsulatum*	Sputum Urine Blood Bone marrow	Smear, culture, animal inoculation, serologic test, skin test, and biopsy
Mucormycosis	Members of the order Mucorales (*Absidia*, *Rhizopus*, and *Mucor*)	Nose Pharynx Stool CSF	Nose, pharynx, stool and CSF culture; biopsy

Disease	Causative organism	Specimen	Examination
Nocardiosis	*Nocardia asteroides*, *Nocardia brasiliensis*	Sputum, Spinal fluid	Sputum and spinal fluid culture and smear; biopsy
Paracoccidioidomycosis	*Paracoccidioides brasiliensis*	Lung, tissue, sputum	Culture, serology
Sporotrichosis	*Sporothrix schenckii*	Skin	Skin culture and biopsy
Tinea pedis (athlete's foot)	*Epidermophytons* and *Candida albicans*	Skin	Hair, skin, and nail scrapings for culture
Tinea capitis (ringworm of scalp)	*Microsporum* (any species) and *Trichophyton* (all except *T. concentricum*)	Skin	Hair, skin, and nail scrapings for culture
Tinea barbae (ringworm of the beard, barber's itch)	*Trichophytons* and *microsporums*	Skin	Hair, skin, and nail scrapings for culture
Tinea cruris (jock itch)	*Epidermophytons* and *Candida albicans*	Skin	Hair, skin, and nail scrapings for culture

(Adapted from Collins RD: Illustrated Manual of Laboratory Diagnosis, 2nd ed. Philadelphia, JB Lippincott, 1975)

4. A culture is done to identify the specific type of fungus. Fungi are slow growing and are subject to overgrowth by contaminating and more rapidly growing organisms. Fungemia is associated with an opportunistic infection and often a blood culture is the earliest suggestion of the causative organism. The use of the DuPont Isolator System, a lysis-centrifugation system, not only shortens the time of detection, but also improves the rate of detection.

5. A fluorescent brightener, Calcofluor white, fluoresces upon excitement with ultraviolet light. This reagent stains fungi, causing them to exhibit fluorescence that can be detected microscopically. The reagent can be used on tissue and has the same sensitivity as KOH. However, it allows for easier and faster detection of fungal elements. Calcofluor white can also be examined by bright-field or phase-contrast microscopy.

6. The latex serology test for cryptococcal antigen detects 95% of *Cryptococcus* meningitis and approximately 67% of desseminated cryptococcosis. Tests to detect antibodies to *Candida* species lack specificity in distinguishing between colonization and deep-seated invasion. Because of this insensitivity, tests for the detection of *Candida* antigen and its metabolites have been developed. These latex tests may be helpful in separating the two groups of patients, even those who are immunosuppressed.

Types of Specimens

1. Skin
2. Nails
3. Hair
4. Ulcer scrapings
5. Pus
6. Cerebrospinal fluid
7. Urine
8. Sputum
9. Blood
10. Bone marrow
11. Stool
12. Bronchial washings
13. Biopsies

Diagnosis of Spirochetal Disease: General Observations

Spirochetes are spiral and curved bacteria. There are four genera of spiral and curved bacteria, which include a number of human pathogens. The genera are *Borrelia*, *Treponema*, *Leptospira*, and *Spirillum* (Table 7-8).

Clinical Considerations

1. *Borrelia*
   (a) *Borrelia* appears in the blood at the onset of various forms of relapsing fever. This genus is responsible for European and American relapsing fever.

(b) *Borrelia vincentii* is the species responsible for ulcerative gingivitis (trench mouth).

2. *Treponema*
   (a) *Treponema pallidum* is the species responsible for venereal and nonvenereal syphilis in humans.
   (b) *Treponema pertenue* is the causative agent of yaws.
   (c) *Treponema carateum* causes pinta (carate).

3. *Leptospira*
   (a) *Leptospira* is the genus of microorganism responsible for Weil's disease (infectious jaundice), swamp fever, swineherd's disease, and canicola fever.
   (b) The organism is widely distributed in the infected person and appears in the blood early in the disease.
   (c) After 10 to 14 days the organisms are present in considerable numbers in the urine.
   (d) Patients with Weil's disease show striking antibody responses, and serologic testing is useful in diagnosis.

4. *Spirillum*
   Streptobacillus moniliformis as well as *Spirillum minus* is the species responsible for rat-bite fever. The condition occurs worldwide, is

TABLE 7-8.
Spirochetal Diseases and Their Laboratory Diagnosis

Disease	Causative Organism	Source of Specimen	Diagnostic Tests
Pinta	*Treponema carateum*	Skin	Skin smear, serologic test
Rat-bite fever	*Spirillum minus* *Streptobacillus moniliformis*	Blood Joint fluid Abscess	Skin, blood, and joint fluid culture and serologic test
Relapsing fever	*Borrelia recurrentis*	Blood	Blood smear and culture and serologic test
Syphilis	*Treponema pallidum*	Skin	Skin smear; TPI and FTA-Ab test
Weil's disease (leptospiral jaundice)	*Leptospira icterohaemorrhagiae*	Urine, blood, CSF	Urine and blood smear; culture-muscle biopsy; serologic test
Yaws	*Treponema pertenue*	Skin	Skin smear and serologic test

(Adapted from Collins RD: Illustrated Manual of Laboratory Diagnosis, 2nd ed. Philadelphia, JB Lippincott, 1975)

common in Japan and Asia, but uncommon in North and South America and most European countries. Cases in the United States have followed bites by laboratory rats.

Diagnosis of Viral and Mycoplasmal Disease: General Observations

Viral diseases are the most common of human infections. Once thought to be confined to the childhood years, viral infections in adults have increasingly been recognized as the cause of morbidity and death. They include infectious diseases such as hepatitis and AIDS and other sexually transmitted diseases; they are considered as possible etiologic agents in cancer, and they affect immunosuppressed patients and the elderly.

Viruses are submicroscopic, filterable, infectious organisms that exist as intracellular parasites. They are divided into two groups according to the type of nucleic acid they contain: ribonucleic acid (RNA) or deoxyribonucleic acid (DNA).

Mycoplasmas are scotobacteria without cell walls and are surrounded by a single triple-layered membrane. They are also known as *pleuropneumonia-like organisms* (PPLO).

Viruses and mycoplasmas are both small, infectious agents that are capable of passing through bacteria-retaining filters. Although smallness is the only property they have in common, viruses and mycoplasmas cause illnesses that are often indistinguishable from each other in clinical signs and symptoms, and both are found together frequently as a double infection. Thus, the serologic (antigen–antibody) procedures that are used commonly in the diagnosis of viral disease are also used for diagnosing cases of mycoplasmal infection (Table 7-9).

Physiologically, mycoplasmas are considered generally as an intermediate disease stage between bacteria and rickettsiae. One species, *Mycoplasma pneumoniae*, is recognized as the causative agent of primary atypical pneumonia and bronchitis. Other species are suspected as possible agents in urethritis, infertility, early abortion, rheumatoid arthritis, myringitis, and erythema multiforme.

Approach to Diagnosis

1. Viral isolation in tissue culture remains the gold standard for the detection of many common viruses.
   - (a) Tissue culture
   - (b) Special media
   - (c) Typing such as: Herpes simplex
   - (d) Identification reagents, immunofluorescence and immunoperoxidase
   - (e) Electron microscope
2. Serology for antigen–antibody detection

TABLE 7-9.

Virus Study Procedures

Disease or Syndrome	Clinical Specimens	Suspected Viral Agents
Nervous System		
Aseptic meningitis	Stool	Enteroviruses (Cox-
Encephalitis	Throat swab	sackie, echo, polio)
Poliomyelitis	CSF	Toga virus
	(Acute and convalescent	*Herpes simplex, Vari-*
	sera)	*cella zoster*, mumps,
		measles
		Cytomegalovirus
Respiratory/Upper	Throat washing or	Adenovirus, rhinovirus,
Respiratory Infec-	swab, stool	enterovirus, myx-
tions		ovirus, respiratory
Croup	Nasopharyngeal swab	syncytial, influenza,
Bronchiolitis	(Acute and convalescent	Parainfluenza
Influenza	sera)	
Viral pneumonia		
Infectious mono-	Serology	Epstein–Barr
nucleosis		
Exanthema and rashes		
Chickenpox	Vesicle swab	*Varicella zoster*
Zoster (shingles)	Throat swab	*Herpes simplex*
Herpes simplex	Stool	Coxsackie A
Herpangina	Urine	Measles
Measles	(Acute and convalescent	Rubella
Rubella	sera)	Enterovirus
Perinatal Infections		
Cytomegalic inclu-	Urine	Cytomegalovirus
sion disease	Throat swab	Rubella
Rubella syndrome	CSF	*Herpes simplex*
Herpes simplex	(Acute and convalescent	
	sera)	
Gastrointestinal		
Diarrhea	Stool (for ELISA or	Rotavirus
	EM) 10–20 g as	Enterovirus
	soon after onset as	Adenovirus
	possible	Norwalk Agent
Myocarditis, peri-		
carditis		
Pleurodynia	Stool	Coxsackie B
Epidemic myalgia	Throat swab	Echovirus
Myopericarditis	Pericardial or pleural	Cytomegalovirus
Lymphadenopathy	fluid	Other etiology
	(Acute and convalescent	
	sera)	
Eye infections	Conjunctival swab or	*Herpes simplex, adeno-*
	scraping	*varicella zoster,*
Hepatitis	Serology	vaccinia, enterovirus
		B, A, and Non A, Non B
		Delta virus

(Adapted from August MJ: Practical aspects of viral diagnosis. J Med Technol 2(8):502, August 1985)

3. The available cell cultures vary greatly in sensitivity to different viruses. It is important to understand that one cell type or species may be more sensitive than another for the detection of virus in low titers. For example: Primary human monkey kidney (1 MK) can be used for adenovirus, enterovirus, herpes simplex, measles, mumps, myxovirus, pox, rubella, and varicella zoster; and human embryonic kidney (HEK) cannot be used for cytomegalovirus or myxovirus.

4. The critical first step in successful viral diagnosis is the timely and proper collection of specimens. The choice of which specimen to collect depends upon the typical signs and symptoms and the virus suspected. The improper choice and collection of specimens is one of the biggest factors in time wasted in obtaining a viral diagnosis.

Specimen Collection

1. As early as possible in the course of the illness; the first 4 days after symptom onset
2. Sampling
   (a) Localized infection
       (1) Direct sampling of affected site (*e.g.,* throat swab or skin scraping)
       (2) Indirect sampling. For example, if target sample is CSF in central nervous system (CNS) infection, the indirect approach is throat swab or stool specimens for culture.
       (3) Sampling from more than one site (*e.g.,* in disseminated disease or nonspecific clinical findings)
       (4) Applicators used to obtain specimens may affect successful recovery of viral agent. Do not use wooden applicators; they are toxic to viruses, as well as chlamydia, bacteria, and mycoplasma.
       (5) Transporting specimens
           (a.) Keep in mind that viral specimens are unstable. Viruses rapidly lose infectivity outside of living cells.
           (b.) Prompt delivery to laboratory is essential. Samples must be refrigerated and placed in a container with wet ice or cold packs for transit.
           (c.) No freezing or thawing of specimens. This diminishes the quantity of viable virus.

Clinical Considerations

1. Herpes simplex virus is the virus most frequently isolated in clinical laboratories today.
2. The most common serologic request is acute viral titers (see p. 483 for complete serology discussion).
3. Average waiting time for viral culture results is 3 to 4 days; more than 70% can be reported in 5 days. Rapid test results (24 hours) are

accurate and available for some viruses such as cytomegalovirus (CMV).

4. Significance of viral cultures:
    (a) Positive viral culture results *diagnostic* for these sources
(1) Autopsy	(5) Other fluids
(2) Blood	(6) Cervix
(3) Biopsy	(7) Eye
(4) CSF	(8) Skin lesions

        Probably diagnostic (diagnostic if confirmed by serology)
(1) Throat	(2) Urine

        Possibly diagnostic: Stool
    (b) In contrast to normal bacterial inhabitants of humans, viruses do not compromise flora at any site. However, bacterial or fungal contamination of specimens can occur.

Diagnosis of Sexually Transmitted Diseases: General Observations

Sexually transmitted diseases are an ever-increasing public health problem and are caused by a variety of etiologic agents (Table 7-10). Some conditions, such as chlamydia and nongonococcal urethritis (NGU), have reached epidemic proportions. Although NGU is nonreportable in the United States, it is estimated that more than 2 million new cases occur each year. Manifestations of infection range from asymptomatic carriers to a spectrum of disease that includes cervicitis, conjunctivitis, endometritis, epididymitis, infertility, pharyngitis, proctitis, lymphogranuloma venereum, salpingitis, trachoma, urethritis and, in the neonate, conjunctivitis and pneumonia. The causative agent of *Lymphogranuloma venereum* (LGV) is *Chlamydia trachomatis*. The primary lesion of LGV is a small, painless vesicle. Other symptoms include pelvic inflammatory disease, inguinal lymphadenopathy, fever, chills, and malaise. Occasionally, a genitoanorectal syndrome, consisting of a bloody, mucopurulent rectal discharge, occurs. Diagnosis is usually made by isolating the causative organism, although complement fixation (CF) and macroimmunofluorescence tests are available.

Suggested Specimens

1. Urine
2. Semen
3. Urethral, vaginal, cervical, or oral swabs
4. Prostatic secretion
5. Tissue biopsy
6. Blood
7. Stool

(*text continues on page 422*)

TABLE 7–10.
Sexually Transmitted Diseases and Their Laboratory Diagnoses

Disease*	Causative Agents†	Diagnosis
Chancroid	*Hemophilus ducreyi*	Culture of lesion or aspirate. Differential diagnosis should include syphilis and herpes culture.
Gonorrhea	*Neisseria gonorrhoeae*	Gram stain of male urethra, culture of male urethra or female cervix, rectum, or pharynx. When indicated, urogenital swab tested for direct antigen.
Granuloma inguinale (Donovanosis)	*Calymmatobacterium granulomatis* (formerly *Donovania granulomatis*)	Wright's or Giemsa stain of lesion, tissue biopsy
Hepatitis B	Hepatitis B virus (HBV)	Serologic testing HB_sAg—most infectious state of disease. HB_sAg: Presence and persistence of infectivity and chronicity usually appear prior to symptoms.
Genital herpes	*Herpes simplex virus* (HSV) types 1 and 2	Culture from unroofed blister, scrapings examined by fluorescent microscopy or cytologic stains
Lymphogranuloma venereum (LGV)	*Chlamydia trachomatis* serotypes L_1, L_2, and L_3	Aspirate of bubo, serologic tests of blood
Molluscum contagiosum	*Molluscum contagiosum* virus	Clinical appearance of lesions (pearly white, painless, umbilicated papules), microscopic exam of scrapings
Chlamydia	*Chlamydia trachomatis* serotypes D–K	Cell culture, urogenital swabs for direct antigen test, or fluorescent microscopy
Candidosis (monilia)	*Candida albicans*	Culture, KOH wet mount
Pelvic inflammatory disease (PID)	*Neisseria gonorrhoeae* *Chlamydia trachomatis*	Clinical symptoms, cervical culture, laparoscopy, or culdocentesis
Pediculosis pubis	*Phthirus pubis* (pubic or crab louse)	Adult lice or nits appear on body hairs.
Scabies	*Sarcoptes scabiei*	Characteristic lesions, scrapings for microscopy
Syphilis	*Treponema pallidum*	Darkfield microscopic exam of primary and secondary lesions for *T. pallidum*. Nontreponemal reagin tests (VDRL, RPR) and specific tests (FTA–ABS, MHA–TP) are used to identify active and latent syphilis.
Trichomoniasis	*Trichomonas vaginalis*	Vaginal, urethral, prostatic secretion examined microscopically in a drop of saline for motile trichomonas; culture; speculum exam reveals foamy, greenish discharge and presence of bright red dots in vaginal wall and cervix

Disease/Condition	Pathogen	Diagnostic Method
Nonspecific urethritis (nongonococcal urethritis–NGU)	*Chlamydia trachomatis* (50% of cases), ureaplasma urealyticum, a human T-strain mycoplasma (*mycoplasma hominis*), *Trichomonas vaginalis, Candida albicans, Herpes simplex virus*	Failure to demonstrate *Neisseria gonorrhoeae* cell culture, culture of genital specimen, tissue, urine
Nonspecific vaginitis	*Gardherella vaginalis*	Wet mount or PAP smear; fishy smell is released when specimen fluid is mixed with 10% KOH. Culture or enzyme immunoassay to RO gonorrhea
Condylomata Acuminata (venereal warts)	Human papilloma DNA virus	Typical clinical lesion; cauliflower-like, soft, pink growths around vulva, anus, labia, vagina, glans penis, urethra and perineum; rule out syphilis
Acquired immuno deficiency syndrome (AIDS)	HIV virus	Serology
Gastrointestinal (giardiasis Amebiasis, shigellosis, camp/bacteriosis, and anorectal infections.	Enteric infections: *Giardia lamblia Entamoeba histolytica Cryptoporidum* spp. *Shigella* spp. *Campylobacter fetus Strongyloides* spp. (worms)	Stool-polyvinyl alcohol fixative or formalin ethyl acetate sedimentation (FES); same as above. Stool stain Rectal stool swab culture Rectal stool swab culture Stool (FES)
	Anorectal: *Neisseria gonorrhoeae Chlamydia trachomatis Treponema pallidum Herpes simplex* virus Human papilloma virus	Anal canal swab Specimen, culture Anal swab or rectal biopsy Dark-field microscopy plus serology, lesion swab, culture Signs and symptoms

* The major diseases are syphilis and gonorrhea.
† The pathogens causing sexually transmitted diseases span the full range of medical microbiology. The only common characteristic of these pathogens is that they may cause genital disease or may be transmitted by genital contact.

421

Common Diagnostic Methods

1. Viral isolation in tissue cell cultures
2. Specific serologic antibody assays and syphilis detection tests
3. Cytologic techniques such as PAP and Zanck smears to demonstrate giant cells of herpes virus infection.
4. Gram's stain
5. ELISA and immunoperoxidase assay to detect causative agent
6. Monoclonal antibodies to detect and identify etiologic agent.

Clinical Considerations

1. Patients with one sexually transmitted disease are frequently infected with other sexually transmitted pathogens.
2. Asymptomatic carriage is more common than generally realized.
3. Tracing of sexual partners is very important.
4. Treatment failure may occur because the patient has been reinfected by a nontreated partner.

DIAGNOSTIC PROCEDURES

Six classes of laboratory tests are used in the diagnosis of infectious diseases: smears and stains, cultures, animal inoculation, tissue biopsy, serologic testing, and skin testing. Cultures and skin testing are described in detail in this chapter. Serologic testing is described in Chapter 8. A brief description of each of these procedures follows.

The Smear

A smear is a specimen for microscopic study that is prepared by spreading a small quantity of material across a glass slide. If the material is to be stained, it is generally fixed to the slide by passing the slide quickly through the flame of a Bunsen burner. Smears can also be fixed in methanol.

The Stain

Smears are most often observed after they have been stained. Stains are salts composed of a positive and negative ion, one of which is colored. Structures in the specimen pick up the stain, thereby making the organism visible under the light microscope. One staining procedure, called the *negative stain*, colors the background and leaves the organisms uncolored. The gross structure of the organisms can then be seen.

Types of Stains: Bacterial stains are of two major types: *simple* and *differential*. A *simple stain* consists of a coloring agent such as gentian violet, crystal violet, carbol-fuchsin, methylene blue, or safranine. A thin smear of organisms is stained and then observed under the oil-immersion lens. A *differential stain* is one in which two chemically different stains are applied to the same smear. Organisms that are physiologically different will pick up different stains.

The *Gram's stain* is the most important of all bacteriologic differential stains; it divides bacteria into two physiologic groups: gram-positive and gram-negative.

The staining procedure has four major steps: (1) staining the smear with gentian or crystal violet; (2) washing off the violet stain and flooding the smear with an iodine solution; (3) washing off the iodine solution and flooding the smear with 95% alcohol; and (4) counterstaining the smear with safranine, a red dye.

In addition to allowing for morphologic study of the bacteria under question, the Gram's stain, as mentioned, divides all bacteria into two physiologic groups according to their ability or inability to pick up one or both of the two stains. The two categories of bacteria (gram-positive and gram-negative) exhibit different properties, which help in their identification.

Other stains besides the Gram's stain are used in examinations of bacteriologic smears. Some, such as the *acid-fast stain*, are used in identifying organisms of the genus *Mycobacterium*. Others are employed in the differentiation of certain structures such as capsules, endospores, and flagella.

Cultures

A culture is the growth of microorganisms or living tissue cells on special media conducive to the growth of this material. Cultures may be maintained in test tubes, petri dishes, dilution bottles, or any other suitable container. The container holds a food (called the *culture medium*) that is either solid, semisolid, or liquid. Each organism has its own special requirements for growth (proper combination of nutritive ingredients, temperature, and presence or absence of oxygen). The culture is prepared in accordance with its food needs. Later, it is either refrigerated or incubated according to the temperature requirements for growth.

Animal Inoculation

Animal inoculation is the means used to isolate bacteria when other means have failed. For example, when tuberculosis is suspected but smears have failed to confirm the disease, guinea pig inoculation is used. The organisms responsible for plague (*Yersinia pestis*) and tularemia (*Francisella tularensis*) may be isolated by animal inoculation. When viruses, certain spirochetes, certain fungi, and some parasites must be identified, animal inoculation is often used.

Tissue Biopsy

At times, microorganisms are isolated from small quantities of body tissue that have been surgically removed in the operating room or in the physician's office. Such tissue is removed using full aseptic technique and is transferred to a sterile container to be transported rapidly to the laboratory for analysis. Generally, the specimens are ground finely in a sterile homogenizer and plated out.

Serologic Testing

Serologic testing, which will be discussed in detail in Chapter 8, is a method for analysis of blood specimens for antigen–antibody reactions. This form of testing is generally valuable in diagnosis only late in the course of the infection. Specimens should be collected immediately after the patient has been admitted to the hospital, and again, 3 to 4 weeks after the onset of the disease.

Skin Testing

Skin testing, which will be described later in this chapter, is used to determine hypersensitivity of a person to the toxic products formed in the body by pathogens. Three types of skin tests are generally employed: scratch tests, patch tests, and intradermal tests.

BLOOD CULTURES

Background

Blood for culture is probably the single most important specimen submitted to the microbiologic laboratory for examination. Blood cultures are collected whenever there is reason to suspect bacteremia or septicemia. Although a mild transitory bacteremia is a frequent finding in many infectious diseases, the persistent, continuous, or recurrent type of bacteremia is indicative of a more serious condition.

Indications for Blood Culture

1. Bacteremia
2. Septicemia
3. Unexplained postoperative shock
4. Postoperative shock following genitourinary tract manipulation
5. Unexplained fever of more than several days' duration
6. Chills and fever in patients with
   (a) Infected burns
   (b) Urinary tract infections
   (c) Rapidly progressing tissue infections
   (d) Postoperative wound sepsis
   (e) Indwelling venous or arterial catheters
7. Debilitated patients undergoing therapy with
   (a) Antibiotics
   (b) Corticosteroids
   (c) Immunosuppressives
   (d) Antimetabolites
   (e) Parenteral hyperalimentation

Note: In typhoid fever and certain other diseases such as tularemia and plague, blood cultures are positive only in certain stages of the disease. Therefore, the clinician should be familiar with the clinical course of the disease, so that the most advantageous time for taking a blood sample may be known.

Procedure for Obtaining Blood Culture

Clinical Alert

In venipuncture, the potential for infecting the patient as a result of the diagnostic procedure is very high. Therefore, aseptic technique must be rigorously followed.

1. The proposed puncture site should be scrubbed with an antiseptic such as Betadine (povidone-iodine) or 70% alcohol.
2. The rubber stoppers of culture bottles should be cleansed with iodine and allowed to air dry. They should then be cleansed with 70% alcohol.
3. Venipuncture should be performed with a sterile syringe and needle; avoid any contamination of the cleansed site.
4. Approximately 5 to 15 ml of blood should be drawn in a 20-ml syringe.
5. After the specimen is obtained, the needle on the syringe should be discarded and replaced with a second sterile needle before the sample is injected into the culture bottles.
6. If two culture bottles are to be inoculated (one anaerobic and one aerobic), the anaerobic bottle should be inoculated first with enough blood to have a 1:10 dilution of a blood:broth mixture. Then the aerobic bottle should be inoculated aseptically to the same dilution.
7. The needle and syringe should be removed from the bottle, and both bottles should be mixed gently. To vent the aerobic bottle, a cotton-plugged needle specially designed for that purpose should be used.
8. Specimens should be properly labeled with the patient's name, age, date, time, number of culture, notation of patient isolation category (if applicable), and any other information the laboratory requires.

Clinical Alert

1. Handle all blood specimens as if they are capable of transmitting disease.

2. After disinfection, *do not probe* the venipuncture site with a finger unless sterile gloves are worn or the finger has been disinfected. Probing is the greatest potential cause of contamination in blood culture.
3. The attending physician should be notified immediately about positive cultures so that appropriate treatment may be started immediately.
4. If a specimen is spilled, and the patient is in blood or body fluid isolation, far more caution must be observed than if the patient is in respiratory isolation.
5. Specimens can be drawn at two or three different sites to exclude a skin-contaminating organism.

Clinical Implications

A. *Negative cultures*

If all cultures, subcultures, and Gram-stained smears are negative, the blood culture may be reported as: *No growth, aerobic or anaerobic, after 3 days' incubation. Further report to follow. Final report: No growth after 7 to 14 days' incubation.*

B. *Positive cultures*

Pathogens most commonly found in blood cultures include the following:

1. *Bacteroides* species
2. *Brucella* species
3. Coliform bacilli
4. Filariae*
5. *Francisella tularenis*
6. *Hemophilus influenzae*
7. *Leptospira* species
8. *Listeria monocytogenes*
9. Malaria*
10. *Neisseria meningitidis*
11. Pneumococci
12. Rickettsiae*
13. *Staphylococcus aureus,*
   S. epidermidis,
   S. saprophyticus
14. *Streptococcus pyogenes*
15. *Salmonella* species
16. Trypanosomes*
17. Gram-negative rods *Eschericia coli,* Enterobactic species, klebsiella species, and so forth.

Interfering Factors

1. Blood cultures are subject to contamination, especially by skin bacteria. These organisms should therefore be identified in the laboratory.
2. Nonfilterable blood is usually due to the presence of abnormal proteins.

---

* Culture is not the ideal method for isolating parasites. Peripheral blood smears are the usual method for detection of parasites.

Special Situation
With patients who have already received antibacterial therapy, certain enzymes may be incorporated into the growth medium to eliminate the activity of the antibacterial agent in the blood.

URINE CULTURES

Normal Values
Negative: less than 10,000 organisms/ml. Any bacteria found are either contaminants from the skin or invading pathogens.

Clinical Alert

1. A bacterial count of less than 10,000 bacteria/ml is not indicative of infection and possibly may be contamination. A count of 100,000 or more bacteria/milliliter indicates infection.
2. Urine cultures of *E. coli* are not definitely significant unless they contain more than 100,000 organisms/ml.

Background
Urine cultures are most commonly used to diagnose a bacterial infection of the urinary tract (kidneys, ureter, bladder, and urethra). Urine is an excellent culture medium for most organisms that infect the urinary tract, grow within the urine in the body, and result in high counts in established untreated infection. The combination of pyuria (pus in the urine) and significant bacteriuria strongly suggests the diagnosis of urinary tract infection.

Collection of Specimens for Culture:
General Principles
1. Early morning specimens should be obtained whenever possible because bacterial counts are highest at that time.
2. A clean voided urine specimen of 3–5 ml should be collected in a sterile container. Specimens may also be collected by catheterization, suprapubic aspiration, or directly from an indwelling catheter. Urine must not be obtained from a urine-collecting bag.

Clinical Alert

Catheterization heightens the risk of introducing infection. Whenever possible, avoid collecting urine by this method. **DO NOT** catheterize when merely a bacteriologic specimen is needed.

---

3. Urine should be taken to the laboratory as soon as possible and examined immediately. When this is not possible, the urine can be refrigerated (maximum 2 hours storage time) until cultured, if necessary. If collected for cytomegalovirus, the urine specimen should be kept at room temperature until taken to the virus laboratory for culture. *If refrigerated, the virus will be destroyed.*

4. Two successive clean-voided or midstream specimens should be collected in order to be 95% certain that true bacteriuria is present.

5. Whenever possible, specimens should be obtained before antibiotics or other antimicrobial agents have been administered.

6. The instruction for collection of all specimens should be the responsibility of professional health personnel (nurse, physician, medical technologist). Failure to isolate a causative organism is frequently the result of faulty collection techniques that can come from misinformation about the collection procedure.

7. Proper supplies and privacy for cleansing and collection should be provided. (Sterile specimen containers and antiseptic sponges should be available.)

8. Properly instructed patients will usually cleanse their pelvis or vulva and perineum at least as well as the health attendant. However, when the patient is unable to follow the procedure, a trained person can cleanse the patient and collect the specimen.

9. The specimen should be covered and labeled with
   (a) Patient's name
   (b) Suspected clinical diagnosis
   (c) Method of collection
   (d) Precise time obtained
   (e) Whether forced fluids or IVs have been administered
   (f) Any specific chemotherapeutic agents being administered

Procedure for Collection of Midstream or Clean-Catch Urine Specimen

Clinical Alert

Urine is an excellent culture medium, which at room temperature allows the growth of many organisms. Collection of specimens, therefore, should be as aseptic as possible. Samples should be taken immediately to the laboratory where they can be examined while still warm. If prompt analysis is not possible, the specimen must be refrigerated (2 hours maximum storage).

1. Women
   (a) Lower undergarments are to be removed.

(b) Patient should thoroughly wash hands with soap and water and then dry them with a disposable towel.

(c) The cap from a sterile container should be removed and placed with its outer surface down in a clean area.

(d) The area around the urinary meatus must be cleaned from front to back with an antiseptic sponge.

(e) With one hand, the patient should spread the labia, keeping them apart until the specimen is collected.

(f) After cleansing, the patient voids. After the first 25 ml has been passed into the toilet bowl, the urine is caught directly into the sterile container without stopping the stream. The patient voids until the container is almost full. The collection cup should be held in such a way that contact with the legs, vulva, or clothing is avoided. Fingers should be kept away from the rim and inner surface of the container.

2. Men

(a) Patient washes as in (b) above.

(b) The foreskin is completely retracted to expose the glans.

(c) The area around the meatus is cleansed with antiseptic sponges.

(d) Patient is to pass the first portion of urine (25 ml) directly into the toilet bowl and then pass a portion of the remaining urine into the sterile specimen container. The patient voids until the container is almost full. The last few drops of urine should not be collected.

3. Infants and children

In infants and young children, urine may be collected in a plastic collection apparatus. Because the collection bag touches skin surfaces and thereby picks up commensals, the specimen must be analyzed as soon as possible.

Clinical Implications

A count of 100,000 or more bacteria per milliliter indicates infection. A bacterial count of less than 10,000 bacteria per milliliter is not indicative of infection and possibly may be contamination. When present in significant titer, the following organisms, present in the urine, may be considered pathogenic.

1. Coliform bacilli
2. Enterococci
3. Gonococcus
4. *Klebsiella* (often)
5. *Mycobacterium tuberculosis*
6. *Proteus* species
7. *Pseudomonas aeruginosa*
8. Staphylococci, coagulase-positive and coagulase-negative
9. Streptococci, beta-hemolytic, usually Groups B and D

10. *Trichomonas vaginalis*
11. *Candida albicans* and other yeasts

Interfering Factors

1. The urine of patients who are receiving forced fluids may be sufficiently diluted to reduce the colony count below 10^5/ml.
2. Bacterial contamination comes from sources such as
   (a) Hair from the perineum
   (b) Bacteria from beneath the prepuce in men
   (c) Bacteria from vaginal secretions from the vulva or from the distal urethra in women
   (d) Bacteria from the hands, skin, or clothing

Patient Preparation

1. Explain the purpose and procedure of the test to the patient.
2. The cleansing procedure must remove contaminating organisms from the vulva, urethral meatus, and perineal area so that bacteria found in the urine can be assumed to have come from the bladder and urethra only.

Clinical Alert

The urine studied for culture should *not* be a sample taken from a urinal or bedpan and should *not* be brought from home. The urine is to be collected directly into a sterile container that will be used for culture.

Special Situation

With suspected urinary tuberculosis, the specimen should consist of three consecutive early morning samples. Special care should be taken in washing the external genitalia to reduce contamination with commensal acid-fast *Mycoplasma smegmatis*.

RESPIRATORY TRACT CULTURES

Four major types of cultures may be used to diagnose infectious diseases of the respiratory tract: (1) sputum, (2) throat swabs, (3) nasal swabs, and (4) nasopharyngeal swabs. At times, the purposes for which certain tests are ordered will overlap. Each of these cultures will be described below.

Normal Values

The following organisms may be present in the nasopharynx of apparently healthy individuals:

1. *Candida albicans*
2. Diphtheroid bacilli
3. *Hemophilus hemolyticus*
4. *Hemophilus influenzae*
5. *Branhamella catarrhalis*
6. *Staphylococcus aureus* (occasionally)
7. Staphylococci (coagulase-negative)
8. Streptococci (alpha-hemolytic)
9. Streptcococci (nonhemolytic)
10. Micrococci

Clinical Alert

1. Twenty percent of normal adults are carriers of *Staphylococcus aureus;* 10% are carriers of Group A hemolytic streptococci.
2. A new 10-minute strep test is being used that gives results after 10 minutes instead of 24 to 48 hours. It shows a false-negative rate of 5% to 10%, about the same as traditional methods. It permits rapid diagnosis and treatment.
3. Both throat and urine cultures are done to detect Epstein–Barr virus (EBV) and CMV.

Sputum

Background
Sputum is *not* material from the postnasal region and is *not* spittle or saliva. A specimen of sputum must be coughed up from deep within the bronchi.

Indications for Collection
Sputum cultures are important in the diagnosis of the following conditions:

1. Bacterial pneumonia
2. Pulmonary tuberculosis
3. Chronic bronchitis
4. Bronchiectasis
5. Suspected pulmonary mycotic infections
6. Mycoplasma pneumonia infection
7. Suspected viral pneumonia

Procedure

1. Sputum must be coughed up from the bronchi.
2. The specimen must be collected in a clear, sterile container, and the container must be capped.
3. The volume of the expectorate need not exceed 1 to 3 ml of purulent or mucopurulent material. This quantity is sufficient for most examinations except tuberculosis testing.
4. The specimen should be examined before delivery to the laboratory to determine whether the specimen is truly sputum and not saliva. Too often the culturing of unsuitable material (saliva) results in misleading information because the true infecting agent has not been observed.

Maintenance and Delivery of Specimen

1. Specimens should not be refrigerated.
2. Specimens should be delivered to the laboratory rapidly, so that organisms are still viable.
3. All specimens should be labeled with the name of the patient, date, room number, and suspected disease.

Patient Preparation

1. The patient should be instructed that this test requires tracheo-bronchial sputum, a substance from the lungs that is brought up by a deep cough.
2. The use of superheated hypertonic saline aerosols for sputum induction is recommended when the cough is not productive. Proper decontamination of the equipment must be carried out.

Clinical Alert

In children or adults who cannot produce sputum, a laryngeal swab may be taken.

Throat Culture (Swab) (Washings)

Indications for Collection

1. Throat cultures are important in the diagnosis of the following conditions:
   (a) Streptococcal sore throat
   (b) Diphtheria
   (c) Thrush (candidal infection of the mouth)

    (d) Tonsillar infection
    (e) Gonococcal pharyngitis
    (f) N-P for *Bordetella pertussis*
2. Throat cultures are useful in establishing the focus of infection in
    (a) Scarlet fever
    (b) Rheumatic fever
    (c) Acute hemorrhagic glomerulonephritis
3. Throat cultures can be used in detecting the carrier state of such organisms as
    (a) Beta hemolytic streptococcus
    (b) *Neisseria meningitidis*
    (c) *Corynebacterium diphtheriae*
    (d) *Staphylococcus aureus*

Procedure
1. The patient must be placed in a good light.
2. A sterile throat culture kit with a polyester-tipped applicator, or swab, is used.
3. A sterile container or tube of culture medium must be available.
4. With the patient's tongue depressed by a tongue blade and the throat well exposed and illuminated, the swab must be rotated firmly and gently over the back of the throat, both tonsils or fossae, and areas of inflammation, exudation, or ulceration.
    (a) Care should be taken to avoid touching the tongue or lips with the swab.
    (b) Because most patients will gag or cough, the collector should preferably wear a mask or stand to the side of the patient.
5. The swab is replaced in the inner tube and the ampule is crushed. The swab is then forced into the released medium. The medium is covered and the specimen is sent immediately to the laboratory.
6. If throat culture cannot be examined within 1 hour, it can be refrigerated.

Procedure for Pediatric Patients
1. Seat the patient in the adult's (parent's) lap.
2. Have the adult encircle the child's arms and chest to prevent the child from moving.
3. The collector should place one hand on the child's forehead to stabilize the head and prevent movement.
4. Proceed with the technique used for collection of the throat and nose culture.

For throat washings have the patient gargle with 5 to 10 ml of sterile saline solution and deposit it in a sterile cup. This provides more material than a throat swab and is more productive for viral isolation.

Nasal Culture (Swab)

Indications for Collection
1. Acute leukemia patients
2. Transplant recipients
3. Intermittent dialysis patients
4. Tracing epidemics

Procedure
Swab both external nares and deeper, moister recesses of the nose. Both nose and throat specimens are preferred for recovery of paramyxoviruses.

WOUND CULTURES

Normal Values
Clinical specimens taken from wounds may be expected to have any of the following microorganisms. The pathogenicity of the organisms is dependent on the quantity present.

1. *Actinomyces* species
2. *Bacteroides* species
3. *Clostridium perfringens* and other species
4. *Escherichia coli*
5. Other gram-negative enteric bacilli
6. *Mycobacterium* species
7. *Nocardia* species
8. *Pseudomonas* species
9. *Staphylococcus* species
10. *Staphylococcus epidermidis*
11. *Streptococcus faecalis*
12. *Streptococcus pyogenes*

Background
Material from infected wounds will reveal a variety of aerobic and anaerobic microorganisms. Because anaerobic microorganisms are the predominant microflora in humans and are constantly present in the upper respiratory tract, gastrointestinal tract, and genitourinary tract, they are also likely to invade other parts of the body, causing severe and often fatal infections.

Clinically significant pathogens are likely to be found in the following specimens:

1. Pus from any deep wound or aspirated abscess, especially if associated with a foul odor
2. Necrotic tissue or debrided material from suspected gas gangrene tissue

3. Material from infections bordering mucous membranes
4. Drainage from postoperative wounds
5. Ascitic fluid

Procedure for Anaerobic Collection Using Aspirated Material
1. Open the collection kit; the container contains carbon dioxide.
2. Remove the sterile syringe (sterile needle, if needed).
3. Aspirate the material; 1 to 3 cc is the preferred sample.

Culture Maintenance
All media must be incubated under strictly anaerobic conditions.

Procedure for Anaerobic Collection Using Swab Sets (Commonly Used Only If Unable To Aspirate Fluid or Pus)
1. Open the collection container, remove the swab, and take a sample by applying the sterile swab directly to the source of the culture.
2. Insert the swab into the container. Break the swab and discard the top portion.
3. Seal the container.
4. Do not touch the swab tip or inner surface of the collection container.
5. Label the specimen with
   (a) Patient's name
   (b) Date of sample
   (c) Source of specimen
   (d) Clinical diagnosis
   (e) Isolation status
   (f) Any other pertinent information required by the laboratory
6. Take the culture in such a way that exposure to oxygen is minimized or excluded.
7. If infection from mycobacteria or fungi is suspected, exudate or tissue should be collected in place of a swab.
8. With cultures of dry wounds, swabs should be moistened in sterile saline before use.

Clinical Alert

A microscopic examination of pus and wound exudates can be very helpful in diagnosis of the pathogenic organism. Consider the following:

1. Pus from streptococcal lesions is thin and serous.
2. Pus from staphylococcal infections is gelatinous.
3. Pus from *Pseudomonas aeruginosa* infections is blue-green.
4. Actinomycosis infections show "sulfur" granules.

The most useful specimens for analysis are pus or excised tissue. Dressings from discharging wounds are also acceptable. If swabs must be used, at least three swabs from one site must be submitted, and these swabs should be serum-coated. Swabs with a light smearing of pus dry out very quickly and are virtually useless.

SKIN CULTURES

Normal Values

The following organisms may be present on the skin of a healthy person. When present in low numbers, certain of these organisms may be considered normal commensals; at other times, when they multiply to excessive quantities, these same organisms may be pathogens.

1. *Clostridium* species
2. Coliform bacilli
3. Diphtheroids
4. Enterococci
5. Mycobacteria
6. *Proteus* species
7. Staphylococci
8. Streptococci
9. Yeasts and fungi

Background

The most common bacteria involved in skin infections are staphylococci, streptococci (Group A), and *Corynebacterium haemolyticum*. The common abnormal skin conditions include

1. Pyoderma
   (a) Staphylococcal impetigo characterized by bullous lesions with thin, amber, varnish-like crusts
   (b) Streptococcal impetigo characterized by thick crusts
2. Erysipelas
3. Folliculitis
4. Furuncles
5. Carbuncles
6. Secondary invasion of burns, scabies, and other skin lesions
7. Dermatophytes, especially athlete's foot, scalp and body ringworm, and "jock itch"

Procedure for Vesicular Lesions or Skin Scrapings

1. Clean the affected site with sterile saline, wipe it gently with alcohol, and allow it to air dry.
2. Aspirate fluid from fresh, intact vesicles with a 25-gauge needle on a tuberculin syringe and flush the contents into the transport medium.

3. If fluid is not present, open the vesicles and use a cotton-, rayon-, or dacron-tipped applicator to swab the base of the lesion to collect infected cells. (Exudate should be absorbed in the culturette.)
4. Place the swab directly into transport medium.
5. To make smears for stains, use a scalpel blade to scrape the base of the lesion. Being careful not to macerate the cells, spread material in a thin layer in a 1 cm circle on a slide.
6. Transport to the laboratory as rapidly as possible for viral cultures.

Clinical Alert

The most useful and common specimens for analysis are skin scrapings, nail scrapings, and hairs (see *Fungal Diseases*).

Clinical Implications

When present in significant quantities on the skin, the following organisms may be considered pathogenic and therefore indicative of an abnormal condition.

1. *Bacteroides* species
2. *Clostridium* species
3. Coliform bacilli
4. Fungi (*Sporotrichum, Actinomyces, Nocardia, Candida albicans, Trichophyton, Microsporum, Epidermophyton*)
5. *Staphylococcus aureus* (coagulase-positive)
6. *Streptococcus pyogenes*
7. *Pseudomonas aeruginosa*

STOOL AND ANAL CULTURES AND SMEARS

Normal Values

The following organisms may be present in the stool of apparently healthy people:

1. *Candida albicans*
2. Clostridia
3. Enterococci
4. *Escherichia coli*
5. *Proteus* species
6. *Pseudomonas aeruginosa*
7. *Anaerobic streptococci*
8. Staphylococci

Clinical Alert

1. *Candida albicans* and *Pseudomonas aeruginosa* in large numbers in the stool is considered pathogenic in the presence of

previous antibiotic therapy. Alterations of the normal flora by antibiotics often change normally harmless organisms into pathogens.
2. *Cryptosporidiosis* is a cause of severe, protracted diarrhea in immunosuppressed patients.

Background

Stool cultures are commonly done to identify parasites, enteric disease organisms, and viruses in the intestinal tract. Of all specimens collected, feces are most likely to contain the greatest number and greatest variety of organisms. In a routine culture, the stool is examined to rule out *Salmonella*, *Shigella*, *Campylobacter*, *Yersinia*, enteropathogenic *Escherichia coli* (in the newborn), and pure cultures of staphylococcus.

A single negative stool culture should not be regarded as confirmation of noninvolvement of infectious bacteria. At least three cultures are usually done if the clinical picture of the patient suggests a bacterial involvement and if the first two cultures are negative. Moreover, after a positive diagnosis has been made, personal contacts of the patient and the convalescent patient should also have three negative stool cultures to prevent spread of infection.

Procedure for Collection

1. Feces should be collected in a dry container free of urine.
2. A freshly passed stool is the specimen of choice. The entire stool should be collected.
3. Only a small amount of stool is needed. A stool the size of a walnut is usually adequate; however, the entire passed stool should be sent for examination.
4. A diarrheal stool usually gives good results (5–10 ml).
5. Stool passed into the toilet bowl must not be used for culture.
6. No toilet paper should be placed in the bedpan or specimen container for it may contain bismuth, which interferes with laboratory tests.
7. Stool should be transferred to a container with tongue blades. The specimen should be labelled and sent immediately to the laboratory.

Clinical Alert

Fecal specimens are far superior to rectal swabs. Often rectal swabs are merely anal and provide little material of diagnostic significance.

Culture Maintenance

1. Examination should be within a few hours of collection.
2. If delays over 18 to 24 hours are suspected, the specimen should be mixed with an equal volume of buffered glycerol-saline.
3. Swabs must be examined immediately to prevent drying out of specimen.

Procedure for Taking Cellophane Tape Test

1. A tape test is indicated in cases of suspected enterobiasis (pinworms).
2. A strip of clear cellophane tape (not micropore or adhesive) is applied to the perineal region. It is then removed and spread on a slide for microscopic examination.
3. A paraffin-coated swab can be used in place of the cellophane tape test. If it is used, it is placed in a covered test tube.
4. Repeated examinations on consecutive days may be necessary.
5. The test for eggs is made preferably in the morning before the patient has defecated or bathed.
6. Test in children: In about one-third of infected children, eggs can also be obtained from beneath the fingernails. Follow the instructions on the kit provided.

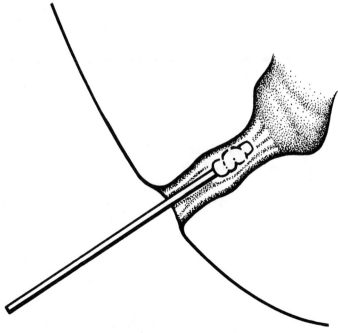

FIGURE 7–1.
Method for obtaining the rectal culture.

Interfering Factors
Feces from patients receiving barium, bismuth, oil, or antibiotics are unsatisfactory for the identification of protozoa.

Patient Preparation for Collection of Stool Specimen
1. The patient should be instructed to defecate into a clean bedpan or a large-mouthed container.
2. The patient should be told not to defecate into the toilet bowl or to urinate into the bedpan or collecting container, because urine has a harmful effect on protozoa.
3. Toilet paper should not be placed in the bedpan or collection container.

Procedure for Taking a Rectal Swab
1. The swab is inserted gently into the rectum (to at least 3 cm) and rotated to obtain a visible amount of fecal material (Fig. 7-1).
2. The swab is placed in a clean container and the cover is closed.
3. The specimen is properly labeled and sent immediately to the laboratory.

Clinical Alert

1. In the hospital, patients with diarrhea should remain in isolation until the cause of diarrhea is determined.
2. When pathogens are found in the stool, the patient usually remains isolated until the stool is formed and antibiotic therapy is completed.

CEREBROSPINAL FLUID (CSF) CULTURES AND SMEARS

Normal Values
No flora are normally present. In healthy persons, the specimen may be contaminated by normal skin flora.

Pathogens Found in CSF
1. *Bacteroides* species
2. Coliform bacilli
3. *Cryptococcus* and other fungi
4. *Hemophilus influenzae* (especially in infants and children)
5. *Leptospira* species
6. *Listeria monocytogenes*
7. *Mycobacterium tuberculosis*
8. *Neisseria meningitidis*
9. Pneumococci
10. Staphylococci
11. Streptococci
12. *Treponema pallidum*

Indications for Collection
1. Viral meningitis
2. Pyogenic meningitis
3. Tuberculosis meningitis
4. Chronic meningitis (due to *Cryptococcus neoformans*)

Explanation of Test
Bacteriologic examination of cerebrospinal fluid (CSF) is an essential step in the diagnosis of any case of suspected meningitis. Acute bacterial meningitis is an infection of the meninges, or membrane covering the brain and spinal cord, and is a rapidly fatal disease if untreated or if given inadequate treatment. Prompt identification of the causative agent is necessary for appropriate antibiotic therapy. Meningitis is caused by a variety of gram-positive and gram-negative microorganisms. Bacterial meningitis can also be secondary to infections in other parts of the body.

It is recommended that a smear and culture be carried out in all CSF specimens from persons with suspected meningitis, whether the fluid is clear or cloudy. (Normal CSF is clear.)

In bacterial meningitis, which is caused by a variety of bacteria, the CSF shows the following characteristics:

1. Purulent (usually)
2. Increased white blood cells
3. Predominance of polymorphonuclear cells
4. Decreased CSF glucose

In meningitis, which is caused by tubercle bacillus, viruses, fungi, or protozoa, the CSF shows the following characteristics:

1. Nonpurulent (usually)
2. Decreased count of mononuclear white cells
3. Normal or decreased CSF glucose

In persons with suspected meningitis, the fluid is generally submitted for chemical and cytologic examinations, as well as for culture.

Procedure
1. The specimen must be collected under sterile conditions, sealed immediately to prevent leakage or contamination, and sent to the laboratory without delay.

Clinical Alert

It is very important that a diagnosis be made as quickly as possible. Because some organisms cannot tolerate temperature changes, it is very important that the culture be done as quickly as possible.

> If a viral etiology is suspected, a portion of the fluid must be immediately frozen for subsequent attempts at isolation of the virus.

2. The specimen should be labeled with the patient's name, age, date, room number, and suspected disease. The laboratory staff should be alerted so that they can prepare to examine the specimen immediately.

Clinical Alert

The laboratory should be given adequate warning that a CSF sample will be delivered. Time is a critical factor; the cells disintegrate if the sample is kept at room temperature for more than 1 hour.

3. The attending physician should be notified as soon as results are obtained so that appropriate treatment can be started.
4. Specimens of CSF can be incubated after collection but can never be refrigerated.

Maintenance of Culture
1. If the specimen cannot be delivered at once to the laboratory for analysis, the container should be kept at 37°C.
2. No more than 4 hours should elapse before laboratory analysis, because of the low survival rate of the organisms causing meningitis, especially *Hemophilus influenzae* and the meningococcus.

Special Situation
In cases of suspected tuberculous meningitis, the specimen may be left standing at 37°C (98.6°F) for an hour to form the characteristic "spider web" clot. This technique is best left for later in the course of the disease, for the clot is often not found early, or it is used as a sign of the progress of chemotherapy.

Clinical Implications
Positive cultures occur in

1. Meningitis
2. Trauma
3. Abscess of brain or ependyma of spine
4. Septic thrombophlebitis of venous sinuses

CERVICAL, URETHRAL, AND ANAL CULTURES AND SMEARS FOR GONORRHEA AND OTHER SEXUALLY TRANSMITTED DISEASES

Procedure for Obtaining Cultures

A. *Female patients*

    1. *Cervical culture:* The cervix is the best site to obtain a culture specimen (Fig. 7-2).

        (a) Moisten the speculum with warm water; do NOT use a lubricant.

        (b) Remove cervical mucus, preferably with a cotton ball held in a ring forceps.

        (c) Insert a sterile, cotton-tipped swab into the endocervical canal; move the swab from side to side; allow several seconds for absorption of organisms by the swab.

FIGURE 7–2.
Method for obtaining the endocervical culture.

Because *Trichomonas vaginalis* may be present in urethral or vaginal discharge, material for culture should be collected as stated previously, but the swab should be placed in a tube containing 0.5 ml of sterile saline and delivered to the laboratory immediately.

Swabs for culture should be transported to the laboratory in Stuart's transport media and held at room temperature until processed. If specimens are not processed within several hours, they should be refrigerated. However, recovery of a pathologic organism may be affected by a delay in processing.

2. *Anal canal culture:* This is the most likely site to be positive when a cervical culture is negative.

Note: The anal canal specimen can be obtained after the cervical specimen without changing the patient's position and without using the anoscope.

(a) Insert a sterile, cotton-tipped swab approximately 1 inch into the anal canal. (If the swab is inadvertently pushed into feces, use another swab to obtain the specimen.)

(b) Move the swab from side to side in the anal canal to sample crypts; allow several seconds for absorption of organisms by the swab.

B. *Male patients*

1. *Urethral culture*

Use a sterile swab to obtain the specimen from the anterior urethra by gently scraping the mucosa (Fig. 7-3).

FIGURE 7–3.
Method for obtaining the urethral culture.

Clinical Alert

If the urethral culture in men is negative, but gonorrhea is still suspected, prostatic massage may increase the number of organisms in urethral discharge.

2. *Anal canal culture*
   Follow the same procedure as in female patients.
C. *Both male and female patients*
   Oropharyngeal culture
   Culture specimens should also be obtained from the oropharynx in persons engaging in oral sex.

Clinical Alert

Repeated culturing for gonococci without detection does not exclude a diagnosis of gonorrhea.

Patient Preparation
1. The patient is to be placed in the dorsal lithotomy position and appropriately draped.
2. The person collecting the specimen should wear sterile, disposable gloves.

SKIN TESTS

Background
Skin testing is done for three major reasons: (1) to detect a person's sensitivity to allergens such as dust and pollen, (2) to determine a person's sensitivity to microorganisms believed to cause disease, and (3) to determine whether a person's cell-mediated, immune function is normal. The test that detects sensitivity to allergens will be mentioned only briefly in this chapter. Most of the discussion will center on tests used in the determination of sensitivity to pathogens.

In general, the following three types of skin tests are used:

1. Scratch tests
   Scratches approximately 1 cm long and 2.5 cm apart are made in rows on a patient's back or forearm. Extremely small quantities of allergens are introduced into these scratches. Positive reaction: swelling or redness at the site within 30 minutes.

2. Patch tests
   A small square of gauze is impregnated with the substance in question and applied to the skin of the forearm. Positive reaction: swollen or reddened skin at the site of the patch after a given period of time.
3. Intradermal tests
   The substance that is being tested is introduced within the layers of skin by a tuberculin syringe fitted with a short-bevel 26- or 27-gauge needle. Positive reaction: red and inflamed area at the site of the injection within a given period of time (*e.g.*, 72 hours in the Mantoux test for tuberculosis).

Skin tests revealing a hypersensitivity to a toxic product from a disease-producing agent may also indicate an immunity to the disease. Positive reactions may additionally indicate the presence of an active or inactive case of the disease under study. The following is a categorization of skin tests according to their nature and purpose:

1. Tests to determine possible susceptibility (or resistance) to infection; for example, Schick test (positive reaction = lack of immunity to diphtheria)
   Dick test (positive reaction = lack of immunity to scarlet fever)
2. Tests to indicate a present or past exposure with the infectious agent; for example, tuberculin test (positive reaction = presence of active or inactive tuberculosis)
3. Tests to show sensitivity to various types of materials to which a person may react in an exaggerated manner; for example, Allergenic extracts such as house dust and pollen (positive reaction to sensitivity to allergen extracts)
4. Tests to detect impaired cellular immunity
   Intradermal skin testing with several common antigenic microbial substances is one way of determining whether the immune function is normal. This would be important in treating leukemias and cancer patients with chemotherapy.
   PPD tuberculin skin tests, mumps virus, *Candida albicans*, skin fungi, and streptokinase–streptodornase. (Negative reaction to any intradermal antigen is indicative of impaired immunity due to abnormal cell-mediated immune function.)

Procedure for Taking Skin Test
1. Most diagnostic skin tests come in an unopened, sterile kit. Follow the manufacturer's instructions carefully.
2. Generally, 0.1 ml of the substance under question is injected intradermally in the volar aspect of the forearm.
3. Positive reaction: redness or swelling of more than 1 cm in diameter. A central area of necrosis is an even more significant finding.

Clinical Alert

Material for diagnostic skin tests may be inadvertently injected subcutaneously rather than intradermally. A subcutaneous injection will yield a false-negative result.

Procedure for Taking Patch Test
1. The skin is cleansed and allowed to dry.
2. Remove the protective cover from a specially prepared adhesive patch or gauze square impregnated with the testing substance and firmly apply it to the forearm or the interscapular region of the back.

Procedure for Taking Scratch Test
The scratch method is especially recommended in patients who give a history of extreme sensitivity.

1. The skin is cleansed with alcohol (or acetone if the patient is allergic to alcohol) and allowed to dry. Sites to be used are the forearm or the interscapular region of the back. The elbow and wrist areas are less reactive and should be avoided.
2. The skin is stretched taut, using the thumb and index finger.
3. Using a sterile lancet to puncture the epidermis, a scratch approximately 1 to 4 mm long is made. The purpose is to raise the skin. The skin should be abraided without drawing blood. In the event that blood is drawn, the site should not be used.
4. One drop of the substance used for testing is applied to the scarification, taking care not to touch the skin with the dropper.
5. A control test should be performed for comparison purposes.

Tuberculin Skin Test (for Detection of Tuberculosis)

Normal Values
Negative or not significant

Explanation of Test
The tuberculin skin test is an intradermal test used to detect tuberculosis infection; it does not distinguish active from dormant infections. Tuberculin is a protein fraction of tubercle bacilli, and when it is introduced into the skin of a person with active or dormant tuberculosis infection, it causes a localized erythema and induration of the skin because of an accumulation of small, sensitized lymphocytes.

The tuberculin test of choice is the Mantoux test, using a needle and syringe.

Multiple puncture tests (TINE) are used for screening in asymptomatic persons.

Indications for Testing
1. Persons with signs (X-ray film abnormality) and/or symptoms (cough, hemoptysis, weight loss, etc.) suggestive of current tuberculosis disease
2. Recent contacts with known tuberculosis cases or persons suspected of having tuberculosis
3. Persons with abnormal chest roentgenograms compatible with past tuberculosis
4. Persons with medical conditions that increase the risk of tuberculosis (silicosis, gastrectomy, diabetes, immunosuppressive therapy, lymphomas, AIDS)
5. Groups at high risk of recent infection with Mycobacterium tuberculosis, such as immigrants from Asia, Africa, Latin America, and Oceania; some inner city and skid row populations; personnel and long-term residents in some hospitals, nursing homes, mental institutions, and prisons

Procedure
A. Intradermal skin test
   1. PPD-t is drawn up into a tuberculin syringe (follow manufacturer's directions carefully), using a ½ inch 26- or 27-gauge needle.
   2. The skin on the volar or dorsal aspect of the forearm is cleansed with alcohol and allowed to dry.
   3. The skin is stretched taut.
   4. The tuberculin syringe is held close to the skin so that the hub of the needle touches it as the needle is introduced. A discrete pale elevation of the skin—a wheal—6 mm to 10 mm in diameter should be produced when the prescribed amount of fluid (0.1 ml) is accurately injected intracutaneously.

Clinical Implications
1. The larger the size of the skin reaction, the more likely it is to represent tuberculosis infection. However, a significant reaction to the skin test does not necessarily signify the presence of the disease.
2. Because a significant reaction does not distinguish between an active and a dormant infection, the stage of infection can be determined from the results of clinical bacteriologic tests of the sputum and from roentgenograms.
3. A significant reaction in a patient who is clinically ill means that active tuberculosis cannot be dismissed as a diagnostic possibility.
4. A significant reaction in healthy persons usually signifies healed tuberculosis or an infection caused by a different mycobacteria.

Clinical Alert

1. Tuberculin should never be transferred from one container to another.
2. Skin tests should be given immediately after the syringe is filled.
3. The greatest value of tuberculin skin testing is in its negative implications. This means that a negative test result in the presence of signs and symptoms of lung disease is strong evidence against active tuberculosis, in the majority of cases.
4. Bacteriologic confirmation of a presumptive diagnosis of tuberculosis must be done.
5. Incidence of tuberculosis is higher among older persons, men, non-whites, and the foreign born.
6. Typical new case: Born in 1930s, infected in 1940s, developed disease in 1980s.
7. Sixteen percent of tuberculosis is extrapulmonary.
8. Transmission of tuberculosis usually requires close, frequent, and prolonged exposure.
9. Diagnosed case of tuberculosis averages nine contacts, of which 21% are infected.

Interfering Factors
1. False-negative results may occur even in the presence of active tuberculosis and whenever sensitized T lymphocytes are temporarily depleted in the body (Table 7-11).

Reading the Test Results
1. The test should be read 48 to 72 hours after infection.
2. The patient should be examined in a good light.
3. The patient should flex his or her forearm at the elbow.
4. The skin should be inspected for induration (hardening or thickening).
5. The examiner's finger should be rubbed lightly from the area of normal skin to the indurated zone.
6. The zone of induration should be circled with a pencil and the diameter measured in millimeters.
7. Little change in size occurs before the fifth day; however, large reactions are still evident at least seven days later.

Interpreting the Test Results
The interpretation of the test is based on the presence or absence of induration.

Negative or not significant reaction: zone less than 5 mm in diameter
Significant reaction: zone 10 mm or more in diameter

TABLE 7–11.
Potential Causes of Falsely Nonsignificant Tuberculin Test Reactions

Factors Related to Person Being Tested
Infections:
  Viral (measles, mumps, chickenpox)
  Bacterial (typhoid fever, brucellosis, typhus, leprosy, pertussis, overwhelm-
    ing tuberculosis, tuberculous pleurisy)
  Fungal (South American blastomycosis)
Live virus vaccinations (measles, mumps, polio)
Metabolic derangements (chronic renal failure)
Nutritional factors (severe protein depletion)
Diseases affecting lymphoid organs (Hodgkin's disease, lymphoma, chronic
  lymphocytic leukemia, sarcoidosis)
Drugs (corticosteroids and many other immunosuppressive agents)
Age (newborns, elderly patients with "waned" sensitivity)
Recent or overwhelming infection with *M. tuberculosis*
Stress (surgery, burns, mental illness, graft-versus-host reactions)

Factors Related to Tuberculin Used
Improper storage (exposure to light and heat)
Improper dilutions
Chemical denaturation
Contamination
Adsorption (partially controlled by adding Tween 80)

Factors Related to Method of Administration
Injection of too little antigen
Delayed administration after drawing into syringe
Injection too deep

Factors Related to Reading Test and Recording Results
Inexperienced reader
Conscious or unconscious bias
Error in recording

Schick Test

Normal Values
See "Clinical Implications."

Background
1. Diphtheria is a respiratory disease caused by the bacterium *Corynebacterium diphtheriae.*
2. A person who is immune to diphtheria will produce antitoxins that
   will circulate in his or her blood in significant quantities.
3. A person who is susceptible to diphtheria will lack (or have very low
   levels of) antitoxins, and therefore will not be able to neutralize the
   diphtheria toxin injected intradermally in the test.

Explanation of Test
1. The Schick test is a means for determining the presence or absence of a significant quantity of diphtheria antitoxins in the blood. The presence of these antitoxins indicates immunity to the disease.
2. If the skin test causes erythema and flaking of the skin at the site of the injection, the person tested is susceptible to diphtheria. This is a positive reaction.
3. A negative reaction, indicated by no flaking or erythema, means that under normal conditions of exposure, the person will not contract diphtheria.
4. The test gives a rough estimate of the quantity of antitoxins circulating in the blood.

Procedure
1. A 0.1-ml quantity of purified diphtheria *toxin* (0.02 of the amount necessary to kill a guinea pig) dissolved in human serum albumin is injected intradermally on the volar surface of the forearm. A 0.1-ml quantity of inactivated diphtheria *toxoid* is injected into the other arm as a control to rule out sensitivity to culture proteins.
2. These areas are examined at 24 and 48 hours and between the third and fourth days.

Interpreting Test Results
1. Positive test: Site of toxin injection begins to redden in 24 hours and increases and reaches a maximum size in about 1 week, when it will be swollen and tender and as large as 3 cm in diameter. There is usually a small, dark red central zone that gradually turns brown and leaves a pigmented area. The area of *toxoid* injection shows no reaction.
2. Negative test: No reaction at either site.

Clinical Implications
1. If the allergic response to the control material parallels that to the toxin in size and duration of reaction, the test is recorded as a negative Schick.
2. If, however, the reaction to the unheated toxin is at least 50% larger and persists longer than the reaction to the control, the individual is both susceptible to the toxin and allergic to the contaminating substances that are not destroyed by heating; a positive Schick is recorded.
3. If a reaction occurs (*i.e.*, a positive test), the person does not have enough antibodies to neutralize the toxin and is therefore susceptible to diptheria. The person has no immunity to diptheria.
4. Persons who have been well immunized with four injections of diptheria toxoid show uniformly negative reactions to the Schick test.
5. If the test is positive in a well-immunized person, this is strong evidence of the person's inability to produce antibodies.

6. A negative test means that the person has immunity to exposure to diptheria.
7. The Schick test has a limited need in the United States.

> **Clinical Alert**
>
> The major significant reservoirs of diphtheria are immunized persons, particularly the elderly whose immunity has waned, and children who have not been immunized.

Dick Test

Normal Values
See "Clinical Implications."

Background
1. Scarlet fever, also called *scarlatina,* is a communicable, hemolytic streptococcal infection caused by *Streptococcus pyogenes.* The condition causes generalized toxemia, a typical rash and scaling of skin, during the recovery period.
2. Occurrence of scarlet fever has been decreasing in recent years.
3. Scarlatinal or erythrogenic toxin is responsible for the rash of scarlet fever.

Explanation of Test
The Dick test is a diagnostic skin test that measures a person's susceptibility to scarlet fever. It also indicates immunity to the disease. A solution of dilute scarlatinal toxin is injected intradermally to detect antibody and to determine immunity to scarlet fever.

Procedure
1. A 0.1-ml dilute solution of scarlet fever (Dick) toxin is injected intradermally on the volvar surface of the forearm.
2. The test area is examined within a 24-hour period.

Interpreting Test Results
1. The test should be read within 18 to 24 hours.
2. Positive reaction: site of injection is very red and markedly swollen (3–5 cm. in diameter). Swollen area has sharply raised edges. A positive test indicates damage done by the injected toxin that has not been neutralized by antibodies present in the body.

3. Negative reaction: no more than a faint pink streak along the course of the needle
4. Slightly positive reaction: faint red area measuring less than 1 cm in diameter; no swelling

Clinical Implications

1. A positive reaction signifies that the person has insufficient circulating antitoxins to the Dick toxin and is susceptible to scarlet fever. A positive test reverts to a negative reaction following infection.
2. A negative reaction signifies that a person is relatively immune to the disease.

Clinical Alert

There are three immunologically rare but distinct toxins that may account for second attacks of scarlet fever.

Mumps Test

Causative Agent

Mumps, the common disease causing swelling and tenderness of the parotid glands, is caused by a myxovirus.

Explanation of Test

An antigen made from infected monkeys or chickens is injected intradermally, and a control material made from noninfected monkeys or chickens is also injected intradermally. A positive mumps skin test may indicate prior or present infection and is, therefore, not effective as a diagnostic tool. The test is used primarily as part of a battery of skin tests for determining immunocompetence.

Interpreting Test Results

1. The test should be read in 48 hours.
2. Positive reaction: erythema and a lesion larger than 10 mm in diameter
3. Negative reaction: No erythema and a lesion less than 10 mm in diameter

Clinical Implications

1. A positive reaction indicates resistance to the mumps virus.
2. A negative reaction indicates susceptibility to the mumps virus.

Blastomycosis (Gilchrist's Disease) Test

Causative Agent
Blastomycosis, a condition characterized by cutaneous, pulmonary, and systemic lesions, is caused by organisms of the genus *Blastomyces*.

Explanation of Test
Blastomycin, an antigen, is injected intradermally. The test is reasonably specific for blastomycosis, but in practice this skin-test antigen is usually injected simultaneously with histoplasmin, coccidioiden, and tuberculin.

Blastomycosis is also diagnosed by the recovery of the organism from pus, sputum, or tissue specimens.

Interpreting Test Results
1. The test should be read in 48 hours.
2. Positive reaction: area of erythema and induration 5 by 5 mm or greater
3. Doubtful reaction: area of induration less than 5 mm in diameter or erythema only
4. Negative reaction: no induration; or erythema less than 5 mm in diameter

Clinical Implications
A positive reaction may be indicative of

1. Past infection
2. Mild, chronic, or subacute infection
3. Improvement in cases of serious symptomatic blastomycosis that previously had been blastomycin-negative

Coccidioidomycosis Test

Causative Agent
Coccidioidomycosis, an infectious fungus disease occurring in both an acute form and a progressive form, is caused by *Coccidioides immitis*.

Explanation of Test
Coccidioidin, an antigen prepared from culture, is injected intradermally. A skin reaction will appear 10 to 21 days after infection, and a sensitivity continues throughout life. Coccidioidomycosis can also be diagnosed by recovery of the causative organism from pus, sputum, or tissue specimens.

Interpreting Test Results
1. The test must be read in 24 to 72 hours. If an immediate reaction occurs, it is nonspecific for coccidioidomycosis and is ignored.

2. Positive reaction: area of erythema and induration of 5 mm or more in diameter. Reaction disappears within 24 to 72 hours.

Clinical Implications
1. The skin test becomes positive in 87% of the cases of coccidioidomycosis during the first week of clinical symptoms and in almost 100% of patients after the first week.
2. A positive reaction persists for many years, but this does not imply that active infection is present. However, when there is a positive reaction during the course of infection in which an earlier test was negative, it can indicate active infection.
3. Documentation of conversion in a person who has been in an endemic area is virtually diagnostic of coccidioidal infection.

Histoplasmosis Test

Causative Agent
Histoplasmosis, a systemic fungus infection of the reticuloendothelial system, is caused by the organism *Histoplasma capsulatum*.

Explanation of Test
Histoplasmin, an antigen prepared from culture, is injected intradermally. Skin reactions to histoplasmin are of relatively little diagnostic value, because anergy may provide false-negative results. Histoplasmosis is also diagnosed by identification of the causative agent in pus, sputum, or tissue specimens.

Interpreting Test Results
1. The test should be read in 24 to 48 hours. If an immediate reaction occurs, it is nonspecific for histoplasmosis and is ignored.
2. Positive reaction: area of erythema and induration of 5 mm or more in diameter
3. Negative reaction: no induration; erythema less than 5 mm in diameter

Clinical Implications
1. A positive test indicates past or present infection.
2. Acutely ill patients may not have a positive reaction.

> **Clinical Alert**
>
> The skin test for histoplasmosis should be given after specimens for complement-fixation tests have been collected. The skin test reagent may induce or increase the titer of complement-fixing antibodies, even in the absence of active histoplasmosis.

BIBLIOGRAPHY

August M: Practical aspects of viral laboratory diagnoses. J Med Technol 2(8):501–506, August 1985

Blair RE et al (eds): Damon Clinical Laboratories Handbook. Stow, OH, Damon Corp., Lexi-Comp, 1989

Benenson AS (ed): Control of Communicable Diseases in Man, 14th ed. Washington DC, American Public Health Association, 1985

Berger RE (ed): Sexually transmitted diseases. Urol Clin North Am 2(1): Feb 1984

Burrows W: Textbook of Microbiology, 22nd ed. Philadelphia, WB Saunders, 1985

Checko PJ: Guidelines for the collection, procession, and interpretation of microbiological specimens in extended care facilities. Infect Control Urol Care 5:27, 1980

Davis BD et al: Microbiology, 4th ed. Philadelphia, JB Lippincott, 1990

Feld R: Q fever. Diagn Clin Test 28:30–32, Mar 1990

Finegold S, Baron E: Bailey and Scott's Diagnostic Microbiology, 6th ed. St. Louis, CV Mosby, 1986

Garcia LS: Parasitology update. Teleconference Network of Texas, April 10, 1990

Halsted CH, Halsted JA (eds): The Laboratory in Clinical Medicine, 2nd ed. Philadelphia, WB Saunders, 1981

Hammerschlag MR et al: When to Suspect Chlamydia. Patient Care 21(18):64–70, 75–76, 78, Nov 15, 1987

Hoeprich PD, Jordan MC: Infectious Diseases, 4th ed. Philadelphia, JB Lippincott, 1989

Hong R: Recurrent infections. Pediatrics in Review II:180–183, 1990

Hsiung GD: Diagnostic Virology. New Haven, CT, Yale University Press, 1982

Isselbacher KJ et al (eds): Harrison's Principles of Internal Medicine, 11th ed. New York, McGraw–Hill, 1987

Kilbourn JP: Bacterial flora of the urinary tract. J Am Med Technol 43:321–332, Nov 1981

Kite P et al: Diagnosis of neonatal bacteremia using combinations of tests. Midwifery 4(3):123–129, Sep 1988

Koneman EW et al (eds): Color Atlas and Textbook of Microbiology, 3rd ed. Philadelphia, JB Lippincott, 1988

Kunin CM: Detection, Prevention, and Management of Urinary Tract Infections, 4th ed. Philadelphia, Lea & Febiger, 1987

Matson C: Streptococcal pharyngitis. Consultant 28(12):87, 90, Dec 1988

McFarlane A: Using the laboratory in infection control. Prof Nurse 4(8):393–394; 396–397, May 1989

Musial CD, Cockerill FR, Roberts GD: Fungal infections of the immunocompromised host: Clinical and laboratory aspects. Clin Microbiol Rev 1:349–361, Oct 1988

Pauker SG: HIV Screening: Nosocomial epedemiologic risks and decision analysis. Law Med Health Care 18(1/2):33–40, Spring–Summer 1990

Sacher RA, McPherson RA: Widmann's Clinical Interpretation of Laboratory Tests, 10th ed. Philadelphia, FA Davis, 1991

Sonnenwirth AC, Jarrett L: Gradwohl's Clinical Laboratory Methods and Diagnosis, 8th ed. St. Louis, CV Mosby, 1980

Statland BE: How illness demographics will affect the lab. MLO 21(7):79–82, 84, 86, Jul 1989

Strampfer MJ et al: Laboratory aids in the diagnosis of bacterial meningitis—Winthrop University Hospital Infectious Disease Symposium. Heart Lung 17(6):605–607, Nov 1988

Wasley G: Laboratory tests: Detecting sexually transmitted diseases. Nurs Times 84(39):59–61, Sep 28–Oct 4, 1988

Washington JA II (ed): Laboratory Procedures in Clinical Microbiology, 2nd ed. New York, Springer–Verlag, 1985

Volk W: Essentials of Medical Microbiology, 3rd ed. Philadelphia, JB Lippincott, 1986

Yannelli B et al: Yield of stool cultures, ova and parasite tests and clostridium difficile determinations in nosocomial diarrheas. Am J Infect Control 16(6):246–249, Dec 1988

Youmans GP: The Biologic and Clinical Basis of Infectious Diseases, 3rd ed. Philadelphia, WB Saunders, 1986

IMMUNODIAGNOSTIC STUDIES

Introduction

Overview
Immunology is the study of antigen–antibody reactions *in vitro*. *Diagnostic immunology*, or *serodiagnostic testing*, uses serologic tests to aid in the diagnosis of infectious disease, immune disorders, allegic reactions, neoplastic disease (tumor-related antigens), and in blood grouping and typing (immunohematology.)

General Principles
1. Tests involve the study of serum proteins with immunologic action.
2. Immunologically active proteins are known as *antibodies/immunoglobulins*.
3. Patient's serum is tested to determine whether it contains antibodies against a particular antigen or immunogen. Immunogens are bacteria, viruses, parasites, fungi, and enzymes.
4. Common serologic methodology is based on a rise in titer of a specific antibody between the *acute phase* (beginning) of an illness and the *convalescent phase* (2–4 weeks later).
5. The formation of antibodies or autoantibodies against an antigenic challenge is identified.

Antigen–Antibody Reaction
The concepts of antigen and antibody are so interdependent that it is impossible to discuss one without the other.

1. *Antigen*/immunogen: any substance that stimulates the formation of antibodies in the body and reacts with them specifically
2. *Antibody*/immunoglobulin: a substance usually appearing in the body as a result of the introduction of an antigen and which reacts specifically with that antigen

The body's antigen–antibody response is the method of natural defense against invading organisms. In autoimmune disorders, the production of autoantibodies or antibodies to self occurs.

Types of Immunologic Tests
Immunologic methods demonstrate that antigen–antibody reactions have taken place. There are five or six major laboratory techniques for demonstrating this reaction. The tests described in this chapter generally fall into one of these categories.

1. *Immunofluorescence tests*
   (a) Immunofluorescent testing is based on the "sandwich" technique.
   (b) When an individual is challenged by a foreign material (antigen), the immune system responds by developing antibodies

against the antigen. These antibodies are known as *immunoglobulins.*

(c) When the antibodies react with the antigens, antigen–antibody complexes are formed.

(d) The antigen–antibody (Ag–Ab) complex can be visualized in this way: A laboratory animal is challenged with human immunoglobulin. The animal recognizes this immunoglobulin as foreign and manufactures antibodies against it.

(e) Antibody molecules are tagged with fluorescent dyes such as fluorescein without interfering with the molecule's function.

(f) The fluorescein-conjugated antibody (antibody plus dye) is allowed to react with the antigen–antibody complexes mentioned in (c). Then the resulting "sandwich" is observed under the microscope in ultraviolet light.

(g) The following are examples of immunofluorescent tests:

(1) Fluorescent treponemal antibody (FTA) test to diagnose syphilis

(2) Indirect fluorescent antibody (IFA) test to diagnose toxoplasmosis, to detect antibodies to Epstein–Barr virus (EBV), herpes simplex virus (HSV) antibody, and antinuclear antibodies (ANA) to name a few

2. *Precipitation tests*

(a) The reaction between a soluble antigen and its antiserum leads to a visible result in the form of precipitation.

(b) Antigen and antibody must be mixed in a favorable ratio for a precipitate to form.

(c) The following are examples of precipitation tests commonly for diagnoses.

(1) Immunodiffusion (ID) for fungal antibodies; coccidioidomycosis, blastomycosis, histoplasmosis

(2) Double-gel diffusion (DGD) for detecting antibodies or antigens such as enterotoxins in suspected cases of food poisoning

(3) Counterimmunoelectrophoresis (CIE) to detect minute amounts of microbial or tissue antigens or antibodies

3. *Agglutination tests*

(a) When a particulate antigen such as a saline suspension of red blood cells mixes with homologous antiserum, cells clump together and settle to the bottom of the fluid.

(b) The following are examples of hemagglutination tests:

(1) Thyroid hemagglutination test

(2) Microhenagglutination test for *Treponema pallidum*

(3) Hemagglutination (HI) and Hemagglutination inhibition (HAI) tests to determine immunity to rubella

(4) Cold agglutinins test

(c) When a small antigen (bacteria, virus, parasite) attached to a larger carrier particle (latex, bentonite, charcoal) mixes with patient's serum, it produces visible agglutination.

(d) The following are examples:

  (1) Rubella screening antibody

  (2) Cryptococcal antibody and antigen

  (3) Cytomegalovirus antibody

  (4) Rapid plasma regin charcoal agglutination

  (5) Bentonite parasitic antibody determination

4. *Complement-fixation test (CF)*

  (a) A patient's serum is incubated with guinea pig complement and the antigen being tested. At the end of incubation, indicator sheep red blood cells are added. *No* hemolysis is a *positive* test. Complement will "fix" or attach to the antigen–antibody complex if it forms. The test is commonly used to diagnose the following

  (1) Histoplasmosis

  (2) Rickettsial disease

  (3) Blastomycosis

  (4) Trichinosis

  (5) Schistosomiasis

  (6) Viral antibodies

  (b) Cytolysis: Cellular antigens and their antibodies in the presence of complement lead to lysis of the cell (*e.g.*, human complement level).

  (c) Immune adherence: Certain microorganisms adhere to nonphagocytic cells in the presence of homologous antimicrobial serum and complement.

5. *Neutralization of toxins tests*

  When exotoxins are formed, they may be neutralized by small quantities of homologous antibodies, also called antitoxins. This neutralization is tested by inoculation of laboratory animals.

6. *Enzyme-linked immunoabsorbent assay (ELISA)* used to detect rubella; hepatitis, antibodies to Lyme disease, HIV, chlamydia, among others. ELISA can be used to assay both antigens and antibodies. (See Table 8-1 of relative sensitivity of tests.)

Collection of Serum for Immunologic Tests

1. *Take two samples.* One sample should be taken at the beginning of the illness (the acute phase), and the other should be taken 3 to 4 weeks later (the convalescent phase). In general, the usefulness of the serologic tests depends on an increase in titer between the acute and the convalescent phase.

  Note: In a few serologic tests, one serum sample may be adequate because (1) presence of antibody indicates an abnormal condi-

TABLE 8–1.
Relative Sensitivity of Tests Measuring Antibody and Antigen

Test	Approximate Detectable Amount (μg/ml)	
	Antibody	Antigen
Precipitation	20.0	1.0
Immunoelectrophoresis	20.0	—
Double diffusion in agar gel	1.0	—
Complement fixation	0.5	—
Radial immunodiffusion	0.05	0.5
Bacterial agglutination	0.01	—
Hemolysis	0.01	—
Passive hemagglutination	0.01	—
Hemagglutination inhibition	—	0.001
Antitoxin neutralization	0.01	—
Radioimmunoassay	0.0005	0.000005
Enzyme-linked immunosorbent assay	0.0005	0.000005
Virus neutralization	0.00005	—

(Hyde RM, Patnode RA: Immunology: The National Medical Series for Independent Study. New York, John Wiley & Sons, 1987, p 83)

tion, or (2) the antibody titer is unusually high. Only one sample is required in the following tests:

(a) Antinuclear antibody
(b) Heterophilic antibody titer
(c) Histoplasmosis CF
(d) Toxoplasmosis (IFA)
(e) Rubella titer
(f) VDRL test

2. *Take the serologic test before skin testing.* Skin testing often induces antibody production and therefore may interfere with the results of the serologic test.
3. *Identify the sample plainly, and provide appropriate clinical data.* The sample should have information on the patient's name, age, suspected diagnosis, vaccinations, therapy, and previous infections.
4. *Send samples to the laboratory before hemolysis occurs.* Hemolysis can interfere with the interpretation of the results. The presence of hemoglobin in serum can destroy complement and can interfere with the determination of complement-fixing antibodies.

Interpreting Results of Immunologic Tests
Certain factors will affect the interpretation of test results, such as the following:

1. History of previous infection by the same organism
2. Previous vaccination (determine how recent it has been)

3. Anamnestic reactions caused by heterologous antigens (An *anamnestic reaction* is the appearance in the blood of antibodies after administration of an antigen to which the patient had developed a primary immune response.)
4. Cross-reactivity
   Antibodies produced by one species of an organism frequently react with an entirely different species.
   Examples
   (a) Tularemia antibodies may agglutinate *Brucella* and vice versa.
   (b) Rickettsial infections may produce antibodies that react with *Proteus* OX19.
5. Presence of other serious conditions
   No immunologic response can be demonstrated in some persons having either agammaglobulinemia (inherited immune deficiency characterized by the lack of production of immunoglubulins) or any illness such as leukemia or advanced cancer that is being treated with immunosuppressant drugs.

Serologic versus Microbiologic Methods

Chapter 7 provided descriptions of many microbiologic tests for diagnosing a disease entity. The best means of establishing the etiology of an infectious diseas is by isolation and confirmation of the pathogen involved.

Serologic methods can aid or confirm microbiologic analysis when

1. The patient is observed late in the course of the disease.
2. Antimicrobial therapy has suppressed growth of the invading organism.
3. Culture methods (viral, bacterial) were ineffective in substantiating growth of the suspected causative agent.

SEROLOGIC TESTS OF INFECTIOUS DISEASES OF BACTERIAL, VIRAL, FUNGAL, AND PARASITIC ORIGIN

Bacterial

Syphilis Detection Tests

Normal Values
Nonreactive: negative

Background
Syphilis is a venereal disease caused by *Treponema pallidum,* a spirochete with closely wound coils approximately 8 to 15 μ long. The untreated disease progresses through three stages that may extend over many years.

Explanation of Tests

The major types of tests used in the diagnosis of syphilis are (1) flocculation or agglutination, (2) fluorescent antibody test (FTA), and (3) hemagglutination tests (Table 8-2).

1. *Flocculation or agglutination test*
   Flocculation reaction is a microscopic clumping of antigen and antibody. Positive results in a test of this type depend on the degree of flocculant material formed in the test substance. The VDRL is an example of a flocculation test in current use. The RPR is a macroscopic agglutination test.
2. *Fluorescent antibody test*
   The FTA-ABS is an example of a fluorescent antibody test in current use.
3. *Hemagglutination tests*
   The TP-MHA is an example of a hemagglutination test in current use.

Testing for Serum Antibody

During the course of the infection, two types of antibodies may form: (1) reagin, and (2) specific treponemal antibody. Different serologic tests are available to show the presence of each of these antibodies.

Tests to show reagin: VDRL and RPR

Tests to show treponemal antibody: FTA, microhemagglutination test for *Treponema pallidum*. In general, the serologic tests for detection of treponemal antibody are used on all reactive VDRL and RPR tests or on physician request.

Interpreting Tests for Syphilis

In interpreting tests for syphilis, the following factors must be considered.

1. Geographical area
2. Ability of patient to produce reagin or treponemal antibodies
3. Stage of the disease

Procedure

1. A venous blood sample is obtained (serum is used).
2. Fasting is usually *not* required.

Clinical Implications

1. These test results are considered *positive* for syphilis antibodies.
   (a) "Reactive"
   (b) "Weakly reactive"
   (c) "Borderline"
2. When the test is positive for syphilis, it is always confirmed. If none of the diseases that cause false positives are present, the diagnosis

TABLE 8–2.
Serologic Tests for Syphilis (STS)

Name of Test	Type/Description	Comments
FTA (fluorescent treponemal antibody)	Syphilitic serum is bound to surface of *Treponema pallidum*	Fluorescent-labeled antibody against human globulin is added to serum. Spirochetes combined with tagged antibody will fluoresce.
FTA-ABS (fluorescent treponemal antibody absorption)	Fluorescent antibody absorbs out antibody to nonpathogenic treponemes	Detects treponemal antibodies; differentiates biologic false positives from true syphilis positives and diagnoses syphilis when definite clinical signs of syphilis are present but other tests are negative
FTA-ABS, IgM only		Used in diagnosis of congenital syphilis; not used as screening test. A positive RPR can be confirmed with this test.
RPR (rapid plasma reagin)	Agglutination	Reagin reacts with lipid antigens; used as screening test; shows presence of reagin; more sensitive than VDRL. Patients treated for syphilis should have baseline RPR
VDRL	Flocculation	Used as a screening test; developed in the Venereal and Research Laboratories of the U.S. Public Health Service; shows presence of reagin
TP-MHA (microhemagglutination assay for *Treponema pallidum* antibodies)	Hemagglutination	Shows presence of treponemal antibody; even more specific than an FTA-ABS
Reiter	Complement-fixation	An antigen–antibody reagin that causes hemolysis; detects the presence of treponemal antibody in the blood; based on the outdated Wassermann test

of syphilis is suggested if the history and symptoms of the patient point to the disease. A single nonreactive test *suggests* the absence of syphilis but does not *prove* it. The test requires repetition if the patient's medical history warrants it.

3. Treatment of syphilis may change both the clinical course and serological pattern of the disease. The effect of treatment during the

three stages in relation to the VDRL, or any test for syphilis that shows the presence of reagin, is as follows:

(a) If the patient is treated adequately before the appearance of the primary chancre, it is probable that the VDRL will remain non-reactive (negative).

(b) If the patient is treated at the seronegative primary stage (*e.g.,* after the appearance of the chancre but before the appearance of reaction or reagin), the VDRL will remain nonreactive.

(c) If the patient is treated in the seropositive primary stage (*e.g.,* after the appearance of reaction) the VDRL usually becomes nonreactive within 6 months.

(d) If the patient is treated during the secondary stage, the VDRL will usually become nonreactive within 12 to 18 months. If the patient is treated 10 or more years after the onset of the disease, the VDRL can be expected to change little, if any. The longer the patient goes untreated, the longer it will take the VDRL to become nonreactive after adequate treatment, *if it ever does.*

4. A negative serologic test may indicate that

(a) The patient does not have syphilis.

(b) The infection is too recent to have allowed the patient to produce antibodies that give the reactions. Repeat tests should be performed 1 week, 1 month, and 3 months later to exclude syphilis in patients with typical symptoms of syphilis.

(c) The patient is temporarily nonreactive after treatment or because of other causes such as drinking of alcoholic fluids.

(d) The syphilis is in a latent or inactive phase.

(e) The patient has a faulty immunodefense mechanism.

(f) The laboratory techniques were inferior.

False-Positive Reactions

A positive reaction does not necessarily mean that the patient has syphilis. Several conditions will give a biological false-positive (BFP) reaction for syphilis (Table 8-3). Biological false-positive reactions are by no means "false." They may reveal the presence of serious diseases other than syphilis. Little is known about the antibody or reaction concerned in the mechanism of BFP reactions. It is believed that reagin (reaction) is an antibody against tissue lipids. Lipids are presumed to be liberated from body tissue in the course of normal wear and tear, and these liberated lipids may induce the formation of antibodies within the same patient.

Interfering Factors

In tests for syphilis that detect reagin

1. Alcohol decreases the intensity of the reaction.
2. Excess chyle in the blood interferes with the reaction. For this reason, the blood sample should be drawn before a meal.

TABLE 8–3.
Nonsyphilitic Conditions Giving Biological False Positives (BFPs) Using VDRL and RPR Tests

Disease	Percentage (Approximate) BFPs
Malaria	100
Leprosy	60
Relapsing fever	30
Active immunization in children	20
Infectious mononucleosis	20
Lupus erythematosus	20
Lymphogranuloma venereum	20
Pneumonia, atypical	20
Rat-bite fever	20
Typhus fever	20
Vaccinia	20
Infectious hepatitis	10
Leptospirosis (Weil's disease)	10
Periarteritis nodosa	10
Trypanosomiasis	10
Chancroid	5
Chickenpox	5
Measles	5
Rheumatoid arthritis	5–7
Rheumatic fever	5–6
Scarlet fever	5
Subacute bacterial endocarditis	5
Pneumonia, pneumococcal	3–5
Tuberculosis, advanced pulmonary	3–5
Blood loss, repeated	?(low)
Common cold	?(low)
Pregnancy	?(low)

Patient Preparation

Instruct the patient not to drink alcohol for 24 hours before taking of a blood sample.

Clinical Alert

1. Sexual partners of patients with primary, secondary, or early latent syphilis should be evaluated for signs and symptoms of syphilis and should have a blood test for syphilis. Social contacts of infants with symptomatic neonatal syphilis should be examined in a similar manner.

2. After treatment, patients with early syphilis should be tested at 3-month intervals for 1 year. The reaction level declines in most patients followed for a year until little or no reaction is detected.

Lyme Disease Test

Normal Values
Indirect fluorescent antibody titer: 1:256; ELISA: nonreactive; 249 antibody response unit
Western blot assay: 5 bands

Explanation of Test
The test is helpful in the diagnosis of Lyme disease caused by a newly discovered spirochete, *Borrelia burgdorferi*. Ticks are the best documented vectors of the spirochete. Patient history of exposure to deer ticks in an endemic area and presence of clinical symptoms are needed owing to variety of clinical pictures. This measurement can be used as an indication of infection or postexposure and is preferred done on serial serum samples.

Types of Tests
Indirect fluorescent antibody, ELISA, Western blot assay (confirmatory)

Procedure
A venous blood sample of 1 ml is obtained.

Interfering Factors
1. False-positive results occur in 21% of persons with high rheumatoid factors.
2. Persons with treponemal disease (syphilis) have considerable cross-reactivity.

Clinical Implications
1. Identification of
    (a) Fifty percent of early Lyme disease and erythema chronica marginatum migrans
    (b) One hundred percent of patients with later complications of carditis, neuritis, arthritis, and patients in remission

Legionnaires' Disease Antibody Test

Normal Values
Negative

Type of Test
Indirect fluorescent antibody

Explanation of Test
This test facilitates the diagnosis of Legionnaires' disease. Etiologic agent is *Legionella pneumophila*. This test is most supportive when serial serum samples are obtained, when used with tissue specimen testing by fluorescent technique, and when the organism is cultured. Serum studies are useful in evaluating epidemic disease.

Clinical Implications
1. There are more than 20 different species of *Legionella*, and testing will be expanded to include new species as reagents become available. The test is species-specific.
2. Evidence of antibody response to this disease requires a fourfold increase in titer to 1:128 or greater.
3. Evidence of previous infection requires a single titer of 1:256 or greater.
4. The most supportive evidence of recent *Legionella* infection is a fourfold rise in titer between acute (within the first week) and convalescent (3 to 6 weeks after appearance of fever) phases.

Chlamydia Antibodies IgG Test

Normal Values
Indirect fluorescent antibody titer ≤1:640

Background
Chlamydia have many features that bacteria have and are susceptible to antibiotic therapy. They require living cells to multiply, as do viruses. There are two species of the genus *Chlamydia: C. trachomatis* and *C. psittaci*. Direct fluorescent test or ELISA on clinical specimens are now preferred over antibody titer.

Type of Test
Indirect fluorescent antibody

Explanation of Test
This test, using paired samples, is helpful in diagnosing *Chlamydia psittaci* and lymphogranuloma venereum (LGV) infections.

Procedure
A venous blood sample of 10 ml is drawn.

Clinical Implications
1. A positive titer could indicate either LGV or psittacosis. Diagnosis of psittacosis should include documentation of previous contact with sick birds (parrots) or employment in pet shops.
2. In women, chlamydia cause
   (a) Pelvic inflammatory disease
   (b) Endometriosis
   (c) Salpingitis
3. In men, chlamydia cause
   (a) Reiter's syndrome
   (b) Epididymitis
4. Perihepatitis (Fitz-Hugh–Curtis syndrome) has been linked with chlamydia.

Interfering Factors
Depending on geographic location, titers of 1:16 or less can be found in the general population.

Streptococcal Antibody Tests: Anti-streptolysin O Titer (ASO), Streptozyme, Anti-Dnase B (ADB) (Streptodornase)

Normal Values
ASO titer: less than 166 Todd units
Streptozyme: positive—presence of antibody (multiple)
Dnase B: normals—0 yr–4 yr ≤170 units
              5 yr–19 yr ≤480 units
              20 yr and over ≤340 units

Background
Streptolysin "O" is a hemolytic factor produced by most strains of Group A beta-hemolytic streptococci. Anti-streptolysin O(ASO) is the specific neutralizing antibody produced after infection with these organisms. ASO appears in the serum from 1 week to 1 month after the onset of a streptococcal infection. Anti-Dnase B (ADB) is another specific antibody formed to inhibit reactions to Group A streptococci.

Explanation of Test
The ASO test is used to diagnose conditions resulting from a streptococcal infection. It is useful in the diagnosis of rheumatic fever and

glomerulonephritis. This test detects antibodies to the exoenzymes of streptococcus Group A, which may develop in rheumatic fever, glomerulonephritis, bacterial endocarditis, scarlet fever, and other related conditions. Serial determinations with a rising titer over a period of weeks are more significant than a single determination.

Types of Tests
1. The ASO test, which is most widely used, will detect antistreptolysin only
2. Streptozyme will detect antibodies to multiple enzymes produced by streptococcus.
3. The ADB test will detect anti-Dnase B.

Procedure
1. A venous blood sample of 10 ml (serum) is obtained and repeated 10 days later.
2. Subsequent testing is advisable two times a week for 4 to 6 weeks following a streptococcal infection.

Clinical Implications
1. The titer that is considered elevated varies, but in general a titer of greater than 166 Todd units is definitely elevated.
2. Both the ASO and ADB tests alone will be positive in 80% to 85% of streptococcal A infections such as streptococcal pharyngitis, rheumatic fever, pyoderma, and glomerulonephritis.
3. When the two tests are run concurrently, 95% of cases of streptococcal infection can be detected.
4. A repeated low titer is good evidence that there is no active rheumatic fever. However, a high titer does not necessarily mean rheumatic fever or glomerulonephritis, yet it does indicate a focus of streptococcal infection. The deciding factors in diagnosis are clinical symptoms and other laboratory tests.
5. The production of ASO is especially high in cases of rheumatic fever and glomerulonephritis. It is characteristic for each of these conditions to show a marked increase of the ASO titer during the symptomless period preceding an attack of the illness; however ADB titers are particularly high in pyoderma.

Interfering Factors
1. An increased titer is sometimes found in healthy carriers.
2. Antibiotic therapy will suppress the streptococcal antibody response.
3. Increased beta-lipoprotein levels inhibit streptolysin O, thereby giving falsely high ASO titer.

> **Clinical Alert**
>
> The ASO test is impractical in patients who have recently received antibiotics or who are scheduled for antibiotic therapy, because the treatment suppresses the antibody response.

Teichoic Acid Antibody Test

Normal Values
Titer of 1:2 or less
Values vary depending on laboratory methods.

Background
Gram-positive bacteria have teichoic acid as an element of cell walls.

Explanation of Test
This test is used to measure teichoic acid antibodies and is helpful in managing patient response to therapy. This antibody is found in some patients with infections caused by *Staphylococcus aureus*.

Procedure
A venous blood sample of 7 ml is obtained.

Clinical Implications
Positive tests are associated with a greater than fourfold increase between acute and convalescent samples. Teichoic acid antibodies are associated with

1. Staphylococcal endocarditis
2. Osteomyelitis

Viral

Infectious Mononucleosis Tests: Routine; Heterophile Antibody Titer Test; Epstein–Barr Virus (EBV) Antibody Tests

Normal Values
Negative titer < 1:80

Background
Normal serum contains heterophile antibodies. A heterophile antibody is one that is capable of reacting with an antigen that is completely unrelated to the antigen originally stimulating its formation. Infec-

tious mononucleosis, caused by the Epstein–Barr virus (EBV), herpes virus family, induces the formation of lymphocytes and monocytes in lymph nodes in increased numbers and in abnormal forms. It also stimulates an increase in heterophile antibody formation. EBV is also known to produce a cytomegalo-virus-like lymphoproliferative disease in renal and liver transplants, in acquired immunodeficiency syndrome (AIDS) and in posttransfusion. In recent years, recognition has been given to an EBV syndrome or chronic fatigue syndrome, which might be found in generally healthy young individuals. Some cases of EBV syndrome become debilitating.

Explanation of Test

Monospot, Mono-test and Monostican are some of the routine diagnostic presumptive tests for infectious mononucleosis. Confirmatory tests are heterophile antibody tests and specific tests for EBV

In the laboratory, the sheep red blood cell is commonly used to detect heterophile antibodies in the serum of patients (not Forssmantype) with suspected infectious mononucleosis. Such patients begin developing heterophile antibodies shortly after the appearance of symptoms, usually during the first 2 weeks. When the clinical picture suggests infectious mononucleosis (IM) with a negative heterophile antibody test, specific tests for EBV can be done. A rise in the EBV titer is diagnostic of IM.

IgM antibodies that are specific for the viral antigen peak (fourfold increase in 25% of patients) and disappear soon after the disease subsides, making a specific diagnosis of infectious mononucleosis possible.

The EBV titers using IFA usually appear after the first week of illness, rise types by the third week and remain for years thereafter. The following four types of antibodies can be detected:

1. Antiviral capsid antigen (VCA); IgG and IgM variety; most commonly used test
2. Antibody to the EBV nuclear antigen (EBNA)
3. IgG antibody to early antigen (EA)

Types of Tests

Indirect fluorescence antibody (IFA) and IFA with use of complement

Procedure

A venous blood sample of 5 ml is obtained.

Clinical Implications

1. A presumptive antibody titer of 1:56 is suspicious. A titer of 1:224 or greater is diagnostic of infectious mononucleosis.
2. Positive reactions last 4 to 8 weeks after the appearance of symptoms.
3. The highest titers are usually found during the second and third week of illness but have no relationship to the severity of the dis-

ease or its prognosis.

4. The clinical symptoms of infectious mononucleosis disappear before the abnormal blood picture disappears.

5. When interpreting the significance of the titer from the presumptive test, certain points are important:
   (a) Ninety percent of the normal adult population have antibodies to antiviral capsid antigen (VCA) and EBA antigens.
   (b) A high incidence of elevated titers is found in infectious mononucleosis and
   (1) Burkitt's lymphoma
   (2) Nasopharyngeal carcinoma
   (3) Hayden's disease
   (4) Lymphocytic leukemia
   (5) Hepatitis A & B
   (6) Pancreatic carcinoma
   (7) Systemic lupus erythematosus (SLE)
   (8) Sarcoidosis
   (9) Izuma fever
   (10) Chronic fatigue (EBV) syndrome

6. The presence of IgM antibodies or of antibodies to VCA and absence of an immune response to EBV nuclear antigen (EBNA) indicate recent infection with EBV.

7. Antiviral capsid antigen (VCA). Both IgM and IgG are present during the acute state and peak during this period. Titers decline by 1 to 2 months. IgG titers decline, but are present at lower levels for a few years. (Good evidence against EBV infection is the persistent absence of antibody to VCA.)

8. Antibody to the EBNA. This antibody is absent during the acute phase and appears weeks to months after most cases.

9. IgG antibody to early antigen EA. Most persons with infectious mononucleosis have a transient EA response. In addition, increased (1:40) EA levels occur in chronic active or reactive EBV infection. This test is also positive in nasopharyngeal carcinoma types 1 and 2.

10. In *chronic fatigue syndrome*, VCA IgG antibody stays elevated for the length of the disease, which could be months, even years. Most characteristically, IgG antibody to EA rises with onset of the syndrome, presenting with several periodical peaks of titer, over the course of illness.

Rubella Antibody Tests

Normal Values
No real normal
HI or HAI: titer <1:10 (<1:8), patient susceptible to rubella virus
HI or HAI: titer 1:10 (1:8) and up, protection against rubella virus
   ELISA: negative, not immune; positive, immune

Latex agglutination: negative, not immune; positive, immune

Background

Rubella virus is the causative agent of German measles, a mild systemic disease characterized by fever and transient rash. It is important to identify exposure to rubella infection and susceptibility status in pregnant women, since infection in the first trimester of pregnancy is associated with congenital abnormalities, miscarriage, or stillbirth in about 3% of infected women. Rubella infection will induce IgG and IgM antibody formation.

Explanation of Test

This test is done to determine immune status and confirm rubella infection. The test is indicated in pregnancy, to identify potential carriers of rubella who may infect women of childbearing age, such as hospital employees responsible for maternal child care, and others such as teachers, dentists, nurses, physicians, and midwives.

Types of Tests

HAI, the classic test, but not state of the art; latex agglutination results within 10 minutes; EIA or ELISA (enzyme immunoassay or enzyme-linked immunoassay).

Procedure

A venous blood sample of 5 ml is obtained.

Clinical Implications

1. Demonstration of an IgG with a fourfold rise in titer between acute and convalescent specimens and the presence of IgM antibody are indicative of a recent rubella infection.
2. Stable titers should not be interpreted as evidence of recent rubella infection.
3. In naturally acquired rubella, IgM and IgG antibodies are present, although IgM is not detectable beyond 8 weeks of onset.
4. In congenital rubella, infants' antibodies on delivery are composed of fetal IgM, fetal IgG, and fetal IgA as well as maternal IgG; mother will have only IgG.

Antibody levels in the infant that are passively acquired will decrease markedly within 2 to 3 months.

Hepatitis Tests

Normal Values

Negative for hepatitis A, hepatitis B, and non-A, non-B hepatitis and Delta (Δ) hepatitis.

Background

There are at least three different types of viral hepatitis: hepatitis A, hepatitis B, and non-A, non-B (NANB) hepatitis. Although these forms are clinically similar, they differ with respect to immunology, epidemiology, prognosis, and prophylaxis (Figs. 8-1 and 8-2).

Hepatitis A (HA), caused by hepatitis A virus (HAV), commonly known as *infectious hepatitis,* has a characteristic short incubation period of 2 to 6 weeks; onset is acute rather than insidious. It is usually transmitted through personal contact, either oral or fecal, although a parenteral mode of transmission is possible, (documented, but rare). Hepatitis A is found more frequently in children or young adults and is not associated with either development of chronic hepatitis or development of the carrier state.

In contrast, hepatitis B, caused by hepatitis B virus (HBV), also called *serum hepatitis,* or *transfusion hepatitis,* may be associated with drug usage, may have a relatively longer incubation period (6 to 26 weeks), and its primary mode of transmission is parenteral. It tends to occur more often in men than in women and is a significant cause of chronic active hepatitis. It is characterized by insidious onset; approximately 10% of hepatitis B patients become carriers.

Delta hepatitis (Δ) is always associated with a coexistent HBV infection; it usually causes severe liver damage. Common diagnosis is made by RIA or ELISA tests that detect antibody or antigen to delta (Δ) agent. Although referred to in the literature, in practice it is relatively uncommon.

Type 1

Epidemic non-A, non-B is similar to hepatitis A and differential diagnosis depends on exclusion of other etiologies of hepatitis, especially hepatitis A, by serologic test.

Type 2

Non-A, non-B, B-like hepatitis is also known as non-B transfusion-associated hepatitis, post-transfusion non-A, non-B hepatitis, or hepatitis C. Differential diagnosis depends on exclusion of hepatitis A and B and on epidemiology.

This type of hepatitis is more common when paid blood donors are used and is the most common posttransfusion hepatitis in the United States. It also causes sporadic community-acquired hepatitis, accounting for 15% to 40% of cases. Recent literature refers to hepatitis C, and tests for antibody (ELISA) to hepatitis C virus (HCV) are available for clinical testing. The presence of HCV antibodies indicates that an individual (donor or patient) has been infected with HCV, may harbor infectious HCV, and may be capable of transmitting NANBH.

Transmission is through contaminated blood or plasma derivation or by use of improperly sterilized syringe and needle. Incubation period is from 2 weeks to 6 months, but most fall within a 6-to-9 week period. Prophylactic immunoglobulin is used for associated needle shots.

(*text continues on page 480*)

Anti-HAV		Interpretation	Immune to further HAV infection	Potentially infectious to others for HAV
Positive	Anti-HAV/IgM Positive	Recent infection with HAV	Yes	Yes—if early in symptomatic phase
				No—if later— 7–10 days after onset of jaundice
	Anti-HAV/IgM Negative	Past infection with HAV at some undetermined time*	Yes*	No
Negative		Infection not due to HAV	No	No

* Anti-HAV positive result can also occur following use of IG. Passively acquired anti-HAV will provide only temporary immunity to HAV. IG does not affect the anti-HAV-IgM result.

FIGURE 8–1.
Interpretation of hepatitis A serologic results.

HBsAg				Interpretation	Immune to further HBV infection	Potentially infectious to others who are susceptible to HBV
Positive	HBsAG positive for at least 6 months	Liver enzymes are elevated		a. Chronic persistent hepatitis (CPH), or	Yes	Yes
				b. Chronic active hepatitis (CAH)*	Yes	Yes
		Liver enzymes are not elevated		a. Chronic carrier of HBV (asymptomatic)†	Yes	Yes
	HBsAG not positive for 6 months or unknown			a. Acute HBV infection if anti-HBc/IgM is positive, or	Yes	Yes
				b. Chronic carrier of HBV if anti-HBc is positive and anti-HBc/IgM is negative	Yes	Yes
Negative	Anti-HBs positive	Anti-HBc positive or unknown		a. Normal immune response to prior infection	Yes	No
		Anti-HBc negative		a. Response to immunization with HBV vaccine, or	Yes	No
				b. Passive immunity after IG, HBIG vaccination	Yes/No‡	No
				c. Normal immune response to prior HBV infection, many years later	Yes	No
	Anti-HBs negative	Anti-HBc positive		a. "Window phase" or convalescence if anti-HBc/IgM is positive, or	Yes	No
				b. "Low level carrier" in nonacute setting§	Yes	No/Yes§
		Anti-HBc negative		a. No evidence of HBV infection	No	No

* Liver biopsy is needed to make definitive diagnosis between CPH and CAH.
† HBeAg and anti-HBe testing is appropriate in this setting: HBeAg positive persons are at higher risk of transmitting disease than persons HBeAg negative and anti-HBe positive.
‡ Passive protection is of limited duration.
§ May be infectious in a transfusion setting. HBsAg level below level of detection or late convalescence with loss of anti-HBs detectability.

FIGURE 8–2.
Interpretation of hepatitis B serologic results.

Explanation of Test

These measurements are used in the differential diagnosis of viral hepatitis. The identification of the virus in serum will aid in determining progress, assessing probability of close contacts developing hepatitis, and help in forming a hepatitis control program.

Differentiation among the major viruses responsible for hepatitis requires the use of specific serological markers in order to characterize the infection. Specific serologic markers are available for the diagnosis of HAV and HBV, whereas the NANB viruses are identified by the exclusion of A and B.

By measuring just three of the seven available hepatitis markers, the viral agent causing the symptoms of acute viral hepatitis can be determined. The first of these markers is the antibody to the HAV, IgM specific (HAV/IgM). This marker first appears between 4 weeks and 6 weeks after innoculation and indicates an acute stage of hepatitis A infection. The other two markers analyzed are the B surface antigen and B core antibody, or B core antibody IgM (where available), which identify the early acute stage of a B-viral infection. The absence of these markers leads to a diagnosis of NANB infection, some other viral infection, or hepatic toxicity. See page 477 for hepatitis C virus (HCV).

Appearance of Hepatitis Viral Markers Following Infection

Serological Marker	Time After Infection	Clinical Implications
Hepatitis A virus		
HAV-Ab/IgM	4–6 wk	Positive for acute state, hepatitis A; develops early in disease
HAV-Ab/IgG	8–12 wk	Indicative of previous exposure and immunity to hepatitis A
Hepatitis B virus		
HBsAg–hepatitis B surface antigen	4–12 wk.	Positive for acute stage, hepatitis B; earliest indicator of the presence of acute infection; also indicative of chronic infection
HBeAg	4–12 wk	Positive for acute active stage with viral replication (infectivity factor); "highly infectious"
HBcAB, hepatitis B core antibody	6–14 wk	This marker may stay in serum for longer time, and together with HBsAB, represents convalescent stage; indicates past infection

(continued)

Appearance of Hepatitis Viral Markers Following Infection
(continued)

Serological Marker	Time After Infection	Clinical Implications
ABcAbIgM	6–14 wk	Indicates acute infection
HBeAb antibody	8–16 wk	Indicates resolution of acute infection
HbsAb antibody	4–10 mo.	Indicative of previous exposure and immunity to hepatitis B, but not necessarily to other types of hepatitis; this is the marker for permanent immunity

The assessment of the HBV involves the use of three markers that are expected to occur during the course of infection.

1. Hepatitis B surface antigen (HBsAg) is present in serum 4 weeks to 12 weeks after infection, denoting the initial acute stage of infection.
2. Shortly after the appearance of the hepatitis B surface antigen, the core antibody (HBcAb) is detectable within a period of 6 weeks to 14 weeks.
3. Finally, 4 months to 10 months after infection, hepatitis B surface antibody (HBsAb) can be detected, indicating *clinical recovery* and *immunity to the B virus.*

Types of Tests
Radioimmunoassay (RIA), ELISA

Procedure
A venous blood sample of 6 ml is obtained or 2 ml for each test.

Clinical Implications
1. HAV-Ab/IgM and HAV-Ab/IgG refer to total antibody to HAV. They are indicators of recent acute as well as past infection and are useful in confirming previous exposure and immunity to hepatitis A.
2. If transfused, blood containing hepatitis virus markers carries a 40% to 70% risk of causing hepatitis. Transfusion of HBsAg-negative blood tends to cause a clinical mild hepatitis.
   Use enteric precautions for hepatitis A.
3. Hepatitis B surface antigen (HBsAg) is found in many patients with chronic active hepatitis, whether or not acute hepatitis has occurred previously. Hepatitis B antigen is frequently found in
   (a) Patients receiving renal dialysis
   (b) Institutionalized patients with Down syndrome

(c) Patients receiving immunosuppressive medication (certain cases)

(d) Lymphocytic leukemia

(e) Hodgkin's disease

(f) Lepromatous leprosy

A small number of seemingly healthy persons with no history of acute illness have HAV and HBV in their blood serum. It may be that in these patients a very mild, subclinical infection has occurred that is more likely to produce a carrier state than an acute illness and subsequent clearing. However, normal subjects will not be positive for anti-HAV/IgM. IgM titers are only positive during the acute episode and generally become negative 4 months after exposure. The presence of HBeAg is an early indicator of acute, active hepatitis B infection representing the most infectious period. It is usually short-lived (3–6 weeks). Persistence of "e" antigen in the acute stage beyond 10 weeks is indicative of progression to chronic carrier state and probable chronic disease.

4. Presence of IgM is an early indicator of acute infection. HBcAb is a lifelong marker that represents past exposure as well as active infection in the acute/chronic period. In the absence of HBsAg and anti-HBs, this hepatitis B core antibody is an important serologic marker to identify recent infection. This situation is referred to as the "core" window. The presence of HBsAB is an indication of clinical recovery and subsequent immunity to HBV virus. It generally appears 1 to 4 months following onset of symptoms, but appearance may be delayed much longer. The presence of HBeAB represents seroconversion from HBeAg to anti-HBe during the acute stage and is prognostic for resolution of infection. The presence of antibody to hepatitis B "e" antigen, along with anti-HBc, can also confirm the recent acute or convalescent stage in the absence of HBsAg and anti-HBs.

5. Use blood and body fluid precautions for hepatitis B and NANB hepatitis.

Clinical Alert

1. Apply enteric precautions (continue for 7 days after onset of jaundice) in hepatitis A. Hepatitis A is most contagious before symptoms and jaundice appear. Gowns and gloves are most useful when gross soiling with feces is anticipated or possible.

2. Apply blood and body fluid precautions for type B hepatitis, including hepatitis B antigen carrier. Precautions apply until patient is HBsAG-negative and the anti-HBs appear. Use caution when handling blood and blood-soiled articles. Take spe-

cial care to avoid needlestick injuries. Pregnant women need special counseling. Gowns are indicated when blood splattering is anticipated. If gastrointestinal bleeding is likely, wear gloves if touching feces. A private hospital room may be indicated if preface bleeding is likely to cause environmental contamination. Wear gloves to start an intravenous infusion or to handle blood-contaminated articles from persons suspected of having hepatitis or known to have hepatitis A.

3. No one who has had a blood transfusion should donate blood for 6 months. This is because a person who acquires hepatitis from a blood transfusion may not develop symptoms for up to 6 months. Persons with a positive test for HBsAg should never be permitted to donate blood or plasma.

4. Sexual contacts of persons with hepatitis B result in a great risk of infection with the disease. HBsAg has been found in most body fluids, including saliva, semen, and cervical secretions.

5. Until a specific diagnosis of hepatitis A is made, blood and body fluid precautions are advisable.

6. Immunization of contacts should be done as soon after exposure as possible. For hepatitis B, both HBIG (or, if unavailable, IG) and HBV vaccine should be administered within 24 hours of high-use needlestick and with 14 days of last sexual contact with an HBsAg-positive person. For hepatitis A, IG should be given within 2 weeks to all household and sexual contacts; in day care, it should be given to all classroom contacts. If diapered children are in the day-care center, IG should be given to all children and staff in the center.

Viral Antibody Tests

Normal Values
Negative respiratory, gastrointestinal, central nervous system, and exanthem virus antibodies
Negative titer: <1:8

Explanation of Test
The following studies are done to establish the diagnosis of various viral diseases: respiratory, gastrointestinal, central nervous system (CNS), and exanthem, on the basis of antibody level. If a specific test for respiratory viral antibodies is ordered, it is done to identify influenza A and B, respiratory syncytial virus, mucoplasma, and adenovirus studies. If a CNS virus antibody test is ordered, it is done to identify infec-

tion with mumps, measles, herpes simplex, lymphocytic, choriomeningitis, or encephalitis.

Types of Tests
Complement-fixation, confirmed by agglutination if necessary

Procedure
Viral studies require two venous blood specimens of 10 ml. The first specimen is obtained during the acute phase of illness, and the second or convalescent specimen is obtained 10 days later. All viral studies require blood serum. Spinal fluid can be used for CNS viral examination.

Clinical Implications
Fourfold increase in antibody titer from acute to convalescent serum should be observed (*e.g.*, 1:8 to 1:32 titer). This change in antibody level implies recent viral infection and is clinically significant.

Rabies Antibody Tests

Normal Values
Indirect fluorescent antibody (IFA) <1:16

Explanation of Test
Serologic testing is done for several reasons, including to diagnose rabies in animals or to determine the adequacy of antibody responses in either pre- or postexposure courses of rabies immunization. The diagnosis of rabies in humans is also confirmed by culture and histologic methods. Direct immunofluorescence to demonstrate the rabies antigen is also a reliable method and is used on brain smears and corneal scrapes. It has also been reported that the rabies antigen can be detected by examination of skin biopsies taken from the nape of the neck.

Serologic Tests Used
1. Complement fixation methods
2. Mouse neutralization
3. Indirect fluorescent antibody
4. Fluorescent focus

Procedure
A venous blood sample of 10 ml is obtained to determine titer in persons who have received the vaccine for preexposure (*e.g.*, employees of animal shelters).

Clinical Implications
A positive response or rise in titer will appear in those who have been successfully immunized with human diploid vaccine.
Rabies titer of 1:16 or greater is considered protective.

Clinical Alert

1. Prevention: Preexposure vaccine (HDVC, human diploid cell rabies vaccine) should be given to high-risk individuals such as veterinarians, wildlife personnel, personnel in quarantine kennels, and those working in special laboratories.
2. Postbite: Give rabies immunoglobulin (RIG) as soon as possible, regardless of interval from exposure, to neutralize virus in the wound. Human diploid cell rabies vaccine in 5 1-ml intramuscular doses should be given in the deltoid. The first dose is given at the same time RIG is given and then 3, 7, 14, and 28 days after the first dose.
3. The animal should be killed and tested as soon as possible. Holding for observation is not recommended.

Antibody to Human Immunodeficiency Virus (HIV); Acquired Immunodeficiency Syndrome (AIDS) Test

Normal Values
Negative: Nonreactive

Explanation of Test
This ELISA test (see p. 462) is used to detect the presence of antibody to human immunodeficiency virus (HIV). It is used to screen blood and blood products that will be used for transfusion. This methodology is also used to test those persons at high risk for the development of acquired immunodeficiency syndrome (AIDS) such as homosexuals, intravenous drug users, and others who have been exposed to infected blood or blood products. AIDS is a clinical syndrome, and the diagnosis must be established clinically. A reactive ELISA test alone cannot be used to diagnose AIDS.

A reactive ELISA test should always be repeated in duplicate using the same blood sample. If repeatably reactive, follow-up testing such as the Western blot (WB) or indirect fluorescent antibody (IFA) test should be performed. These tests are more specific. A positive WB or IFA is considered a confirmatory test for the presence of antibody to HIV.

Procedure
A venous blood sample is obtained.

Interfering Factors
1. Nonreactive HIV test results occur during the acute stage of the infection when the virus is present but antibody development is not sufficient to be detected. The virus may be present for up to 6 months before antibody can be detected. During this stage, the test for HIV antigen may confirm an HIV infection.
2. Test kits for HIV are manufactured to be extremely sensitive. As a result, nonspecific reactions may occur with some specimens when the person has been previously exposed to the human cells or media in which the HIV is grown for manufacture of the test kit (*e.g.*, prior pregnancy or blood transfusion).

Clinical Implications
1. A positive test should be repeated and confirmed by other tests.
2. A positive ELISA that fails to be confirmed by Western blot or IFA should not be considered negative, especially in the presence of symptoms and/or signs of AIDS. Repeat testing in 3 to 6 months is suggested.
3. A positive result may occur in noninfected persons due to unknown factors.
4. A negative test tends to rule out AIDS as a diagnosis for high-risk patients with illness but who do not have the characteristic opportunistic infection or tumor.
5. An HIV infection is described as a continuum of conditions ranging from the acute, transient, mononucleosis-like syndrome associated with seroconversion, to asymptomatic HIV infection to symptomatic HIV infection and, finally, to AIDS. AIDS is end-stage HIV infection.
6. Recognizing HIV infection as a disease is important. Drugs are being tested to determine whether they halt or slow the disease process in infected asymptomatic individuals. Treatments for the infections and malignancies that occur in AIDS patients are more effective and less toxic when started early in the course of HIV infection.

Clinical Alert
1. Results should not be given by telephone. Use of the computer for transmission of results varies in medical facilities. Check with your facility for the current regulation regarding use of the computer for HIV test results.

2. All results, both positive and negative, must be in the medical records. Precautions must be taken to maintain the confidentiality of the results. People will be more likely to undergo testing voluntarily if they believe that inappropriate disclosure of HIV testing information, which could result in the loss of jobs, housing, or insurance coverage, will not occur.
3. The physician must sign a legal form stating that the patient has been informed of the risks of testing.
4. A person who has antibodies to HIV is presumed infected with the virus, and appropriate counseling and medical evaluation should be offered.
5. Positive test results must be reported to the state public health authorities following the regulations established in each state.

Patient Preparation
1. An informed consent must be signed by any person who is being tested for AIDS. The consent must accompany the specimen to the laboratory, or if the patient goes to the laboratory for the venipuncture, the consent must accompany the patient. (See Appendix for sample form.)
2. It is essential that counseling precede and follow the administration of an HIV antibody test. The test should not be performed without the subject's prior knowledge. The informed-consent process should include a discussion of the clinical and behavioral implications of the test results, including the accuracy of the test and the encouraging of behavioral changes (*e.g.*, sexual contact, shared needles, or blood transfusion). The person tested must also be aware of other people to whom the test results must be given, such as those health care workers who have legitimate access to patient charts.
3. Infection control measures are the same as for hepatitis B and hepatitis non-A, non-B. (See Appendix for universal precautions.)

Herpes Simplex Antibodies IgG and IgM

Normal Values
Some level of antibody can be found in the normal population.

Background
Herpes simplex virus (HSV) has become quite prevalent in the past few years; it is often the most common cause of sexually transmitted disease.

Explanation of Test

This test is used to determine the infectious status of pregnant patients in their last days of gestation because the virus could be transmitted to the infant via the birth canal. The detection of HSV infections provides for quick antiviral therapy and is useful for patient counseling and epidemiologic considerations. Testing for HSV antibody has been widely used in bone marrow recipients and donors.

Types of Tests

Immunofluorescent antibody test, ELISA

Procedure

1. A venous blood sample is obtained.
2. Paired samples should be used to demonstrate an increase in titer.

Clinical Implications

1. The presence of IgM antibodies or a fourfold or greater increase in IgG titer is indicative of recent infection.
2. Antibodies for HSV appear approximately 4 to 6 weeks after infection, then decline, but remain at a persistent stable level. There is a crossmatching between the virus types one and two, and distinguishing one from the other may be difficult.

Cytomegalovirus Antibody

Normal Values

Negative

Background

Cytomegalovirus (CMV) is a ubiquitous human viral pathogen belonging to the family of herpes virus. Infection with CMV is usually asymptomatic and can persist in the host as a chronic or latent infection. Cytomegalovirus has been linked with sexually transmitted infections. Blood banks routinely screen units for CMV antibody, thus resulting in CMV-negative and CMV-positive blood reports (used in previously positive patients).

Explanation of Tests

Test is to determine presence of CMV antibody in various groups of patients: congenitally infected newborns, immunocompromised patients (transplantations, AIDS), and sexually active adults presenting with mononucleosis-like disease.

Antibody titers must be evaluated in view of history of the patient, presence of clinical symptoms, and results of viral culture.

Type of Tests

IFA, ELISA, latex agglutination

Procedure
1. A venous blood sample is obtained.
2. Post-transplantation titers are to be collected in weekly intervals (particularly in bone-marrow follow-up).

Clinical Implications
1. Infants who acquire CMV during a maternal primary infection are prone to develop severe cytomegalic inclusion disease (CID). CID may be fatal or may cause neurologic sequelae, such as mental retardation, deafness, microcephaly, or motor dysfunction.
2. Transfusion of CMV-infected blood products or transplantation of CMV-infected donor organs may result in interstitial pneumonitis in an immunocompromised recipient.
3. Seroconversion or a significant rise in titer may indicate recent infection, but it cannot differentiate between primary or recurrent antibody response.

Human T-cell Lymphotrophic Virus-I (HTLV) Antibody

Normal Values
Negative

Explanation of Test
This test is done to detect the presence of antibody to human T-cell lymphotropic virus-1. This retrovirus has been associated with adult T-cell leukemia (ATL) and demyelinating neurologic disorders. The presence of HTLV-1 antibodies in an asymptomatic person means that the person should not donate blood. This finding does not mean that the person has leukemia or a neurologic disorder or that they will develop.

Procedure
A venous blood sample is obtained.

Clinical Implications
1. Positive results (antibodies to HTLV-1) are found in a person with HTLV-1 infection. Transmission of infection to recipients of HTLV-1 infected blood is well documented.
2. The finding of antibodies to HTLV-1 has no relationship to the presence of antibodies to HIV-I and does not imply any risk of AIDS.
3. HTLV-1 is endemic in the Caribbean, Southeastern Japan, and some areas of Africa.
4. In the United States, HTV-1 has been detected in persons with ATL, intravenous drug users, healthy persons, and donated blood products. Transmission can also occur through breast milk, sexual contact, and sharing of contaminated needles and syringes among intravenous drug abusers (Leavelle, 1990).

> **Clinical Alert**
>
> Repeatedly positive tests are confirmed by Western blot assay.

Fungal

Fungal Antibody Tests (Histoplasmosis, Blastomycosis, Coccidioidomycosis)

Normal Values
Negative
Complement-fixation (CF) titer < 1:8
Immunodiffusion-negative

Background
Certain species of fungi are associated with human respiratory diseases acquired by inhalation of spores from sources such as dust, soil, and bird droppings. Serologic tests may be used for diagnosis of these conditions.

Fungal diseases may be categorized as either "superficial" or "deep." For the most part, the superficial mycoses are limited to the skin, mucous membranes, nails, and hair. The deep mycoses involve the deeper tissues and internal organs. Histoplasmosis, coccidioidomycosis, and blastomycosis are three diseases caused by the deep mycoses.

The following are brief descriptions of the fungal diseases:

1. Coccidioidomycosis (desert fever, San Joaquin fever, valley fever) is contracted from inhalation of soil or dust containing spores of *Coccidioides immitis.*
2. Blastomycosis is an infection caused by organisms of the genus *Blastomyces.*
3. Histoplasmosis is a granulomatous infection caused by *Histoplasma capsulatum.*

Types of Tests
Complement-fixation, immunodiffusion

Explanation of Test
These tests are used to detect serum precipitin antibodies and complement-fixing antibodies present in the fungal diseases coccidioidomycosis, blastomycosis, and histoplasmosis.

Procedure
A venous blood sample of at least 7 ml is obtained (serum is used).

Clinical Implications
Antibodies to coccidioidomycosis, blastomycosis, and histoplasmosis appear early in the disease (from the first to fourth weeks) and then disappear.

Interfering Factors
1. Antibodies against fungi may be found in the blood of apparently normal people.
2. In tests for blastomycosis, there may be cross-reactions with histoplasmosis.

Candida Antibody Test

Normal Values
Negative. Precipitins are found on occasion in normal population.

Background
Candidiasis is usually caused by *Candida albicans* and affects the mucous membranes, skin, and nails. Compromised individuals are most likely to have invasive disease.

Explanation of Test
Identifying this antibody is helpful when the diagnosis of systemic candidiasis cannot be shown by culture or tissue sample. Clinical symptomology must be present for the test to be useful.

Types of Tests
Counterimmunoelectrophoresis (CIE) for *Candida* antigen and antibody; antigen particularly valuable on CSF and urine; latex agglutination

Procedure
A venous blood sample of 7 ml is drawn.

Clinical Implications
1. A titer greater than 1:8 in latex agglutination is indicative of systemic infection.
2. A fourfold rise in titer of paired blood samples 10 to 14 days apart indicates acute infection.
3. Patients on long-term intravenous therapy commonly have disseminated infection by *Candida albicans*.
4. Vulvovaginal candidiasis, common in late pregnancy, can transmit candidiasis to the infant via the birth canal.

Interfering Factors
1. Approximately 25% of the normal population tests positive.
2. Cross-reaction can occur with latex agglutination (LA) testing in cases involving cryptococcosis and tuberculosis.

3. Positive results can be obtained with mucocutaneous candidiasis or severe vaginitis.

Aspergillus Antibody Test

Normal Values
Negative

Background
The aspergilli, especially *Aspergillus fumigatus*, *A. flavus*, and *A. niger*, are associated with pulmonary infections and invasive fatal disease in immunosuppressed patients. Manifestations of infection with aspergillus include allergic bronchopulmonary disease, mycetoma of the lung, endophthalmitis, and disseminated disease involving the brain, kidney, heart, and bone.

Explanation of Test
This test is used to detect antibodies present in aspergillosis infections.

Types of Tests
Immunodiffusion

Procedure
A venous blood sample of at least 2 ml is obtained; it can be done on CSF.

Clinical Implications
Positive tests are associated with

1. Pulmonary infection in compromised patients
2. Infection of prosthetic heart valves with aspergillus
3. If the serum exhibits one to four bands, aspergillosis is strongly suggested. The presence of weak bands suggests early disease or hypersensitivity pneumonitis.

Cryptococcus Antibody Test

Normal Values
Negative

Background
Cryptococcus neoformans, a yeastlike fungus, causes an infection that is thought to be acquired by inhalation into the lungs. The organism has been isolated from several sites in nature, especially weathered pigeon droppings. Knowledge of unusual exposure by affected patients is not

recognized. Symptoms include fever, headache, dizziness, ataxia, somnolence, and, occasionally, cough.

Explanation of Test
This test is used to detect antibodies present in *Cryptococcus* infections. It appears that 50% of patients have a predisposing condition, such as lymphoma, sarcoidosis, or steroid therapy. Infection with *C. neoformans* has long been known to be associated with Hodgkin's disease and other malignant lymphomas. Infection with *C. neoformans* in conjunction with malignancy occurs to such a degree that some researchers have raised a question of an etiologic relationship between the two diseases.

Types of Tests
Latex agglutination for antigen or antibody

Procedure
A venous blood sample of 1 ml or 2 ml of spinal fluid is obtained.

Clinical Implications
Positive tests are associated with infections of the lower respiratory tract by inhalation of aerosols containing *C. neoformans* cells disseminated by the fecal droppings of pigeons.

Parasitic

Toxoplasmosis (TPM) Antibody Tests; Indirect Fluorescent Antibody (IFA) Tests

Normal Values
Normals:

Titer <1:16: no previous infection (*except* for ocular infection)
Titer 1:16–1:256: prevalent in general population
Titer >1:256: suggests recent infection
Titer >1:1024: indicates active infection
Rising titer of greatest significance

Background
Toxoplasmosis is a disease caused by the sporozoal parasite *Toxoplasma gondii*. It may be a severe generalized disease or a granulomatous disease of the CNS. The condition may be either congenital or postnatal, and is found in man as well as domestic (cats) and wild animals. Humans may acquire infection by ingestion of inadequately cooked meat or other contaminated material.

Congenital toxoplasmosis may lead to fetal death. Symptoms of subacute infection may also appear shortly after birth or months and even years later. Complications of congenital toxoplasmosis include hydrocephaly, microcephaly, convulsions, and chronic retinitis.

It is believed that one quarter to one half of the adult population is asymptomatically infected with toxoplasmosis. The Centers for Disease Control therefore recommend that physicians consider serologic testing of their pregnant patients for detection of this disease.

Explanation of Test
The IFA test helps to differentiate toxoplasmosis from infectious mononucleosis. Antibodies appear in 1 to 2 weeks and peak at 6 to 8 months. It is also a valuable screening test for latent toxoplasmosis.

Procedure
A venous blood sample of 5 ml is obtained (serum is tested).

Clinical Implications
The IFA test may be considered positive under any of the following conditions:

1. Titer of 1:256 or higher indicates recent exposure or current infection.
2. Any titer in a newborn infant
3. Titer of 1:1024 or greater is significant and may reflect active disease.
4. Titer of 1:16 or less may be seen in ocular toxoplasmosis.

Amebiasis (*Entamoeba histolytica*) Antibody Detection

Normal Values
Negative

Explanation of Test
Entamoeba histolytica, the causative agent of amebiasis, is a pathogenic parasite found in the intestine. The *E. histolytica* test is used to detect the presence or absence of specific serum antibodies to this parasite. The usual definitive method of diagnosis of amebiasis is stool examination. However, the absence of detectable organisms in the stool does not necessarily rule out the disease, because antibiotic therapy, oil enemas, and barium make a stool identification impossible.

Types of Tests
1. Indirect hemagglutination
2. Latex agglutination
3. Counterimmunoelectrophoresis (CIE)

Procedure
A venous blood sample of 5 ml is obtained (serum is tested).

Clinical Implications

1. Indirect hemagglutination—positive 1:128 and greater—indicates active or recent infection.
2. A positive test may reflect only past, not current, infections.
3. Positive results occur in
   (a) Amebic liver abscess
   (b) Amebic dysentery
4. In persons currently infected, titer range from 1:256 to 1:2048.
5. Titer of 1:32 or less generally exclude presence of disease.

Mixed

TORCH Test

Normal Values
Negative

Background
TORCH is an acronym that stands for *Toxoplasma*, rubella, cytomegalovirus, and herpes simplex virus. These etiological agents are frequently implicated in congenital or neonatal infections that are not clinically apparent and may result in serious impairment of the central nervous system. Congenital infection can be confirmed serologically by the demonstration of specific IgM-associated antibodies in the infant blood.

Explanation of Test
These measurements are performed on both mother and newborn infant to test for exposure to agents involved in congenital infection of the newborn. The test is used in the differential diagnosis of acute, congenital, and intrapartum infections caused by *Toxoplasma gondii*, rubella virus, cytomegalovirus, and herpes virus disorders. The presence of IgA or IgM in newborns reflects actual fetal production. High levels of IgM at birth indicate fetal response to an antigen. In this instance an intrauterine infection should be considered. TORCH is more useful in excluding a possible infection than proving etiology.

Procedure
A venous or cord blood sample of 3 ml is obtained.

Clinical Implications

1. Persistence of rubella antibody in an infant beyond 6 months is highly suggestive of congenital infection. Congenital rubella is characterized by neurosensory deafness, heart anomalies, cataracts, growth retardation, and encephalitic symptoms.
2. Diagnosis of toxoplasmosis is established by sequential examina-

tion, rather than by a single positive test. Sequential examination reveals rising antibody titers, changing titers, and conversion of serologic tests from negative to positive. A titer of 1:256 suggests recent infections. About one third of infants who acquire infection *in utero* will show signs of cerebral calcifications and chorioretinitis at birth. The remainder of infected infants will be born asymptomatic.

3. A marked and persistent rise in complement-fixing antibody titer over time is consistent with rubella in infants before 6 months of age.

4. Presence of antibodies in CSF, with signs of herpetic encephalitis and the persistence of antibody levels in herpes virus type 2 or 1 in a newborn showing no obvious external lesions is consistent with a diagnosis of herpes simplex.

Cold Agglutinins (Acute and Convalescent Studies)

Normal Values
Normal: ≤1:16

Background
Cold agglutinins are usually I_gM autoantibodies that cause the agglutination of the patient's own red blood cells at temperatures in the range of 0 to 10°C. These antibodies, with maximum activity at temperatures below 37°C, are termed *cold* and are found in the blood of normal persons in small amounts.

In cases of suspected primary atypical pneumonia, there is a titer rise 8 to 10 days after onset, a peak in titer 12 to 25 days, and a decrease in titer 30 days after onset. Up to 90% of those with severe illness will have a positive titer.

Explanation of Test
The test is used most commonly to diagnose primary atypical pneumonia caused by *Mycoplasma pneumoniae* and certain hemolytic anemias (cold agglutination disease). Diagnosis depends on the demonstration of a fourfold or higher increase in antibody titers between an acute blood serum sample taken as early as possible in the course of the infection and a blood serum sample taken in convalescence, 7 to 10 days after the acute sample. Both frequency of positive reactions and the elevation of the titer appear to be directly related to the severity of the infection.

Procedure
A venous blood sample of 10 ml is obtained. The specimen should be collected and transported to the lab at 37°C. When this is not possible,

the sample should be prewarmed to 37°C for at least 15 minutes before the serum is separated from the cells.

Because cold agglutinins will attach themselves to the red blood cells and, therefore, will not be present in the serum for testing, these precautions are necessary.

Clinical Implications
1. High titers are commonly associated with the following conditions:
    (a) Atypical pneumonia
        (1) Mycoplasma pneumonia
        (2) Influenza A and B
    (b) Congenital syphilis
    (c) Severe hemolytic anemia of cold variety—paroxysmal cold hemoglobinurias
    (d) Cirrhosis
    (e) Lymphatic leukemia
    (f) Malaria
    (g) Peripheral vascular disease
    (h) Cold hemagglutinin disease
2. In patients with a titer in the tens of thousands, agglutination of red blood cells may occur within their blood vessels after exposure to cold, causing such conditions as the following:
    (a) Frostbite
    (b) Focal gangrene
    (c) Raynaud's syndrome
    (d) Anemia
3. More important than any single high titer is the rise in titer during the course of illness. The titer will usually decrease by the fourth to sixth week after onset of illness.
4. Chronically increased titers are associated with
    (a) Hemolytic anemia
    (b) Cold agglutinin disease
    (c) Cold hemoglobinemia
    (d) Severe Raynaud's phenomenon (sometimes leading to gangrene in cold weather)
    (e) Lymphatic leukemia
5. Transient increases in titers are associated with
    (a) Mycoplasma atypical pneumonia
    (b) Infectious mononucleosis
    (c) Congenital syphilis
    (d) Hepatic cirrhosis
    (e) Trypanosomiasis

Interfering Factors
1. A high titer of cold agglutinins can interfere with typing and cross-matching.

2. High titers sometimes appear spontaneously in older persons. The high antibody titer may persist for years.
3. Antibiotic therapy may interfere with the development of cold agglutinins.

C-Reactive Protein (CRP) Test

Normal Values
<0.8 mg/dl

Background
During the course of an inflammatory process—whether due to infection or to tissue destruction—an abnormal specific protein, CRP, appears in the blood. This protein is virtually absent from the serum of healthy persons. CRP appears rapidly in the blood in response to many injurious stimuli. Almost any disease that brings about an inflammatory condition of any tissue will result in quantities of CRP being present in the blood and body fluids (*e.g.*, peritoneal fluid and synovial fluid).

CRP is thought to be synthesized mainly in the liver and is found in large amounts in inflammatory body fluids such as peritoneal, pleural, pericardial, and synovial. It is considered to be a transport protein for certain polysaccharides. From recent studies, it appears that a major function of CRP in health and disease involves its ability to interact with the complement system.

Explanation of Test
The CRP test is an antigen–antibody reaction test that is a nonspecific method for evaluating the severity and course of inflammatory diseases and those conditions in which there is tissue necrosis, such as myocardial infarction, malignancies, and rheumatoid arthritis. The presence of CRP in the blood serum can be detected 18 to 24 hours after the onset of tissue damage. This is a useful test in following the progress of rheumatic fever under treatment and in the interpretation of the sedimentation rate. It is also valuable in monitoring the surgical wound healing process, especially in internal incisions, burn patients, and kidney transplant care.

Procedure
A venous blood sample of 10 ml is obtained.

Clinical Implications
1. A positive reaction indicates the presence of an active inflammation, but not the cause of the process. The results of the test must be used in association with clinical judgment.

2. The test is positive with the following conditions:
   (a) Rheumatic fever
   (b) Rheumatoid arthritis

   > **Note:** The test becomes negative with successful treatment, indicating that the inflammatory reaction has disappeared, even when the sedimentation rate continues.

   (c) Lupus erythematosus (disseminated)
   (d) Myocardial infarction
   (e) Malignancy (active, widespread)
   (f) Bacterial and viral infections (acute)
   (g) After surgery with no complications, will decline by fourth postoperative day.
3. Demonstration of the presence of CRP has added significance over and above the finding of an elevated erythrocyte sedimentation rate (ESR), which may be influenced by changed physiologic states.
4. CRP tends to increase before rises in antibody titer and ESR. Levels of CRP tend to decrease sooner than ESR levels.

Patient Preparation
1. Instruct the patient to fast for 8 to 12 hours before test if laboratory requires fasting. (Check the policy of the laboratory being used.)
2. Water is permitted.

IMMUNOLOGIC TESTS FOR AUTOIMMUNE DISEASES AND RELATED DISORDERS OF THE IMMUNE SYSTEM

Protein Electrophoresis

Normal Values for Serum Protein Electrophoresis (SPE)
Total protein: 6.3–7.9 g/dl
Albumin: 3.1–4.3 g/dl
Alpha-$_1$-globulin: 0.1–0.3 g/dl
Alpha-$_2$-globulin: 0.6–1.0 g/dl
Beta-globulin: 0.7–1.4 g/dl
Gamma-globulin: 0.7–1.6 g/dl

Normal Values for Urine Protein Electrophoresis

Description Report
The principle of electrophoresis is based on the fact that a charged particle placed in an electrical field will migrate toward one of the electrodes of the field depending on (1) the electrical charge on the particle; (2) the size of the particle; (3) the strength of the electrical field; and (4) the nature of the medium used to support the particle

during the migration process. Typically, although not exclusively, the use of electrophoretic techniques enjoys its greatest current applicability in the separation of proteins.

Proteins are large molecules composed of amino acids. Amino acids are molecules capable of existing either as positively or negatively charged particles, depending on the pH of the solution in which they reside. Because of their ability to exist as positive ions in acidic solutions and negative ions in basic solutions, amino acids are said to be amphoteric. For all practical purposes, the amphoteric characteristics of proteins can be considered to be very similar to those of the amino acids of which they are composed. Amino acids or proteins have one other feature that contributes to their unique properties as ampholytes: there is a pH value at which the number of positive charges and negative charges on the molecule balance each other. This point, called the *isoelectric point*, is such that if a protein is placed in a solution at the pH of its isoelectric point, that protein has no net charge and, thus, will not migrate in an electrical field. The higher the pH value above the isoelectric point, the greater the net negative charge on the protein and the further it will migrate toward the positive electrode when placed in a direct current electrical field. On the other hand, the lower the pH of the solution below the isoelectric point of the protein, the greater the net positive charge on the protein and the further it will migrate toward the negative electrode when placed into a direct current electrical field.

Proteins can be separated into five factors by standard electrophoretic techniques: albumin, and alpha 1, alpha 2, beta, and gamma globulins. High-resolution buffers allow separation into 10 to 12 serum components. Abnormalities are encountered in a variety of disease states (Fig. 8-3).

Description of Factors: Alpha 1, Alpha 2, Beta, and Gamma Globulins

Alpha-1 Globulins

Alpha-1 lipoprotein: transports lipids, fat-soluble vitamins, and hormones

Alpha-1 antitrypsin: inhibits trypsin and chymotrypsin; acute-phase reactant; subject to genetic control

Alpha-acid glycoprotein: inactivates progesterone; acute-phase reactant

Thyroxine-binding globulin: binds thyroxine

Alpha-2 Globulins

Alpha-2 macroglobulin: inhibitor of plasmin and trypsin; growth-factor activity; binds insulin

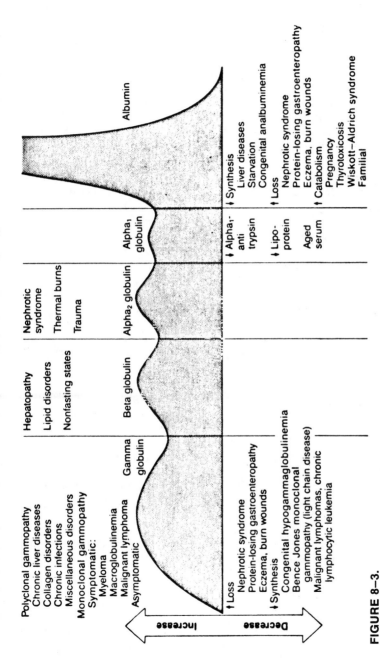

FIGURE 8–3.
Correlation of serum protein electrophoresis patterns with clinical disorders. (After Ritzmann SE, Daniels JC: Serum protein electrophoresis. In Race GJ [ed]: Tice's Practice of Medicine, Vol. 2. New York, Harper & Row, 1974)

Alpha-2 lipoprotein: transports lipids, particularly triglycerides

Haptoglobin: binds hemoglobin; prevents loss of iron from body; acute-phase reactant

Ceruloplasmin: oxidase activity; has role in metabolism of copper

Cholinesterase: hydrolyzes acetylcholine

Prothrombin: essential factor in blood coagulation system

Alpha-HS glycoprotein: unknown

Zn-alpha 2 glycoprotein: unknown

G-globulin: unknown; occurs in multiple molecular forms

Beta Globulins

Beta lipoprotein: transports lipids, lipid-soluble vitamins and hormones

Transferrin: transports iron; defense against certain infectious agents

Hemopexin: binds heme

Plasminogen: lysis of fibrin in blood clots

Complement: activity involves a large number of proteins that contribute to the natural phagocytic property of blood

$Beta_2$-glycoprotein: unknown

Fibrinogen: essential factor in blood coagulation system

Gamma Globulins

Immunoglobulin G: Antibody functions against viruses, bacterial toxins, Rh antibodies, nuclear antibodies, anti-insulin, and ragweed antibodies

Immunoglobulin A (serum): Antibodies such as antibacterial agglutinins, antinuclear and anti-insulin antibodies; the predominant immunoglobulin in body fluids and secretions

Immunoglobulin M: Antibodies such as the ABO isoagglutinins, cold agglutinins, antibodies to gram-negative bacteria, Wasserman antibody, antithyroglobin, and others

Immunoglobulin D: Antibody occurs in large quantities on the membrane of human B cells and may, as an antigen receptor, be involved in B-cell activation.

Immunoglobulin E: Antibody is associated with such immediate hypersensitivity reactions as anaphylaxis and atopy and with immunity to certain helminthic parasites.

Explanation of Test

Measurements are done to identify various disorders such as dysproteinemias, hypogammaglobulinemias, and some inflammatory states. The correlation of specific electrophoretic patterns with certain disorders is helpful in identifying various clinical diseases.

Procedure
1. A venous blood sample of 10 ml is obtained.
2. One hundred milliliters from a 24-hour urine collection are submitted if a urine protein electrophoresis is to be run simultaneously.

Clinical Implications
1. Decreased alpha-1 antitrypsin is associated with juvenile pulmonary emphysema.
2. Increased alpha-1 acid glycoprotein is associated with chronic inflammatory, degenerative, and some malignant diseases.
3. Increased alpha-2 globulins are associated with altered vascular permeability as in nephrotic syndrome and acute inflammatory diseases. Most other increases are due to either haptoglobin, alpha-2 macroglobulin, or both.
4. Rarely are there increases or decreases in the beta globulins without the alteration being related to some disorder in the gamma globulin function.
5. Increases of gamma globulins are associated with antibodies in which one or more of the immunoglobulins are elevated. Decreases may be seen in genetic deficiencies of immunoglobulin production or immunosuppression.

Clinical Alert

1. Rarely is any single type of electrophoretic analysis used by itself to determine any of the gammopathies. It is necessary to use immunoelectrophoresis, bone marrow studies, and clinical findings to verify the data.
2. Normally, little protein is excreted in the urine, but relatively large amounts may escape in various disease states. In lipoid nephrosis, there is selective proteinuria (*i.e.*, primarily albumin escapes). In nonselective proteinuria, such as in glomerulonephritis, all the serum proteins tend to appear in the urine. Urine protein electrophoresis is used to primarily identify Bence–Jones proteins, which migrate in the beta- and gamma-globulin regions.

Quantitative Immunoglobulins: IgG, IgA, and IgM

Normal Values
The following values refer to the serum concentrations of immunoglobulins:

IMMUNOGLOBULINS (IgG, IgA, and IgM)

Normal Values
IgG: 700–1,500 mg/dL for males and females ≥ 18 years of age
IgA: 60–400 mg/dL for males and females ≥ 18 years of age
IgM: 60–300 mg/dL for males and females ≥ 18 years of age

PEDIATRIC NORMALS
(*Results reported in mg/dL*)

Total IgG
  (Men and Women)
        0–4   months: 141–930
        5–8   months: 250–1,190
        9–11 months: 320–1,250
        1–3   years: 400–1,250
        4–6   years: 560–1,307
        7–9   years: 598–1,379
        10–12 years: 638–1,453
        13–15 years: 680–1,531
        16–17 years: 724–1,611

IgA
  (Men and Women) (ranges ±2 SD)
        0–4   months: 5–64
        5–8   months: 10–87
        9–14 months: 17–94
        15–23 months: 22–178
        2–3   years: 24–192
        4–6   years: 26–232
        7–9   years: 33–258
        10–12 years: 45–285
        13–15 years: 47–317
        16–17 years: 55–377

IgM
  (Men)
        0–4   months: 14–142
        5–8   months: 24–167
        9–23 months: 35–200
        2–3   years: 41–200
        4–17   years: 47–200

IgM
  (Women)
        0–4   months: 14–142
        5–8   months: 24–167
        9–23 months: 35–242
        2–3   years: 41–242
        4–17   years: 56–242

Background
Immunoglobulin is a general term for antibody. Five classes of immunoglobulins—IgG, IgA, IgM, IgD, and IgE—have been isolated in humans. Each of the immunoglobulins bears a structural similarity to

the other antibody molecules. The basic functions of immunoglobulins are to neutralize toxic substances (antigens) entering the body, to allow for phagocytosis, and to kill microbial organisms.

A brief description of three major immunoglobulins, IgG, IgA, IgM, and their properties follows (see Fig. 8–4 and Table 8–4):

IgG

1. Major immunoglobulin in normal human serum, accounting for approximately 75% to 80% of the total
2. Four subclasses of IgG have been identified based on heavy chain differences: IgG_1, IgG_2, IgG_3, and IgG_4.
3. Occurs as the major antibody in secondary immune responses (after IgM)

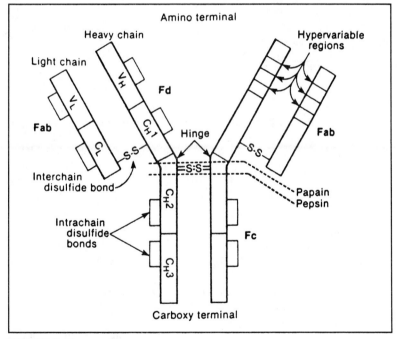

FIGURE 8–4.
Basic unit (monomer) of IgG molecule consisting of four polypeptide chains linked covalently by disulfide bonds (S–S). V = variable region; C = constant region; L = light chain; H = heavy chain. (From Hyde RM and Patnode RA: Immunology—The National Series for Independent Study, p 32. A Wiley Medical Publication. New York, John Wiley & Sons, 1987. Harwal Publishing Co, Media, PA)

TABLE 8–4.
Structural Characteristics of Immunoglobulins

	IgG	IgA	IgM	IgD	IgE
H chain	γ	α	μ	δ	ε
H chain subclasses	$\gamma_1, \gamma_2, \gamma_3, \gamma_4$	α_1, α_2	μ_1, μ_2	—	—
Molecular weight	150,000	160,000–400,000	900,000	180,000	190,000
S value	7	7–18	19	7	8
Valence	2	2–8	10	2	2
J chain	—	+	+	—	—
Gm allotypes	+	—	—	—	—
Am allotypes	—	+	—	—	—
Km allotypes	+	+	+	+	+
L chain	κ, λ	κ, λ	κ, λ	κ, λ	κ, λ

H chain, heavy chain; S value, sedimentation coefficient of a protein as determined by ultracentrifugation; Gm, genetic marker on the γ chain; Am, genetric marker on the α chain; Km, genetic marker on the χ chain; L chain, light chain.
(Hyde RM, Patnode RA: Immunology: The National Medical Series for Independent Study. New York, John Wiley & Sons, 1987)

4. IgG is important in phagocytosis (opsonization), because phagocytic cells (*e.g.*, macrophages, neutrophils) have receptors for the Fc fragment of IgG, primarily IgG_1 and IgG_3.
5. IgG molecules are capable of fixing complement, except for IgG_4.
6. IgG is the only immunoglobulin that can cross the placenta and, therefore, is responsible for protection of the newborn during the first months of life.

IgA
1. Present in both serum and body fluids and thus takes two forms: serum IgA and secretory IgA
2. Serm IgA accounts for 10% to 15% of the total human immunoglobulin.
3. Secretory IgA is the predominant immunoglobulin in various secretions (*e.g.*, saliva, tears, colostrum and bronchial, genitourinary, and intestinal secretions).
4. IgA may occur as a monomer, as is usually the case in serum; in secretory fluids, IgA consists of two monomeric units plus J chain and secretory component.
5. Serum IgA is approximately 85% subclass IgA_1; secretory IgA is present as the IgA_2 heavy-chain isotype.
6. Secretory IgA protects the mucous membranes in the respiratory and gastrointestinal tract as the first line of defense against inva-

sion by microorganisms at the point of entrance into the internal environment.

IgM

1. Constitutes 5% to 10% of total human immunoglobulin
2. Predominant antibody in the early (primary) immune response to most antigens and the predominant antibody produced by the fetus
3. Possesses antibody activity against gram-negative organisms and rheumatoid factors
4. Forms the natural antibodies such as the ABO blood group
5. Is the most efficient immunoglobulin at fixing complement in lytic reactions and enhancing phagocytosis.
6. Does not cross the placenta and is, therefore, usually absent in the newborn. It is observed approximately 5 days after birth.

Explanation of Test

If there is a monoclonal protein or M component present on serum protein electrophoresis (SPE), a quantitative measurement of IgG, IgA, and IgM can virtually identify the specific immunoglobulin. IgD and IgE are present in trace amounts.

Quantitative immunoglobulins are useful in monitoring the course of a disease and its treatment. Normal concentrations of the serum immunoglobulins vary with age.

Procedure

1. A venous blood sample of 10 ml is usually obtained.
2. Check with the individual laboratory requiring the sample. Quantities needed may vary from laboratory to laboratory.

Clinical Implications

A. IgG
   1. Increases in
      (a) Chronic granulomatous infections
      (b) Infections of all types
      (c) Hyperimmunization
      (d) Liver disease
      (e) Malnutrition (severe)
      (f) Dysproteinemia
      (g) Disease associated with hypersensitivity granulomas, dermatologic disorders, and IgG myeloma
      (h) Rheumatoid arthritis
   2. Decreases in
      (a) Agammaglobulinemia
      (b) Lymphoid aplasia
      (c) Selective IgG, IgA deficiency
      (d) IgA myeloma

   (e) Bence–Jones proteinemia
   (f) Chronic lymphoblastic leukemia
B. **IgA**
   1. Increases in
      (a) Chronic, nonalcoholic liver diseases, especially primary biliary cirrhosis (PBC). PBC is a progressive disease most commonly seen in women in the second half of their reproductive period.
      (b) Obstructive jaundice
      (c) Wide range of conditions that affect mucosal surfaces
      (d) Asparaginase treatment
      (e) Exercise
      (f) Alcoholism
      (g) Subacute and chronic infections
   2. Decreases in
      (a) Ataxia-telangiectasia
      (b) Chronic sinopulmonary disease
      (c) Congenital deficit
      (d) Late pregnancy
      (e) Prolonged exposure to benzene
      (f) Abstinence from alcohol after a period of 1 year
      (g) Drugs and dextrin immunosuppressive therapy
      (h) Protein-losing gastroenteropathies
      (i) Immunologic deficiency states

> **Clinical Alert (for IgA)**
>
> Persons with IgA deficiency are predisposed to autoimmune disorders and can develop antibody to IgA with possible anaphylaxis occurring if transfused.

C. **IgM**
   1. Increases (in adults) in
      (a) Waldenström's macroglobulinemia
      (b) Trypanosomiasis
      (c) Actinomycosis
      (d) Carrión's disease (bartonellosis)
      (e) Malaria
      (f) Infectious mononucleosis
      (g) Lupus erythematosus
      (h) Rheumatoid arthritis
      (i) Dysgammaglobulinemia (certain cases)

Clinical Alert

In the newborn, a level of IgM above 20 mg/dl is an indication of in utero stimulation of the immune system and stimulation by the rubella virus, the cytomegalovirus, syphilis, or toxoplasmosis.

2. Decreases in IgM
   (a) Agammaglobulinemia
   (b) Lymphoproliferative disorders (certain cases)
   (c) Lymphoid aplasia
   (d) IgG and IgA myeloma
   (e) Dysgammaglobulinemia
   (f) Chronic lymphoblastic leukemia

Immunoelectrophoresis (IEP)

Normal Values
Descriptive report of abnormality, if present

Background
Monoclonal immunoglobulins consist of heavy and light chains. The five classes of heavy chains are designated by Greek letters: γ in IgG, α in IgA, μ in IgM, δ in IgD and ε in IgE. There are two types of light chains— κ (kappa) and λ (lambda). Monoclonal proteins consist of IgG κ, IgG λ, IgA κ, IgA λ, and so forth. Immunoelectrophoresis of the serum is necessary to identify the presence or absence of a monoclonal protein and to determine its heavy-chain and light-chain types.

The presence of a monoclonal protein in the serum of urine suggests a neoplastic process; a polyclonal increase in immunoglobulins is seen in chronic liver disease, chronic connective tissue disease, or infection.

In multiple myeloma, 99% of patients will have a monoclonal protein in the serum or urine. Macroglobulinemia of Waldenström is characterized by the presence of a monoclonal IgM protein in the serum in all cases.

A monoclonal light chain (κ or λ), Bence–Jones protein, is found in the urine of approximately 75% of patients with multiple myeloma. Approximately 75% of patients with Waldenström's macroglobulinemia will have a monoclonal light chain in the urine. Heavy-chain fragments as well as free light chains may be seen in the urine of patients with multiple myeloma or amyloidosis.

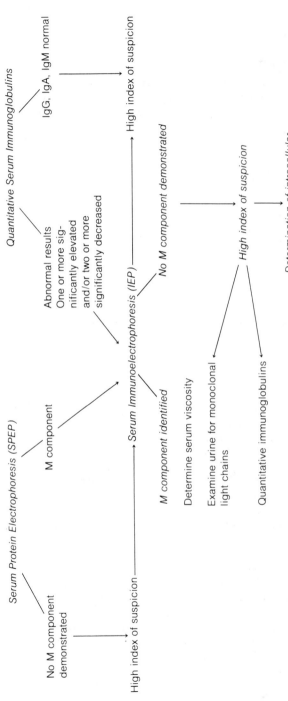

FIGURE 8–5.

Approach to the laboratory evaluation of monoclonal gammopathies. Immunoelectrophoresis should be performed if the serum protein electrophoresis and/or serum immunoglobulin concentrations are abnormal as noted or if there is a high index of suspicion due to the patient's clinical presentation. Quantitative immunoglobulins and serum viscosity are useful measurements for monitoring the patient. Monoclonal light chains in the urine (≥200 mg/24 hours) suggest a malignant condition. This approach supplements hematopathologic and clinical information. (From Henry JB [ed]: Todd, Sanford, Davidsohn's Clinical Diagnosis and Management by Laboratory Methods, 17th ed. Philadelphia, WB Saunders, 1984)

Explanation of Test

IEP should be performed if the serum protein electrophoresis (SPE) and/or quantitative immunoglobulin concentrations are abnormal. IEP is a sensitive procedure to detect and identify the heavy-chain class and light-chain type of the monoclonal protein (see Fig. 8–5).

Procedure

A venous blood sample of 15 ml is obtained. The patient should be fasting. Age of patient should be noted because this procedure is seldom indicated in patients less than 30 years of age. Monoclonal proteins are rarely identified in this age group.

Submit 25 ml from a 24-hour urine collection if a urine IEP is to be run simultaneously. Again, patient's age should be noted.

Total Hemolytic Complement (CH50)

Normal Values

25–70 units/ml

Background

Complement (C) is a complex cascade system in which inactive proteins become active and interact in a sequential system very much like the clotting system. The complement system is very important as part of the body's defense mechanism against infection. Activation of complement results in cell lysis, release of histamine from mast cells and platelets, increased vascular permeability, contraction of smooth muscle, and chemotaxis of leukocytes. These inactive proteins make up about 10% of the globulins in normal blood serum. The complement system is also interrelated with the coagulation, fibrinolytic, and kinin systems. Complement is critical during infection in its capacity to mediate the inflammatory response. The action of complement is not always beneficial, however. The potent reactions mediated by this complex system are not always normally contained. In the presence of gram-negative bacteremia, the complement can escape its built-in control mechanisms, causing severe damage to the body in the process. It is not clear how this happens, but it is known that complement abnormalities develop before shock occurs.

Explanation of Test

This test is used as a screen for certain autoimmune diseases and is a prognostic aid in the successful treatment of others. Measurement of complement activity is used to estimate the extent of immune complex formation, and should detect all inborn and most acquired complement component deficiencies. Serial measurements are valuable in monitoring the course of disease and treatment in systemic lupus erythematosus, rheumatoid arthritis, and glomerulonephritis. It is a useful adjunct to specific tests for rheumatoid factor and systemic lupus erythematosus when immune complexes appear to be the primary mediators of tissue injury.

Procedure

A venous blood sample of 10 ml is obtained. A joint fluid specimen of at least 1 ml can also be collected in a tube with no additives and brought immediately to the laboratory.

Clinical Alert

Complement deteriorates at room temperature and serum or fluid samples should be brought to the laboratory as soon as possible. Separate serum from clot and freeze at −70°C until test is performed. Both blood and fluid must be processed and frozen within 2 hours after the time of collection from the patient. Failure to process in this manner may lead to falsely decreased functional activity levels.

Clinical Implications

1. *Increased values* are associated with most inflammatory responses.
   (a) Pyogenic infections
   (b) Acute gout
   (c) Myocardial infarction
   (d) Nonspecific polyarthritis
   (e) Diabetes, especially if associated with proliferative retinopathy (usually normal in diabetic nephropathy)
   (f) Ulcerative colitis
2. *Decreased values* are associated with
   (a) Specific deficiency of a complement component
      (1) Hereditary defect of an important complement component. Patients deficient in C2 may have autoimmune disorders such as lupus erythematosus, and C1q deficiency may cause agammaglobulinemia.
      (2) Lack of one of the inhibitors of the complement system such as occurs in hereditary angioedema
   (b) Complement consumption by activation of the alternative pathway as in certain infectious diseases, which can cause complement exhaustion or decrease
      (1) Gram-negative septicemia
      (2) Acute glomerulonephritis
      (3) Subacute bacterial endocarditis

(c) Complement consumption due to activation of proteolytic enzymes and tissue damage as in

(1) Systemic lupus erythematosus
(2) Acute glomerulonephritis
(3) Serum sickness
(4) Acute vasculitis
(5) Severe rheumatoid arthritis
(6) Membranoproliferative glomerulonephritis
(7) Hepatitis
(8) Cryoglobulinemia

C3 Complement Component

Normal Values
75–150 mg/dl

Background
C3 comprises 70% of the total protein in the complement system and is essential to the activation of both classical and alternative pathways. Along with the other components of the complement system, C3 may be used up in the complement cascade of reactions that occur in some antigen-antibody reactions. C3 is synthesized in many tissues, including liver, macrophages, fibroblasts, lymphoid cells and skin.

Explanation of Test
This test is ordered when it is suspected that individual complement component concentrations are abnormally reduced. This is one of three tests frequently ordered; Clq and C4 are the other two. Of these three, C3 is the most commonly requested component of complement. It has been shown that there is a good correlation between most forms of nephritis, the degree of severity of nephritis, and C3 levels. This is particularly true with acute poststreptococcal nephritis and for patients with systemic lupus erythematosus and nephritis. C3 may be nonspecifically elevated in acute-phase reactions and occasionally nonspecifically depressed in liver disease. Most active diseases with immune complex formation are associated with moderate to marked decreased C3 levels.

Procedure
A venous blood sample of at least 2 ml is obtained.

Clinical Implications
Decreased levels are associated with

1. Severe recurrent bacterial infections due to C3 homozygous deficiency
2. Absence of C3b inactivator factor
3. Acute glomerulonephritis

4. Immune complex disease
5. Active systemic lupus erythematosus
6. Membranoproliferative glomerulonephritis
7. Autoimmune hemolytic anemia
8. Occasional drug reactions
9. Nephritic rheumatoid arthritis
10. Disseminated intravascular coagulation (DIC) disorder

Increased levels are found in numerous inflammatory states as an acute-phase response.

Clinical Alert

Patients with low C3 levels are in danger of shock and death.

C4 Complement Component

Normal Values
10–30 mg/dl

Background
C4 is another of the components of the complement system in the cascade activation pathway. C4 may be bypassed in the alternative complement pathway when immune complexes are not involved, or it may be used up in the very complicated series of reactions that follow many antigen–antibody reactions. C4 is synthesized in lung and bone.

Explanation of Test
This is one of the follow-up tests done when there is a suspicion that total complement levels are abnormally decreased, as in rheumatoid disease investigation. This value is a determination of only one of the components of the complement system. The other tests are C1q and C3.

Procedure
A venous blood sample of at least 2 ml is obtained.

Clinical Implications
Decreased levels are associated with

1. Acute systemic lupus erythematosus
2. Early glomerulonephritis
3. Immune complex disease
4. Cryoglobulinemia
5. Inborn C4 deficiency
6. Hereditary angioneurotic edema

Increased levels are associated with a variety of malignancies.

C'1 Esterase Inhibitor (C'1 INH)

Normal Values
8–24 mg/dl

Background
C'1 esterase inhibitor of the activated first component of the complement system is an antigen; lack of this antigen causes the esterase level
to rise during an attack of hereditary angioneurotic edema (HAE). The
primary function of this inhibitor is to act as a regulatory brake on the
complement activation process.

Explanation of Test
This determination is an important tool in diagnosing HAE. This disorder is caused by a low concentration of C'1 esterase inhibitor or by an
abnormal structure of the protein. Affected persons are apparently heterozygous for the condition. It is important to differentiate persons
with HAE from those suffering from the more prevalent, less serious,
allergic and nonfamilial angioneurotic edema.

Procedure
A venous blood sample of at least 1 ml is obtained.

Clinical Implications
Decreased values are associated with HAE, a genetic disease characterized by acute edema of subcutaneous tissue, gastrointestinal tract, or
upper respiratory tract. During acute attacks of the disease, C4 and C2
components can be markedly reduced.

Clinical Alert

Prednisolone and transfusions of fresh frozen plasma have been
successfully used to treat HAE.

T and B Cell Lymphocyte Surface Markers; T-Helper/T-Suppressor Ratio

Normal Values
T and B Surface Markers
Percent T cells (CD2): 60%–88%
Percent Helper cells (CD4): 34%–67%
Percent Suppressor cells (CD8): 10%–42%
Percent B cells (CD19): 3%–21%

Absolute Counts
Lymphocytes: 0.66–4.60 thou/μL
T cells: 644–2201 cells/μL
Helper cells: 493–1191 cells/μL
Suppressor T cells: 182–785 cells/μL
B cells: 92–392 cells/μL

Lymphocyte Ratio
T_H/T_S Ratio >1.0

Background

Lymphocytes can be divided into two categories, T and B cells, according to their primary function within the immune system. In the body, T and B cells work together to help provide protection against infective agents, foreign tissue, and oncogenic agents, and they play a vital role in regulating self-destruction or autoimmunity.

The majority of circulating lymphocytes are T cells having a life span of months to years. B cells comprise 10% to 30% of the lymphocytes and have a life span measured in days.

A. *B cells (antibody)*
   1. They are considered "bursa or bone marrow dependent," and are responsible for humoral immunity (in which antibodies are present in the serum).
B. *T cells (cellular)*
   1. They are thymus-derived and are responsible for cellular immunity.
   2. T cells are further divided into T-helper (T_H) cells and T-suppressor (T_S) cells.

Explanation of Test

This test is done to evaluate the immune system by identifying the specific cells involved in the immune response. A number of disease states are characterized by abnormalities in the number and percent of T helper, T suppressor and B lymphocytes. Measurement of T and B lymphocytes can be a valuable diagnostic aid in the classification of lymphocytic leukemia, lymphoma, and immunodeficiency diseases, including AIDS; in the assessment of immunocompetence in chronic infections, viral versus immune hepatitis; in the diagnosis and treatment of autoimmune disorders; in the monitoring of patients following chemotherapy and radiotherapy; and in the assessment of immune status following renal, heart, and bone marrow transplants. The cell types present in patients' blood can be identified with monoclonal antibodies specific for cell markers using an instrument called a flow cytometer. In the flow cytometer, cells are passed single file in front of a finely focused Argon laser beam (Fig. 8–6). As the cells pass the beam, light is scattered. The amount of light that is scattered is dependent upon the

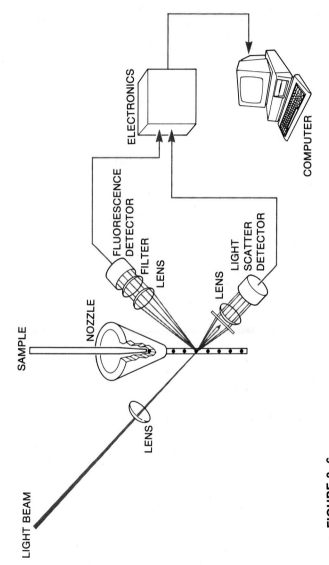

FIGURE 8–6.
Schematic diagram of a flow cytometer.

size of the cell (forward light scatter) and the granularity (90 light scatter). The flow cytometer is equipped with detectors for light scatter and fluorescence intensity as well as a series of filters for directing the light scatter to the appropriate detector. The light energy is converted into electrical energy that is digitized and translated by a computer to a graphic display. Based upon the cell size and granularity, the cells can be identified as lymphocytes, monocytes, or granulocytes.

Procedure

A venous blood sample of 20 ml is obtained. The sample must not be refrigerated or frozen.

Clinical Implications

1. A decrease in B cells is associated with
   (a) *Primary*
      (1) Transient hypogammaglobulinemia of infancy
      (2) X-linked hypogammaglobulinemia
      (3) Selective deficiency of IgG, IgA, IgM
   (b) *Secondary*
      (1) Lymphomas
      (2) Nephrotic syndrome
      (3) Multiple myeloma
2. Decrease in T cells is associated with
   (a) *Primary*
      (1) DeGeorge's syndrome
      (2) Nezelof's syndrome
   (b) *Secondary*
      (1) Hodgkin's or other malignant disease
      (2) Acute viral infection such as measles (transient decrease)
3. Combined decrease in B and T cells is associated with
   (a) *Primary*
      (1) Autosomal or sex-linked recessive cause
      (2) Wiskott–Aldrich syndrome
      (3) Immunodeficiency with ataxia and telangiectasis
   (b) *Secondary*
      (1) Radiation   (2) Aging
4. T cells increase in Graves' disease, and B cells increase in active lupus erythematosus and chronic lymphocytic leukemia.
5. Standard immunosuppressive and cytotoxic drug therapy usually decreases lymphocyte totals.
6. In AIDS, the T_4/T_8 ratio decreases (<1) due to a loss of T-helper lymphocytes.
7. Certain cell subsets or clusters of differentiation (C-D) (see Table 8-5)

TABLE 8–5.
Transplant Profile

Marker	Distribution	Purpose of Assay
T11 (CD2)	Pan-T	Decreases to <10% of pre-treatment level after successful antirejection therapy
T3 (CD3)	Mature T	See T11; assess effectiveness of therapy with OKT3
T4 (CD4)	Helper/inducer	Decreases in viral infection
T8 (CD8)	Suppressor/cytotoxic	Increases in viral infection
B1 (CD20)	Mature B	See 12; increased in lymphoma; account for B cells in lymphocyte gate
12*	HLA-DR	Percent positive >>B1+ cells in acute viral infection
MO1 (CD11)	Monocyte/granulocyte	Assists gating; account for monocytes, neutrophils, and NK cells in lymphocyte gate
MIgG†		Controls for nonspecific binding of IgG subclass reagents
MIgM†		Controls for nonspecific binding of IgM subclass reagents

* 12 normally expressed on B cells and monocytes. In viral infection and rejection, activated T8 and T4 cells express 12 as well.
† Pooled mouse immunoglobulin.
(Keren DF: Flow Cytometry in Clinical Diagnoses. Chicago, American Association of Clinical Pathologists Press, 1989)

Thyroid Antibody Tests (Antithyroglobulin and Antimicrosomal)

Normal Values
<1:100 by gelatin and/or hemagglutination for both antithyroglobulin and antimicrosomal antibodies

Background
Antibodies to thyroid gland components have been found in a variety of thyroid disorders. There are a number of autoantibodies involved, including one reaction against thyroglobulin and another against the microsomal component of thyroid epithelial cells. It has been suggested that the long-acting thyroid stimulator (LATS) may also be an autoantibody.

Thyroid antibodies are seldom found in serum of normal patients. However, 5% to 10% of the normal population may exhibit low titers of the thyroid antibodies with no symptoms of disease. The incidence is higher in women and increases with age. The presence of thyroid antibodies may also be indicative of previous autoimmune disorders. Patients with low thyroid antibody titers should be tested periodically, because the presence of the antibody may be an early sign of autoimmune disease.

In active cases of thyroid autoimmune disease and in some cases of thyrotoxicosis, moderate (1:1600) to high (1:25,600) antibody titers may be observed. The detection of very high (greater than 1:25,600) antibody titers in a patient with a firm, hard, fast-growing, symmetric goiter strongly suggests Hashimoto's goiter.

The presence and concentration of these antibodies in the circulation and their serologic detection can play a great role in evaluation and treatment of such disease states. Tests for thyroid autoantibodies are recommended in the differential diagnosis of patients with Hashimoto's disease (chronic thyroiditis) and Graves' disease (hyperthyroidism). They are also associated with primary myxedema, nontoxic goiter, carcinoma of the thyroid, de Quervain's disease, juvenile lymphocytic thyroiditis, Sjögren's syndrome, pernicious anemia, Addison's disease, myasthenia gravis, and diabetes mellitus.

Explanation of Test

These studies detect thyroid antibodies that are elevated in certain thyroid diseases such as Hashimoto's disease. When tests for both thyroglobulin antibodies and thyroid microsomal antibodies are done in combination, the specificity for detection of thyroid autoimmune antibodies is greatly increased and is more sensitive than a single test used for detection.

Procedure

A venous blood sample of 10 ml is obtained.

Clinical Implications

1. High titers of both antibodies are found in
   (a) Hashimoto's disease (hypothyroid)
   (b) Lymphadenoid goiter
2. Combination high titers are not found in
   (a) Nontoxic goiter
   (b) Thyroid cancer
   (c) de Quervain's subacute thyroiditis

Antithyroglobulin Antibody Test

Normal Values
Titer: <1:100

Background
In certain destructive diseases of the thyroid, intact thyroglobulin may be released from the thyroid gland, stimulating antibody formation. These antibodies may be responsible for further destruction of this gland.

Explanation of Test
This test is used in the differential diagnosis of thyroid diseases such as Hashimoto's thyroiditis and cancer of the thyroid.

Procedure
A venous blood sample of at least 2 ml is obtained.

Clinical Implications
1. Increased antithyroglobulin antibodies are associated with
   (a) Hashimoto's thyroiditis—80% of patients
   (b) Active cases of thyroid autoimmune diseases and thyrotoxicosis (sometimes). High levels of 1:1600 to 1:25,600 will be detected.
   (c) A titer in the millions strongly suggests Hashimoto's disease
   (d) Occasionally found in
      (1) Myxedema
      (2) Granulomatous thyroiditis
      (3) Nontoxic nodular goiter
      (4) Thyroid carcinoma
   (e) Other autoimmune diseases such as
      (1) Sjögren's syndrome
      (2) Systemic lupus erythematosus
      (3) Rheumatoid arthritis
      (4) Autoimmune hemolytic anemia
2. Low titers may be associated with pediatric Hashimoto's disease.

Interfering Factors
About 10% of the population may have low titers of thyroid antibodies with no incidence of disease.

Antimicrosomal Antibody Test

Normal Values
Titer: <1:100

Background

Microsomes are normally present within the cytoplasm of epithelial cells surrounding the thyroid follicle. Microsomes can escape from the follicular cells. Once free, they act as antigens giving rise to specific antibodies with cytotoxic effects on these follicular cells.

Explanation of Test

This measurement is very specific for the detection of thyroid microsomal antibodies, which are present in approximately 80% of persons with Hashimoto's thyroiditis.

Procedure

A venous blood sample of at least 2 ml is obtained.

Clinical Implications

Positive reactions are associated with

1. Hashimoto's thyroiditis in 80% of cases
2. Juvenile lymphocytic thyroiditis in 90% of cases
3. Myxedema
4. Granulomatosis thyroiditis
5. Nontoxic nodular goiter
6. Thyroid cancer in 20% of cases
7. Other autoimmune diseases such as
    (a) Sjögren's syndrome
    (b) Systemic lupus erythematosus
    (c) Rheumatoid arthritis
    (d) Autoimmune hemolytic anemia

Interfering Factors

Antibodies are present in 5% to 10% of healthy persons.

Raji Cell Assay

Normal Values

Negative

Background

Circulating immune complexes have been implicated in numerous immunopathologic disorders. The demonstration of complexes may prove useful in predicting the clinical course of systemic lupus erythematosus (SLE).

Explanation of Test

This assay is based on the ability of immune complexes to bind Raji cells (a human lymphoblastoid cell line) through C3 receptors. Immune complexes bound to the surface of the Raji cells can be assayed by the addition of radiolabeled anti-IgG antibody.

Procedure
A venous blood sample of 10 ml is obtained.

Clinical Implications
1. Immune complexes that can be detected using this method include those found in
   (a) Autoimmune disorders
       (SLE)
   (b) Viral infections
   (c) Parasitic infections
   (d) Disseminated malignancy
   (e) Microbial infections
   (f) Drug reactions
2. Other disorders include
   (a) Cryoglobulinemia
   (b) Celiac disease
   (c) Dermatitis herpetiformis
   (d) Crohn's disease
   (e) Ulcerative colitis
   (f) Cirrhosis
   (g) Sickle cell anemia

Anti-SS-A and Anti-SS-B Antibody Tests

Normal Values
Negative for SS-A and SS-B antibodies

Explanation of Test
The purpose of this measurement is to detect SS-A (Ro) and SS-B (La) antibodies that are produced in Sjögren's syndrome. This syndrome may manifest itself with symptoms that are similar to those of connective tissue disorders such as rheumatoid arthritis, systemic lupus erythematosus, or progressive systemic sclerosis. However, no immunologic test is diagnostic for Sjögren's syndrome. SS-A and SS-B antibody detection is particularly useful when an "ANA negative" case of SLE is expected.

Procedure
A venous blood sample of 10 ml is obtained.

Clinical Implications
1. SS-B antibodies are associated with primary Sjögren's disease, an immunologic abnormality associated with decreased secretion of exocrine glands. Fifty percent of these patients will have rheumatoid arthritis.
2. SS-A antibodies may be found in Sjögren's syndrome alone or in Sjögren's syndrome associated with systemic lupus erythematosus.
3. Persons with both Sjögren's syndrome and rheumatoid arthritis have neither anti-SS-A nor anti-SS-B antibodies. These patients tend to develop antibodies against the Epstein–Barr virus associated with rheumatoid arthritis nuclear antigen (RANA).

4. Autoantibodies against salivary duct antigens have been detected in 50% of cases.

Anti-Smooth Muscle Antibody (ASMA) Test

Normal Values
Negative
If positive, serum will be titered.

Background
This autoantibody is associated with liver and bile duct autoimmune diseases. Apparently, these disorders are not caused by any organism or external agent; the immune response itself is believed responsible.

Explanation of Test
This measurement is helpful in differentiating chronic active hepatitis and primary biliary cirrhosis from other liver diseases in which anti-smooth muscle antibodies (ASMAs) are seldom present, such as systemic lupus erythematosus.

Procedure
A venous blood sample of at least 2 ml is obtained.

Clinical Implications
1. ASMAs are found in
   (a) Chronic active hepatitis, a progressive disease of unknown etiology found predominantly in young women and having factors characteristic of both acute and chronic hepatitis (80% of patients). If this disease is associated with a positive antinuclear antibody test, the disease is often called *lupoid hepatitis.*
   (b) Biliary cirrhosis
2. When ASMAs are found in acute diseases such as viral infections and infectious mononucleosis, they are frequently of the IgM class.
3. When ASMAs are found in chronic hepatitis, the antibodies are of the IgG class.
4. These antibodies are seldom present in
   (a) Extrahepatic biliary obstruction
   (b) Drug-induced liver disease
   (c) Viral hepatitis
   (d) Hepatoma
5. More than 20% of patients with intrinsic asthma have ASMAs.
See Table 8–6 regarding prevalence of autoantibodies in liver disease.

TABLE 8–6.
Prevalence of Autoantibodies in Liver Disease

Disease	Anti-Smooth Muscle (%)	Antimitochondrial (%)	ANA
Chronic active hepatitis	70–90	30–60	60
Chronic persistent hepatitis	45	15–20	15–30
Acute viral hepatitis	10–30	5–20	20
Acute alcoholic hepatitis	0	0	0
Biliary cirrhosis	30	60–70	5
Cryptogenic cirrhosis	15	30	0
Alcoholic (Laennee's) cirrhosis	0	0	0
Extrahepatic biliary obstruction	5–10	5–10	5

(Adapted from Whittingham MB, Irwin J, Mackay IR et al: Gastroenterology 51:499, 1966; and Husby G, Skrede J, Blomhoff JP: Scand J Gastroenterol 12:297, 1977)

Antimitochondrial Antibody (AMA) Test

Normal Values
Negative
If positive, serum will be titered.

Background
Antimitochondrial antibody (AMA) is non-organ and non-species specific and is directed against a lipoprotein in the inner mitochondrial membrane. The AMAs are predominantly of the IgG class; however, they have not been proven directly to cause liver cell or bile duct destruction.

Explanation of Test
This measurement is an important aid in the diagnosis of primary biliary cirrhosis (PBC). PBC is a progressive disease most commonly seen in women in the second half of their reproductive period. These antibodies are also associated with autoantibodies and with autoimmune disease.

Clinical Implications
1. A titer of 1:160 or greater is present in 79% to 94% of patients with primary biliary cirrhosis.

2. High titers are also associated with
   (a) Long-standing hepatic obstruction
   (b) Chronic hepatitis
   (c) Cryptogenic cirrhosis
3. No titer is found in extrahepatic jaundice
4. Increased titer is occasionally found in
   (a) Systemic lupus erythematosus
   (b) Rheumatoid arthritis
   (c) Thyroid disease
   (d) Pernicious anemia
   (e) Idiopathic Addison's disease

Antiparietal Cell Antibody (APCA) Test

Normal Values
Negative
If positive, serum will be titered.

Background
The disruption of normal intrinsic factor production or function due to autoimmune processes can lead to pernicious anemia. Antibodies to two antigens of the gastric parietal cell, antiparietal cell antibodies (APCAs), and intrinsic factor antibodies are found in pernicious anemia.

Explanation of Test
This measurement is helpful in diagnosing chronic gastric disease and differentiating autoimmune pernicious anemia from other megaloblastic anemias. Persons with other anemias will not have detectable APCAs.

Procedure
A venous blood sample of at least 2 ml is obtained.

Clinical Implications
1. The APCAs occur in serum of 80% to 90% of patients with autoimmune pernicious anemia.
2. Occasionally present in patients with
   (a) Gastric ulcer
   (b) Gastric cancer
   (c) Atrophic gastritis
   (d) Thyroid disease
   (e) Diabetes mellitus

Interfering Factors
In normal children, there is a 2% incidence of APCAs and up to a 10% to 20% incidence in the elderly.

Antiglomerular Basement Membrane (AGBM) Antibody Test

Normal Values
Negative

Background
Antibodies specific for renal structural components such as the glomerular basement membrane of the kidney can bind to respective tissue-fixed antigens, producing an immune response.

Explanation of Test
This test is primarily used in the differential diagnosis of glomerular nephritis induced by antiglomerular basement membrane antibodies (AGBMs) from other types of glomerular nephritis. The AGBMs cause about 5% of glomerular nephritis, and about two thirds of these patients may also develop pulmonary hemorrhage (Goodpasture's syndrome).

Procedure
A venous blood sample of 5 ml is obtained.

Clinical Implications
The AGBM antibodies are detected in

1. Anti-GBM glomerular nephritis
2. Tubulointerstitial nephritis
3. Anti-GBM Goodpasture's syndrome

Acetylcholine Receptor (AChR) Binding Antibody Test

Normal Values
Negative or ≤0.03 nmol/L

Background
Acetylcholine receptor antibodies (AChRs) appear in myasthenia gravis, and it is believed that this disease involves destruction by the muscle cells of acetylcholine receptors bound by antibody at the skeletal muscle motor endplate.

Explanation of Test
This test is considered by many authorities to be diagnostic for myasthenia gravis in patients with symptoms. It is also helpful in managing patient response to immunosuppressive therapy.

Procedure
A venous blood sample of at least 2 ml is obtained. Notify the laboratory if any immunosuppressive drugs have been given.

Clinical Implications
1. The AChR antibodies are found in approximately 90% of persons with myasthenia gravis and confirm the autoimmune nature of the disease.
2. Patients who have only eye symptoms tend to have lower titers than those with generalized symptoms.

Interfering Factors
False-positive binding occurs in amyotrophic lateral sclerosis patients who have been treated with snake venom.

Allergens–IgE Antibodies; RAST

Normal Values
Result of test is reported as negative or positive by comparison with a negative control tested simultaneously.

Background
A large number of substances have been found to have allergic potential. Measurable allergen-specific antibodies can be identified only by radioallergosorbent tests (RAST). It is recommended that the patient's serum first be screened with a selected panel of six allergens and then followed, if appropriate, by an extended panel of additional allergens. Check with the laboratory for an up-to-date listing because additional antigens are continually being added. (More than 100 from these categories: grasses, trees, molds, venoms, weeds, animal danders, foods, house dust, mites, antibiotics, and insects.)

Explanation of Test
The purpose of this study is to test for reaction to certain respiratory and food allergy stimulants. The RAST tests measure the increase and quantity of allergen-specific immunoglobulin-E antibodies. These measurements are used in persons, especially children, with extrinsic asthma, hay fever, and atopic eczema and are an accurate and convenient alternative to skin testing. Although more expensive, they do not cause hypersensitivity reactions.

Procedure
A venous blood sample of 4 to 10 ml is obtained for each group of six RAST tests.

Clinical Complications
1. Detection of an allergen-specific IgE antibody indicates immediate hypersensitivity to an allergen.
2. A positive RAST is diagnostic of allergy to a particular allergen or allergens, irrespective of the level of total IgE.
3. A positive test is more than 400% of the control.

Thermoproteins

Thermoproteins are plasma or urinary proteins that exhibit abnormal activity at temperatures above or below 37°C. Three types of thermo-proteins are cryoglobulins (see below), pyroglobulins (p. 530), and Bence–Jones protein (p. 165). Thermoproteins are usually found in association with systemic disorders such as multiple myeloma, Waldenström's macroglobulinemia, proliferative lymphoreticular disorders, connective tissue diseases, chronic infections, and essential thermoproteinemia. Clinically, the spectrum of disorders ranges from asymptomatic disorders to life-threatening illnesses.

Cryoglobulin Test

Normal Values
Negative
If positive after 1 or 7 days, immunoelectrophoresis of the cryoprecipitate is performed to identify the protein complex.

Background
Cryoimmunoglobulins are protein complexes that undergo reversible precipitation at low temperatures and redissolve upon warming in the body or in the laboratory.

Explanation of Test
This test is helpful in providing additional diagnostic information in the identification of certain disorders such as malignant B-cell diseases, collagen disorders, acute and chronic infections, and primary cryoglobulinemia in persons with cold hypersensitivity. Detection of cryoglobulins is insensitive, but highly specific, for immune complexes.

Procedure
A venous blood sample of 15 ml is obtained. Keep the specimen at 37°C until the cells are separated.

Clinical Implications

Cryoglobulins are associated with

1. Multiple myeloma
2. Chronic lymphocytic leukemia
3. Waldenström's macroglobulinemia
4. Lymphosarcoma (possibly)
5. Rheumatoid arthritis
6. Sjögren's syndrome
7. Systemic lupus erythematosus
8. Polyarteritis nodosa
9. Syphilis
10. Kola-azar
11. Leprosy
12. Subacute endocarditis
13. Infectious mononucleosis
14. Cytomegalovirus disease
15. Sarcoidosis
16. Poststreptococcal glomerulonephritis
17. Cirrhosis of liver
18. Hemolytic anemia
19. Essential cryoglobulinemia
20. Ulcerative colitis

Pyroglobulin Test

Normal Values

Negative

Background

Pyroglobulins are abnormal proteins that present in some instances of monoclonal gammopathies. These proteins precipitate or gel when blood serum is heated to 56°C.

Explanation of Test

The determination of this thermoprotein is one of the diagnostic measures used in identifying monoclonal gammopathies. The monoclonal peak (M peak) is produced by a single family of clones of abnormal plasma cells.

Procedure

A venous blood sample of 10 ml is obtained.

Clinical Implications

Pyroglobulins may be associated with

1. Myeloma
2. Lymphoma
3. Polycythemia vera
4. Systemic lupus erythematosus

Anti-Ribonucleoprotein (RNP) Antibody Test (Antibody to Extractable Nuclear Antigens)

Normal Values

Negative

Explanation of Test
This determination to detect autoantibodies to ribonucleoprotein is helpful in the differential diagnosis of systemic rheumatic disease and is a useful follow-up test for collagen vascular autoimmune disorders.

Procedure
A venous blood sample of 10 ml is obtained.

Clinical Implications
1. These antibodies are associated with a wide variety of rheumatic disorders.
   (a) Systemic lupus erythematosus   (c) Sjögren's syndrome
   (b) Progressive systemic sclerosis   (d) Discoid lupus
2. A high level of RNP antibodies is an outstanding feature of mixed connective tissue disease. Other types of antinuclear antibody are not seen.

Anti-Smith (Sm) Antibody Test
(Antibody to Extractable Nuclear Antigens)

Normal Values
Negative

Explanation of Test
This test is highly diagnostic of systemic lupus erythematosus and is a follow-up for collagen vascular autoimmune disease. The Smith antigen is a glycoprotein and a nonhistone acidic nuclear protein.

Procedure
A venous blood sample of 10 ml is obtained.

Clinical Implications
Antibodies to the Sm antigen occur in systemic lupus erythematosus and are a specific marker for the disease.

Antiscleroderma (Scl-70) Antibody Test

Normal Values
Negative

Explanation of Test
This is a follow-up test for collagen vascular autoimmune disease. This test is highly diagnostic for scleroderma. The Scl-70 antibody is rarely present in other rheumatic diseases such as mixed connective tissue disease, systemic lupus erythematosus, rheumatoid arthritis, and Sjögren's syndrome.

Procedure
A venous blood sample of 10 ml is obtained.

Clinical Implications
The appearance of Scl-70 antibody is known as a marker for scleroderma or progressive systemic scleroses.

Rheumatoid Factor (RA Factor)

Normal Values
0–69 IU/ml (nonreactive)

Background
The blood of many persons with rheumatoid arthritis contains a macroglobulin type of antibody that has been called *rheumatoid factor* (RF).
Rheumatoid factor has the property of an antibody. There is some
evidence indicating that rheumatoid factors are antigammaglobulin
antibodies; however, until a specific antigen eliciting the production of
RF is discovered, the exact nature of RF can only be speculated. Even
more uncertain is the role that RF plays in rheumatoid arthritis. Although RF may cause or perpetuate the destructive changes associated
with rheumatoid arthritis, it may be incidental to these changes or
may even serve some beneficial purpose. Rheumatoid factor is not limited to blood from patients with rheumatoid arthritis but may sometimes be found in serum from patients with a variety of other diseases.
However, the incidence and values of rheumatoid factors are higher in
patients with rheumatoid arthritis than in patients with other diseases.
It has been proposed that the antiglobulins in rheumatoid arthritis
result from chronic stimulation by an unknown antigen, perhaps microbial in origin.
    Rheumatoid arthritis is essentially a clinical diagnosis, and seven
of the following criteria must be met, one of which is this blood
test, #8:

1. Morning stiffness for at least 6 weeks
2. Pain on motion or tenderness in at least one joint for at least 6
   weeks
3. Swelling in at least one joint for at least 6 weeks
4. Swelling in at least one other joint for at least 6 weeks
5. Symmetrical joint swelling with simultaneous involvement of the
   same joint on both sides of the body
6. Subcutaneous nodules
7. X-ray changes, including bony decalcification
8. Positive blood test for rheumatoid factor
9. Poor mucin precipitate from synovial fluid

10. Characteristic histologic changes in synovium
11. Characteristic histologic changes in nodules

Explanation of Test
Methods of testing for rheumatoid factor are both qualitative and quantitative.
Rheumatoid factors are antibodies directed against the Fc fragment of IgG. These are usually IgM antibodies but may also be IgG or IgA.

Procedure
A venous blood sample of 10 ml is obtained.

Clinical Implications
1. When a patient with a positive test improves, the test will remain positive, except in a small number of patients whose titers were initially low.
2. A positive RA factor test often supports a tentative diagnosis of early rheumatoid arthritis (*e.g.*, in a young adult in whom a distinction must be made between RA and rheumatic fever) and may lend credence to a diagnosis of inactive rheumatoid arthritis in a patient with a compatible history but only a mild deformity and no obvious synovitis at the time of examination.
3. Elevated values occur in a variety of diseases other than rheumatoid arthritis, including lupus erythematosus, endocarditis, tuberculosis, syphilis, sarcoidosis, cancer, viral infections, diseases affecting the liver, lung, or kidney, Sjögren's syndrome, and in patients with skin and renal allografts.
4. Absence of RA factor does not exclude the diagnosis of rheumatoid arthritis.

Interfering Factors
The result is normally higher in older patients and when multiple vaccinations and transfusions have been administered.

Antinuclear Antibody (ANA) Test

Normal Values
Negative
If positive, pattern will be reported and serum will be titered.

Background
The diagnosis of systematic lupus erythematosus (SLE) is often difficult because the clinical setting in SLE patients is extremely varied and may mimic several connective tissue diseases such as rheumatoid arthritis and other systemic autoimmune disorders. SLE is characterized by a profuse production of different autoantibodies, of which some

are pathogenic. A multisystem disease, SLE can affect every organ system in the body (especially the kidney) and varies in its clinical manifestations from patient to patient and even in a given patient from time to time.

One of the most useful laboratory techniques in the diagnosis of SLE is the IFA test for detection of antinuclear antibodies (ANAs). Antinuclear antibodies are gamma globulins that react with nuclei of all organs of man or animals. These ANAs usually belong to more than one immunoglobulin class. An effective fluorescent ANA test detects approximately 95% of cases of SLE.

Explanation of Test
This test is used to detect the presence of antinucleoprotein factors associated with certain autoimmune diseases. A particular pattern is associated with SLE; another antibody pattern correlates with scleroderma, Sjögren's syndrome, Raynaud's disease, and so forth. See following table on immunologic specificity of antinuclear antibodies for this disease and pattern association.

Although the titer of ANA may not correlate with the clinical course of the disease in all cases, most SLE patients produce high ANA titers with homogeneous and peripheral (RIM) staining patterns. In addition, speckled and nucleolar patterns may be associated with SLE at lower frequencies.

Antigen Type	Associated Diseases	Pattern
N-DNA	SLE	RIM and/or homogeneous
SS-DNA	Rheumatic and non-rheumatic diseases	RIM and/or homogeneous
DNP	SLE, drug-induced LE	RIM and/or homogeneous
Histone	SLE	Homogeneous
SM	SLE	Speckled
RNP	Mixed connective tissue disease (MCTD)	Speckled
SS-B	Sjögren's syndrome	Speckled
Scl-70	Scleroderma	Speckled
Nucleolar	Scleroderma with Raynaud's phenomenon	Nucleolar
Centromere	Scleroderma with CREST syndrome	Discrete speckled
Unknown	Unknown	Atypical discrete speckled

ANA: A Diagnostic Test Kit. Davis, CA, Antibodies Incorporated, 1983)

Procedure
A venous blood sample of 10 ml is obtained.

Clinical Implications
1. A test is positive at a titer of 1:10 or 1:20, depending on the laboratory.

2. Appearance of a positive result does not necessarily indicate a disease process because ANAs are present in some apparently normal persons.
3. Some positive reactions have been reported to be related to patients with connective tissue disease or to persons who may develop such a disease at a later time.
4.

Condition	Percent Positive	Normals	Percent Positive
SLE	99	Men aged 20–60	3
Lupoid hepatitis	99	Women aged 20–60	7
Scleroderma	73	Both sexes over 80	49
Rheumatoid arthritis	60		
Discoid lupus	47		
Sjögren's disease	43		
Dermatomyositis	33		
Polyarteritis	22		

5. Additional confirmatory tests for SLE include (1) anti-SM, (2) CH50, and (3) kidney and/or skin biopsy.
6. A negative test for total antinuclear antibody is strong evidence against the diagnosis of SLE.

Interfering Factors
1. A number of drugs may cause positive tests for ANAs. Patients receiving procainamide or hydrolazine, for example, may develop ANAs at increased titers even though they may not exhibit any clinical features of SLE.

Follow-up Tests for Positive ANA
1. Anti-double-stranded DNA
2. Antibodies to extractable nuclear antigens (anti-RNP, anti-Smith)
3. Anti-SSA, also known as Ro
4. Anti-SSB, also known as La
5. Antiscleroderma Scl-70
6. Anticentromere, also known as CREST antibody

Anti-ds-DNA Antibody Test

Normal Values
70 units (ELISA)
1:20 (IFA)

Background
The pathogenic mechanisms in SLE and related diseases are not entirely known. There is strong evidence for viral etiology in certain ani-

mal models of SLE; in man, the evidence is only indirect. Genetic factors also appear to be significant, and family clustering of these diseases has been reported with significant associations to certain HLA phenotypes. Environmental factors such as exposure to sunlight and certain chemicals may also be important. It is well known that drugs such as procainamide and hydralazine can cause SLE-like diseases.

Although the etiology and pathogenesis of SLE and related autoimmune diseases are not completely understood, the primary mechanism of tissue injury is the formation of antigen–antibody immune complexes. Not all ANAs are pathogenic. For the few that are harmful, such as antibody to native (double-stranded, ds) DNA, the pathogenicity depends on such factors as immunoglobulin class, ability to activate complement, size of the immune complex, site of tissue deposition, and so forth. Studies of immune complex–mediated tissue injury in the kidney have shown a clear relationship between deposition of immune complexes and the presence of glomerular disease.

Explanation of Test

The anti-ds-DNA test is done specifically to identify or differentiate native (double stranded, ds) DNA antibodies found in 40% to 60% of patients with SLE during the active phase of their disease from other non-native DNA antibodies found in other rheumatic diseases. The presence of antibodies to ds-DNA generally correlates with lupus nephritis. An anti-ds-DNA test is valuable in supporting a diagnosis, monitoring disease activity and response to therapy, and establishing a prognosis for SLE.

Procedure

A venous blood sample of 10 ml is obtained.

Clinical Implications

1. The titer of the anti-ds-DNA may decrease with successful therapy and increase in an acute recurrence of SLE.
2. DNA-anti-ds-DNA immune complexes play a role in the pathogenesis of SLE through the deposit of the complexes in the kidney and other tissues.

Interfering Factors

1. If the Farr assay, a radioimmunoassay method, is performed, and detection of single-stranded as well as double-stranded DNA occurs, the specificity of the test for antibody to ds-DNA is questionable. Antibodies to single-stranded DNA (ss-DNA) are nonspecific in that they have been reported in association with various other rheumatic diseases.

Anticentromere Antibody Test

Normal Values
Negative
If positive, serum will be titered.

Explanation of Test
A variant of scleroderma called CREST syndrome, which is characterized by calcinosis, Raynaud's phenomenon, esophageal dysfunction,
sclerodactyly and telangiectasia, is characteristically associated with
the presence of anticentromere antibody in approximately 90% of patients. The presence of this antibody is detected using a fluorescence
technique in which tissue culture-grown cells (Hep-2) in appropriate
stages of cell division are employed.

Procedure
A venous blood sample of 10 ml is obtained.

Clinical Implications
Positive results are associated with the CREST syndrome in scleroderma.

Anti-Insulin Antibody Test

Normal Values
<3% binding of labeled beef and pork insulin by patient's serum

Background
Diabetics may form antibodies to the insulin they are given. For this
reason, larger doses are required, because the insulin is not available
for glucose-depressant function when insulin is partially complexed
with the antibodies. These insulin antibodies are immunoglobulins
called *anti-insulin AB* and act as insulin-transporting proteins. The
most common type of anti-insulin AB is IgG, but it is found in all five
classes of immunoglobulins in insulin-treated patients. These immunoglobulins, especially IgE, may be responsible for allergic manifestations; IgM may cause insulin resistance.

Explanation of Test
This insulin–antibody level is helpful in determining the most appropriate therapeutic agent in diabetic patients and the cause of allergic
manifestations. It is also used to identify insulin resistance, a state in
which the daily insulin requirement exceeds 200 units for more than 2
days and may be associated with elevated anti-insulin antibody titers
and insulin-binding capacity.

Procedure
A venous blood sample of at least 2 ml is obtained.

Clinical Implications
Elevations are associated with insulin resistance and allergic manifestations to insulin.

Antimyocardial Antibody Test

Normal Values
Negative
If positive, serum will be titered.

Background
The role of antimyocardial antibodies in cardiac disorders is not clearly established, but there appears to be a significant association between the presence of these antibodies and heart disease. The antibodies are found following cardiac surgery and myocardial infarction and may precede clinical evidence of myocardial injury.

Explanation of Test
This test may be valuable in the differential diagnosis of coronary heart disease and in detecting minimal myocardial damage when the results of other tests are inconclusive.

Procedure
A venous blood sample of 5 ml is obtained.

Clinical Implications
These antibodies are present

1. Following cardiac surgery
2. In myocardial infarction; less frequently in coronary insufficiency without infarction
3. In rheumatic fever
4. In chronic rheumatic diseases
5. In streptococcal infections

Antisperm Antibody Test

Normal Values
Negative

Background
The mechanism by which antisperm antibodies reduce male fertility is related neither to orchitis nor oligospermia. The majority of infertile

men have blocking of the efferent ducts in the testes, and a physical explanation thus exists for reduced sperm counts. It is likely that, as in vasectomy, reabsorption of sperm from blocked ducts results in the formation of autoantibodies to sperm.

Explanation of Test

This test to detect sperm antibodies is done in investigations of infertility. It is known that antibodies directed toward various sperm antigens can result in reduced fertility in men. However, the precise nature of the immune response against sperm antigens and the particular type of antibody responsible is unknown.

Procedure

Specimen Required

Testing fluid preference for men suspected of sperm antibodies is semen. In cases in which sample production may present difficulties, a serum sample can be tested. Testing fluid preference for women is serum. This is due to difficulties encountered with appropriate cervical mucus collection.

Serum: 2.0 ml of serum from the individual suspected of having sperm antibodies. Send specimen *frozen* in plastic vial on dry ice.

Semen: Contents of ejaculate of semen. Send specimen *frozen* in plastic vial on dry ice.

Cervical Mucus: 1.0 ml of cervical mucus. Send specimen *frozen* in plastic vial on dry ice.

Clinical Implications

Antisperm antibodies are associated with

1. Blocked efferent ducts in the testes
2. Vasectomy. Antibodies and probable cellular immunity to sperm develop in most men as a result of the interaction of sperm antigens with the immune system.
3. In some studies in women, approximately 75% of women with primary infertility had sperm agglutinins. However, 11% to 15% of pregnant women also had the same sperm antibody titers.

Clinical Alert

The potential adverse consequences of an immune response to sperm include possible systemic effects in other organ systems and possible interference with fertility after reversal of vasectomy.

Alpha₁-Antitrypsin (AAT) Test

Normal Values
126–226 mg/dl
If result is <140 mg/dl, phenotype will be determined.

Background
Alpha₁-antitrypsin is a protein produced by the liver. It is believed that this protein inhibits protease released into body fluids by dying cells. Deficiency of this protein is associated with pulmonary emphysema and liver disease. Human blood serum is known to contain at least three inhibitors of protease, two of which are best known as alpha₁-antitrypsin and alpha₂-macroglobulin. Total antitrypsin levels in blood are composed of approximately 90% AAT and 10% alpha₂-macroglobulins.

Explanation of Test
This test is a nonspecific method of diagnosing inflammation, severe infection, and necrosis. This measurement is important in the diagnosis of respiratory disease and cirrhosis of the liver because of the direct relation this protein has been shown to have in pulmonary and other metabolic disorders. It appears that pulmonary problems such as emphysema may be brought about by the inability of antitrypsin-deficient persons to ward off the action of endoproteases. Those who are deficient in AAT develop emphysema at a much earlier age than other emphysema patients.

Procedure
1. A venous blood sample of 5 ml is obtained.
2. Fasting is required if the patient has elevated cholesterol or triglyceride levels.

Clinical Implications
1. The following should facilitate an adequate interpretation of levels of AAT:
    (a) High levels: generally found in normal persons
    (b) Intermediate levels: found in persons with a predisposition to pulmonary emphysema
    (c) Low levels: found in patients with obstructive pulmonary disease and in children having cirrhosis of the liver
2. *Increased levels* indicate the following:
    (a) Acute and chronic inflammatory disorders
    (b) After infections of typhoid vaccine
    (c) Cancer
    (d) Thyroid infections
    (e) Use of oral contraceptives

   (f) Stress syndrome
   (g) Hematologic abnormalities
3. *Decreased levels* are associated with these progressive diseases:
   (a) Early-onset, chronic pulmonary emphysema in adults
   (b) Liver cirrhosis in children
   (c) Pulmonary disease
   (d) Severe hepatic damage
   (e) Nephrotic syndrome
   (f) Malnutrition

Interfering Factors
Serum levels may increase normally by 100% in pregnancy.

Patient Preparation
1. Instruct the patient about fasting, if necessary.
2. Water is permitted.

Clinical Alert

Persons with deficient AAT levels should be counseled to avoid smoking and occupations where significant levels of air pollutants such as fumes and dust can lead to respiratory inflammation. Because AAT deficiencies are inherited, genetic counseling may be indicated.

BLOOD BANKING OR IMMUNOHEMATOLOGY TESTS

These tests are done to prevent transfusion and transplant reactions, to identify such problems as hemolytic disease of newborns, and to determine parentage. Immunohematology testing identifies highly reactive antigens present in nucleated blood cells and their respective serum antibodies. Each individual's blood cells demonstrate a unique combination of antigens. Almost all body fluid tissues contain ABH blood group-like substances. They are also found in animals, bacteria, and plants. The related factors in the blood group system are inherited independently of each other according to Mendelian laws.

Testing of Donated Blood and Blood Processing

Testing of Recipient and Donor Blood
Required testing for all donated blood and blood processing includes several determinations:

1. ABO red cell groups
2. Rh factors
3. Antibody screen
4. Test for hepatitis B surface antigen (HB₅Ag)
5. Test for non-A, non-B hepatitis: Alanine aminotransferase (ALT)
6. Test for hepatitis C virus (anti-HVC)
7. Test for syphilis (VDRL)
8. Test for acquired immune deficiency syndrome (HIV)
9. Test for adult t-cell leukemia/lymphoma (HTLV-I)

> **Note:** Tests for acquired immunodeficiency syndrome, hepatitis, syphilis, and T-cell leukemia are explained in this chapter. ALT test is in Chapter 6.

Required testing for potential whole-blood recipient or packed red cells recipient includes the following examinations:

1. ABO red cell group
2. Rh factor
3. Antibody screen
4. Crossmatch for compatibility between donor cells and recipient serum

For plasma administration, no crossmatch is needed but compatible ABO typing should be done.

Platelets and granulocytes should be tested for HLA compatibility. (HLA means *histocompatibility locus A*). These antigens are found in most tissues of the body and also on blood cells. As a result of previous transfusions or pregnancy, some patients will develop antibodies against these antigens and may have a transfusion reaction, if transfused with incompatible blood.

Additional Testing and Processing Considerations for Donated Blood

An overview of the concepts of autologous and directed donations, cytomegalovirus tests, and irradiation of blood products and their importance to blood banking/testing is presented below.

1. *Autologous donations* (origin of the donation and blood recipient are one and the same) are blood products donated by the patient, for his or her own use. Many patients undergoing elective surgery have opted to donate their own blood prior to scheduled surgery because of the concern over transfusion-transmitted diseases.
2. *Homologous* (origin of donation and blood recipient are not one and the same) *donations* are the regular blood products donated by one individual for use by another individual(s).
3. *Directed donations.* The public fear of AIDS and other transfusion-transmitted diseases has led to demands from possible recipients of blood components that they be allowed to choose the donors to be used for their transfusions. Laws have been passed in several states

establishing this as a procedure that must be followed in non-emergent situations if requested by a potential blood recipient or blood donor. Most hospitals and blood centers do provide this service. Policy and testing procedures must be the same as for a homologous blood donor (usual method of donating blood). Patients using their own blood (autologous donors) need not meet the usual criteria for regular (homologous) blood donors.

(a) There is no upper or lower age limit.

(b) There are no weight requirements.

(c) Pregnant women can donate.

(d) Hematocrit should be 33% or greater. Phlebotomy below this level can be done with approval of the patient's physician.

(e) Donations can be more frequent. Phlebotomy can be done every 3 days, and the last phlebotomy should be done 72 hours before the scheduled surgery. The patient's physician may recommend iron supplements to maintain adequate hemoglobin levels and to replace lost red cells.

4. *Cytomegalovirus testing.* Cytomegalovirus testing is done for certain groups of patients who may be at risk for transfusion-associated CMV infections. Transfusion-associated CMV infection was first seen as a mononucleosis syndrome following cardiopulmonary bypass surgery. This was thought to be related to the use of fresh blood during the surgery and the use of fresh blood has since decreased. Clinical symptoms of CMV transfusion-transmitted infection include pneumonitis, hepatitis, retinitis, or disseminated disease. This generally occurs in immunosuppressed patients, especially in premature infants weighing less than 1200 g at birth, bone marrow transplant patients, organ transplants, and some immunocompromised oncology patients. To prevent transfusion-associated CMV infections, CMV antibody testing is done, and these patients should receive CMV-seronegative blood and blood products (see p. 488 in viral tests).

5. *Irradiation of blood products* Sometimes, blood products are irradiated (prior to transfusion) in certain immunosuppressed patients. Graft-versus-host disease (GVHD) is a rare complication following transfusion of severely immunosuppressed patients such as bone marrow transplant patients and patients undergoing chemotherapy or irradiation. Graft-versus-host disease occurs if donor lymphocytes from blood or blood products engraft and multiply in severely immunodeficient recipients. The engrafted lymphocytes react against the tissues of the host recipient. Clinical symptoms include skin rash, fever, diarrhea, hepatitis, bone marrow suppression, and infection, usually progressing to a fatal outcome. Graft-versus-host disease can be prevented by exposing the blood products to 1500 to 5000 rads of Cesium 137 in the laboratory. This

exposure renders 85% to 95% of the lymphocytes in a unit of blood, platelet, or granulocyte concentrate incapable of engrafting, but it does not affect the red cells, platelets, or granulocytes.

Blood Groups; ABO Red Cell Groups

Normal Values

Antigen Present on Red Blood Cell	Antibodies Present in Serum	Major Blood Group Designation	Distribution in United States	
None	Anti-A, anti-B	O (universal donor)*	O	46%
A	Anti-B	A	A	41%
B	Anti-A	B	B	9%
AB	None	AB (universal recipient)†	AB	4%

Named universal donor *because the person has no antigens on red blood cells and therefore is able to donate to all blood groups.*
†*Named* universal recipient *because the person has no antibodies in serum and therefore is able to receive blood from all blood groups.*

Explanation of Test

Blood typing is a test required of all blood donors and all potential blood recipients. The main purpose of this test is to prevent the transfusion of incompatible blood products.

Human blood is grouped according to the presence or absence of specific chemical structures called *blood group antigens*. These antigens, which are found on the surface of the red blood cells, are substances capable of inducing the body to produce antibodies. Since 1900, more than 300 distinct antigens have been recognized on the red cell surface. However, compatibility of the ABO group is the foundation on which all other pretransfusion testing rests. The ABO system is now known to include several antigenic manifestations and many antibody specificities. In a strict sense, it is incorrect even to refer to the serologic findings as one system.

The red blood cell membrane is crowded with antigenically active molecules. Specific sugars, in specific linkage conformation, determine the antigenic activities called *A* and *B*. The presence of one sugar, N-acetylgalactosamine, gives the molecule A activity; a different sugar, galactose, determines B activity. The backbone molecule, without the added galactose or N-acetylgalactosamine, has antigenic activity called *H*. This H substance, as well as H gene activity, is essential to the expression of the ABO antigens. Group A contains red blood cells with the A antigen; group B, with the B antigen; AB, with both A and B antigens; O cells contain neither A nor B antigens.

In general, patients are given blood of their own ABO group, for antibodies against the other blood antigens may be found in the blood serum. These antibodies are designated anti-A or anti-B, according to the antigen they act against. Under normal conditions, a person's blood serum will *not* contain the antibody that is able to destroy its antigen. For example, a person with antigen A will *not* have anti-A in his serum, but he may have anti-B antibodies. Therefore, in addition to detecting antigens on red cells, it is necessary to test the patient's blood for the presence of specific antibodies to confirm ABO grouping.

Clinical Alert

To prevent a transfusion reaction, a situation that could be extremely dangerous and potentially fatal, a patient's blood group must be determined *in vitro* before any blood is administered.

Before a blood transfusion is begun, two professional persons must check the recipient's identified blood group with the donor type to be used in the transfusions. A blood group change or suppression may be induced by cancer or leukemia.

Procedure
A venous blood sample of 10 ml is obtained.

Rh Factors; Rh Typing

Normal Values
Whites: 85% Rh-positive (*i.e.*, have the Rh antigen)
    15% Rh-negative (*i.e.*, lack the Rh antigen)
Blacks: 90% Rh-positive
    10% Rh-negative

Background
Human blood may be classified as Rh-positive or Rh-negative, depending on the presence or absence of Rh antigen on the red cell membrane. The Rh antigen, first discovered in 1939, has been extensively studied since 1943. The Rh antigen now called Rh_o (D) is, after the A and B antigen, the most important antigen in transfusion practice. Different systems of naming these antigens have been developed, and each system has its particular merits. The two nomenclatures used most frequently are given below.

Comparison of Terms Used in Rh System*

	Weiner	Fisher-Race
	Rh_o	D
	rh′	C
	rh″	E
	hr′	c
	hr″	e
	hr	f(ce)
	rh^G	G

---

* *The term* Rh factor, *without qualification, means* Rh_o $(D = Rh:1)$.
Rh-positive *means* RH_o *(D) positive.*

Explanation of Test

The Rh system is composed of antigens tested for in conjunction with the ABO group. $D(Rh_o)$ factor is often the only factor for which testing is done. When this factor is not present, further typing is done to identify any of the less common Rh factors before the person is identified as Rh-negative. Rh-negative individuals may develop antibodies against Rh-positive antigens if they are challenged by either a transfusion of Rh-positive blood or a fetomaternal bleed from an Rh-positive fetus.

To determine the presence or absence of Rh antigen, the red blood cells are tested with anti-D sera. Agglutination of the cells indicates presence of antigen D. Absence of agglutination indicates absence of the antigen. There are three different ways to type blood for the Rh factor.

1. Saline tube test
2. Slide test
3. Modified tube test
   (a) Serum-suspended cells
   (b) Saline-suspended cells

Need for Rh Typing

Rh typing must be conducted because

1. The administration of Rh-positive blood to an Rh-negative person may sensitize the person to form anti-D.
2. The administration of D-positive blood to a recipient having anti-D in the serum could be fatal.
3. One must identify Rhig (Rh immunoglobins) candidates. Rh immunoGlobulin is a concentrated solution of IgG anti-D derived from human plasma. A 1-ml dose contains 300 μg and is sufficient to counteract the immunizing effects of 15 ml of packed red cells or 30 ml of whole blood.
   (a) Rh-negative, pregnant women with Rh-positive partners may carry Rh-positive fetuses. Cells from the fetus may pass through the placenta to the mother and cause production of antibodies

in the maternal blood. The maternal antibody, in turn, may pass through the placenta into the fetal circulation and cause destruction of fetal blood cells. This condition, called *hemolytic disease of the newborn* (formerly called *erythroblastosis fetalis*), may cause reactions ranging from anemia (slight or severe) to death *in utero.* This condition can be prevented if an Rh-negative woman receives RhIG antepartum at 28 weeks' gestation and a postpartum injection of RhIG shortly after delivery of an Rh-D positive infant. Postpartum Rh immunization can occur despite an injection of RhIG if more than 30 ml of fetal blood have entered the mother's circulation. The American Association of Blood Banks recommends that a postpartum specimen of all Rh-D negative women (at risk of immunization) be examined to detect a fetal maternal hemorrhage larger than 30 ml.

(b) Rh typing must also be done in patients who have had abortions or miscarriages.

Clinical Implications

1. The significance of Rh factors is based on their capacity to immunize in transfusions or pregnancies. The Rh_o (D) factor is by far the most antigenic, and the other Rh factors are much less likely to produce isoimmunization. The following general conditions must be met in immunization to Rh factors:
   (a) The blood factor must be absent in the immunized person.
   (b) The blood factor must be present in the immunizing blood.
   (c) The blood factor must be of sufficient antigenic strength.
   (d) The amount of incompatible blood must be large enough to induce antibody formation.

   Factors other than Rh_o (D) may induce formation of antibodies in Rh-positive persons, if conditions in no. 1 are met.

2. Antibodies for Rh' (C) are frequently found together with anti-Rh_o (D) antibodies in the Rh-negative, pregnant woman whose fetus or child was type Rh-positive and possessed both factors.

3. With exceedingly rare exceptions, Rh antibodies do not occur without preceding antigenic stimulation as in
   (a) Pregnancy and abortions
   (b) Blood transfusions
   (c) Deliberate immunization, most commonly of repeated IV injections of blood for the purpose of harvesting a given Rh antibody.

Rh Antibody Titer Test

Normal Values
Normal is zero, no antibody

Explanation of Test

This antibody study is performed on a blood specimen to obtain the Rh-antibody level in a pregnant woman who is Rh-negative but whose partner is Rh-positive. If the Rh-negative woman is carrying an Rh-positive fetus, the antigen from the blood cells of the fetus causes antibody production in the serum of the mother. The firstborn child usually shows no ill effects, but with subsequent pregnancies the antibodies in the mother's serum increase and are sufficient to cause destruction of the red cells of the fetus (hemolytic disease of the newborn).

Procedure

A venous blood sample of 10 ml is obtained.

Clinical Implications

If the Rh-antibody titer in the pregnant woman is greater than 1 : 64, an exchange transfusion is considered.

Rosette Test

Normal Values

Qualitative-negative

Explanation of Test

The Rosette test is performed to detect a fetomaternal bleed that exceeds 30 ml of whole blood so as to provide sufficient protection for the Rh-D negative mother against immunization to Rh-D positive fetal cells. The Rosette technique has an accuracy of 97%.

Procedure

A venous blood EDTA sample of 7 ml is obtained shortly after delivery. In the laboratory, a suspension of red cells from the Rh-D–negative mother is mixed with anti-D, incubated and washed to remove unbound antibody, and then mixed with Rh-D positive cells, centrifuged, and examined microscopically for the presence of rosettes or mixed-field agglutinates.

Clinical Implications

1. When the test sample contains few or no Rh-D–positive fetal cells, rosetting or agglutination is not observed, and the fetomaternal bleed was less than 30 ml, one dose of RhIG is sufficient to prevent immunization (Table 8–7).
2. When rosetting is observed, there is a possibility of a fetomaternal bleed of greater than 30 ml and a quantitative test is required to determine the number of doses of RhIG necessary to prevent immunization.

TABLE 8–7.
Recommendations for Dose of RhIG in Massive Fetomaternal Blood Based on the Acid Elution Test

Fetal cells (%)	Fetomaternal Hemorrhage Volume (ml whole blood)		Vials of RhIG to Inject
	Average	*Range**	
0.3–0.5	20	<50	2
0.6–0.8	35	15–80	3
0.9–1.1	50	22–110	4
1.2–1.4	65	30–140	5
1.5–2.0	88	37–200	6
2.1–2.5	115	52–250	6

* The range provides for the poor precision of the acid separation elution test. These recommendations are based upon one vial needed for each 15 ml of red blood cells or 30 ml of whole blood.

Kleihauer–Betke Test

Normal Values
Quantitative

Explanation of Test
The Kleihauer–Betke test is a quantitative test to determine the amount of fetomaternal hemorrhage in an Rh-D negative mother and the number of injections of RhIG necessary to prevent immunization.

Procedure
A venous blood EDTA sample of 7 ml is obtained shortly after delivery.

The Kleihauer–Betke stain is based on the fact that at a low pH, hemoglobin A in mother's cells is eluted from red blood cells fixed on blood smears, whereas hemoglobin F in infant's cells resists elution, and this can be demonstrated by subsequent staining with erythrocin B. Fetal cells will stain a dark reddish-pink, whereas adult cells will appear white to light pink.

Crossmatch (Compatibility Test)

Normal Values
Compatibility is shown by the absence of clumping or hemolysis when serum and cells are appropriately mixed and incubated in the labora-

tory. (The major crossmatch is that between recipient serum and donor cells; the minor crossmatch is that between recipient cells and donor serum.)

Background

The primary purpose of the crossmatch, or compatibility test, is to prevent a transfusion reaction. The compatibility test includes the *major crossmatch* and the *minor crossmatch*. (The minor crossmatch is not usually done anymore.)

1. Major crossmatch is done to detect antibodies in the recipient's serum that may damage or destroy the cells of the proposed donor (Table 8–8). Of the two tests, the major crossmatch is the more important.
2. Minor crossmatch is done to detect antibodies in the donor's serum capable of affecting the red blood cells of the recipient. Because donor antibodies will be greatly diluted *in vivo* by the recipient's plasma, these antibodies are considered to be of minor importance.
3. The type and screen is a group of tests performed on the blood that will determine the ABO and Rh_o (D) type as well as the presence or absence of unexpected antibodies on the recipient. The type and screen is a safe substitute for the routine 1- and 2- unit crossmatch in those operative procedures that usually do not require transfusion (*e.g.*, cholecystectomy). However, in the unlikely event that blood is needed, a major crossmatch must be performed prior to transfusion.

(*text continued on page 553*)

TABLE 8–8.
Antibodies Found in Crossmatching

Blood Grouping System	Antibody	Description
Rh-hr	Anti-D	Rh1
		May cause severe hemolytic disease of newborn
	Anti-C	Rh2
		Often found with anti-D, -Ce(rh_i) or -C^w
	Anti-E	Rh3
		Often found with anti-c
	Anti-c	Rh4
		Often found with anti-E
	Anti-e	Rh5
		Often found with anti-C
	Anti-C^w	Rh8
	Anti-V	Rh10
		Alternate antigen names: ce^s, hr^v

(*continued*)

TABLE 8–8.
(continued)

Blood Grouping System	Antibody	Description
Kell	Anti-K	K1
		Some non-red cell immune
		Occasional Kell system antibodies may not react
	Anti-k	K2
		Antigen may be depressed by the presence of Kp^a
	Anti-Kp^a	K3
		Few non-red cell immune
	Anti-Kp^b	K4
	Anti-Js^a	K6
		Few non-red cell immune
	Anti-Js^b	K7
Duffy	Anti-Fy^a	Some antibodies exhibit dosage.
	Anti-Fy^b	Some antibodies may bind complement.
Kidd	Anti-Jk^a	Antibodies may exhibit dosage.
		May cause severe delayed hemolytic transfusion reactions
Kidd	Anti-Jk^b	Antibody titers may drop rapidly below detectable levels.
		Antibodies may require anti-C3 for detection.
Lutheran	Anti-Lu^a	Antibody gives mixed-field–like agglutination
	Anti-Lu^b	
MN	Anti-M	Common antibody
		Seldom clinically significant or implicated in HDN
		May be pH-dependent or exhibit dosage
	Anti-N	Rare antibody
		Rarely causes HDN
		Formaldehyde-induced anti-N commonly found in dialysis patients
	Anti-S	Antibody may be enhanced if incubated below 37°C before AHG.
	Anti-s	
	Anti-U	Autoanti-U identified as rare cause of WAIHA
Lewis	Anti-Le^a	Frequently found in serum of pregnant women
	Anti-Le^b	Neutralized by soluble antigen
	-Le^{bh}	Anti-Le^b often found with anti-Le^a
	-Le^{bL}	Anti-Le^b usually made by Le(a-b-) individuals
P	Anti-P_1	Antigen strength variable; neutralized by soluble antigen
	Anti-P	Biphasic hemolytic IgG autoantibody in PCH
		Alloantibody is usually potent IgM hemolysin.
	Anti-PP_1P^k (Tj^a)	

(continued)

TABLE 8–8.

(continued)

Blood Grouping System	Antibody	Description
Xg	Anti-Xg^a	X-linked
Colton	Anti-Co^a	Rare antibodies
	Anti-Co^b	
Dombrock	Anti-Do^a	Incidence of Do^a lower in blacks, American Indians, and Orientals
	Anti-Do^b	Infrequently reported antibodies
Diego	Anti-Di^a	Di^a antigen frequency higher in Orientals and American Indians
	Anti-Di^b	
Wright	Anti-Wr^a	IgM and IgG forms of antibody reported
		Frequently occurring antibody
Vel	Anti-Vel	Antibodies usually IgM
		Antigen strength variable
		Binds complement
Sid	Anti-Sd^a	Antigen weaker during pregnancy
		Wide variation of antigen expression
		Agglutinates have refractile, mixed-field appearance.
HLA associated	Anti-Bg$_a$	Antigen strength variable
	-Bg$_b$	Antibodies often found in multitransfused or multiparous patients
	-Bg$_c$	
	-Bg	Antibodies characteristically weakly reactive
		Bg/HLA Bg^a/HLA-B7
		associations: Bg^b/HLA-B17
		Bg^c/HLA-A28
Cartwright	Anti-Yt^a	Antibody not uncommon in Yt(a-) individuals
	Anti-Yt^b	Rare antibody usually found in combination with other antibodies
HTLA (high titer low avidity)	Anti-CH^a	Antigen strength variable
	-Rg^a	Antibodies characteristically weakly reactive
	-Kn^a	
	-McC^a	
	-Yk^a	
	-Cs^a	
	-Gy^a	
	-Hy	
	-JMH	
I	Anti-I	Most frequent cold autoagglutinin
		Anti-I in CHD has wide thermal range, high titer; binds complement; seen as alloantibody in i adults
	Anti-i	Antibody seen in serum of patients with infectious mononucleosis
		Rare cause of CHD
		Antigen very weakly expressed on the cells of most adults

(Adapted from Baxter Healthcare Corporation, Dade Division. Miami, FL, Baxter Healthcare Corporation, 1987)

Explanation of Test

Crossmatching in the laboratory must be done to detect the following:

1. Different types of antibodies, such as
   (a) High-protein medium-acting antibodies
   (b) Saline-acting antibodies
   (c) Antibodies recognizable only with the antiglobulin technique

---

Clinical Alert

Even the most carefully performed crossmatch will not detect all possible sources of incompatibility.

Procedure

A venous blood sample of 10 ml is obtained.

Clinical Implications

1. A *transfusion reaction* will occur when incompatibile blood is transfused, specifically if antibodies in the recipient's serum would cause rapid destruction of the red blood cells of the proposed donor.
   (a) Certain antibodies, though not causing immediate red cell destruction and transfusion reaction, may nevertheless reduce the normal life span of transfused incompatible cells, necessitating subsequent transfusions.
   (b) Obviously, the patient will derive maximum benefit from red cells that survive longest in his circulation.
2. The probable benefits of each blood transfusion must be weighed against risks such as the following:
   (a) Hemolytic transfusion reactions due to infusion of incompatible blood, which can be fatal
   (b) Induction of febrile or allergic reactions
   (c) Transmission of infectious disease, especially hepatitis
   (d) Stimulation of antibody production, which could complicate later transfusion or childbearing

---

Clinical Alert

1. The most common cause of hemolytic transfusion reaction is the administration of blood to the wrong recipient because of improper patient identification and labeling of donor blood. The error, then, is often one of negligence.

2. Assess for the following *symptoms of transfusion reaction:*
    (a) Feeling of heat along the vein into which blood is transfused
    (b) Constricting pain in chest and lumbar region of back
    (c) Flushing of face
    (d) Hemoglobinuria
    (e) Generalized oozing of blood
    (f) Bleeding from operative wounds
    (g) Allergic reactions such as local erythema, hives, and itching
3. After massive blood transfusions, assess for
    (a) Hypocalcemia   (d) Increased oxygen affinity
    (b) Potassium intoxication   (e) Hypothermia
    (c) Increased blood ammonia   (f) Hemosiderosis
4. Document any signs and symptoms of transfusion reaction and follow-up interventions.

Coombs' Antiglobulin Test

Normal Values
Direct Coombs' test negative, done on red blood cells
Indirect Coombs' test negative, done on serum

Explanation of Test
The Coombs' test is used to show the presence of antigen–antibody complexes by its direct method, or it may be used to detect the presence of antibodies that react only with the aid of a potentiating medium, by its indirect method.
A. *Direct Coombs' test*
    1. Detects the presence of antigen–antibody complexes on the red blood cell membrane (*in vivo*) or red blood cell sensitization
    2. Diagnoses the following conditions:
        (a) Hemolytic disease of the newborn when the red cells of the infant are sensitized, thus exhibiting antigen–antibody complexes *in vivo*
        (b) Acquired hemolytic anemia when the patient may have produced an antibody that coats his own cells (auto-sensitization *in vivo*)
        (c) Transfusion reaction when the patient may have received incompatible blood that has sensitized his red cells

(d) Red blood cell sensitization caused by drugs
B. *Indirect Coombs' test*
1. Detects presence of antibody in serum (*e.g.*, a major crossmatch)
2. Reveals presence of anti-Rh antibodies in mother's blood during pregnancy
3. Is valuable in detecting incompatibilities not found by other methods

Procedure
A venous blood sample of 10 ml is obtained.

Clinical Implications
A. *Direct Coombs' test*
1. Positive test in
(a) Autoimmune hemolytic anemia (most cases)
(b) Transfusion reaction
(c) Patients receiving cephalothin therapy (75% of cases) and some penicillin
(d) Also drugs such as alpha-methyldopa (Aldomet)
2. Negative test in
Nonautoimmune hemolytic anemias
B. *Indirect Coombs' test*
1. Positive test in
(a) Presence of specific antibody, usually as a result of a previous transfusion or pregnancy
(b) Presence of a nonspecific antibody, as in cold agglutination disease and drug-induced hemolytic anemia

Interfering Factors
A number of drugs may cause a positive direct Coombs' test.

Clinical Alert
Antibody identification is done when the antibody screen or direct antiglobulin tests are positive. This is a procedure by which unexpected blood group antibodies are classified. These tests are important in pretransfusion testing so that the appropriate antigen-negative blood can be selected and in the diagnosis of hemolytic disease of the newborn and autoimmune hemolytic anemia. Specimen collection includes obtaining venous blood samples of 7 ml of whole blood with EDTA added and 20 ml of clotted blood. Notify the laboratory of diagnosis, history of recent and past transfusions, pregnancy, and any drug therapy.

Leukoagglutinin Test

Normal Values
Negative

Background
Leukoagglutinins are antibodies that react with white blood cells and are responsible for some febrile, nonhemolytic transfusion reactions. Patients with this type of transfusion reaction should be transfused with leukocyte-poor blood.

Explanation of Test
This study is done after a reaction occurs when compatible blood has been given. When blood containing leukoagglutinins is infused, the donor plasma contains an antibody that reacts with recipient white cells and produces an acute clinical syndrome of fever, dyspnea, cough, and pulmonary infiltrates. In severe cases, cyanosis and hypertensive episodes have also been described. Patients who have been immunized by multiple previous transfusions, during pregnancy, or during allografts often suffer from febrile, nonhemolytic transfusion reactions due to the transfused incompatible leukocytes. This type of reaction must be distinguished from hemolytic reactions before further transfusions can be safely administered.

Procedure
A venous blood sample of 10 ml is obtained.

Clinical Implications
1. Agglutinating antibodies may appear in the donor's plasma if tested.
2. When the agglutinating antibody is in the recipient's plasma, although febrile reactions are common, no pulmonary manifestations occur when incompatible leukocytes are transfused.
3. Febrile reactions are more common in pregnant patients and those with a history of multiple transfusions.

Clinical Alert

1. Febrile reactions can be prevented by separating white cells from the donor blood before transfusion.
2. Patients whose blood contains leukoagglutinins should be notified and generally transfused with leukocyte-poor blood to avoid or reduce the chance of future febrile nonhemolytic transfusion reactions.

Platelet Antibody Detection Tests

Normal Values
PLAI: negative
ALTP: negative
PAIgG: negative
Platelet hyperlysibility: negative
Drug-dependent platelet antibodies: negative

Explanation of Test
Platelet antibody detection studies are aids to diagnosis in posttransfusion purpura, alloimmune neonatal thrombocytopenic purpura, idiopathic thrombocytopenia purpura, paroxysmal hemoglobinuria, and drug-induced immunologic thrombocytopenia.

Procedure
Ten milliliters to 30 ml of venous blood is required for specific assays. Check with your laboratory.

Interfering Factors
Positive reactions may be produced by alloantibodies resulting from previous blood transfusions in pregnancies. Such antibodies are usually specific for HLA antigens expressed in platelets and other cells. Whenever possible, samples for platelet antibody testing should be obtained before transfusion.

Clinical Implications
1. Antiplatelet antibody, usually having anti-PLAI specificity, is detected in posttransfusion purpura.
2. A persistent or rising antibody titer in pregnancy is associated with neonatal thrombocytopenia.
3. PLAI incompatibility between mother and fetus appears to account for more than 60% of alloimmune neonatal thrombocytopenic purpura. A finding that the mother is PLAI-negative and the father is PLAI-positive provides presumptive evidence for the diagnosis.
4. Platelet-associated IgG antibody is present in 95% of idiopathic (autoimmune) thrombocytopenic purpura (both acute and chronic). In patients who are responding to steroid therapy or who are undergoing spontaneous remission, increased circulatory times correlate with decreased PAIgG levels.
5. The platelet hyperlysibility assay measures the sensitivity of platelets to lysis. This test is positive in paroxysmal hemoglobinuria and is specific for that diagnosis.
6. In drug-induced immunologic thrombocytopenia, antibodies reactive only in the presence of the inciting drug can be detected. Quinidine and quinine most commonly cause this type of thrombocyto-

penia as well as chlordiazepoxide, sulfa drugs, and diphenyl-hydantoin. Gold-dependent antibodies and heparin-dependent platelet IgG antibodies can be detected by direct assay. (In approximately 1% of persons receiving gold therapy, thrombocytopenia develops as a side effect. Thrombocytopenia is a well-known side effect of heparin, and an immune mechanism may be the cause.)

Note: Platelet typing is also done. Compatibility tests of platelets assure that hemostatically effective platelets can be transfused to indicated patients as in aplastic anemia and malignant disorders. This is important because most patients transfused repeatedly with platelets from random donors become partially or totally refractory to further transfusion as a consequence of alloimmunization.

Platelet typing can also be helpful in providing additional evidence to support a diagnosis of post-transfusion purpura. Platelets are routinely typed for PLAI, HLH-A2, and PLEI. It is recognized that platelets matched for HLA antigens will generally produce satisfactory post-transfusion improvement. It has been reported that a standard platelet count performed 1 hour from the end of a transfusion of fresh platelet concentrate is a sensitive indicator of the presence or absence of clinically important antibody against HLA antigens.
Specimen requirements vary:

30 ml of venous blood when platelet count is 50,000 to 100,000/ mm^3

20 ml of venous blood when platelet count is 100,000 to 150,000/ mm^3

10 ml of venous blood when platelet count is >150,000/mm^3

Human Leukocyte Antigen (HLA) Test

Normal Values
Normals are not applicable. Requires clinical correlation.

Background
The major histocompatibility antigens of man belong to the HLA system, are present on all nucleated cells, and can be detected most easily on lymphocytes. Each antigen is produced under genetic control by a gene that shares a locus on the chromosome with another gene, one paternal and one maternal (two alleles). More than 27 antigens have been identified. The HLA complex, located in the short arm of chromosome number six, is a major histocompatibility complex in man and controls many important immune functions.

Explanation of Test
This test is done to determine the leukocyte antigens that are present on the surface of human cells. When transplantation is contemplated, HLA typing is used to identify the degree of histocompatibility between a donor and the recipient. By matching donors and potential recipients who have compatible lymphocytes and similar HLA types, it is possible to prolong transplant survival and reduce the likelihood of rejection episodes. This test is also used as an aid in diagnosing certain rheumatoid diseases, particularly ankylosing spondylitis. HLA-B27, one of the HLA antigens, is found in 90% of patients with this disease. The presence of a certain HLA antigen may be associated with an increased susceptibility to a specific disease, but it does not mandate the development of that disease in the patient. However, 8% of North American Caucasians are HLA-B27 positive, and these people have a 120 times greater risk of developing ankylosing spondylitis than those who are HLA-B27 negative.

Procedure
A heparinized venous blood sample of 10 to 24 ml is obtained. The HLA type is determined by testing the patient's lymphocytes against a panel of defined HLA antiserums directed against the currently recognized HLA antigens. When viable human lymphocytes are incubated with a known HLA cytotoxic antibody, an antigen–antibody complex will be formed on a cell surface. The addition of serum containing complement kills the cells, which are then recognized as possessing a defined HLA antigen.

Clinical Implications
1. Association between particular HLA antigens and various disease states includes
   (a) Ankylosing spondylitis: HLA-B27 (found in 90% of patients with this disorder)
   (b) Multiple sclerosis: HLA-B27 + Dw2 + A3 + B18
   (c) Myasthenia gravis: HLA-B8
   (d) Psoriasis: HLA-A13 + B17
   (e) Reiter's syndrome: B27
   (f) Juvenile insulin-dependent diabetes: Bw15 + B8
   (g) Acute anterior uveitis: B27
   (h) Graves' disease: B27
   (i) Juvenile rheumatoid arthritis: B27
   (j) Celiac disease: B8
   (k) Dermatitis herpetiformis: B8
   (l) Autoimmune chronic active hepatitis: B8
2. Four groups of cell surface antigens, HLA-A, HLA-B, HLA-C, and HLA-D, appear to constitute the strongest barriers to tissue transplantation.

3. If a putative father presents a phenotype (two haplotypes, one from father and one from mother) with no haplotype or antigen pair identical to one of the child's, he is excluded as the father. If one of the putative father's haplotypes is the same as one of the child's, he may be the father. The chances of his being properly identified as the father increase with the rarity of the haplotype in the population. If the haplotype is a very common one in the population, the possibility increases that another man with the same haplotype may be the father. Knowing the incidence of haplotype in the population, the probability can be calculated that the nonexcluded man is the father, with the degree of certainty diminishing as the incidence of the haplotype increases in the population.

Clinical Alert

HLA testing is best used as an adjunct to diagnosis and should not be regarded as diagnostic by itself.

Lymphocytotoxic Antibody Screen

Normal Values
Negative

Explanation of Test
This test is done to detect antibodies that will prevent rejection of renal transplant.

Procedure
A venous blood sample is obtained.

Clinical Implications
1. Positive results are reported as percentage reactivity and are indicative in the recipient of a renal transplant of preformed antibodies against donor antigens.

TUMOR MARKERS

Physical examination and standard radiologic techniques can be expected to detect a tumor 1 cm^3 in volume. This tumor mass would have completed 30 doublings (two thirds of its growth) and would contain a billion (10^9) cells. Tumor cells capable of forming metastases are likely to have been released into the bloodstream or regional lymphatics. Thus, research has been focused on the identification of certain tumor-related substances that might allow (1) early detection of malignancy, (2) assessment of prognosis, and (3) evaluation of changing tumor burden.

These tumor markers, if broadly defined, may include genetic markers (abnormal chromosomes or oncogenes), enzymes, hormones, oncofetal antigens, glycoproteins, or tumor antigens on cell surfaces, and substances produced in response to tumor growth (cell reactive protein, circulating immune complexes, and others).

One must keep in mind that these markers lack specificity for cancer in general and none is pathognomonic for one type of neoplasm. The diagnostician must still rely heavily upon history, physical examination, and radiographic techniques for the staging of cancer. Tumor marker studies do not replace biopsy and pathologic examination of tissue. Table 8–9 displays clinical markers in current use.

Antigenic determinants are expressed on the surface of normal T and B lymphocytes and myeloid cells during various stages of development. Malignant cells can express the same antigens; determination of these antigens can allow one to draw conclusions as to the origin of the malignant cell.

The nomenclature is confusing and ever-changing. The following is a small sample of cell-surface markers and their usefulness.

Cell-Surface Markers

CD Designation	Other Designations	Recognized Component or Other Comment
CD_3	Leu$_4$	CD_3 complex or T cells
CD_4	T_4, Leu 3a	HIV receptor, designates helper T cells
CD_4	Leu 9	Early T-cell marker
CD_8	T_8	Designates suppressor T cells
CD_{10}	CALLA (common acute lymphoblastic leukemia antigen, J$_5$)	CALLA-positive cells denote a better prognosis than CALLA negative cells.
CD_{13}	M_7	Granulocyte/monocyte marker
CD_{15}		Granulocyte/monocyte marker
CD_{19}	B_4	Early B-cell marker
CD_{20}	B_1	B-cell marker
CD_{25}	TAC	IL-2 receptor
CD_{33}	MY9	Granulocyte/monocyte marker

(Fourth International Workshop and Conference on Human Leukocyte Differentiation Antigens, 1989. Blood 74 (4): 1448–1450, 1989)

Note: There is an absence of discussion on oncogenes or chromosomal abnormalities. Chromosomal abnormalities and oncogenes are not discussed in this section (see Chap. 11). The reader is also referred to the following reference for a discussion of the preceding as tumor markers: Rosen N, Israle M: Genetic abnormalities as biological tumor markers. Semin Oncol 14 (2): 213–231, Jun 1987.

(text continues on page 565)

TABLE 8–9.

Tumor Markers

Tumor markers are substances produced and secreted by tumor cells and found in serum of persons with cancer. This table includes tumor-related antigens as well as enzymes and hormones. Refer to Chapter 6 for complete listing of normal values.

Name of Test Clinical Marker in Current Use and Selected Normal Values	Type of Cancer in Which Tumor Marker May Be Found	Conditions Other Than Cancer That Are Associated With Abnormal Values
1. Carcinoembryonic antigen (CEA), NL 0 2.5 ng/ml; up to 10 ng/ml in smokers. Initially isolated in endodermally derived adenocarcinoma and fetal gastrointestinal tissue.	1. Colon, lung, metastatic breast, pancreas, stomach, prostate, ovary, bladder, limbs, neuroblastoma, leukemia, osteogenic carcinoma	1. Inflammatory bowel disease, pancreatitis, gastritis, bronchitis, pulmonary infections, colonic polyps, chronic renal failure, cirrhosis
2. Alpha-fetoprotein (AFP). 10 ng/ml. A 70,000 mw glycoprotein, produced by fetal liver, yolk sac, and intestinal epithelium, AFP disappears from the blood soon after birth and doesn't appear in healthy people thereafter.	2. Embryonal cell carcinoma of testis, yolk sac tumors, teratocarcinomas, gastric cancer, lung cancer, hepatocellular carcinoma (**never** elevated in pure seminoma); can cross react with lutinizing hormone (LH); increased with gonadal failure. Half-life is 3–6 days.	2. Fetal distress, neural tube defects, hepatitis, primary biliary cirrhosis, partial hepatectomy, atoxia telangectasia, Wisklott–Aldrich syndrome
3. Chorionic gonadotropin B-HCG, NL, 1 mg/ml. Produced normally by placental syncytiotrophoblast. Levels peak at 10 weeks' gestation.	3. Gestational trophoblastic disease, seminomatous and nonsemimatous testis cancer; less valuable in lung, gastrointestinal cancer, melanoma, lymphproliferative diseases. Half-life is 12–20 hr.	

	Marker	Associated cancers	Other causes of elevation
4.	Calcitonin (CT). Malignant C-cell tumors often produce increased calcitronin levels.	Thyroid, lung, or breast, pancreas, hepatoma; renal cell carcinoid	Zollinger–Ellison syndrome, pernicious anemia, chronic renal failure, pseudohypoparathyroidism, apudomas, alcoholic cirrhosis, Paget's disease, pregnancy.
5.	Prostatic acid phosphatase (PAP). Increased PAP values are probably due to increased metabolism and catabolism of cancer cells. NL < 4. Depends on age. Increasing level with increasing stage of cancer.	Prostate leukemia carcinomas	Osteoporosis, renal osteopathy, hepatic cirrhosis, pulmonary embolism, prostate surgery, prostatic massage, benign prostate hypertrophy, chronic prostatitis
6.	Tissue polypeptide antigen (TPA). NL 80–100 units/L in serum. May be detected in urine, washings and effusions.	Gastrointestinal, genitourinary tract, breast, lung, thyroid	Hepatitis, cholangitis, cirrhosis, diabetes, pneumonia, or urinary infections
7.	Ca 125 (ovarian cancer 125). NL 35 units/ml.	Ovary, fallopian tube, cervical cancer, endometrial vulvar carcinoma, pancreas	Can be elevated in benign gynocologic diseases or even healthy women; cirrhosis
8.	Prostate-specific antigen (PSA). NL 0–4.0 ng/ml. More sensitive than PAP; level correlates with stage of disease	Prostate cancer	Benign prostate hypertrophy prostate massage, prostate surgery
9.	Neuron-specific enolase (NSE). Produced by neurons and neuroendocrine cells of the central and peripheral nervous system; can be used to stain tissue to aid in diagnosis	9A. Neuroblastomas. 9B. APUD system tumors. (i) Small cell lung cancers (ii) Pancreatic islet cell (iii) Medullary thyroid (iv) Pheochromocytoma	
12.	Lactate dehydrogenase (LDH); increased isoenzymes I and II	Acute lymphocytic leukemia, non-Hodgkins lymphoma, Ewing's sarcoma, neuroblastomic carcinoma of testis	Cellular injury, hemolysis

(continued)

TABLE 8–9.
(continued)

Tumor markers are substances produced and secreted by tumor cells and found in serum of persons with cancer. This table includes tumor-related antigens as well as enzymes and hormones. Refer to Chapter 6 for complete listing of normal values.

Name of Test Clinical Marker in Current Use and Selected Normal Values	Type of Cancer in Which Tumor Marker May Be Found	Conditions Other Than Cancer That Are Associated With Abnormal Values
13. Alkaline phosphatase–originates in osteoblasts, lining of hepatobiliary tree and intestinal tract, placenta.	13. Osteosarcoma, hepatocellular carcinoma, metastatic tumor to liver; primary or secondary bone tumors	13. Paget's disease; nonmalignant liver disease
14. Monoclonal proteins (M proteins). Immunoglobulins, whole or pieces, that are produced by B lymphocytes. Normal vs. abnormal immunoglobulins are detected by serum protein electrophoresis (SPEP) or urine protein electrophoresis (UPEP).	14. Multiple myeloma, macroglobulinemia, amyloidosis CLL, B-cell lymphomas, CML multiple solid tumors	14. Cold agglutinin disease, mixed cryoglobulins, Sjögren's syndrome, Gaucher's disease, lichen myxedematosus cirrhosis, renal failure sarcoid
15. Beta-2 microglobulin NL 4 to 12 mg/ml; part of the HLA antigen system	15. Multiple myeloma, other B-cell neoplasms, lung cancer, hepatomas, breast cancer	

(NL = Normal limit)

BIBLIOGRAPHY

Antibodies Incorporated: Antinuclear Antibody (ANA) Test Kit [pamphlet]. Davis, CA, Antibodies Incorporated, 1983

Antibodies Incorporated: ANA: A Diagnostic Tool [booklet]. Davis, CA, Antibodies Incorporated, 1983

Baltimore D, Wolff S: Confronting AIDS—Update 1988. Washington, DC, Institute of Medicine, National Academy of Sciences, 1988

Bates SE, Lango DL: Use of serum tumor markers in cancer diagnoses and management. Semin Oncol 15:102–138, 1987

Beckman Instruments: The Immunoglobulins. Brea, CA, Beckman Instruments, 1989

Belongia E et al: A Clinician's Guide to AIDS and HIV Infection in Wisconsin. Madison, WI, State of Wisconsin Department of Health and Social Services, 1987

Beneson A et al: HIV Testing: Model Performance Evaluation Program. Atlanta, Centers for Disease Control, 1990

Ciba-Geigy: Immunology of systemic lupus erythematosus and related rheumatic diseases (vol 39). West Caldwell, NJ, Ciba-Geigy, 1987

Committee on Standards, American Association of Blood Banks: Standards for Blood Banks and Transfusion Services, 12th ed. Arlington, VA, American Association of Blood Banks, 1987

Deodhar S: Laboratory Tests for Antinuclear Antibodies: Clinical Applications in the Diagnosis and Management of Systemic Lupus Erythematosus and Other Rheumatic Diseases. San Juan Capistrano, CA, Nichols Institute, 1983

Henry JB (ed): Todd, Sanford, Davidsohn's Clinical Diagnosis and Management by Laboratory Methods, 17th ed. Philadelphia, WB Saunders, 1984

Huestis DW et al: Practical Blood Transfusion, 4th ed. Boston, Little, Brown & Co, 1988

Hyde RM, Patnode RA: Immunology: The National Medical Series for Independent Study. New York, John Wiley & Sons, 1987

Kallestad Publications: The laboratory evaluation of the complement system. Lab Commun 2: 1982

Keren DF: Flow Cytometry in Clinical Diagnosis. Chicago, ASCP Press, 1989

Kickler TS: Platelet-compatability testing: An update. Lab Manage: Sept 1987

Measel JW: Clinical application of flow cytometry. Diagn Clin Test 27: July 1989

Miller LE et al: Manual of Laboratory Immunology, 2nd ed. Philadelphia, Lea & Febiger, 1991

Leavelle DE (ed): Interpretive Handbook: Interpretive Data for Diagnostic Laboratory Tests. Rochester, MN, Mayo Medical Laboratories, 1990

Ritzman SE: Protein Abnormalities, vol 1. New York, Alan R Liss, 1982

Rose NP, Friedman H, Foley JE (eds): Manual of Clinical Laboratory Immunology, 3rd ed. Washington, DC, American Society for Microbiology, 1986

Sheehan C: Clinical Immunology: Principles and Laboratory Diagnosis. Philadelphia, JB Lippincott, 1990

Walker RH: Technical Manual, American Association of Blood Banks, 10th ed. Arlington, VA, American Association of Blood Banks, 1990

Widmann FK: An Introduction to Clinical Immunology. Philadelphia, FA Davis, 1989

NUCLEAR MEDICINE STUDIES

Introduction

Radionuclide studies are performed in a department of nuclear medicine. The success of a particular study depends on the existence of detectable differences in the concentrations of administered radioactive materials in normal and abnormal tissue in areas of the body under study.

Radionuclide imaging is used mainly to allow visualization of organs and regions within organs that cannot be seen on a simple radiograph. Space-occupying lesions, especially tumors, stand out particularly well. Generally, these lesions are represented by areas of reduced radioactivity; however, in some instances, such as in bone scanning, areas of increased activity represent pathology.

Radionuclide describes an unstable nucleus with its orbital electrons. In an attempt to reach stability, the radionuclide emits one or more types of radiation, the most common examples being alpha particles, beta particles, and gamma electromagnetic radiation. In nuclear medicine, with the exception of therapy, gamma radiation is used in diagnostic procedures. Gamma radiation is easy to detect and is the least ionizing type.

Principles of Nuclear Imaging

In general, gamma rays are used for imaging organ systems and provide an indication of how well an organ system functions. Computerized radiation detection equipment, particularly *scintillation detectors*, show the presence of gamma rays by giving off a light flash, or scintillation. The imaging device outlines and photographs the organ under study and provides information on its size, shape, position, and functional activity. The nuclide scan should be thought of as an approximate form of organ measurement. However, some measurements are specific, such as those obtained in nuclear cardiology, where very reliable and accurate information, such as ejection fractions, can be obtained.

The radioactive materials used in nuclear medicine in diagnostic imaging are called *radiopharmaceuticals*. These radiopharmaceuticals will distribute throughout tissues, organs, and organ systems, depending on their tissue specificity and how they are administered. Radiopharmaceuticals are more likely to concentrate in one organ or one organ system than another. Within these organs, the radioactive material shows distributions in normal tissue that differ from those in diseased tissue. The following are examples of tissue specificity in radiopharmaceuticals used in nuclear medicine imaging:

Organ Tissue	*Radiopharmaceutical**
Abscess imaging	^{111}In white blood cells or Technetium 99m (^{99m}Tc) white blood cells
Bone	^{99m}Tc Methylene diphosphonate (MDP)
Brain	^{99m}Tc exametazime or ^{123}Iofetamine
Cisternography	^{111}In Diethylene triamine pentaacetic acid (DTPA)
Heart scan—MUGA	^{99m}Tc Red blood cells
Heart scan—MI	^{99m}Tc Pyrophosphate
Hepatobiliary	^{99m}Tc Iminodiacetic acid analogs
Kidney scan	^{99m}Tc Dimercaptosuccinic acid (DMSA)
Kidney glomerular filtration rates	^{99m}Tc DTPA
Liver	^{99m}Tc Sulfur colloid
Lung perfusion	^{99m}Tc Macroaggregated albumin
Lung ventilation	^{133}Xenon gas or ^{81m}Krypton gas
Radioiodine uptake	^{123}Iodine or ^{131}Iodine
Renogram	^{131}I-Hippuran
Spleen	^{99m}Tc Sulfur colloid
Thallium stress	^{201}Thallium chloride
Thyroid	^{99m}Tc Pertechnetate or ^{123}Iodine
Tumor (gallium)	^{67}Gallium citrate

Radiopharmaceutical development in the future will use monoclonal antibody technology. Radioactive antibodies will travel to specific sites within the body for the detection of breast, ovarian, lung, gastrointestines, and pancreatic malignancies.

In the nuclear medicine in vitro laboratory, radionuclides are utilized in numerous ways. They may be tagged to proteins and used in competitive protein binding studies. They also may be labeled to antibodies or antigens and used in radioimmunoassay (RIA) studies. Radioimmunoassay methods have a high degree of sensitivity and specificity to detect substances within the body in trace quantities. This may be as low as a picogram or one trillionth of a gram. The type of substances detected include hormones, antibiotics, carcinogens, drugs, vitamins, and immunoglobulins.

Manufacture of Radionuclides

Radionuclides can be manufactured in a variety of ways. Two of the more common methods are as follows:

1. A substance to be made radioactive is placed inside a reactor, where several processes may take place, one of which is the bombardment of the material by neutrons liberated by the fission process. The radioactive substances gives off energy in the form of particles of electromagnetic radiation.
2. The other method involves the use of cyclotrons. A source of particles is placed in the cyclotron and exposed to high energies. The particles are directed to a target material producing an altered nucleus, which is unstable. The cyclotron can produce a variety of useful radionuclides with short half-lives that are free of contaminants, which is not the case with the nuclear reactor. It might be added that the major disadvantage of the cyclotron is its high cost per unit compared to the nuclear reactor. The end product, however, is the same—an unstable nucleus attempting to return to a stable state.

Imaging Used in Nuclear Medicine

There are two major types of imaging. The first is known as *hotspot imaging,* in which an increased area of uptake of the radiopharmaceutical is compared to its normal distribution. The bone scan is an example of hotspot imaging. The other type is *coldspot imaging,* in which an area of decreased uptake of the radiopharmaceutical is compared to the background. Examples of coldspot imaging are liver scanning and lung scanning.

Today there are several types of imaging devices used in the field of nuclear medicine. The most basic imaging device is the gamma camera. This instrument is placed over the target area, where it views the entire field at once. For routine imaging, it does not move, nor does it require the patient to move. A picture is constructed similar to that used in time photography. The major limitation of the gamma camera is that it is two dimensional and suffers from a lack of depth perception. Today, gamma cameras have achieved the third dimension through single photon emission computed tomography (SPECT/ECT) camera systems. The single gamma photon emitted from the injected radiopharmaceutical is computed to be located in a designated tomograph. (**Note:** Tomography is the process of obtaining a picture of a specific segment or slice in the body.) Along with improvements in radiopharmaceuticals, SPECT has increased the specificity, sensitivity, and diagnostic ability of nuclear medicine imaging. Another form of tomographic imaging is positron emission tomography (PET) (see p. 621 for discussion).

The following are *uses of SPECT/ECT:*

1. Brain and cerebral blood flow with blood–brain barrier penetrating agent
2. Liver

3. Spleen
4. Cardiac infarct
5. Lungs
6. Indium, white blood cells for inflammation
7. Bone for special areas such as spine, knees, hips, temporomandibular joint (demonstrates a higher degree of lesion detection beyond other conventional approaches).
8. Heart thallium increases sensitivity and specificity for detecting coronary artery disease.

Dual photo scanners are gaining acceptance in the evaluation of bone density of the lumbar spine, hip, and wrist. They are being used in the early diagnosis of osteoporosis. The device uses low-level radiation and is linked to a computer to determine mineral content of the bone. The resulting data can help determine the strength of the bones and risk of fracture. No radionuclides are administered to the patient, however. The test is mentioned here only because it is often done in the department of nuclear medicine.

The computed results of conventional imaging may be recorded in the following ways:

1. Gray-scale photo images. These are recorded on special single-emulsion film; the varying count rate appears as lighter or darker shades of gray, thus using the complete spectrum of the gray scale. It gives a differential display of count and rate, whereas the black and white dot scan either records or does not record.
2. Color imaging. Color imaging involves a more complicated procedure than those described above and usually requires some sort of computer processing. It is especially useful to those clinicians who are not used to gray-scale imaging.
3. Cine mode. By linking a computer to the scintillation camera, sequential pictures (or frames) are obtained and stored. After computer data processing, the frames are viewed in a cinematic mode, in which the movement of the radiopharmaceuticals portray a specific organ's function.

General Procedure for Nuclear Medicine Scans
1. A radiopharmaceutical is administered orally or intravenously to the patient.

   Note: Before administration of the radionuclide, a blocking agent that is not radioactive may be administered to prevent tissues other than the organ under study from concentrating the radioactive substance. Examples of blocking agents include

   (a) Lugol's solution, administered orally when iodine-tagged isotopes are used, except in thyroid studies

    (b) Potassium perchlorate, administered orally to patients who are allergic to iodine. Blocks choroid plexus in brain.
2. A sufficient time interval is allowed for the radioactive material to follow its specific metabolic pathway in the body and to concentrate in the specific tissue to be studied.
3. An imaging device outside the body records the position and concentration of the penetrating radiation that emerges from the radionuclide.
4. Total length of examining time depends upon the following:
    (a) Radiopharmaceutical used and time variable to allow for concentration in tissues
    (b) Type of imaging equipment used
    (c) Patient positioning
    (d) Different or additional views based upon patient history and nuclear medicine physician protocols

Limitations of Procedure
Localizing tumors by scanning can be difficult when normal tissues surrounding the lesion absorb the radionuclide and produce fuzzy or ambiguous outlines.

Benefits and Risks
Benefits and risks should be explained prior to testing. Patients retain the radioactivity for relatively short periods of time. The radioactive energy does dissipate on its own, and some of the radiation will be eliminated in urine and feces.

Technetium, which is the most commonly used tracer, is significantly reduced in 6 hours and is virtually gone from the patient's body in 24 hours. Other tracers such as iodine and thallium take approximately 8 and 3 days, respectively, for half of the energy to dissipate.

Patients need to know that once the energy has been eliminated, they are no longer carrying the radioactivity. A radiation hazard to the patient always exists. In all radionuclide procedures, the value and importance of the information gained must be weighed against the potential hazard of radiation to the patient. If a nuclide study will advance the solution of a difficult problem, or provide information that cannot be obtained in any other way, then it should be done. For example, some of the following factors may be considered:

1. If a liver scan can be used to demonstrate hepatic metastases in a patient with lung carcinoma, thus sparing the patient from an unnecessary thoracotomy, the procedure is indicated.
2. In almost all instances, radionuclide imaging exposes the patient to less radiation than would be received undergoing a similar procedure with diagnostic radiographs.

3. With a nuclear medicine scan, metastatic disease to the bone can be found 6 months to a year before it can be detected with the usual bone radiograph. Also to be noted, the total body radiation from an injection of a bone agent tagged to technetium-99m (^{99m}Tc) is about one ninth as much as the unavoidable natural radiation that a person receives in 1 year from the ground and stars. In fact, this dosage is less than that received from a radiograph of the chest.

Clinical Considerations

The following information should be obtained prior to diagnostic testing:

1. Menstrual history of women of child-bearing age. Pregnancy is a contraindication to radionuclide studies.
2. Whether a mother is breastfeeding her baby: This is very important because radionuclide studies are contraindicated in nursing mothers. The mother may be advised to stop nursing for a set period of time (*e.g.*, 2–3 days with ^{99m}Tc).
3. History of allergies. Certain patients may have adverse allergic reactions to some of the radionuclides.
4. Knowledge of recent exposure to radionuclides: A history of any recent examination in which radionuclides were administered should be recorded and a body background taken in the nuclear medicine department. If for any reason it is suspected that a patient may have had an unreported examination in which a radionuclide was administered, again, a body background should be taken, because a previous study could seriously interfere with the clinician's interpretation of the current study.
5. Presence of any prostheses in the body. These must be recorded on the patient's history because certain devices can shield the gamma energy.
6. Current medication, treatment, or diagnostic measures (*e.g.*, telemetry, oxygen, and urine collection)
7. Age and current weight. This information is used to calculate the amount of the radioactive substance to be administered prior to imagery. If the patient is under 18, notify the examining department prior to testing. This information is vital for a technologist to perform any nuclear medicine procedure.
8. Other special considerations regarding the patient's well-being should be communicated to the examining department, such as
   (a) Transportation, such as cart, wheelchair
   (b) If patient is on telemetry
   (c) Requires oxygen
   (d) Requires urine collection
   (e) Any allergies
   (f) An intravenous or nasogastric tube
   (g) If patient is a diabetic
   (h) Pertinent medications

Clinical Alert

Premenopausal women should be advised to practice effective birth control during the testing period. These tests may be harmful to a fetus. Nuclear medicine needs to be notified if the patient may be pregnant or is breast-feeding.

9. Thyroid scans need to be completed before radiographic examinations using contrast medicine (intravenous pyelogram, gallbladder, cardiac catheterization, and myelograms) are performed.
10. If possible, any medication containing iodine should not be given until thyroid scans are concluded. Notify the attending physician if thyroid studies have been ordered, together with interfering radiographs or medications.

Follow-Up Care
1. Advise the patient to empty his or her bladder when imaging is completed, to decrease radiation exposure time.
2. Documentation is important and should include assessment and education of the patient and significant others, how the patient tolerated the procedure, and the total examining time. (See Chap. 1, p. 10.)

Part One
Nuclear Scans

Kidney Scan

Normal Values
Normal size, shape, position, and function of kidneys

Explanation of Test
This test is done to determine anatomic outlines and renal plasma flow in each kidney. It is also used to detect renal masses and to localize the kidney before needle biopsy. It can reveal positive evidence of renal disease when other tests are normal. The scan will also reveal lesions produced by vascular occlusion in the kidney. Parenchymal, tubular,

and glomerular function can be ascertained with a number of renal imaging agents. Radioactive substances such as ^{99m}Tc, DMSA, gluco-heptonate (GH), or DTPA are injected intravenously and a short time later will be concentrated and held in the kidneys. ^{99m}Tc DMSA and ^{99m}Tc GH are used primarily for anatomic visualization, whereas ^{99m}Tc DTPA is used to demonstrate glomerular filtration. Scanning will dem-onstrate the size, shape, and position of the kidneys as well as the distribution of the radioisotope in the kidneys. Renal scans and reno-grams can be done simultaneously, giving both morphologic and func-tional data about the kidneys. The iodine-sensitive or azotemic patient who cannot tolerate an intravenous pyelogram can be evaluated in this way. In many instances, this study will be accompanied by a diagnostic ultrasound procedure.

Procedure
1. Scanning of the kidney area is done 30 minutes to 1 hour after the intravenous injection of the radionuclide. A renal blood flow and a 10-minute postinjection static film are taken in the sitting position.
2. Scans of the kidneys are then repeated at a later time or may be done at several different time intervals after the initial injection. This will depend on the patient's condition and the pharmaceutical used.
3. The patient must remain still during the delayed scans for 30 min-utes or more, and usually, a prone position is used for this part of the procedure. Most often, both kidneys are scanned at the same time; however, they can be done separately.
4. In many nuclear medicine departments, this information is then processed by computer for further interpretation.

Clinical Implications
1. Abnormal results indicate
   (a) Space-occupying "cold" or nonfunctioning areas caused by tumors, cysts, or abscesses
   (b) Congenital abnormalities
   (c) Nonfunctioning kidneys
   (d) Infarction
   (e) Status of postrenal trans-plant
   (f) Severe renal insufficiency
2. In patients with uremia, the size, shape, and location of the kidneys can be demonstrated when no visualization occurs in the intrave-nous pyelogram.

Patient Preparation
1. Explain the purpose and procedure of the test.
2. Alleviate any fears the patient may have about radionuclide proce-dures.

Renogram

Normal Values
Right and left kidney blood flow is compared in healthy persons; flow is
equal in both kidneys.
In 10 minutes, 50% of the isotope should be excreted.

Explanation of Test
This test is done to study the function of both kidneys and is used to
detect renal parenchymal or vascular disease as well as defects in excretion. This is a dynamic study; blood flow is recorded as it is occurring. The test is indicated under the following conditions:

1. To detect the presence or absence of unilateral kidney disease
2. For long-term follow-up of patients with hydroureteronephrosis
3. To determine if recognized nephroureteral dilation represents significant obstruction
4. To study the hypertensive patient to determine a renal basis for the
   disease
5. To study the hypertensive obstetrical patient
6. To study the azotemic patient and the patient in whom urethral
   catheterization is contraindicated or impossible
7. To evaluate obstruction in the upper urinary tract
8. To study the kidney when an intravenous pyelogram cannot be
   done because of allergy to iodine

The radioactive drug ^{131}I-hippuran is the nuclide administered intravenously and is used to measure effective renal plasma flow. The
placement of the radiation detectors over the kidneys permits the monitoring of the uptake and the disappearance of the radioactivity. This
information is usually displayed with a chart recording or entered into
a computer. The shape of this wave may be correlated with several
measures of renal function such as tubular secretion and excretion.

Procedure
1. The patient is usually placed in an upright position in front of the
   recording device.
2. The radiopharmaceutical hippuran is injected intravenously. An
   intravenous diuretic may also be administered.
3. Imaging with the camera is started immediately upon injection.
4. A urine sample or a blood specimen may be obtained at the end of
   the procedure. Bladder catheterization is necessary in persons with
   suspected distal ureteral obstruction.
5. Total examination time is approximately 30 minutes.

Clinical Implications
Abnormal pattern results may be indicative of

1. Hypertension
2. Obstruction due to stones or tumors
3. Renal failure
4. Decreased renal function
5. Diminished blood supply

Patient Preparation

1. Explain the purpose and procedure of the test.
2. The patient should eat and be well hydrated with two to three glasses of water (unless contraindicated) before undergoing the scan (10 ml of water per kilogram of body weight).
3. Alleviate any fears the patient may have concerning radionuclide procedures.

Clinical Considerations

A renogram may be performed in pregnant women when it is imperative that renal function be ascertained.

> **Clinical Alert**
>
> The test should not be done immediately after intravenous pyelogram because the patient needs to be at least normally hydrated.
>   Severe impairment of renal function or massive enlargement of the collecting system may impair drainage even without true obstruction.

Thyroid Scan

Normal Values

Normal or evenly distributed concentration of radioactive iodine; normal size, position, shape, site, weight, and function of thyroid; absence of nodules

Explanation of Test

This test systematically measures the uptake of radioactive iodine (either ^{131}I or ^{123}I) by the thyroid. It is requested for the evaluation of thyroid size, position, and function. It is used in the differential diagnosis of masses in the neck, base of the tongue, or mediastinum. Thyroid tissue can be found in each of these three locations. In many instances, ^{99m}TC may be used in place of iodine for visualizing the thyroid.

    Benign adenomas may appear as nodules of increased uptake of iodine ("hot" nodules), or they may appear as nodules of decreased intake ("cold" nodules). Malignant areas generally take the form of cold nodules. The most important use of thyroid scans is the functional assessment of these thyroid nodules.

Iodine (and, consequently, radioiodine) is actively transported by the thyroid gland, where it is incorporated into the production of thyroid hormone. The radioactivity of the gland is scanned by a gamma camera, and this information is then transformed into a film, thus outlining the normal thyroid and demonstrating any areas of abnormality.

A thyroid scan performed with iodine is usually done in conjunction with a radioactive iodine uptake study, which is usually performed at 6 and 24 hours postdose when ^{131}I is used. The uptake and scan are performed the same day when ^{123}I is used (one 24-hour uptake may still be required with ^{123}I). For a complete thyroid workup, thyroid hormone levels are usually measured by taking a blood specimen and performing radioimmunoassay tests as directed by the physician. Some physicians may also require a thyroid ultrasound examination as part of a complete workup.

Procedure

1. The patient either swallows radioactive iodine in either a tasteless capsule or a liquid or has the radionuclide injected intravenously (for ^{99m}Tc).
2. Usually, the neck area is counted for uptake 6 or 24 hours later (or both). The area is scanned at 24 hours when ^{131}I is used and at 2 to 6 hours when ^{123}I is used.
3. The patient lies on his or her back on the examining table with the neck hyperextended.
4. Normal scan time is 20 minutes.

Clinical Implications

1. Cancer of the thyroid most often presents itself as a nonfunctioning cold nodule, which indicates a focal area of decreased uptake.
2. Some abnormal results are
   (a) Hyperthyroidism, represented by an area of diffuse increased uptake
   (b) Hypothyroidism, represented by an area of diffuse decreased uptake
   (c) Graves' disease, represented by an area of diffuse increased uptake
   (d) Autonomous nodules, represented by focal area of increased uptake
   (e) Hashimoto's disease, represented by mottled areas of decreased uptake

Interfering Factors

1. Ingested iodine and contrast diagnostic substances can interfere with a thyroid scan for up to 6 months. For this reason, thyroid scans should be completed before radiographic examinations using contrast media are performed.
2. Radioactive technetium is used when gallbladder radiograph or intravenous pyelogram has been done previously.

Limitations of Test

Measurements of free serum thyroxine (free T_4) and free triiodothyronine (free T_3) by RIA are much more reliable tests for function of the thyroid.

Patient Preparation

1. Instruct the patient about the purpose, procedure, and special restrictions of the test.
2. Because the thyroid gland responds to small amounts of iodine, the patient may be requested to refrain from iodine intake for at least 1 week before the test. Patients should consult with a physician first. Restricted items include the following:
   (a) Certain thyroid drugs
   (b) Weight-control medicines
   (c) Multiple vitamins
   (d) Some oral contraceptives
   (e) Gallbladder and other radiographic dyes containing iodine
   (f) Cough medicine
   (g) Iodine-containing foods, especially kelp, and "natural" foods
3. Alleviate any fears the patient may have about radionuclide procedures.

Clinical Alert

1. Thyroid scans are contraindicated in pregnancy. Thyroid testing in pregnancy is limited to blood testing.
2. This study should be completed before thyroid-blocking contrast agents for radiographs are administered and before thyroid or iodine drugs are given.
3. Occasionally, scans are done purposely with iodine or some thyroid drug in the body. In these cases, the doctor is testing the thyroid response to drugs. These stimulation and suppression scans are usually done to determine the nature of a particular nodule and to determine if the tissue is functioning or nonfunctioning.

Parotid or Salivary Gland Scan

Normal Values
No evidence of tumor type activity or blockage of ducts
Normal size, shape, position of glands

Explanation of Test
This study is helpful in the evaluation of swelling masses in the parotid region. This scan is done to detect blocked ducts of the parotid and submaxillary glands, and tumors of parotid or salivary glands, and to diagnose Sjögren's syndrome in rheumatoid arthritis. The radionuclide injected intravenously ^{99m}Tc pertechnetate. One of the limitations of the test is that it cannot furnish an exact preoperative diagnosis.

Procedure
1. A radionuclide (^{99m}Tc) is injected intravenously. Scanning is done immediately. There are three phases to imaging: blood flow; uptake or trapping mechanism, secreting capability.
2. The patient is examined in a sitting position.
3. Pictures of the gland are taken every few minutes for 30 minutes (two anteroposterior and one oblique).
4. If a secretory function test is being done to detect blockage of the salivary duct, three fourths of the way through the test, the patient is asked to suck on a lemon slice. If the salivary gland is normal, it will cause the gland to empty. This is not done in tumor detection.
5. Total test time is 45 to 60 minutes.

Clinical Implications
1. The reporting of a hot nodule amidst normal tissue that accumulates the radionuclide is associated with tumors of the ducts as in
   (a) Warthin's tumor
   (b) Oncocytoma
   (c) Mucoepidermoid tumor
2. The reporting of a cold nodule amidst normal tissue that does not accumulate the radionuclide is associated with
   (a) Benign tumors, abscesses, or cysts, which are indicated by smooth, sharply defined outlines
   (b) Adenocarcinoma, which is indicated by ragged, irregular outlines
3. The reporting of diffuse decreased activity such as an obstruction, chronic sialadenitis, or Sjögren's syndrome.
4. The reporting of diffuse increased activity such as acute parotitis.

Patient Preparation
1. Explain the purpose and procedure of the test.
2. There is no pain or discomfort involved.

3. Alleviate any fears the patient may have concerning radioisotope procedures.

Liver Scan

Normal Values
Normal size, shape, and position within the abdomen; normal size of cardiac impression on liver; normally functioning liver, reticuloendothelial system

Explanation of Test
This test is used to demonstrate the functions, anatomy, and size of the liver. Alterations in function may indicate an obstruction, hepatitis, hepatic abscesses, and the cause of jaundice. It is helpful in determining the cause of right upper quadrant pain, and in the detection of metastatic disease, cirrhoses, ascites, infarction due to trauma, and liver damage due to radiation therapy. The majority of liver scans still continue to be performed as part of a search for metastatic disease and in the differential diagnosis of jaundice.

A radioactive material, ^{99m}Tc-labeled sulfur colloid, is injected intravenously. Liver imaging is done using SPECT, which gives a three-dimensional result of the radiopharmaceutical distributions. ^{99m}Tc labeled to a patient's own red blood cell is the radiopharmaceutical most specific for detection of hemangioma in the liver.

Liver/Lung Combination Scan
There may be times when a liver/lung scan may be ordered in combination with a white blood cell or gallium scan to identify tumor masses or abscess formation in the subdiaphragmatic area. Procedure and patient preparation are the same as for a liver scan and lung scan.

Limitations of Test
This procedure provides limited information on hepatic parenchymal cell function.

Procedure
1. The chosen pharmaceutical is injected intravenously.
2. After administration of the radionuclide, the patient lies on his or her back on an examining table for anterior pictures to determine liver uptake.
3. The entire study usually takes 80 minutes from injection to finish.
4. See also *Gallbladder Scan.*
5. Under certain conditions, the study can be performed without emission computed tomography (ECT) at the bedside or in the emergency room.

Clinical Implications

Abnormal results will reveal abnormal patterns in

1. Cirrhosis
2. Hepatitis
3. Trauma
4. Hepatomas
5. Sarcoidosis
6. Metastasis
7. Cysts
8. Perihepatic abscesses
9. Hemangiomas
10. Adenomas
11. Ascites

Heart Scans (Cardiac Isotope Imaging)

Normal Values

Normal heart: no areas of ischemia; blood flow equal throughout myocardium; normal ejection fractions and velocity

Normal stress test: electrocardiogram (ECG) and blood pressure normal

Normal nitro test: blood pressure within expected limits

Normal shunt scan: pulmonary transit times and normal sequence or chamber filling

Explanation of Test

More than one type of myocardial scan may be performed. These scans are noninvasive and involve the intravenous injection of a radiopharmaceutical followed by imaging. These studies are indicated in the investigation of coronary artery disease, heart chamber dimensions and functional capabilities, angina, aneurysm, infarct, cardiomyopathy, atypical chest pain, and pre- and postsurgical evaluation. New treatments have stimulated assessment of posttraumatic contusion.

1. *PYP heart scan* (hotspot, myocardial infarct imaging)
   Technetium-99m stannous pyrophosphate is the radioactive imaging agent used to demonstrate the general location, size, and extent of myocardial infarction 24 to 96 hours after suspected myocardial infarction and as an indication of myocardial necrosis, to differentiate between old and new infarcts. In some instances, the test is sensitive enough to detect an infarct 12 hours to 6 days after its occurrence. Acute infarction is associated with an area of increased radioactivity or hotspot on the myocardial image. This test is useful when ECG and enzyme studies are not definitive. PYP scans are commonly done the day before heart surgery and again postoperatively.
2. *Monoclonal antibody labeling*
   Imaging with monoclonal antibodies requires the intravenous administration of radiolabeled antimyosin antibodies. These permit

identification of an infarct site. It is more accurate in localizing the site than ^{99m}Tc, which is influenced by radiotracer uptake in the spine and ribs.

3. *Thallium stress heart scans*

Thallium-201 (^{201}TI) is the radioactive imaging agent used in conjunction with a bicycle ergometer or treadmill stress ECG test to diagnose ischemic heart disease and allows differentiation of ischemia and infarction. It will reveal wall motor defects and heart pump performance during increased oxygen demands. These scans are also done before and after streptokinase treatment for coronary artery thrombosis. When thallium is injected at the time of maximum stress and is followed by imaging, areas of myocardial ischemia can be detected.

Thallium-201 is a physiologic analog of potassium. The myocardial cells extract potassium, as do other muscle cells.

Myocardial thallium activity is also dependent on blood flow. For this reason, when thallium-201 is injected during peak exercise, the normal myocardium will have much greater thallium activity than the abnormal myocardium, with maximum concentration normally occurring in about 10 minutes. Thus, cold spots indicate a decrease or absence of flow.

A test that is abnormal during exercise but returns to normal function 4 hours after exercise indicates ischemia.

The scan for infarction will remain abnormal after rest.

Hypertrophy produces an increase in uptake.

A completely normal thallium stress study may eliminate the need for cardiac catheterization in the evaluation of chest pain and nonspecific abnormalities of the ECG. The use of SPECT imaging can more accurately localize regions of ischemia.

4. *DPY-thallium/Persantine scans*

Dipyridamole/Persantine imaging is indicated in persons unable to exercise to achieve desired cardiac stress and maximum cardiac vasodilation. These medications have been shown to have an effect similar to that of exercise on the heart.

Persons who are candidates are those with lung disease, peripheral vascular disease with claudication, amputation, spinal cord injury, multiple sclerosis, morbid obesity, and patients taking beta blockers.

Persantine and DPY tests are also valuable as significant predictors of cardiovascular death, reinfarction, and risk of postoperative ischemia events; these tests can also be used in reevaluation of unstable angina.

The major disadvantage of DPY and Persantine imaging is the lack of information that would be provided by the ECG response to exercise.

5. *Gated equilibrium heart scan resting (multigated acquisition, MUGA); Ejection fractions*
   This method is similar to routine imaging except that scintillation events are distributed into not one, but multiple images during acquisition. *Gated* refers to the synchronizing of the imaging equipment and computer with the patient's ECG so that images are free of motion or blur. "First-pass studies" refers to the image's mode when the bolus of radiopharmaceutical first passes through the right heart, lungs, and left heart.
   The distribution is regulated by synchronizing the recording of cardiac images with the ECG. This technique provides a means of obtaining information about cardiac output, end systolic volume, end diastolic volume, ejection fraction, ejection velocity, and regional wall motion of the ventricles. By using a computer, wall motion of the ventricles can be portrayed in a cinematic mode to visualize contraction and relaxation. This method of determining heart wall motion and ejection fraction (that portion of the ventricular volume ejected in systole) could only be measured by angiography before use of this technique. This scan may also be performed with stress testing.

6. *Nitro test*
   This procedure is an adjunct to MUGA studies to see the effect of drug intervention (using nitroglycerine) on heart performance.

7. *Heart shunt*
   This angiographic study of the chambers of the heart using jugular vein injection of ^{99m}Tc is helpful in the study of heart chamber disorders, especially in the investigation of left-to-right and right-to-left shunts. Children are the usual candidates for this procedure.

   8. *Three-dimensional image reconstruction*
   This specialized test requires a positron-emitting tracer and positron tomographic cameras. The formidable equipment required (a cyclotron and expensive detection equipment) restricts the use of this test in the average institution.

Procedure for PYP Heart Scan

1. This myocardial scan involves a 30-minute to 3-hour waiting period for the patient after the intravenous injection of the radionuclide. During this waiting period, the radioactive material will accumulate in the heart muscle.

2. The imaging period takes 15 to 30 minutes, during which time the patient must lie quietly on an examining table.

Procedure for Thallium Stress Heart Scan

1. Before the stress test is begun, an intravenous line is started, and ECG leads and blood pressure cuff are attached.

2. When the cardiologist has determined that the patient has reached

maximum heart stress using the treadmill or bicycle ergometer (10 to 30 minutes), an injection of radioactive thallium is given. The patient then lies down on the scanning table.

3. The scanning is begun immediately, and pictures are taken. The imaging period is about a half hour. A repeat scan is done approximately 4 hours later at rest to check redistribution.

Procedure for MUGA
1. This scan may be performed with or without stress testing and is usually performed in conjunction with heart wall motion study.
2. The test could be performed at bedside if necessary.
3. The patient's own red blood cells become labeled with ^{99m}Tc stannous pyrophosphate.

Procedure for Nitro Test
1. A cardiologist should be present.
2. A resting MUGA is done for a baseline study.
3. Nitroglycerine is given, another scan is taken, nitroglycerine is given again, and scans are taken until the level of blood pressure desired by the cardiologist is reached.
4. Total study time is 1.5 hours.

Procedure for Heart Shunt
1. A radionuclide is injected in the external jugular vein to ensure a compact bolus.
2. The patient lies on his or her back with the head slightly raised.
3. The total patient time is approximately 30 minutes; the actual scan time 5 minutes.
4. A resting MUGA is performed with *each* shunt study.

Procedure for Persantine Thallium
1. Persantine is infused intravenously over a 4-minute period prior to administration of thallium.
2. Blood pressure, heart rate, and ECG are monitored for any changes during persantine infusion. Aminophylline will be given if vital signs change radically.

Procedure for DPY
1. After infusion and injection of DPY and thallium, precise positioning of the patient is done to ensure that the heart is visible in all of the 64 images acquired.
2. DPY may be given orally in some instances.
3. Under certain conditions, the DPY procedures can be done at bedside. When tomographic views are obtained in the nuclear medicine department, results are more sensitive and specific.

Clinical Implications
1. Abnormal myocardial scans will reveal perfusion defects associated with
   (a) Ischemic heart disease
   (b) Location and extent of myocardial infarction
   (c) Progress of disease (estimated)
2. Larger perfusion defects have a much poorer prognosis than small defects.
3. When a scan is entirely normal in a person admitted with a diagnosis of "rule out myocardial infarction," this is an indication that an acute infarction is not present.
4. Specific and significant abnormalities in the stress ECG or myocardial scan are usually indications for cardiac catheterization or further studies.
5. Abnormal MUGA studies are associated with
   (a) Congestive cardiac failure
   (b) Change in ventricular function due to infarction
   (c) Persistent arrhythmias from poor ventricular function
6. Abnormal heart shunts reveal
   (a) Left-to-right shunt   (c) Mean pulmonary transit time
   (b) Right-to-left shunt

Patient Preparation
1. Explain the purpose and procedure of the test.
2. Fasting is necessary for at least 2 hours, and no smoking is permitted for 2 hours before and during the entire stress thallium test.
3. Advise the patient that the exercise stress period will be continued for 45 to 60 seconds after injection to allow the thallium to be cleared during a period of maximum blood flow.
4. Tests can be done at bedside in the acute phase of infarction if equipment is available.
5. A legal permit must be signed by the patient (parents or guardian of child) for a heart shunt scan.
6. No discomfort is experienced during the thallium series test (only feelings associated with stress testing).

Interfering Factors
1. False-positive infarct avid (PYP) scans can occur in chest wall traumas, recent cardioversion, and unstable angina.
2. Neither PYP nor thallium studies are reliable in the evaluations of nontransmural infarction.
3. Long-acting nitrates affect coronary blood flow. For this reason, such medications should be discontinued 8 to 12 hours prior to testing.
4. Injection of DPY in the upright or standing positions or with isometric handgrip may increase myocardial uptake.

5. Gated and PYP studies will interfere with other nuclear tests such as liver, bone, or lung scan if they are done on the same day.

Clinical Alert

1. The stress study is contraindicated on patients who
   (a) Have a combination of right and left bundle branch block
   (b) Have left ventricular hypertrophy
   (c) Are using digitalis and quinidine
   (d) Are hypokalemic (because the results are difficult to evaluate)
2. Some defects seen immediately afterexercise in a patient without infarction will disappear if imaging is repeated 2 to 3 hours later. Those defects that persist at the time of repeat imaging (4–24 hours later) are associated with the presence of a myocardial scar.
3. Contraindications to persantine imaging are severe coronary artery disease and angina at rest.
4. Adverse short-term effects of DPY occur in 30% to 40% of patients and include nausea, headache, dizziness, facial flush, vomiting, angina, ST-segment depression, and ventricular arrhythmia.

Lung Scans; Ventilation and Perfusion

Normal Values
Normal functioning lung
Normal pulmonary vascular supply
Normal gases exchanged

Explanation of Test
Lung scan is done for three major purposes: to detect the percentage of the lungs functioning normally; to diagnose and locate pulmonary emboli; and to assess the pulmonary vascular supply by providing an estimate of regional pulmonary blood flow. It is a simple method for following the course of embolic disease, because an area of ischemia will persist after apparent resolution on a radiograph of the chest. In the case of pulmonary emboli, the blood supply beyond an embolus is restricted. Imaging will reveal poor or no visualization of the affected area. Only three tests are positive immediately following pulmonary embolus: pulmonary arteriogram, measurement of physiologic dead space, and lung scan. Assessment of the adequacy of pulmonary artery

perfusion in areas of known disease can also be done reliably. As soon as a pulmonary embolism is suspected, a ventilated perfusion study should be considered and, if possible, should be performed within 2 days of the acute event.

There are three types of lung scans: (1) the ventilation scan, in which the movement of air or lack of air in the lungs may be demonstrated; (2) the perfusion scan, in which the blood supply to the tissues in the lungs can be demonstrated; and (3) the inhalation scan, in which droplets of radioactive material can be administered by a positive-pressure ventilator. The aerosol is then breathed through a mouthpiece or facemask. A normal aerosol scan looks much like a perfusion scan except that the trachea and major airways are more visible.

Krypton-81m or xenon[133] gas is used in the ventilation lung scan. When inhaled, radioactive gas follows the same pathway as the air in normal breathing. In some pathologic conditions affecting ventilation, there will be significant alteration in the normal ventilation process. The ventilation scan is performed with the lung perfusion scan and is significant in the diagnosis of pulmonary emboli. When the ventilation scan is performed in conjunction with the lung perfusion scan, it is helpful in diagnosing bronchitis, asthma, inflammatory fibrosis, pneumonia, chronic obstructive pulmonary disease, and lung cancer.

The lung perfusion study is usually performed after the ventilation scan. Following the intravenous injection of a macroaggregated albumin labeled with technetium, assessment of pulmonary vascular supply is done by scanning.

Certain limitations exist with these tests. With a positive chest film and a positive scan, the differential possibilities are multiple: pneumonia, abscess, bullae, ateliosis, and carcinoma, among others. A pulmonary arteriogram is still necessary before an embolectomy can be attempted.

Clinical Alert

Pulmonary perfusion imaging is contraindicated in patients with primary pulmonary hypertension or right-to-left heart shunts.

Procedure

1. The patient is asked to breathe for approximately 4 minutes through a closed, nonpressurized ventilation system. During this time, a small amount of radioactive gas will be administered into the system.
2. Breath-holding will be required for a brief period some time during the examination.

3. The examining time is 10 to 15 minutes. When performed with a lung perfusion scan, 30 to 45 minutes is the testing time (used in differential diagnosis of embolism).
4. The perfusion scan immediately follows the ventilation study.

Clinical Implications
Abnormal ventilation and perfusion patterns may indicate the possibility of

1. Tumors	4. Atelectasis	7. Inflammatory fibrosis
2. Emboli	5. Bronchitis	8. Chronic obstructive pulmonary disease
3. Pneumonia	6. Asthma	9. Lung cancer

Interfering Factors
False-positive scans occur in vasculitis, mitral stenosis, pulmonary hypertension, and when tumors obstruct a pulmonary artery with airway involvement.

Patient Preparation
1. Explain the purpose and procedure of the test.
2. Alleviate any fears the patient may have concerning nuclear medicine procedures.
3. It is important that a record of a recent radiograph of the chest be available.
4. The patient must be able to follow directions for breathing and holding his or her breath.

Brain Scan Imaging

Normal Values
Normal extracranial and intracranial blood flow
Normal distribution, with highest uptake in the gray matter, basal ganglia, thalamus, and peripheral cortex; central white matter and ventricles show less activity

Explanation of Test
Radionuclide brain imaging using ^{99m}Tc-labeled complexes such as DTPA and pertechnetate were used for the diagnosis of pathologic abnormalities such as tumors, cerebrovascular aneurysms, and hematomas. With the advent of computed tomography (CT) and magnetic resonance imaging (MRI), this form of imaging has generally become obsolete. However, when coupled with the radionuclide angiogram, technetium-labeled complexes have clinical utility in children in such cases as hydrocephalus, encephalitis, and brain death.

Recent developments in radiopharmaceuticals and SPECT have rejuvinated brain imaging. ^{123}I Iofetamine and ^{99m}Tc Exametazime are radiopharmaceuticals used to cross the blood–brain barrier. The blood–brain barrier is not a specific anatomic structure but a complex system including capillary endothelium with closed intracellular clefts, a small or absent extravascular fluid space between endothelium and glial sheaths, and the membrane of the neurons themselves. Also, SPECT technology allows for numerous slices, providing depth resolution from different angles. These developments have permitted nuclear medicine to evolve into a physiologic and functional neuroimaging modality. Although PET scanning is more effective in functional diagnosis, SPECT is less expensive and more available.

Procedure
1. The radionuclide is injected intravenously.
2. Imaging usually begins within a half hour of administration and takes about 1 hour to complete.
3. With the patient in the supine position, SPECT images are obtained around the circumference of the head.
4. With administration of iodoamphetamines, some departments require a dark and quiet environment.

Clinical Alert

Assess for medication history of MAO inhibitors. ^{123}I-Iofetamine should not be used during or 14 days after administration of MAO inhibitors.

Clinical Implications
1. Abnormal patterns are indicative of altered radionuclide distribution in cases such as
   (a) Alzheimer's disease
   (b) Stroke
   (c) Dementia
   (d) Seizure disorders
   (e) Epilepsy
   (f) Systemic lupus erythematosus
   (g) Huntington's disease
   (h) Parkinson's disease
   (i) Pyschiatric diagnosis (schizophrenia)
2. The cerebral blood flow in the presence of brain death will show a very distinct image of no tracer uptake in the anterior or middle cerebral arteries or the cerebral hemisphere along with the presence of uptake in the scalp.

Interfering Factors
1. Any patient motion, such as coughing or leg movement, can alter cerebral alignment.

2. Sudden distractions or loud noises can alter the distribution of ^{123}I-Iofetamine.

Patient Preparation
1. Explain the purpose and procedure of the test.
2. Reassure the patient that the test is safe, nontoxic, and painless.
3. Because precise head alignment is crucial, advise the patient to remain quiet and still.
4. Obtain a careful neurologic history prior to testing.

Gallbladder/Hepatobiliary Scan

Normal Values
Normal concentration pattern revealing normal size, shape, and function of gallbladder and ducts, and upper intestine

Explanation of Test
This study, using ^{99m}Tc-labeled iminodiacetic acid (IDA) agents (*e.g.,* ^{99m}Tc-disida or disofenin tracers), is done to evaluate the gallbladder and biliary tract. It is indicated in the evaluation of acute cholecystitis and obstructive jaundice. Following the intravenous administration of the radionuclide, the substance will be excreted rapidly from the blood by the polygonal cells of the liver. The transit through the liver cells to the biliary tract is rapid, 10 to 30 minutes, and significant uptake occurs in the normal gallbladder.

Limitations of Test
Radionuclides have a short transit time through the liver, with the advantage of a low radiation dose, but the scan must be done quickly, because the radioisotope, excreted by the hepatic parenchymal cells, is concentrated in the gallbladder and excreted into the gastrointestinal tract.

Procedure
1. The radionuclide is injected intravenously.
2. Imaging starts immediately after injection and usually takes 1 hour.
3. Delayed views are usually done at 2, 4, and 24 hours, in the event of the discovery of severe parenchymal disease where bile duct obstruction is not noted. In these cases, bowel activity is generally detected somewhere between 24 and 48 hours after injection. It is important to note that contributions from the right kidney may be mistaken for bowel activity. Also, 24 hours or longer may be indicated for a delayed view in cases of complete obstruction or other hepatobiliary disease.

Clinical Implications
1. Abnormal concentration patterns will reveal unusual bile communications.
2. Determine if the jaundiced patient is a surgical or nonsurgical candidate.
3. Gallbladder visualization excludes the diagnosis of acute cholecystitis with a high degree (close to 100%) of certainty.

Interfering Factors
1. Patients with high serum bilirubin levels (>10 mg/dl) may have less reliable test results.
2. Patients on total parenteral nutrition (TPN) or long-term fasting may not have gallbladder visualization.

Patient Preparation
1. Explain the purpose and procedure of the test.
2. Fasting is required for 2 hours prior to testing.
3. If the patient has been without food for 48 hours or TPN, sincalide may be given intravenously 1 hour prior to testing to reduce cystic bile spasm and enhance gallbladder visualization.

Bone Scan

Normal Values
No areas of greater or lesser concentration of radioactive material in bones

Explanation of Test
This test is used primarily to evaluate and follow up persons with known or suspected metastatic disease, and the majority of bone scans continue to be for this reason. Breast, prostate, lung tumors and lymphomas tend to metastasize to bone. Bone scans will demonstrate lesions 3 to 6 months before they appear in radiographs.

This scan is commonly used in the evaluation of patients with unexplained bone pain, and patients with primary bone tumors, arthritis, osteomyelitis, abnormal healing of fractures, fractures, shin splints, and compression fractures of the vertebral column. It is also used for patients with chronic renal failure in whom it is necessary to detect soft-tissue calcification; and in pediatric patients with hip pain (Legg–Calvé–Perthes disease). It is also done to identify suitable bone biopsy sites, to evaluate those areas difficult to demonstrate radiographically, such as the sternum and the scapula, and to help determine the age and metabolic activity of traumatic injuries and infection.

Other indications are to evaluate candidates for knee and hip prostheses, to diagnose aseptic necroses and vascularity of the femoral head, and for presurgical assessment of viable bone tissue when amputation is necessary. Evaluation of prosthetic joints and internal fixation devices that are suspected of becoming loose or infected is also done.

Temporomandibular Joint Bone Scanning

This test is done to confirm the clinical impression of internal derangement of the temporomandibular joint (TMJ). The TMJ is the most actively used joint in the body. Single photon emission computed tomography has a sensitivity of 94% and a specificity of 70%.

A bone-seeking radiopharmaceutical is used to image the skeletal system. An example would be ^{99m}Tc-labeled phosphate injected intravenously. Imaging usually begins 2 to 3 hours after injection. The examiner will look for the distribution and concentration of the pharmaceutical in the bone. Abnormal pathology such as increased blood flow to bone and increased metabolism will concentrate the radiopharmaceutical at a higher or lower rate than the normal bone. The radiopharmaceutical mimics the calcium physiology and, therefore, will concentrate more heavily in the areas of increased metabolic activity.

Procedure for Bone Scan

1. Radioactive ^{99m}Tc phosphate is injected intravenously.
2. A 2- to 3-hour waiting period is necessary for the radiopharmaceutical to concentrate in the bone. During this time, the patient may be asked to drink four to six glasses of water.
3. Before the scan begins, the patient is asked to urinate, because a full bladder will mask the pelvic bones.
4. The scan takes about 30 to 60 minutes to complete. The patient must be still during scanning. The table or the scanner will slowly move the patient under and over a sensitive radiation detector.

Procedure for TMJ Bone Scan

1. A radionuclide ^{99m}Tc methylene diphosphonate is injected intravenously.
2. Scanning begins 3 hours after administration.
3. SPECT bone imaging as well as lateral plane views are done.
4. During SPECT, the patient must remain immobile for 21 minutes while the detector rotates around the person.

Interfering Factors

1. False-negative bone scans occur in multiple myeloma of bone. When this condition is known or suspected, the scan is an unreliable indicator of skeletal involvement.
2. Patients with follicular thyroid cancer may harbor metastatic bone marrow disease, but these lesions are often missed by scans.

Clinical Implications

Abnormal concentrations indicate the following:

1. Very early bone disease and healing. This is detectable by radioisotopic scan long before it is visible on radiographs. The latter are positive for bone lesions only after 30% to 50% decalcification (bone calcium decreased) has occurred.
2. Many disorders can be detected but not differentiated by this test (*e.g.*, cancer, arthritis, benign bone tumors, fractures, osteomyelitis, Paget's disease, and aseptic necroses). The findings must be interpreted in the light of the whole clinical picture, because any process inducing an increased calcium excretion rate will be reflected by an increased uptake in the bone.
3. Breast cancer–positive bone scan finding in the preoperative period depends on the staging of the disease, and these scans are recommended prior to initial therapy. *Stages 1* and *2*: 4% will have positive bone scan. *Stage 3*: 19% will have positive bone scan. Yearly bone scans should be done for follow-up.
4. Multiple myeloma is the only tumor that shows better detectability with a plain radiograph than with a radionuclide scan.
5. Multiple focal areas of increased activity in the axial skeleton are commonly associated with metastatic bone disease. The reported percentage of solitary lesions due to metastasis varies on a site-by-site basis. With a single lesion in the spine or pelvis, the cause is more likely to be due to metastatic disease than one occurring in the extremities or ribs.

Clinical Implications of TMJ

Increased uptake with hot areas associated with increased osteoblastic activity about the margins of a displaced joint occur in

1. TMJ disk displacement
2. Bite abnormality
3. Congenital deformity of the mandible

Clinical Alert

1. The flare phenomenon occurs in patients with metastatic disease who are receiving a new therapy. In some persons, the bone scan may show increased activity or new lesions in persons with clinical improvement. It is due to a healing response in prostate and breast cancer within the first few months of a new treatment. These lesions should show marked improvement on scans 3 to 4 months later.
2. Radiographic correlation is necessary to rule out a benign process when solitary areas of increased or decreased uptake occur.
3. The TMJ examination should be deferred in women who are pregnant or who are breastfeeding infants.

Patient Preparation

1. Instruct the patient about the purpose and procedure of the test and his or her involvement. Alleviate any fears concerning the procedure. Advise the patient that frequent drinking and activity in the first 6 hours help to reduce excess radiation to the bladder and gonads.
2. The patient can be up and about during the waiting period.
3. If the patient is in pain or debilitated, assist him or her to void before the test. Otherwise, give a reminder about emptying the bladder before the test.
4. A sedative should be ordered and administered to any patient who will have difficulty lying quietly during the scanning period.

Gallium (^{67}Ga) Scans (Liver, Bone, Brain, Breast Scans)

Normal Values

No evidence of tumor-type activity

Explanation of Test

This test is used to detect the presence, location, and size of tumors, adhesions, abscesses, and inflammation in body cavities, primarily in the liver, bone, brain, and breast. It is most useful in differentiating malignant from benign lesions and determining the extent of invasion of known malignancies. The lymph nodes are also scanned for involvement. These studies are used to help stage bronchogenic cancer, Hodgkin's and non-Hodgkin's lymphomas. Gallium scans may also be used to record tumor regression following radiation or chemotherapy, thereby noting the body response to therapy. The radionuclide injected intravenously is gallium citrate (^{67}Ga).

Areas of the body most often examined by this method are the lymph system, liver, bone, brain, and breast. Only 5% pathologic activity is necessary for detection by this technique, whereas 45% activity is required for radiographic examination. The underlying mechanism for the uptake of ^{67}Ga is not well understood. Uptake in some neoplasms may depend on the presence of transferrin receptors in tumor cells but this is only speculation.

Procedure

1. If imaging of the abdomen is to be performed, a laxative is usually given the evening before the scanning.
2. Laxatives, suppositories, or tap water enemas are often ordered before scanning. The patient may eat breakfast the day of imaging.
3. The radionuclide is injected 24 to 72 hours before imaging.

4. The patient must lie quietly without moving during the scanning procedure. Anterior and posterior views of the entire body are done.
5. Additional imaging may be done at 24-hours intervals to differentiate normal bowel activity from pathologic concentrations.

Clinical Implications
1. An abnormal gallium concentration usually implies the existence of underlying pathology, as in
   (a) Malignancy, especially lung, testes, and mesothelioma
   (b) Stages of lymphomas, melanoma, hepatoma, soft-tissue sarcomas, primary tumors of bone and cartilage, neuroblastomas and leukemia
   (c) Abscesses
   (d) Tuberculosis
   (e) Thrombosis
   (f) Abscessed sarcoidosis
2. Further diagnostic studies are usually done to distinguish benign from malignant lesions.
3. Tumor uptake of ^{67}Ga varies with tumor type, among persons with tumors of some histologic types, and even with tumor sites in a given patient.
4. Tumor uptake of ^{67}Ga may be significantly reduced following effective treatment.
5. Although ^{111}In white blood cell imaging is more specific for abscess localization, gallium imaging is still used as a multipurpose screening procedure.

Interfering Factors
1. A negative study cannot be definitely interpreted as ruling out the presence of disease (40% false-negative results in gallium studies).
2. It is difficult to detect a single, solitary nodule such as in adenocarcinoma. Lesions smaller than 2 cm can be detectable. Tumors near the liver are difficult to detect, as is interpretation of ileac nodes.
3. Because gallium does collect in the bowel, there may be an abnormal concentration in the lower abdomen. For this reason, enemas are ordered before testing.
4. Degeneration or necrosis of tumor and antineoplastic drugs immediately before scans cause false-negative results.

Patient Preparation
1. Explain the purpose and procedure of the test.
2. Reassure the patient that there is no pain involved.
3. Alleviate any fear the patient may have about radionuclide procedures.
4. Usually, no change need be made in eating habits before testing. However, some departments expect their patients to eat a low-residue lunch and clear liquid supper the day before examination.

5. The usual preparation includes oral laxatives beginning on the day of injection and continuing until imaging is completed and/or enemas or suppositories prior to the examination. These preparations clean normal gallium activity from the bowel.
6. Actual scanning time is 1 to 2 hours.

Clinical Alert

Breast-feeding should be discontinued for at least 4 weeks following testing.

---

^{131}I Total Body Scan

Normal Values

No functioning extrathyroid tissues outside of the thyroid gland

Explanation of Test

This study using ^{131}I or ^{123}I is done to search for any functioning thyroid tissue anywhere in the body. It is helpful in determining the presence of metastatic thyroid cancer and the amount and location of residual tissue following thyroidectomy. The procedure is occasionally performed in conjunction with thyroid therapy using ^{131}I for thyrocarcinoma.

Procedure

1. A radionuclide is administered orally in a capsule form.
2. Imaging will take place 24 to 72 hours after administration.
3. Imaging can take as long as 2 to 3 hours to perform.
4. Sometimes, thyroid-stimulating hormone (TSH) is administered intravenously before the radionuclide is given. This stimulates any residual thyroid tissue so it will take up enough ^{131}I or ^{123}I to be detected.

Clinical Implications

Abnormal uptake of iodine reveals

1. Areas of extrathyroid tissue such as
    (a) Stroma ovarii
    (b) Substernal thyroid
    (c) Sublingual thyroid
2. Residual tissue following thyroidectomy
3. Metastatic thyroid cancer

Clinical Alert

1. When possible, this test should be performed before any other radionuclide procedures and before using any iodine contrast medium, surgical preparation, or other form of iodine.
2. The test is most effective when endogenous TSH levels are high, in order to stimulate radioiodine uptake by metastatic neoplasm.

Patient Preparation
1. Explain the purpose and procedure of the test.
2. Advise the patient that the imaging process may take a long time.

Bone Marrow Scan

Normal Values
Normal reticuloendothelial and red blood cells and normal distribution of bone marrow

Explanation of Test
This study, using the radionuclide indium chloride, is used in determining the site of bone marrow biopsies, and is indicated in the differential diagnosis of myeloproliferative disorders, in detection of focal defects in bone marrow, and in differentiation of acute from chronic hemolysis and of bone infarction from osteomyelitis in sickle cell disease. It is also helpful in staging lymphoma, Hodgkin's disease, and metastatic cancer in the bone marrow.

Procedure
1. A radionuclide is injected intravenously, and imaging of the whole body follows 48 hours after injection of indium chlorine. If technetium sulfur colloid is used, scanning usually begins 1 hour after injection.
2. The patient must lie quietly on the scanning table during the entire examination. The body, from head to foot, is scanned.
3. Total imaging time is 1.5 hours.

Clinical Implications
Abnormal filling patterns reveal

1. Bone marrow depression following radiation therapy
2. Bone marrow depression following chemotherapy
3. Extended marrow activity in polycythemia vera

4. Extended marrow activity in chronic hemolytic anemia
5. Nonvisualization in myelofibrosis

Patient Preparation

Explain the purpose and procedure of test. Reassure the patient that no discomfort will be experienced during the test. Instruct the patient to void before imaging occurs.

Cisternography; Cerebrospinal Fluid Flow Scan

Normal Values

Unobstructed cerebrospinal fluid (CSF) flow and normal reabsorption

Explanation of Test

This study, in which a radionuclide (usually ^{111}In DTPA) is injected by lumbar puncture, is a sensitive indicator of altered flow and reabsorption of CSF. In the treatment of hydrocephalus, it aids in the selection of the type of shunt and pathway as well as in the prognosis of both shunting and hydrocephalus.

Procedure

1. A sterile lumbar puncture is performed after the patient has been positioned and prepared (see p. 248 for procedure). At this time, a tracer dose of radionuclide is injected into the cerebrospinal circulation.
2. The patient must lie flat after the puncture; the length of time depends on the physician's order.
3. Imaging will be done at 2 to 6 hours after injection, then again at 24 hours, 48 hours, and 72 hours in some cases.
4. Examining time is 1 hour for each scan.

Clinical Implications

Abnormal filling patterns reveal

1. Hydrocephalus
2. Subdural hematoma
3. Spinal mass lesions
4. Posterior fossa cysts
5. Third ventricle tumor
6. Parencephalic and subarachnoid cysts
7. Shunt patency
8. Diagnosis and localization of rhinorrhea and otorrhea

Patient Preparation

1. Explain the procedures for both lumbar puncture and cisternography.

2. Advise the patient that it may take as long as 1 hour for each scan.
3. The patient must be taken by cart to the nuclear medicine department for the first scan, because of the preceding lumbar puncture.

Patient Aftercare
1. Follow instructions for lumbar puncture (see p. 248).
2. Be alert to complications of lumbar puncture such as meningitis, allergic reaction to anesthetic, bleeding into spinal canal, and herniation of brain tissue.

Spleen Scan

Normal Values
Normal size of spleen, cell function, and blood flow to spleen
The amount of uptake in the spleen should always be less than the liver.

Explanation of Test
This examination is performed to demonstrate anatomic changes in the spleen. Spleen imaging is accomplished by the use of a radioactive nuclide colloid such as ^{99m}Tc sulfur colloid. The amount of this pharmaceutical taken up by the spleen is dependent upon the blood flow to the spleen and its cell function. Resulting images allow the examiner to determine the size and condition of the spleen. This scan may also be used to demonstrate space-occupying lesions or accessory spleens, to visualize the infiltration of Hodgkin's or metastatic disease, and to evaluate trauma cases to rule out infarct. This procedure is performed in conjunction with a liver scan. Spleen imaging may be performed using SPECT.

> **Clinical Alert**
>
> 1. It is essential that the nuclear medicine department know the purpose of the examination.
> 2. Additional views may be required for accurate diagnosis, as in trauma and suspected infarct.

Procedure
1. A patient history is obtained and recorded.
2. The radiopharmaceutical is injected intravenously.
3. A 10- to 20-minute wait is required to allow the injected radiopharmaceutical to be absorbed in the reticuloendothelial cells.
4. A minimum of three views is obtained. On some occasions, additional oblique views may be required.

5. Total examining time is approximately 80 minutes from injection to conclusion. The time involved will vary depending on the patient's ability to cooperate and the size and condition of the spleen. The ability of the cells to accumulate the radiopharmaceutical will also affect the imaging time.

Clinical Implications
Abnormal concentrations reveal

1. Unusual splenic size
2. Infarction
3. Ruptured spleen
4. Accessory spleen
5. Tumors
6. Metastatic spread
7. Leukemia
8. Hodgkin's disease

Spleens greater than 14 cm in size are abnormally enlarged; those less than 7 cm are abnormally small. Areas of absent radioactivity or holes in the spleen scans are associated with abnormalities that displace or destroy normal splenic pulp.

Patient Preparation
1. Explain the purpose, procedure, benefits, and risks of the test. Radiation exposure is about 0.5 to 2.0 rads to the liver, slightly less to the spleen, and about 0.05 rads to the entire body. The whole body dose is about equal to 1 year of natural background radiation.
2. A thorough history must be obtained.
3. Whenever possible, schedule the scan before any test using barium as a contrast.
4. The test can be performed when a trauma case or when a ruptured spleen is suspected, at bedside, or in the emergency room. Electroconvulsive therapy must be done in the department of nuclear medicine.

Interfering Factors
1. Possible artifacts may occur if the images are taken immediately after the administration of barium for radiologic colon examinations. Barium is a dense material and may attenuate some of the gamma radiation from ^{99m}Tc sulfur colloid, which is the pharmaceutical most often used.
2. About 30% of persons with Hodgkin's disease with spleen involvement will have a normal spleen scan.

Adrenergic Tumor Scan; ^{131}MIBG

Normal Values
No evidence of tumor sites

Normal salivary glands, urinary bladder, and vague shape of liver and spleen can be seen.

Explanation of Test

The purpose of this study is to obtain images that aid in identifying sites of certain tumors that produce excessive amounts of catecholamines: pheochromocytomas; paragangliomas; neuroblastomas; carcinoid tumors; or medullary carcinoma of the thyroid gland. This is accomplished by venous injection of a radionuclide ^{131}Iodine meta-iodobenzylguanidine (^{131}MIBG) followed by scans on the first, second, and third days or the second, third, and fourth days of the study.

This test is done to identify tumor sites when a reasonable probability exists (evidence of hormones and metabolites of norepinephrine and epinephrine) that pheochromocytomas are present. When laboratory tests do indicate a functional paraganglioma, it is sometimes difficult to locate the tumor anatomically. The recent development of radionuclides that are selectively taken up by paragangliomas, as in this study, has improved localization. Generally, three views are sufficient for a search: (1) anterior display of the pelvis and lower abdomen; (2) posterior display of abdomen and lower chest; and (3) upper chest and head. If metastasis is suspected, then the upper legs, the humeri, and all of the head are examined as well.

It is known that pheochromocytomas develop in cells that make up the adrenergic portion of the autonomic nervous system. A large number of these well-differentiated cells is found in adrenal medullas, paraspino-sympathetic ganglia, and periaortic organs of Zuckerkandl. In addition, a few cells are located elsewhere, as in the urinary bladder and heart, and in association with nerves, usually thought to be primarily parasympathetic, such as the vagus. Adrenergic tumors have been called paragangliomas when found outside the adrenal medulla, but many refer to all neoplasms that secrete norepinephrine and epinephrine as pheochromocytomas. Because the only definite and effective therapy is surgery to remove the tumor, identifying the site using this test, as well as CT scans and ultrasound, is an essential goal of treatment.

Procedure

1. The radionuclide ^{131}MIBG is injected intravenously.
2. Scans will be done on the second, third, and fourth days in most instances (day 1 being the day of injection). Occasionally only one day of imaging will be necessary, whereas in a few patients, imaging will be required on the sixth and seventh days. Scanning will be done from the urinary bladder to the mastoid area when searching for a primary tumor.
3. Scanning time each day is approximately 30 minutes.

Clinical Implications

1. Abnormal results give substance to the "Rough Rule of Ten." This means that
   (a) Ten percent are in children.
   (b) Ten percent are familial.
   (c) Ten percent are bilateral in the adrenal glands.
   (d) Ten percent are malignant.
   (e) Ten percent are multiple, in addition to bilateral, tumors.
   (f) Ten percent are extrarenal.
2. Over 90% of primary pheochromocytomas occur in the abdomen.
3. Pheochromocytomas in children often represent a familial disorder.
4. Bilateral adrenal tumors often indicate a familial disease and vice versa.
5. Multiple extrarenal pheochromocytomas are often malignant.
6. The presence of two or more pheochromocytomas almost always indicates malignant disease.

Interfering Factors
Barium interferes.

Patient Preparation

1. Explain the purpose and procedure, benefits and risks. Radioactive exposure is comparable to CT scan of the adrenal glands or conventional radiograph of the kidneys and adrenal glands. Obtain patient's signed legal consent form.
2. To prevent uptake of radioactive iodine by the thyroid gland, Lugol's solution or potassium iodine will be given for a period of time before the test as well as after the test. For example, a common protocol is 2 days before injection of radionuclide and 10 days after the injection.
3. Scans will usually be taken up to and including three successive days after injection. Occasionally, patients will require imaging on 4 days. Even though most pheochromocytomas are readily defined on all 3 days, in some patients the tumor may not be seen on any day but will be best portrayed on day 3; in others, the opposite will occur; the pheochromocytomas will be seen only on day 1.

Patient Aftercare

1. Check the patient for discomfort or bruising at the site of injection.
2. Follow-up tests include
   (a) Kidney and bone nuclear scans to give further orientation to abnormalities discovered in ^{131}I-MIBG tests.
   (b) CT scans if MIBG scans have failed to locate the tumor.
   (c) Ultrasound of pelvis if the tumor produces urinary symptoms.

Abscess Scan
(WBC Inflammatory Imaging—^{111}In Scan)

Normal Values
No signs of localization of leukocytes

Explanation of Test
This test, in which a sample of the patient's own leukocytes (white blood cells) has been isolated, labeled with indium oxine and reinjected, is used for the localization of abscess formation. The study is indicated in persons with signs and symptoms of a septic process, fever of unknown origin, and suspected intra-abdominal abscess. It is also helpful in determining the cause of complications of surgery, injury, or inflammation of gastrointestinal tract and pelvis. The test results are based on the fact that any collection of labeled white cells outside the liver, spleen, and functioning bone marrow indicates an abnormal area to which the white blood cells are being attracted. This procedure is 90% sensitive and 90% specific for inflammatory disease or abscess formation.

Procedure
1. A venous blood sample of 40 ml is obtained for the purpose of isolating and labeling the white blood cells. This laboratory process takes about 3 hours to complete.
2. The white blood cells are labeled with radioactive ^{111}In and injected intravenously.
3. After a waiting period, the patient returns for imaging at 24 and 48 hours.
4. Imaging time is about 1 hour each time.

Clinical Implications
Abnormal concentrations indicate

1. Abscess formation
2. Acute and chronic osteomyelitis and infection of orthopedic prostheses
3. Active inflammatory bowel disease

Interfering Factors
1. False-negative reactions are known to occur when the chemotactic function of the white blood cell has been altered as in hemodialysis, hyperglycemia, hyperalimentation, steroid therapy, and long-term antibiotic therapy.
2. Gallium scans up to 1 month prior can interfere.
3. False-positive scans occur in the presence of gastrointestinal bleed-

ing and in upper respiratory infections and pneumonitis when patients swallow purulent sputum.

Clinical Considerations

If the patient does not have an adequate number of white blood cells, then donor cells can be used. It is possible in some instances to do a successful study in persons who have less than 1000 white blood cells/cm.

Patient Preparation

1. Explain the purposes, procedure, benefits, and risks.
2. Assess for a history of recent gallium scan.
3. If the patient is premenopausal, instructions are to be given to the patient to use effective birth control while being tested because the test may be harmful to the fetus.

Risks

Fetal radiation should be avoided whenever possible. The radiation dose to the fetus from this test is equal to the radiation from one abdominal radiograph.

Meckel's Diverticulum Scan

Normal Values

Normal blood flow in abdomen
Normal distribution of radiopharmaceutical
No evidence of ectopic tissue

Explanation of Test

This test is indicated in both children and adults with gastrointestinal bleeding of unknown etiology and undetermined abdominal pain and persistent guaiac-positive stools with normal barium radiographs. Meckel's diverticulum can be difficult to detect by standard radiographic techniques. The radionuclide ^{99m}Tc pertechnetate is taken up by the gastric mucosa following intravenous administration. This procedure detects the presence of abnormally situated gastric mucosa. Meckel's diverticulum frequently contains gastric mucosa that can be responsible for hyperacidity, causing bowel wall erosion and hemorrhage.

Procedure

1. Preferably, prior to the procedure, the patient should receive cimetidine orally every 6 hours for 24 hours. Cimetidine inhibits acid secretion and allows for a better scan. However, even without cimetidine administration, the scan can be performed.
2. The radiopharmaceutical is injected intravenously.
3. There are two phases to imaging

(a) Blood flow in the abdomen
(b) Periodic imaging to determine uptake of radiopharmaceutical in duodenum
4. Total examining time is 60 minutes.

Interfering Factors
Barium in the small or large bowel may mask radionuclide concentration.

Clinical Implications
Abnormal distributions indicate presence of Meckel's diverticulum, which is a remnant of the omphalomesenteric duct. Only about 2% of the population will develop this disorder of the duodenum, and of this population, 25% will exhibit symptoms.

Clinical Considerations
A determination should be made that no recent barium studies have been done.

Patient Preparation
1. Explain the purpose and procedure of the test.
2. The patient should be NPO for at least 2 hours prior to the examination.

Parathyroid Scan

Normal Values
No areas of increased perfusion or uptake ratios in parathyroid and thyroid

Explanation of Test
This test is done primarily for presurgical localization of parathyroid adenomas in clinically proven cases of primary hyperparathyroidism. It is helpful in demonstrating intrinsic or extrinsic parathyroid adenoma. Two tracers, thallium and technetium, are used prior to imaging.

Procedure
1. The radionuclide thallium is injected, and 20 minutes later imaging is done. This image is stored in the computer.
2. Without moving the patient, technetium is injected and a second image is obtained and computerized. Computer processing involves subtracting the technetium-visualized thyroid structures from the thallium accumulation in a parathyroid adenoma.
3. Total examination is 30 to 45 minutes.

Interfering Factors

Recent ingestion of iodine in food, medication, and recent tests with iodine content may reduce the effectiveness of the study.

Clinical Implications

Abnormal concentrations reveal parathyroid adenoma, both intrinsic and extrinsic, but cannot differentiate between benign and malignant parathyroid.

Clinical Considerations

Pregnancy is a relative contraindication. However, if primary hyperparathyroidism and surgical exploration is essential prior to delivery, the study may be performed.

Patient Preparation

1. Explain the purpose and procedure of the test.
2. Assess for the recent intake of iodine. However, this finding is not a specific contraindication to performing the study.
3. Inform the patient that the radiation exposure from this study is less than most fluoroscopic radiographs.
4. The thyroid should be carefully palpated because thallium may accumulate in thyroid adenomas.

Scrotal Scan Testicular Imaging

Normal Values

Normal blood flow to scrotal structures with even distribution and concentration of radiopharmaceutical

Explanation of Test

This test is performed on an emergency basis in the evaluation of acute, painful testicular swelling. It is used in the differential diagnoses of torsion of acute epididymitis and in the evaluation of injury, trauma, tumors, and masses. The radiopharmaceutical ^{99m}Tc pertechnetate is used prior to imaging. The images obtained differentiate scrotal lesions associated with increased perfusion from those that are primarily ischemic.

Procedure

1. The patient lies on his back under the nuclear camera. The penis is gently taped back onto the lower abdominal wall.
2. A small tracer dose of radionuclide is injected intravenously.
3. Imaging is performed in two phases: first as a dynamic blood flow study of the scrotum and second, as an assessment of distribution of radiopharmaceutical in the scrotum.
4. Total examining time is 30 to 45 minutes.

Clinical Implications
Abnormal concentrations reveal:

1. Tumors
2. Hematomas
3. Infection
4. Torsions (with reduced blood flow)

The nuclear scan is most specific soon after the onset of pain, before abscess is a clinical consideration.

Patient Preparation
1. Explain the purpose, procedure, benefits, and risks of the test. There is no discomfort involved in testing.
2. If the patient is a child, a parent should accompany the boy. The examining department prefers the father.

Gastrointestinal Blood Loss Scan

Normal Values
No sites of active bleeding

Explanation of Test
This test has been documented as very sensitive in the detection and location of acute gastrointestinal bleeding that occurs distal to the ligament of Treitz. (Gastroscopy is the procedure of choice in diagnosing upper gastrointestinal bleeding). Prior to the refining of this diagnostic technique, barium enemas were used to identify lesions that reflect the site of bleeding, but these examinations are not specific and frequently miss small sites of bleeding such as that caused by diverticular disease and angiodysplasia. This scan is also indicated for detection and localization of recent hemorrhage, both peritoneal and retroperitoneal, as well as documentation and location of sites of pulmonary hemorrhage. In addition, this procedure is frequently done prior to angiography. For example, if a right lower quadrant bleed is detected, then the angiogram will begin by studying the superior mesenteric artery; if a left lower quadrant bleed is detected, then the inferior mesenteric artery will be the beginning point. ^{99m}Tc sulfur colloid is the radiopharmaceutical of choice for suspected active bleeding. Because liver and spleen rapidly clear this agent from the vasculature, the detection of bleeding by extravasation of the radiopharmaceutical into the bowel occurs. For intermittent bleeding, ^{99m}Tc red blood cells is more useful in delayed imaging up to 24 hours after injection.

Procedure
1. Radiopharmaceutical ^{99m}Tc sulfur colloid or ^{99m}Tc red blood cells is injected.

2. Imaging is begun immediately and continued every few minutes, often with delayed images 2, 6, and sometimes 24 hours later, when necessary, to identify the location of active bleeding.
3. Images are obtained anteriorly over the abdomen at 5 minute intervals. If the study is negative at 1 hour, repeat images can be obtained throughout a 24-hour period without reinjection of radiopharmaceutical.
4. Total examining time varies.
5. Reexamination can be performed any time of the day or night, during a 24-hour period. Active bleeding must be occurring at the rate of 0.5 to 1 ml/minute to locate the bleeding site.

Clinical Considerations
1. This test is contraindicated in those who are hemodynamically unstable. In these instances, angiography or surgery should be the procedures of choice.
2. Assess patients for signs of active bleeding during the examining period. The procedure will be performed by the department of nuclear medicine any time during a 24-hour period.

Clinical Implications
Abnormal concentration of red blood cells with areas of radioactivity greater than the background activity are associated with

1. Approximate geographic location of active gastrointestinal bleeding, both peritoneal as well as retroperitoneal.
2. Nongastrointestinal sites of hemorrhage, such as in the lungs, can also be identified, up to 24 hours postinjection.

Interfering Factors
Presence of barium in gastrointestinal tract may obscure the site of bleeding. This is because of the high density of barium and the inability of the technetium to penetrate the barium.

Patient Preparation
1. Explain the purpose and procedure, benefits and risks of the test.
2. Determine whether or not the patient has received barium as a diagnostic agent in the last 24 hours. If the presence of barium in the gastrointestinal tract is questionable, an abdominal radiograph may be ordered.
3. Advise the patient that delayed repeat images may be necessary if barium is present. Also, if active bleeding is not seen on initial scans, additional images must be obtained for as long as 24 hours after injection, whenever the patient has clinical signs of active bleeding.

Part Two
Radionuclide Laboratory Procedures
(Other Than Radioimmunoassay
[RIA] Studies)

Introduction

Minute quantities of radioactive materials may be detected in blood, feces, urine, other body fluids, and glands. Therefore, very small amounts of radioactive substances may be administered to patients, and then their body fluids and glands may be assayed for concentrations of radioactivity.

One procedure checks the ability of the body to absorb the administered radioactive compound. An example of this type of study is the Schilling test. Another procedure such as radioactive iodine uptake or blood volume determination tests the ability of the body to localize or dilute the administered radioactive substance.

The use of radionuclides in analysis depends on the fact that the radioactive atoms of a substance such as iodine react chemically just as nonradioactive iodine does, but the radionuclide can be readily detected because of its radioactivity.

Part II of this chapter includes a sampling of tests that employ the use of radionuclides in the study of disease. Imaging may or may not be part of these procedures.

Schilling Test

Normal Values

Excretion of 7% or more of test dose of cobalt-tagged vitamin B_{12} in urine

Explanation of Test

This 24-hour urine test is used to diagnose pernicious anemia (one form of macrocytic anemia) and malabsorption syndromes. It is an indirect test of intrinsic factor deficiency, evaluates ability to absorb vitamin B_{12} from the gastrointestinal tract, and is based on the anticipated urinary excretion of radioactive vitamin B_{12}.

In this test, the fasting patient is given an oral dose of vitamin B_{12} tagged with radioactive cobalt (^{57}Co). An intramuscular injection of vitamin B_{12} is given to saturate the liver and serum protein-binding sites, which allows radioactive vitamin B_{12} to be excreted in the urine. A 24-hour urine specimen is then collected.

The amount of the excreted radioactive B_{12} is determined and expressed as a percentage of the given dose. Normal persons will absorb (and therefore excrete) as much as 25% of the radioactive B_{12}, for they can absorb vitamin B_{12} from the gastrointestinal tract. Patients with pernicious anemia absorb little of the oral dose and thus have little radioactive material to excrete in the urine.

Procedure
1. The patient must fast for 12 hours before the test. (Breakfast is delayed 3 hours after vitamin B_{12} doses are administered.)
2. A tasteless capsule of radioactive B_{12} labeled with ^{57}Co is administered orally by a nuclear medical technologist.
3. Then a nonradioactive B_{12} is given by intramuscular injection by an registered nurse or nuclear medical technologist.
4. Total urine is collected for 24 to 48 hours from the time the patient receives the injection of vitamin B_{12}.
   (a) Obtain a special 24-hour urine container from the laboratory. No preservative is needed.
   (b) Take care that there is no contamination of the urine with stool.
   (c) Follow the procedure for 24-hour urine collection (see Chap. 3).
   (d) In presence of renal disease, a 48-hour collection may be necessary.

Clinical Implications
1. An abnormally low value (*e.g.*, <7%) or borderline (7%–10%) allows two interpretations:
   (a) Absence of intrinsic factor
   (b) Defective absorption in the ileum
2. When the absorption of radioactive vitamin B_{12} is low, the test must be repeated with intrinsic factor to rule out intestinal malabsorption (confirmatory Schilling test).
   (a) If the urinary excretion then rises to normal levels, it indicates a lack of intrinsic factor, suggesting the diagnosis of pernicious anemia.
   (b) If the urinary excretion does not rise, malabsorption is considered the cause of the patient's anemia.

Interfering Factors
1. Renal insufficiency may cause reduced excretions of radioactive vitamin B_{12}. If renal insufficiency is suspected, a 48- to 72-hour urine collection is advised, because eventually nearly all the absorbed material will be excreted and urine specific gravity and volume are checked.

2. The single most common source of error in performing the test is *incomplete collection of urine*. Some laboratories may require a 48-hour collection to allow for a small margin of error.
3. Urinary excretion of B_{12} is depressed in elderly patients, diabetics, patients with hypothyroidism, and those with enteritis.

Patient Preparation
1. Explain the purpose and procedure of the test.
2. A random sample urine specimen is usually obtained before the B_{12} doses are administered.
3. Give a written reminder to the patient about fasting and collection of a 24-hour urine specimen. Water is permitted during the fasting period.
4. Food and drink are permitted after the doses of vitamin B_{12} are given. The patient is encouraged to drink as much as can be tolerated during the entire test.
5. Be certain the patient receives the nonradioactive B_{12}. If the intramuscular dose of vitamin B_{12} is not given, the radioactive vitamin B_{12} will be found in the liver, instead of the urine.

Clinical Alert

1. No laxatives are to be used during the test.
2. Bone marrow aspiration should be done before the Schilling test, because the vitamin B_{12} administered in the test will destroy the diagnostic characteristics of the bone marrow.

Total Blood Volume Determination; Plasma Volume; Red Cell Volume

Normal Values
Total blood volume: 55–80 ml/kg
Red cell volume: 20–35 ml/kg (greater in men than in women)
Plasma volume: 30–45 ml/kg

Note: Because adipose tissue has a sparser blood supply than lean tissue, the patient's body type can affect the proportion of blood volume to body weight, which is why test findings should always be reported in milliliters per kilogram.

Explanation of Test
The purpose of this test is to determine circulating blood volume, to help evaluate the bleeding or debilitated patient, and to determine the

origin of hypotension in the presence of anuria or oliguria when dehydration may be the cause. This determination is one way to monitor blood loss during surgery; it is used as a guide in replacement therapy following blood or body fluid loss and in the determination of whole body hematocrit. The results are useful in determining the most appropriate blood component for replacement therapy (*e.g.*, whole blood, plasma, or packed red cells).

Total blood volume determinations are of value in the following situations:

1. To evaluate gastrointestinal and uterine bleeding
2. To aid in the diagnosis of hypovolemic shock
3. To aid in the diagnosis of polycythemia vera
4. To determine the required blood component for replacement therapy, as in persons undergoing open heart surgery

These tests will reveal an increased or decreased plasma volume red cell mass. A sample of the patient's blood is mixed with a radioactive substance, incubated at room temperature, and reinjected. Another blood sample is obtained 15 minutes later. The most commonly used tracers in blood volume determination are serum albumin tagged with ^{131}I or ^{125}I and patient or donor red blood cells tagged with ^{51}Cr. The combination of procedures or total blood volume is the only true blood volume. Other volume studies are plasma volume and ^{51}Cr red cell volume, which may be done separately.

The plasma volume is used to establish a vascular baseline, to determine changes in plasma volume before and after surgery, and to evaluate fluid and blood replacement in gastrointestinal bleeding and burn and trauma cases.

The ^{51}Cr red cell volume study is done to see what percentage of the circulating blood is composed of red cells. This procedure is performed in connection with red cell survival, gastrointestinal blood loss, or ferrokinetic studies.

Procedure
1. Record the patient's height and current weight.
2. Venous blood samples are obtained, and one sample is mixed with a radionuclide.
3. Fifteen to 30 minutes later, the blood is reinjected.
4. About 15 minutes later, another venous blood sample is obtained.

Clinical Implications
1. A normal total blood volume with a decreased red cell content indicates the need for a transfusion of packed red cells.
2. Polycythemia vera may be differentiated from secondary polycythemia.
   (a) Increased total blood volume due to an increased red cell mass

suggests polycythemia vera. The plasma volume is most often normal.
(b) Normal or decreased total blood volume due to a decreased plasma volume suggests secondary polycythemia. The red cell volume is most often normal.

Clinical Alert

If intravenous blood component therapy is ordered for the same day, the blood volume determination should be done before the intravenous line is started.

Patient Preparation
1. Explain the purpose and procedure of the test.
2. The patient should be weighed just before the test if possible.

Red Blood Cell (RBC) Survival Time Test

Normal Values
Normal half-time ^{51}Cr red blood cell survival is approximately 28 days. However, a normal value is determined by the nuclear medicine physician/radiologist. In the body, red blood cells live about 100–120 days.
Chromium-51 in stool: <3 ml./24 hr.

Explanation of Test
This blood test has its greatest use in the evaluation of known or suspected hemolytic anemia and is also indicated when there seems to be an obscure cause for anemia, to identify accessory spleens, and to determine abnormal red cell production and destruction. A sample of the patient's red blood cells is mixed with a radioactive substance (^{51}Cr), incubated at room temperature, and reinjected. Blood specimens are drawn at the end of a 24-hour period and at regular intervals for at least 3 weeks. After counting the specimens, the results are plotted and the red cell survival time calculated. Results are based on the fact that disappearance of radioactivity from the circulation corresponds to the disappearance of the red blood cells, thereby determining overall erythrocyte survival.

Scanning of the spleen is often done as part of this test. Red blood cell survival is usually ordered in conjunction with blood volume determination and radionuclide iron uptake and clearance tests. When stool specimens are collected for 3 days, the test is often referred to as the gastrointestinal blood loss test, which is different from the study on page 607.

Procedure

1. A venous blood sample of 20 ml is obtained.
2. Ten to 30 minutes later, the blood is reinjected after being tagged with a radionuclide, ^{51}Cr.
3. Blood samples are usually obtained the first day, again at 24, 48, 72, and 96 hours, then at weekly intervals for 3 weeks. Time may be shortened depending on the outcome of the test. As part of this procedure, a radioactive detector may be used over the spleen, sternum, and liver to assess the relative concentration of radioactivity in these areas. This external counting helps to determine if the spleen is taking part in excessive sequestration of red blood cells as a causative factor in anemia.
4. In some instances, a 72-hour stool collection may be ordered to detect gastrointestinal blood loss. At the end of each 24-hour collection period, the total stool is to be collected by the department of nuclear medicine. This test can be completed in 3 days.

Clinical Implications

1. Shortened red cell survival may be the result of blood loss, hemolysis, and removal of red blood cells by the spleen, as in
   (a) Chronic lymphatic leukemia
   (b) Congenital nonspherocytic hemolytic anemia
   (c) Hemoglobin C disease
   (d) Hereditary spherocytosis
   (e) Idiopathic acquired hemolytic anemia
   (f) Paroxysmal nocturnal hemoglobinuria
   (g) Elliptocytosis
   (h) Pernicious anemia
   (i) Megaloblastic anemia of pregnancy
   (j) Sickle cell anemia
   (k) Sickle cell hemoglobin C disease
   (l) Uremia
2. Prolonged red cell survival time may be the result of abnormality of red cell production as in thalassemia minor.
3. If hemolytic anemia is diagnosed, further studies are needed to establish whether red blood cells have intrinsic abnormalities or whether anemia results from immunologic effects of the patient's plasma.
4. Results will be normal in
   (a) Hemoglobin C trait
   (b) Sickle cell trait
   (c) Elliptocytosis without hemolysis or anemia

5. Half of the radioactivity of plasma may not disappear for 7 to 8 hours.

Patient Preparation

1. Explain the purpose and procedure of the test. Emphasize that this test requires a minimum of 2 weeks of the patient's time with trips to the diagnostic facility for venipunctures.
2. If stool collection is required, advise the patient of the importance of saving all stool and that stool be free of urine contamination.

Clinical Alert

1. The test is usually contraindicated in an actively bleeding patient.
2. Record and report signs of active bleeding.
3. Transfusions should not be given when the test is in progress. If it is necessary to do so, notify the nuclear medicine department to terminate the test.

Radioactive Iodine (RAI) Uptake Test

Normal Values

1%–13% absorbed by thyroid gland after 2 hr ⎫ Values are
5%–20% absorbed by thyroid gland after 6 hr ⎬ laboratory
15%–40% absorbed by thyroid gland after 24 hr ⎭ dependent

Explanation of Test

This direct test of the function of the thyroid gland measures ability of the gland to concentrate and retain iodine. When radioactive iodine is administered, it is rapidly absorbed into the bloodstream. This procedure measures the rate of accumulation, incorporation, and release of iodine by the thyroid. The rate of absorption of the radioactive iodine (which is determined by an increase in radioactivity of the thyroid gland) is a measure of the ability of the thyroid gland to concentrate iodide from the blood plasma. The radioactive isotopes of iodine usually used are either ^{131}I or ^{123}I.

This procedure is indicated in the evaluation of hypothyroidism, hyperthyroidism, thyroiditis, goiter, pituitary failure, and posttreatment evaluation. The patient who is a candidate for this test may have a lumpy or swollen neck or complain of pain in the neck, be jittery and ultrasensitive to heat, or may be sluggish and ultrasensitive to cold. The test is more useful in the diagnosis of hyperthyroidism than in hypothyroidism.

Procedure

Note: The test is usually done in conjunction with a thyroid scan and assessment of thyroid hormone levels (see p. 376).

1. A fasting state is preferred. A good history and listing of all medications is a must for this test.
2. A liquid form or a tasteless capsule of radioiodine is administered orally. However, it can be administered intravenously if a quick test is desired. The patient is usually instructed not to eat for 1 hour after administration of radioiodine.
3. Two, 6, and 24 hours later, the amount of radioactivity is measured by a scan of the radioactivity in the thyroid gland. There is no pain or discomfort involved.
4. The patient will have to return to the laboratory at the designated time, for the exact time of measurement is crucial in determining uptake.

Clinical Alert

1. This test is contraindicated in pregnant or lactating women, in children, and in infants.
2. Whenever possible, this test should be performed before any other radionuclide procedures are done, before any iodine medications are given, and before any radiographs using iodine contrast medium are done.

Clinical Implications

1. Increased uptake (*e.g.*, 20% in 1 hour, 25% in 6 hours, 45% in 24 hours) suggests hyperthyroidism.
2. Decreased uptake (*e.g.*, 0% in 2 hours, 3% in 6 hours, 10% in 24 hours) may be caused by hypothyroidism, but it is not diagnostic for it.
   (a) If the administered iodine is not absorbed, as in severe diarrhea or intestinal malabsorption syndromes, the uptake may be low, even though the gland is functioning normally.
   (b) Rapid diuresis during the test period may deplete the supply of iodine, causing an apparently low percentage of iodine uptake.
   (c) In renal failure, the uptake may be high, even though the gland is functioning normally.

Interfering Factors

1. The chemicals, drugs, and foods that interfere with the test by *lowering uptake* are
   (a) Iodized foods and iodine-containing drugs such as Lugol's solu-

tion, expectorants, saturated solutions of potassium iodide, (SSKI), and vitamin preparations that contain minerals (1–3 weeks' duration time for the effect of these substances in the body)

(b) Radiographic contrast media such as Diodrast (iodopyracet), Hypaque (sodium diatrizoate), Renografin, Lipiodal, Ethiodol, Pantopaque (isophendylate), Telepaque (iopanoic acid) (1 week to a year or more in duration). Consult with nuclear medicine laboratory for specific times.

(c) Antithyroid drugs such as propylthiouracil and related compounds (2–10 days' duration)

(d) Thyroid medications such as cytomel, desiccated thyroid, thyroxine synthroid (1–2 weeks' duration)

(e) Miscellaneous drugs—thiocyanate, perchlorate, nitrates, sulfonamides, orinase, corticosteroids, PAS, isoniazid, Butazolidin (phenylbutazone), Pentothal (thiopental), antihistamines, ACTH, aminosalicylic acid, amphenone, cobalt, coumarin anticoagulants. Consult the diagnostic department for duration times, which may vary.

2. The compounds and conditions that interfere by *enhancing uptake* are

(a) TSH
(b) Pregnancy
(c) Cirrhosis
(d) Barbiturates
(e) Lithium carbonate
(f) Phenothiazines (1 week)
(g) Iodine deficient diets
(h) Renal failure

Patient Preparation

1. Explain the purpose and procedures of the test, which takes 24 hours to complete.
2. Advise that iodine intake is restricted for at least 1 week before testing.

Thyroid-Stimulating Hormone (TSH) Test

Normal Values

TSH: less than 5 μU/ml (laboratory dependent)

In normal persons, TSH, T_4, and RAI uptake are increased within 8 to 10 hours after TSH is given.

Explanation of Test

This test measures the response of the thyroid gland to an injection of TSH. This examination is used in conjunction with the RAI uptake test. It is done to differentiate primary from secondary hypothyroidism, to determine the level of thyroid gland activity, especially borderline thyroid function, and to evaluate thyroid hormone therapy. It is indicated in the evaluation of hypopituitarism and to demonstrate the presence of normal suppressed thyroid tissue in persons with autonomous hyperfunctioning nodules. The thyroid gland may have impaired RAI uptake because of intrinsic disease (primary hypothyroidism) or insufficient stimulation by the pituitary gland (secondary hypothyroidism). Patients who have a decreased amount of functioning thyroid gland, as in subtotal thyroidectomy radiation therapy or thyroiditis, may have a normal RAI uptake and still fail to respond to TSH stimulation. Such persons have a low thyroid reserve and need continued observation to prevent myxedema.

Procedure
1. *Day 1*: Patient receives 10 units TSH intramuscularly.
2. *Day 2*: Background counts over thyroid are taken and 10 more units of TSH are administered intramuscularly. Radioactive iodine is also given at this time. (Either ^{123}I or ^{131}I may be used.)
3. Patient returns in 2 to 6 hours for uptake.
4. *Day 3*: A 24-hour thyroid uptake and thyroid scan are performed.

Clinical Alert

The TSH should be administered by a physician because the patient may have a reaction to this hormone.

Clinical Implications
1. No response to TSH is seen in the following conditions:
   (a) Primary untreated hypothyroidism (increase ranges from 3 times normal to 100 times normal in severe myxedema)
   (b) Chronic Hashimoto's thyroiditis
2. The TSH positive response is seen in the following conditions (secondary hypothyroidism):
   (a) Hypothalamic hypothyroidism
   (b) Pituitary hypothyroidism

Interfering Factors
Iodine intake will invalidate radioiodine uptake results.

Patient Preparation
1. Explain the purpose and procedure of the test, which takes several days to complete. Check with the appropriate department for the protocols to be used.
2. Advise that iodine intake is restricted for at least 1 week before testing.
3. Inform the patient that TSH is given intramuscularly.

Perchlorate Suppression Study/Iodide Washout Test

Normal Values
In normal persons, the uptake of radioactive iodine will not change appreciably following the administration of perchlorate.

Explanation of Test
The perchlorate test is used to evaluate patients with suspected Hashimoto's disease or to demonstrate an enzyme deficiency within the thyroid gland. The procedure is used to identify defects in the iodide organification process within the thyroid. This study is based on the fact that potassium perchlorate competes with and displaces the iodide ions that are not organified. Perchlorate also stops the further trapping of iodide at the time of administration. Iodine is concentrated within the thyroid gland and quickly becomes bound to the protein thyroglobulin after becoming organified. The administration of perchlorate will stop any further trapping of iodide as well as the release of any unbound iodide within the thyroid gland, thus stopping the normal process. When iodine is trapped within the gland, it becomes synthesized with amino acids to form thyroxine, and the perchlorate will not remove the iodine from the gland. In the case of a patient with enzyme deficiency, the perchlorate will remove any unbound iodide from the gland as well as prevent further trapping. Patients with an enzyme deficiency will show a drop in their uptake greater than 15% after the administration of perchlorate.

Procedure
1. A complete patient history is taken.
2. Body background is measured for residual radiation by imaging.
3. A small tracer dose of radioactive iodine is administered orally. (Either ^{123}I or ^{131}I may be used.)
4. An uptake is performed at 1 and 2 hours after administration.
5. After the 2-hour uptake is performed, the patient is given 400 mg to 1 g of potassium perchlorate orally.
6. Uptakes are performed every 15 minutes for the first hour post-dose perchlorate and then 30 minutes thereafter for the next 2 to 3 hours.
7. Uptakes performed after the administration of perchlorate are compared to the 2-hour uptake before perchlorate.
8. The results are recorded on linear graph paper as counts over the thyroid versus time in minutes of the uptake.

Clinical Implications
Abnormal results reveal

1. Enzyme deficiency within a thyroid gland
2. Hashimoto's disease

Note: Both disease processes will interfere with the organification process.

Patient Preparation
1. Explain the purpose and procedure of the test.
2. The patient should be fasting for this procedure.
3. Advise that no form of iodine should be ingested for at least 1 week before testing; this includes medications, foods, and contrasts used in radiographs.

[131]I Thyroid Cytomel Suppression Test

Normal Values
Euthyroid patients with normal thyroid uptakes can expect a depression of the second uptake of at least 50% following Cytomel.

Explanation of Test
This test measures the response of the thyroid metabolic system to the administration of oral triiodothyronine. The uptake of iodine by a normal thyroid gland will decrease following the administration of oral triiodothyronine.

A patient who has a high initial uptake due to iodine deficiency or a dyshormonogenesis condition, or who is recovering from a subacute thyroiditis, will have a sharp decline, usually about one half the baseline value, after the administration of Cytomel. Some patients will not be suppressed by the administration of Cytomel. In most instances, those patients will be hyperthyroid due to a toxic goiter (Graves' disease), a toxic multinodular goiter, or a toxic autonomously functioning thyroid adenoma. In some instances, a nonhypothyroid patient will not suppress after administration of Cytomel. An example would be a person with euthyroid Graves' disease.

Procedure
1. A careful patient history must be taken before the administration of Cytomel.
2. If the physician agrees that the Cytomel will not have an adverse effect, the patient is started on 75 g to 100 g/day for a period of 5 to 10 days (25 μg every 8 hours for 5 days).
3. The patient must return to the nuclear medicine department 1 day before the last dose of Cytomel is taken.
4. On that day, a body background is taken for residual radioactive iodine from the previous uptake and recorded.
5. A new tracer dose of radioactive iodine is given and amount, date, and time are recorded. (Either ^{123}I or ^{131}I may be used.)
6. The patient returns after the last dose of Cytomel is taken, and an

uptake is performed (2- and 6-hour uptakes are usual after radioiodine is given).

Clinical Implications

1. The euthyroid patient who is iodine deficient will normally have a high uptake initially and a decreased second uptake following the administration of Cytomel.
2. A patient with a hyperthyroid condition demonstrating a high initial uptake will show no appreciable change on the second uptake following the administration of Cytomel.
3. Other abnormal findings
   (a) TSH-dependent tissue will be suppressed.
   (b) Autonomous nodules will not be suppressed.
   (c) Patients with thyroid cancer may or may not be suppressed.
   (d) Thyroid tissue destroyed as a result of therapy or disease will remain unchanged.
   (e) A scan of the thyroid performed before and after the administration of Cytomel will demonstrate an autonomous nodule or tissue because it is unaffected by TSH.

Patient Preparation

1. Explain the purpose and procedure of the test, including the time involved and the proper administration of Cytomel.
2. Advise the patient not to consume any products containing iodine or take any medication that would affect this study.

Part Three
Positron Emission Tomography (PET)

Normal Values

Normal patterns of tissue metabolism based on oxygen, glucose, and fatty acid utilization, protein synthesis, and blood volume and flow

Explanation of Test

Positron emission tomography (PET) is the combined use of positron-emitting isotopes and emission-computed axial tomography to measure regional tissue function (see p. 569 for SPECT). Like a CT scan, the PET scanner, which is shaped like a giant tire, does transverse imagery. The injected or inhaled radionuclide will emit radioactivity in the form of positrons that are identified and transformed into a visual display by a computer. The most commonly used positron-emitting radiolabels are oxygen 15 and fluorene 18-fluorodeoxyglucose.

The PET studies are noninvasive tests used most commonly to determine physiologic function of the brain and heart. However, the technique is applicable to the examination of all parts of the body for the diagnosis and staging of disease and monitoring therapy. Unlike MR and CT scans, PET can provide physiologic, anatomic, and biochemical data. Although PET is more sensitive than SPECT, it is considerably more expensive. At this time, use of the PET is mainly in large medical centers with a large number of experimental studies being done.

Uses of PET

Positron emission tomography may be used for a variety of physiologic activities, including

1. Blood flow
2. Tissue metabolism
3. Blood volume
4. Tissue density

Because brain studies are the most common procedures performed, a discussion of PET will be limited accordingly.

Procedure for Brain Studies

1. An intravenous line will be inserted into both hands or arms—one is for injecting the radionuclide, the other is for drawing blood samples.
2. The patient will sit in a reclining couch next to the scanner. A radionuclide is injected intravenously into an arm vein. Scanning will begin 45 minutes later if the brain is to be examined. This is the period of time needed for the radioactive substances to concentrate the brain tissue.
3. If a mental activity such as speech or reading is to be checked, the patient will be asked to do letter recognition activities or read. Some reasoning or remembering functions will be determined by asking the patient to recite the Pledge of Allegiance to himself, to think of words beginning with a specific letter.
4. The patient will be blindfolded and ears plugged with cotton to remove stimuli.
5. The test takes 45 to 60 minutes to complete. At the present time, it takes three to five persons to operate the scanner and cyclotron for just one test.

Clinical Implications

A. Abnormal results are associated with several brain disorders.
   1. In epilepsy focal areas with increased metabolism have been seen during the actual stage of epilepsy, and decreased oxygen utilization and blood flow during the interictal stage. It is proving to be the best test for locating damaged brain tissues in

persons with severe forms of epilepsy. In these cases, it is possible to remove this tissue surgically with greater precision.

2. Profound striatal hypometabolism in Huntington's disease
3. In stroke, an extremely complex pathophysiologic picture is being revealed: anaerobic glycolysis, depressed oxygen utilization, and decreased blood flow. In a cerebrovascular aneurysm, if the patient cannot speak, the test can determine if part of the brain that controls speech is still viable.
4. In dementia the hypothesis of chronic cerebral anoxia has been refuted and instead is beginning to reveal focal disturbances of protein synthesis in this disease. Positron emission tomography is used to differentiate Alzheimer's disease and other types of dementia from depression in older persons.
5. In schizophrenia, some studies using labeled glucose indicate reduced metabolic activity in the frontal region. The PET scans can also distinguish the developmental stages of cranial tumors and give information about operability of such tumors.
6. In brain tumors, data have been collected concerning oxygen use and blood flow relationships for these tumors. Gliomas have relatively good perfusion in comparison to their decreased oxygen utilization. The high uptake of ^{18}FDG in gliomas is reported to correlate with the tumor's histological grade.

B. Other clinical implications are as follows:

1. Heart: In coronary artery disease, during exercise-induced ischemia, focal disturbances of cation extraction occur in the myocardium. These changes persist beyond the time the ECG changes have reverted to normal and angina pain has ceased. The PET scans can be used to monitor heartbeat and is one of the best ways to determine how much of the heart has been damaged.
   (a) Future use as a screening tool for coronary artery disease
   (b) Study of the metabolic state of the heart to determine the rate at which fatty acids are used for energy (a crucial factor in the development of myopathies)
   (c) PET may provide more information than other modalities concerning the state and extent of myocardial infarctions.
2. Lungs: Presence of chronic pulmonary edema. In pneumonia, it has been possible to measure uptake of C-labeled erythromycin. The concentration of antibiotic at the site of infection is related to minimum inhibitory concentration of the microorganisms.
3. Breast: Tumors show a relatively high rate of vascularity.

Interfering Factors

Excessive anxiety can ruin test results when brain function is being tested.

Clinical Considerations

1. Diabetics should take final pretest dose of long-acting insulin prior to eating a meal 3 to 4 hours before testing. After that time, no insulin or any other drug that alters glucose metabolism should be taken.
2. Tranquilizers cannot be given before the test because they alter glucose metabolism.
3. Thorough preparation for the testing experience will make the difference between a successful or unsuccessful outcome and production of usable results.

Patient Preparation

1. Advise the patient to abstain from alcohol, caffeine, and tobacco for 24 hours.
2. Explain the purpose, procedure, benefits, and risks of the test. The level of radiation is short-lived and approximate to that from 5 to 6 radiographs of the chest and less than a quarter of the radiation absorbed during a CT scan of the brain. Repeat or sequential studies can be carried out over short periods of minutes to hours.
3. Advise the patient that lying as still as possible during the scan is necessary. However, the patient is not to fall asleep or count to pass the time.
4. Use measures to reduce anxiety and help the patient manage stress, such as progressive relaxation and breathing techniques.

Patient Aftercare

1. The patient is cautioned not to stand up too quickly after the test is completed to prevent postural hypertension.
2. Advise that urination should occur soon after the scan to clear the radiopharmaceutical from the bladder.

BIBLIOGRAPHY

Bernier DR, Christian PE, Langan JK, et al: Nuclear Medicine Technology and Techniques, 2nd ed. St. Louis, CV Mosby, 1989

Burks J, et al: Radiation exposure to nursing personnel from patients receiving diagnostic radionuclides. Heart Lung 2:217–220, May/June, 1982

Chard T: An Introduction to Radioimmunoassay and Related Techniques. New York, Elsevier Biomedical Press, 1982

D'Agincourt L: PET's diagnostic prowess widens its clinical appeal. Diagn Imag 11(10):90–99, October, 1989

Early PJ, Sodee DB: Principles and Practice of Nuclear Medicine. St. Louis, CV Mosby, 1985

Freeman LM (ed): Current concepts in diagnostic nuclear medicine. Mediphysics 3(4), 1986; 4(2), 1987; 4(3), 1987

Freeman LM (ed): Advances in functional neuroimaging. Mediphysics 1(20), 1988; 1(4), 1988; 2(3), 1989

Harbert J, Rocha A: Textbook of Nuclear Medicine, vol 2. Clinical Applications. Philadelphia, Lea & Febiger, 1984

Maisey MN, Fogelman E: An Atlas of Clinical Nuclear Medicine. St. Louis, CV Mosby, 1988

McDonagh A: Getting your patient ready for a nuclear scan. Nursing '91 21(2):53–57, February, 1991

Plankey EL, Plankey MW: Prep talk: A nuclear approach to cancer detection. Am J Nurs 9(6): June, 1990

Porth CM: Pathophysiology: Concepts of Altered Health States, 3rd ed. Philadelphia, JB Lippincott, 1990

Syncor International Corporation, Product Information of Pharmaceuticals, 1982

Watson LR et al: Adjunctive use of ultrasonography in the management of kidney stones treated by ESWL. Appl Radiol 19(4):19–23, April, 1990

COMMON X-RAY STUDIES

Introduction

General Principles

X-ray studies (also known as *radiographs* or *roentgenograms*) are used to examine the soft and bony tissues of the body. X-rays (roentgen rays) are electromagnetic vibrations of very short wavelength produced when fast-moving electrons hit various substances. They are similar to light rays except that their wavelength is only 1/10,000 the length of visible light rays. Because of their short wavelength, x-rays have the ability to penetrate very dense substances and to produce an image or shadow that can be recorded on photographic film. The entire principle of radiography depends on differences in density between various body structures, which produce shadows of varying intensity on the x-ray film.

In x-ray examinations, a high-voltage electric current is passed through a "target" made of tungsten in a vacuum tube. Less than 1% of the high-speed electrons (cathode rays) are transformed into x-rays; the rest of the energy is transformed into heat.

X-rays travel in straight lines at the speed of light. When a beam of rays passes through matter, its intensity is reduced by absorption. The greater the density of matter, the greater the degree of absorption. A photographic film is affected by x-rays, just as it is affected by light. The sensitive silver emulsion of the film undergoes a chemical change when it has been exposed to radiation. The film is subsequently processed by development and fixation, resulting in an image that is black, white, and various tones of gray. This image will be an accurate representation of the variable densities of the tissue through which the beam has passed. Third generation x-ray equipment uses high-resolution techniques, TV screens, digital magnetic records, and laser driven printers that produce much sharper pictures of bones and organs.

Use of Contrast Media

Many radiographic techniques can use the natural contrasts that exist in body tissue—air, water (in soft tissue), fat, and bone. The lungs and gastrointestinal tract normally contain gases; certain body structures are encased in a fatty envelope, and bone has naturally occurring mineral salts. However, diagnosis of certain pathologic conditions at times requires the visualization of details not revealed through plain film radiography. These details can be highlighted through administration of *contrast media*, which can be inserted orally, rectally, or through injection.

The ideal contrast medium should be harmless, inert, and should not interfere with any physiologic function. It may be either radiopaque (not permitting the transmission of x-rays) or radiolucent (permitting the transmission of x-rays but still offering some resistance).

However, there is really no safe contrast media; any foreign material put into the body can cause reactions.

Certain contrast media are used routinely in radiographic studies.

1. Barium sulfate (radiopaque)
   (a) Used in gastrointestinal studies
   (b) Prepared in a colloidal suspension
   (c) Effectively demonstrates small filling defects
2. Organic iodides (radiopaque)
   (a) Examples: sodium diatrizoate, meglumine diatrizoate, metrizamide and the new, "nonionic" agents
   (b) Used for studies of the kidney, liver, blood vessels, urinary bladder, and urethra
   (c) Water-soluble iodide used in myelography (study of the spinal cord after contrast media have been injected)
3. Iodized oils (radiopaque)
   Used in myelography, bronchography (study of the lung after contrast media have been injected), and lymphangiograms
4. Oxygen, helium, air, carbon dioxide, nitrous oxide, and nitrogen (radiolucent substances)
   Used for visualization of the brain, joints, subarachnoid space, pleural space, peritoneal cavity, and pericardial space

Adverse Reactions to Contrast Media

The administration of contrast media can sometimes cause allergic reactions in certain persons. The degree of reaction may range from mild (causing such symptoms as nausea and vomiting) to severe (causing cardiovascular collapse, central nervous system depression, and death, if untreated).

Table 10–1 indicates the range of possible adverse reactions to iodine contrast media.

Clinical Considerations When Iodine Contrast Media Is Used

1. The highest incidence of side effects occurs in patients 20 to 49 years of age; the lowest incidence, after 70 years of age.
2. The patient who has had an allergic reaction to iodine contrast media should have this fact noted on his or her medical records. Such a patient possibly can have subsequent adverse reactions; the risk rises three to four times, although the second reaction is not necessarily more severe. The patient should also be told that he or she has had an allergic response to a specific substance.
3. Check to see when the patient last had a full meal before sending him or her to the x-ray department. Except in an extreme emergency, iodine contrast media should never be administered intravenously sooner than 90 minutes after eating. In most instances, the patient should be given nothing by mouth (NPO) the night before any radiographic testing employing iodine contrast media.

TABLE 10–1.
Signs and Symptoms of Reactions to Iodinated Contrast Media

Cardiovascular	Respiratory	Cutaneous	Gastrointestinal	Neurological	Urinary
Pallor	Sneezing	Erythema	Nausea	Anxiety	Flank pain
Diaphoresis	Coughing	Feeling of	Vomiting	Headache	Hematuria
Tachycardia	Rhinorrhea	warmth	Metallic taste	Dizziness	Oliguria
Bradycardia	Wheezing	Parotitis	Abdominal cramps	Agitation	Albuminuria
Palpitations	Acute asthma	Urticaria	Diarrhea	Vertigo	WBCs in blood
Arrhythmia	attack	Pruritis	Paralytic ileus	Slurred speech	Acute renal
Acute pulmonary	Laryngospasm	Pain at injection		Disorientation	failure
edema	Cyanosis	site		Stupor	
Shock	Laryngeal	Angioneurotic		Coma	
Congestive heart	edema	edema		Convulsions	
failure	Apnea				
Cardiac arrest	Respiratory				
	arrest				

(*Sources: Abrams HL [ed]: Abrams Angiography, 3rd ed. Boston, Little Brown & Co, 1983. Abrams HL, Skuras J [eds]: Radiographic Contrast Agents. Rockville, MD, Aspen Publishers, Inc., 1989. Tortorice MR: Fundamentals of Angiography. St. Louis, CV Mosby, 1982)*

4. Be aware that death from an allergic reaction can occur if severe symptoms go untreated. Staff in attendance must be able to give cardiopulmonary resuscitation.
5. Promptly administer oral antihistamines per the physician's order if mild to moderate reactions to iodine contrast substances occur.
6. When coordinating x-ray testing that uses contrast media, keep in mind that iodine and barium do not mix.
7. Some physiologic change can be expected whenever an iodine contrast substance is injected, as in an intravenous pyelogram (IVP). The types of changes that can be seen are hypotension, hypertension, tachycardia, or arrhythmias. For this reason, always check the blood pressure, pulse, and respiration before and after these tests.
8. Instruct patients that large amounts of fluids should be taken to promote frequent urination to flush the iodine from the body.
9. Assess for these additional contraindications to iodinated contrast:
   (a) Patients with sickle cell anemia—use may increase sickling effect
   (b) Patients with syphilis—use may lead to nephrotic syndrome
   (c) Patients in long-term steroid therapy—some of drug may be rendered inactive by contrast
   (d) Patients with pheochromocytoma—use may produce a sudden, perhaps fatal, rise in blood pressure
   (e) Patients with hyperthyroidism

Clinical Alert

1. Prevent the need for repeat examination through careful preparation. Because any diagnostic radiogram has some risk, there is a great responsibility to monitor and guide patients carefully. This responsibility is amplified when examinations using contrast media are employed.
2. Risks are involved in repeated x-ray testing and use of contrast media. There is really no safe contrast medium; any foreign material put into the body can cause reactions. For example, in cancer diagnosis, the benefit of early detection outweighs the dangers of cumulative radiation. In a person undergoing a workup for cancer, the risks of x-ray testing should be deemphasized to help reduce anxiety that can be overwhelming in these persons. However, the facts about risk must be given because the patient has a legal right to this information.

Clinical Considerations when Barium Contrast Is Used

There is always a danger when introducing barium sulfate or similar contrast media into the gastrointestinal tract.

1. Barium radiography may interfere with many other abdominal examinations. There are a number of studies, including other x-rays, tests using iodine, ultrasound procedures, radioisotope studies, tomograms, computerized scanning, and proctoscopy, that must be scheduled prior to barium studies. Consult with the x-ray department for the best sequencing of barium studies with other ordered examinations.
2. Emphasize that a laxative should be taken after a procedure is completed if barium sulfate is used during the examination.
3. Elderly, inactive persons should be checked for impaction. The first sign of impaction in the elderly may be fainting.
4. Observe and record stools for color and consistency to determine that the barium has been evacuated. Stools should be checked for at least 2 days. Stools will be light in color until all barium has been expelled. Outpatients should be given a written reminder to inspect stools for 2 days.
5. Avoid giving narcotics, especially codeine, when barium x-rays are ordered because there is a tendency for these drugs to interfere with the elimination of barium from the gastrointestinal tract.
6. Be prepared for complications. Barium may aggravate acute ulcerative colitis or cause an obstruction in the bowel, ranging from partial to complete obstruction.
7. Barium should *not* be used as a contrast for intestinal study when a bowel perforation is suspected. Leakage of barium through a perforation may cause peritonitis. Iodinated contrasts should be used when perforations are suspected.

There are special clinical considerations for ostomy patients undergoing bowel preparation for contrast x-ray testing of the gastrointestinal tract (barium enema, colon x-ray, upper gastrointestinal series, and gallbladder study/oral cholecystogram).

1. A successful outcome depends upon communication of specific, objective information that differs from the standardized information usually given by a radiology department.
2. In most cases, the standard dietary restrictions and medications will apply, but modifications are made in procedures involving mechanical bowel cleansing with enemas, and physiologic cleansing with laxatives.

Clinical Alerts for Patients With Ostomies

1. An enema and laxatives should never be given to a person with an ileostomy in preparation for x-ray filming or endoscopy. Administering an enema would put the person with an ileostomy at risk for dehydration and electrolyte imbalance. However, a person with a sigmoid colostomy needs an enema for x-ray or endoscopy. For this reason, it is very important to identify the type of stoma the patient has because not all colostomies need irrigation. For example, a person with an ascending right-sided colostomy will normally pass a liquid, pasty stool that is high in water content and digestive enzymes; such a patient may have laxatives, and no enema.
2. Notify the radiology staff that the person has an ostomy, so that department can be prepared.
3. Advise patients, both hospitalized and outpatient, to have extra pouches with them during tests, especially if the pouch needs to be removed for the procedure.

See page 653 for specifics of barium enema preparation for ostomies, ileostomies, and colostomies.

Xeroradiography: Overview
Xeroradiography differs from traditional x-ray examinations in that the image is created on a photoconductive surface of selenium rather than on a silver halide film. The selenium plate is housed in a cassette to protect it from rough handling and from light.

Xeroradiography is a photoelectric process; traditional film radiography is primarily a photochemical process. This relatively new technique uses the technology of the office copier to process x-ray images on paper.

Several distinct advantages exist in the use of this method: it offers a very high degree of resolution; small point densities can be easily distinguished because of greater contrast, and the xeroradiographs are easily interpreted.

Xeroradiography has been found useful in radiography of the extremities and especially in soft-tissue studies. Radiographic study of the breast is the prime use of this technique. Patient exposure during a xeromammogram is less than 1 radiation absorbed dose (rad).

Computed Tomography (CT): Overview
Computed tomography (CT), also called CT scanning and computerized axial tomography (CAT), uses x-rays similar to those used in conventional radiography but with a special machine having a scanner

system. The x-rays in conventional radiography pass through the body, and an image of bone, soft tissues, and air is projected onto film. In CT scans, a computer provides rapid complex calculations determining the degree of multiple x-ray beams that are not absorbed by all the tissue in its path. The single most valuable function of CT scanning is to provide the geography and characteristics of tissue structures within solid organs. Because it is basically an anatomic technique, which measures the attenuation coefficient of tissue, it is not useful for measurement of tissue perfusion, metabolism, or vessel blood flow. For this reason, it is not the best technique to evaluate small atrioventricular malformations, early ischemic disease of the brain, or subdural hematomas.

Digital Radiography and Fluorography: Overview
Digital radiography is similar to CT in that it is a computer-based imaging modality with exceptionally high spatial resolution. An ordinary x-ray beam contains far more information about body structure and physiology than it is possible to record in x-ray film, and some information is lost. The lost information includes the compression of three-dimensional data to two dimensions, some decrease in spatial resolution, a reduction in ability to visualize soft tissue, organs, and vascular structures, and the inability to obtain accurate information about blood flow, volume, and ejection fractions. This information is regained to a great extent by digital radiography. Images may be computer-enhanced or otherwise manipulated. Digital storage of the data allows for instant recall of radiological images for review.

Digital Subtraction Imaging: Overview
Digital subtraction angiography (DSA) is a computer-aided method that results in an image of arterial anatomy that is free from the superimposition of surrounding osseous anatomy. Digital subtraction images are produced in this way: Basically, a fluoroscopic image is converted from analog to digital form; the image is stored digitally as a matrix, with a varying number of picture elements (pixels); after each image is converted to digital form, the first image or mask is subtracted from the object image, pixel by pixel. As in CT, the number of pixels into which the image is divided influences the quality of the image, the complexity of the computer needed, and the speed at which images can be processed.

Limitations
1. The patient risk is about the same as that of a conventional intravenous urography (IVU) examination.
2. For examination of the abdomen and lower extremities, inadequate field size necessitates multiple iodine injections.
3. This procedure is not for everyone. It is well suited for many per-

sons in the 40 to 65 age group. It is not appropriate for the extremely sick or for those with preinfarction angina.

Advantages
1. The 120 ml required by standard angiography is reduced to 30 ml. This reduces the risks of contrast toxicity and injury to the blood vessels.
2. Contrast can be infused through a smaller catheter, a no. 5 French rather than a no. 8. The likelihood of complications following the procedure is less and enables the procedure to be done on an outpatient basis in many cases.
3. Improved recording. Digital system records on disks for less than 1 minute.
4. Computer measurements of percentage of blocking can be made.
5. High-quality, computer-enhanced images filtered in real time can be instantly replayed on a TV monitor. This information can be taped and stored on standard video cassettes.
6. Can enhance standard arteriograms. For example, using this technique, the small blood vessels are hard to visualize with a standard arteriogram. In addition, selective studies can be performed with a much smaller amount of contrast.

Magnetic Resonance Imaging, MR, NMR: Overview
Magnetic resonance (MR), formerly called nuclear magnetic resonance (NMR), is a new noninvasive, nonionic technique that produces cross-sectional images of the human anatomy obtained by exposure to magnetic energy sources, but without using radiation. A description is given in this chapter because, although it is not an x-ray method, it is a diagnostic service offered by many x-ray departments in larger medical centers. This versatile device is used primarily in three diagnostic areas: to study blood flow and determine the condition of blood vessels; for *in vivo* spectroscopy to infer tissue pH and energy state; and in whole body imaging to detect tumors, sites of infection, and differentiation of diseased tissues from healthy tissues. The MR machines are essentially large magnets fitted with a group of field control coils. Atomic nuclei, when placed in a magnetic field and stimulated by a particular radio frequency, emit measurable radio signals that are influenced by the type and condition of tissue composed of these nuclei. These radio signals are detected and converted to a visual display on a computer monitor or etched on magnetic tape for later playback on a video screen. (See Chap. 15 for complete explanation of testing.)

Angiography: Overview
Angiography is a method of using x-ray examinations to study the vascular structures of the body. This method involves the injection of

an organic contrast solution (such as iodine) by a catheter inserted into the femoral artery (the usual site, but the brachial artery is also used). The catheter is placed selectively into the artery under fluoroscopic control by the radiologist performing the examination. After satisfactory x-ray films have been obtained, the catheter is removed and direct pressure is held on the puncture site until bleeding is controlled. The patient is usually instructed to remain at complete bed rest for approximately 6 hours.

The terms given to the variety of studies performed are based on the vascular structure to be studied and the method of injection. *Arteriography* refers to contrast studies of arterial vessels. Venous structures can also be seen in later stages of these examinations. *Venography* is a contrast study of peripheral or central veins. *Lymphography* is a contrast study of lymph vessels and nodes. *Angiocardiography* is an investigation of the interior of the heart using a contrast solution. During this examination, the great vessels such as the pulmonary arteries can be seen. *Aortography* refers to a contrast study of either the thoracic aorta (*thoracic aortography*) or the abdominal aorta (*abdominal aortography*) and *lumbar aortography*.

Angiographic examinations may also be named by the route of injection. For example, *renal arteriography* is performed by inserting a catheter into the abdominal aorta and then into the renal artery. In *peripheral arteriography*, an injection may be made directly into the vessel under study, such as the femoral artery. The injection may also be done by the venous method. For example, in venous aortography, a large bolus of contrast medium is injected into a peripheral vein. As the contrast flows through the right side of the heart, lung, and left side of the heart, x-ray films are taken.

Indications for Angiography
1. Examination of cervical carotid arteries
2. Examination of intracranial arteries
3. Before transsphenoidal hypophysectomy
4. Postoperative evaluation
5. Detection of superior sagittal sinus thrombosis
6. Identification of renal and iliac arteries in relation to an abdominal aortic aneurysm
7. Accurate screening examination for renovascular hypertension. In this instance, the study can be performed before a routine IVP using the same dose of contrast material.
8. Periodic reevaluation of arterial angioplasty
9. Vascular integrity can be confirmed in traumatic lesions.
10. Vascular grafts can be followed for patency.

Risks of Radiation

Exposure of the human body to x-rays carries certain risks. These risks are of two types: genetic and somatic. If the genital organs are exposed to radiation, the reproductive cells (specifically, the DNA within the chromosomes) may undergo mutations. These mutations can cause changes in the offspring of the patient. Somatic changes (those occurring in body tissue other than the reproductive cells) may occur in parts of the patient's body receiving excessive doses of radiation or receiving repeated exposure.

The dangers of exposure to radiation arise not only from the absorption of relatively large amounts of radiation received over a short period of time but also from the cumulative effects of very small amounts received over months or years. Moreover, the cumulative effects of radiation may not become evident for several years. Radiation can increase the risk of cancer after a latent period of many years.

A woman in the first trimester of pregnancy especially is at risk. A developing embryo or fetus that is exposed to high levels of ionizing radiation is very likely to be born with abnormalities (see Tables 10–2, 10–3, and 10–4).

Safety Measures
Certain precautions must be taken to protect medical/nursing personnel, patients, and any technical staff assisting in the x-ray examination from unnecessary exposure to radiation.

General Precautions
1. Patients, radiologists, and other staff in the radiology laboratory should wear lead aprons and gloves when not occupying a shielded booth during x-ray exposure.
2. The x-ray tube housing should be checked periodically to prevent leakage.
3. The patient's medical records should be carefully checked to determine the frequency of diagnostic radiologic examinations and the dosage received with each study.
4. X-ray tubes should have additional layers of aluminum to act as filtering devices that will reduce the exposure to radiation without sacrificing detail.
5. Fast film as well as a screen enhancing the action of x-rays should be used.
6. Adjustable or fixed cones as well as diaphragms can be used to reduce exposure to the lowest possible level. These devices will restrict the area being radiated, avoiding excessive peripheral exposure.
7. The gonads should be shielded on all patients capable of producing children unless the examination is of the abdomen or the gonad area.

TABLE 10–2.
Estimated Mean Dose to Uterus/Embryo From Common X-Rays and Scans

Beam Radiation*	Dose Equivalent (rem)
Skull	<0.01
Chest	<0.01
Upper GI series	0.048
Barium enema	0.822
Cholecystogram	<0.02
Intravenous pyelogram	0.814
Abdomen, KUB	0.263
Lumbosacral spine	0.639
Pelvis	0.194
Hip	0.128

Radionuclide Scans†	Dose Equivalent (rem)
Liver (4mCi ^{99m}Tc)	0.028
Bone (20mCi ^{99m}Tc)	0.500
Gallium (5mCi ^{67}Ga)	1.250
Thyroid (5mCi ^{99m}Tc)	0.135

* For the type of radiation used in hospitals, rads and rems are interchangeable. Radiation dose absorbed by the body is measured in rems or rads (mrem or nrad).
† Adapted from Kereiakes JG, Rosenstein M: Handbook of Radiation Doses in Nuclear Medicine and Diagnostic X-Ray. Boca Raton, FL, CRC Press, 1980, p 211, and Husak V, Wiedermann M: Radiation absorbed dose estimates to the embryo from some nuclear medicine procedures. Eur J Nucl Med 5(3):205–207, 1980.

TABLE 10–3.
Estimated Genetic Effects of Radiation per Million Liveborn Offspring*

Genetic Disorder	Incidence	Additional Effects of Exposure of 1 rem/30-Year Generation	
		First Generation	*Later Generations*
Autosomal dominant and X-linked	10,000	5–65	40–200
Irregularly inherited	90,000	Very few	20–900
Recessive	1,000	Very few	Very slow increase
Chromosomal aberrations	6,000	<10	Slight increase

* Adapted from National Research Council Committee on the Biological Effects of Ionizing Radiation: The Effects on Populations of Exposure to Low Levels of Ionizing Radiation, (BEIRIII). Washington, DC, National Academy Press, 1980, p 85

TABLE 10–4.

Understanding Radiation Risks; Gonad and Bone
Marrow Doses of Common X-Ray Procedures

Gonad dose is estimated amount of radiation absorbed by
the ovaries and testes. Exceeding this dose may have genetic effects. Bone marrow dose is estimated amount of
radiation absorbed by bone marrow.

Relatively High Gonad Dose—Adult (over 100 mrad)	Moderate Gonad Dose—Adult (10–100 mrad)	Low Gonad Dose—Adult (less than 10 mrad)
Lumbar spine, lumbo-sacral vertebrae	Stomach and upper gastrointestinal tract	Head (including cervical spine)
Pelvis	Cholecystography, cholangiography	Dental (full mouth)
Hip and femur (upper third)	Femur (lower two thirds)	Arm (including forearm and hand)
Urography	Dorsal spine	Bony thorax (ribs, sternum, clavicle, shoulder)
	Abdomen	
Retrograde pyelography		Dorsal spine
Urethrocystography		
Lower gastrointestinal tract		Lower leg, foot
		Chest (heart, lung) including mass miniature radiography)
Abdomen		
Obstetric abdomen		
Pelvimetry		
Hysterosalpingography		

Relatively High Bone-Marrow Dose—Adult (400–2000 mrad)	Moderate Bone-Marrow Dose—Adult (50–400 mrad)	Low Bone-Marrow Dose—Adult (less than 50 mrad)
Pelvimetry	Retrograde pyelography	Femur, hip
Lower gastrointestinal tract	Urethrocystography	Head, chest, heart, lung

(continued)

TABLE 10–4.
(continued)

Relatively High Bone-Marrow Dose— Adult (400–2000 mrad)	Moderate Bone-Marrow Dose— Adult (50–400 mrad)	Low Bone-Marrow Dose—Adult (less than 50 mrad)
Urography	Hysterosalpingography Stomach and upper gastrointestinal tract Lumbar or dorsal spine, lumbosacral Pelvis, abdomen Cholecystography, cholangiography Bony thorax (ribs, sternum, clavicle, shoulder)	Dental (full mouth) Extremities (hand, foot)

Precautions to Be Used With Pregnant Patients

1. Women of childbearing age who possibly could be in the first trimester of pregnancy should *not* have x-ray examinations. A brief menstrual history should be taken to determine if the woman is or could be pregnant. If any doubt exists about whether the woman is pregnant, she should *not* risk having the examination until a pregnancy test is done.
2. Pregnant patients (at any time during the pregnancy) should avoid radiographic studies of the pelvic region, lumbar spine, and abdomen, or procedures involving serial film or fluoroscopy.
3. If films are made for obstetric reasons, *repeat films* should be avoided.
4. If x-ray studies are made of body parts other than the pelvic area (*e.g.*, of the teeth), the woman should wear a lead apron to cover the abdominal and pelvic regions.

Responsibilities in Ordering and Scheduling X-Ray Examinations

All radiology requisitions should include the correct spelling of the patient's name, age, and diagnosis. The purpose and procedure of the x-ray examination should be carefully explained to the patient. Written instruction sheets with directions for the x-ray examination are most beneficial.

When a complete gastrointestinal series is scheduled for the same day, the order of x-ray examination is as follows: (1) gallbladder x-ray; (2) barium enema; (3) upper gastrointestinal x-ray.

Barium studies should be scheduled *after* gallbladder studies because the barium will interfere with the results of the gallbladder x-rays. Thyroid scans and ^{131}I uptake tests must be performed prior to the gallbladder x-ray because the oral iodine contrast will adversely alter nuclear test results.

X-ray examinations that do not require preparation and that can be ordered when the radiology department and the patient agree on a mutual time are chest x-ray, extremity x-rays, KUB (kidney, ureter, bladder) x-rays, and mammograms.

Chest Radiography

Normal Values
Normal chest
Normal bony thorax (all bones present and in position, symmetry, and
    shape)
Normal soft tissues
Normal mediastinum
Normal lungs (proper number of lobes, position, and alteration)
Normal pleura
Normal heart (aortic arch and abdominal arteries)

Explanation of Test
The chest x-ray is the radiograph requested most frequently. This examination is very important in the diagnosis of cancer, tuberculosis, and other lung diseases, pulmonary disease, and diseases of the mediastinum and bony thorax. The chest x-ray is also a record of the presence or absence of disease on the date it was taken, and any x-ray studies that follow this date determine progress or development of the disease. This study can also give valuable information on the condition of the heart, lungs, gastrointestinal tract, and thyroid gland. It is also important that a chest x-ray be done after the insertion of chest tubes and subclavian catheters to determine the position of these devices and possible pneumothorax. In addition, positions of other devices such as nasogastric tubes and enteric feeding tubes are easily determined. Without x-ray or fluoroscopy, it cannot be ascertained that enteral feeding tubes are positioned beyond the pylorus.

Procedure
1. Routine radiography consists of anterior, posterior, and lateral (front, back, and side) views of the chest. It is usually performed with the patient in a standing position. Upright films of the chest are of utmost importance, because films taken with the patient supine will not demonstrate fluid levels. This is especially important to observe when testing persons confined to bed.
2. Clothing is removed to the waist.

3. The patient is asked to take a deep breath and exhale; then he or she is required to take a deep breath and hold it while the picture is taken.
4. The procedure takes only a few minutes.

Clinical Implications

1. Abnormal results will indicate these conditions of the lungs:
   - (a) Aplasia
   - (b) Hypoplasia
   - (c) Cysts
   - (d) Lobar pneumonia
   - (e) Bronchopneumonia
   - (f) Aspiration pneumonia
   - (g) Pulmonary brucellosis
   - (h) Viral pneumonia
   - (i) Lung abscess
   - (j) Middle lobe syndrome
   - (k) Pneumothorax
   - (l) Pleural effusion
   - (m) Atelectasis
   - (n) Pneumonitis
   - (o) Congenital pulmonary cysts
   - (p) Pulmonary tuberculosis
   - (q) Sarcoidosis
   - (r) Pneumoconiosis (*e.g.*, asbestosis)
   - (s) Westermark's sign indicates decreased pulmonary vascularity, sometimes thought to suggest pulmonary embolus
2. Abnormal results will indicate these conditions of the bony thorax:
   - (a) Scoliosis
   - (b) Hemivertebrae
   - (c) Kyphosis
   - (d) Trauma
   - (e) Sarcoma
   - (f) Bone destruction

Interfering Factors

An important consideration in interpreting chest radiographs is whether the film is in "full inspiration." Certain conditions do not allow the patient to inspire fully. The following conditions should be considered when radiographs are evaluated:

1. Obesity
2. Severe pain
3. Congestive heart failure
4. Scarring of lung tissue

Chest Tomography

Normal Values

Same as for chest x-ray

Explanation of Test

Chest tomograms are particularly useful in the study of patients with pulmonary tuberculosis, the compressed lung beneath a thoracoplasty, and study of lung abscess. They are also used to outline detailed anatomy of the lung, mediastinum, and thoracic structures in which an abnormality is observed in the chest film and to outline the vascular pattern in emphysema, pulmonary hypertension, and pulmonary vascular abnormalities.

Clinical Implications
Abnormal results will reveal the following:

1. Cavities and nodular infiltration in tuberculosis that is not visible on routine x-ray films
2. Bronchiectasis associated with tuberculosis
3. Outline of tumor in patients with bronchogenic carcinoma
4. Calcium in small parenchymal nodules
5. Site of a bronchial occlusion

Radiography and Tomography of the Paranasal Sinuses

Normal Values
Normal sinuses are radiolucent because of their air content. The paranasal sinuses are paired cavities lined by mucous membranes that arise as outpouchings from the nasal fossa and extend into the maxillary, ethmoid, sphenoid, and frontal bones. They are named according to the bones in which they develop.

Explanation of Test
Radiographs of the sinuses are used to detect the unilateral or bilateral diseases that may affect them and that may cause detectable alterations. Tomograms of the sinuses are usually done to outline foreign bodies, to determine the presence or extent of bony tumor involvement, and to determine the extent and location of fractures of the bony walls of the sinuses and nasal bones.

Procedure
1. If possible, the patient should be in an upright sitting position during the examination of the sinuses. This will allow demonstration of fluid levels when they are present.
2. The patient is usually required to have his or her head placed in a padded vice headbrace that restricts movement but is comfortable.
3. The examination may take 10 to 15 minutes to complete.

Clinical Implications
Abnormal results will reveal the following:

1. Acute sinusitis
2. Chronic sinusitis
3. Cysts (retention and nonsecreting)

4. Mucocele
5. Polyps
6. Tumors of the bone and soft tissue
7. Allergic reactions
8. Trauma
9. Foreign bodies

Patient Preparation
Explain the purpose and procedure of the test.

Cardiac Radiography

Normal Values
Normal size and shape of heart, aorta, pulmonary arteries, and pulmonary vascularity

Explanation of Test
Diagnosis of cardiovascular disorders may involve a wide range of diagnostic procedures. There are, however, three routine radiographic imaging techniques that are used for the evaluation of the heart. They are as follows:

1. Plain film radiography
2. Fluoroscopy
3. Cardiac series

The heart may also be evaluated by more sophisticated radiographic studies (*e.g.*, cardiac catheterization) or by procedures that are discussed in more detail in other chapters (*e.g.*, ultrasound studies, radioisotope scans).

Use of Routine Procedures
Plain-film radiography

1. Routine screening technique with all suspected cardiac patients
2. Useful for determining cardiac size

Fluoroscopic examination

1. For assessing heart motion and dynamics
2. For determining whether calcification exists in heart
3. For investigating suspected pericardial effusion
4. For verifying position of pacemaker electrodes
5. For guiding movement of catheter in cardiac catheterization

Cardiac series
This radiographic procedure is a four-view examination. Generally, the patient will be asked to swallow barium during the following views:

1. Posteroanterior view
2. Lateral view
3. Right anterior oblique view
4. Left anterior oblique view

Cardioangiography (angiography of the heart)
   This procedure is technically quite difficult and places the patient at risk. A large quantity of contrast material must be introduced rapidly into the blood vessels, and films must be exposed rapidly so that the blood vessels can be visualized. A radiopaque contrast material containing iodine is injected directly into one of the heart chambers, the greater vessels, or the coronary arteries by a catheter (see section on *cardiac catheterization* in Chap. 15 for more information).

Note: Cardioangiography is the most invasive and thus the most potentially dangerous of all the diagnostic procedures. In many medical facilities, the technique is being replaced by CT scanning, echocardiography, or digital subtraction.

Orthopedic Radiography

Normal Values
Normal osseous and soft-tissue structures

Explanation of Test
Orthopedic x-ray testing is a general radiographic examination of a particular bone, group of bones, or a joint of the body. The bony or osseous system has five functions of radiologic significance. They are support of the body, locomotion, housing of red marrow, calcium storage, and protection of underlying vessical structures.
   The success of orthopedic x-ray examinations depends upon good immobilization of the part being studied. In order to produce a thorough study of the body part, at least two projections are required, usually 90 degrees to one another. For examination of more complex structures such as the spine and skull, multiple projections are required, thus increasing the length of time of the examination.

Procedure
1. The patient is not required to fast.
2. During the examination, the patient may sit, stand, or lie on an examining table. Typically, the body part is examined from several different positions, which may require some manipulation of the body part.
3. Jewelry, clothing with zippers, snaps, and so forth, which will interfere with the examination of the part, must be removed.

4. Medical hardware used to stabilize a traumatized area must sometimes be removed. This is done only with the consent of the attending physician and possibly requires assistance of the nursing staff.

Clinical Implications
Abnormal results are indicated by the following pathology:

1. Fractures
2. Dislocations
3. Arthritis
4. Osteoporosis
5. Osteomyelitis
6. Degenerative joint disease
7. Hydrocephalus
8. Sarcoma
9. Aseptic necrosis
10. Paget's disease
11. Gout
12. Acromegaly
13. Metastases
14. Myeloma
15. *Osteochondrosis, i.e.,* Legg–Calvé–Perthes, Osgood–Schlatter
16. Bone infarcts
17. Histiocytosis X
18. Bone tumors (benign and malignant)

Interfering Factors
Radiographic examination of the lumbosacral spine, coccyx, or pelvis must be completed prior to an barium studies. Jewelry, dense articles of clothing (*i.e.*, belts), zippers, buttons, snaps, and other metallic objects can interfere with a thorough examination of a body part. These articles should be removed prior to the radiologic examination.

Patient Preparation
Explain the purpose and procedure of the test.

Clinical Alert

Orthopedic radiography can provide information about soft-tissue structures, such as the presence of swelling or calcifications. However, radiography alone cannot be used to assess the condition of cartilage, tendons, or ligaments.

Abdominal Plain Film or KUB (Kidney, Ureters, Bladder)

Normal Values
Normal abdominal structures

Explanation of Test
This radiographic study, which does *not* use contrast media, is done to diagnose intra-abdominal diseases such as nephrolithiasis, intestinal

obstruction, soft-tissue masses, or a ruptured viscus. It is also the pre-liminary step in the examination of the gastrointestinal tract, the gall-bladder, or the urinary tract. The study is done before an IVP or before any renal study. It is also useful in the study of abnormal accumula-tions of gas and of ascites within the gastrointestinal tract and of the size, shape, and position of the liver, spleen, and kidneys. This type of study is also called a "scout film" and was formerly called the "flat plate."

Procedure

1. The patient is not required to fast.
2. During the test the patient lies on his or her back on an x-ray table. The patient may also have a second film taken when he or she is standing or sitting.
3. If the patient cannot sit or stand, he or she is asked to lie on the left side with the right side up.
4. There is no discomfort involved, and the test takes only a few min-utes.

Clinical Implications

Abnormal results reveal the following:

1. Calcium in blood vessels, lymph nodes, cysts, tumors, or stones
2. Ureters cannot be defined, but calculi may be detected along the course of the ureters.
3. The shadow cast by the urinary bladder can often be identified, especially when it contains urine of a high specific gravity along with fusion anomalies and horseshoe kidneys.
4. Abnormal size, shape, and position of kidney
5. Presence of appendicolithiasis
6. Presence of foreign bodies
7. Abnormal fluid; ascites

Interfering Factors

Because of the interference of barium, this examination should be done before any barium studies.

Patient Preparation

Explain the purpose and procedure of the test.

Clinical Alert

Abdominal plain films are not useful with conditions such as esophageal varices and bleeding peptic ulcer.

Gastric Radiography (Including Upper GI Examination)

Normal Values
Normal size, contour, motility, and peristalsis of the stomach.

Explanation of Test
This x-ray and fluoroscopic examination is done to visualize the form and position, mucosal folds, peristaltic activity, and motility of the stomach.

Preliminary film without contrast media is useful in detecting perforation, presence of metallic foreign substances, thickening of the gastric wall, and displacement of the gastric air bubble, indicating a mass outside of the stomach wall.

The use of an oral contrast substance such as barium sulfate or Gastrografin (diatrizoate meglumine) will demonstrate a hiatal hernia, pyloric stenosis, gastric diverticulitis, undigested food, gastritis, congenital anomalies (*e.g.*, dextroposition and duplication), and diseases of the stomach (*e.g.*, gastric ulcer, cancer, and stomach polyps).

If this examination includes the esophagus, duodenum, and upper part of the jejunum, it is called the *upper GI examination.*

Procedure
1. The patient lies on the examining table in the x-ray department while a preliminary film is made.
2. The patient swallows the chalky contrast substance while standing in front of the fluoroscopy machine. All the chalky substance must be swallowed.
3. The contrast agent swallow is followed by x-ray filming; 24-hour films may also be taken.
4. Examining time is 45 minutes.

Clinical Implications
Abnormal results reveal the following:

1. Congenital anomalies
2. Gastric ulcer
3. Carcinoma of stomach
4. Gastric polyps
5. Gastritis
6. Foreign bodies
7. Gastric diverticula
8. Pyloric stenosis
9. Hiatal hernia
10. Volvulus of the stomach

Note: The normal contour may be deformed by intrinsic tumor or consistent filling defects as well as stenosis accompanied by dilatation.

Interfering Factors
1. Because of poor physical condition of the patient, examination is sometimes difficult, and it may be impossible to visualize adequately all parts of the stomach.

2. Retention of food and fluid residues may cause difficulty and lead to errors.

Patient Preparation
1. Explain the purpose and procedure of the test. Give a written reminder.
2. No food or liquid is permitted from midnight until the examination is completed.

Patient Aftercare
1. Provide fluids, food, and rest after the test.
2. Administer laxatives if ordered. If barium sulfate or diatrizoate meglumine is used during the examination, a laxative should be taken after the procedure.
3. Observe and record stools for color and consistency to determine that all of the barium has been evacuated.

Radiography and Fluoroscopy of the Small Intestine

Normal Values
Normal contour, position, and motility of the small intestine.

Explanation of Test
This radiographic and fluoroscopic study is done to diagnose diseases of the small bowel (*e.g.*, ulcerative colitis, tumors, active bleeding, or obstruction). The patient swallows a contrast material such as barium sulfate or meglumine diatrizoate to aid in the diagnosis of Meckel's diverticulum, congenital atresia, obstruction, filling defects, regional enteritis, lymphoid hyperplasia, tuberculosis of small intestine (malabsorption syndrome), sprue, Whipple's disease, intussusception, and edema. This test is usually scheduled in conjunction with an upper GI examination.

The mesenteric small intestine begins at the duodenojejunal junction and ends at the ileocecal valve. The mesenteric small intestine is not included routinely as part of the upper GI study.

Procedure
1. A preliminary plain-film study is made while the patient lies on the examining table.
2. While in a standing position in front of the fluoroscopy machine, the patient swallows a chalky contrast material. (All of the chalky substance must be swallowed.)
3. The contrast agent swallow is followed by x-ray filming. Timed films are taken, usually every 30 minutes
4. Examining time is variable. The examination is not completed until the ileocecal valve has filled with contrast. This may take several minutes (for those patients having a bypass) or several hours.

Clinical Implications
Abnormal results indicate

1. Anomalies of the small intestine
2. Errors of rotation
3. Meckel's diverticulum
4. Atresia
5. Neoplasms
6. Regional enteritis
7. Tuberculosis
8. Malabsorption syndrome
9. Intussusception
10. Round worms (ascariasis)
11. Intra-abdominal hernias

Interfering Factors
1. Delays in motility in the small intestine can be due to
   (a) Use of morphine
   (b) Severe or poorly controlled diabetes
2. Increases in motility in the small intestine can be due to
   (a) Fear
   (b) Excitement
   (c) Nausea

Patient Preparation
1. Explain the purpose and procedure of the test. Give a written reminder.
2. Advise the patient that no food or liquids are permitted from midnight until the examination is completed.
3. Do not give laxatives or enemas to an ileostomy patient.

Patient Aftercare
1. Provide fluids, food, and rest after the examination.
2. Administer laxatives if ordered. If a barium sulfate swallow is used during the examination, a laxative should be taken after the examination is finished. Do not give laxatives to an ileostomy patient.
3. Check stools for color and consistency to determine that all the barium has been evacuated.

Barium Enema Radiography of the Colon; "Air-Contrast" Study

Normal Values
Normal position, contour, filling, rate of passage of barium, movement, and patency of colon.

Explanation of Test

This examination of the large intestine, or colon, uses x-ray films and fluoroscopy to visualize the position, filling, and movement of the divisions of the colon. It is an aid in determining the presence or absence of disease such as diverticulitis, cancer, polyps, colitis, any form of obstruction, and active bleeding. Barium or Hypaque is used as a contrast medium and instilled through a rectal tube. The radiologist observes the barium through a fluoroscope as it flows into the large intestine. X-ray films are taken.

For a satisfactory examination, the colon must be cleansed thoroughly of fecal matter. This is most important if a search is being made for a source of bleeding. The accurate identification of small polyps is possible only when there are no confusing shadows caused by retained lumps of stool.

If polyp formation is suspected, an air-contrast colon examination may be ordered. The procedure for this test is basically the same as for the barium enema. However, it does require that more complex radiographs be taken in several positions. A "double contrast" of air and barium is instilled into the colon under fluoroscopy.

Procedure

1. In the x-ray department, the patient is asked to lie on his or her back while a preliminary film is made.
2. The patient lies on his or her side, and the barium is introduced by enema. When barium is given by rectal enema in the x-ray department, it goes through the rectum, up through the sigmoid, descending, transverse, and ascending colon, up to the ileocecal valve. Barium contrast opacifies the bowel mucosa and outlines the haustra folds of the large intestine.
3. The patient is instructed to retain barium until x-ray films are taken. Following fluoroscopic examination, which includes several "spot films," conventional x-ray films are taken. After completion of the films, the patient is asked to go into the bathroom to expel the barium. After evacuation, another film is made.
4. Total examining time may be up to 1¼ hours.

Clinical Implications

1. Abnormal results indicate
   - (a) Lesions
   - (b) Obstructions
   - (c) Megacolons
   - (d) Fistulae
   - (e) Inflammatory changes
   - (f) Diverticulae
   - (g) Chronic ulcerative colitis
   - (h) Stenosis
   - (i) Right-sided colitis
   - (j) Hernias
   - (k) Polyps
   - (l) Intussusception
   - (m) Carcinoma

2. Size, position, and motility of the appendix can be determined by this examination; however, a diagnosis of chronic appendicitis *cannot* be made from x-ray findings. A diagnosis of appendicitis is made from the presence of typical signs and symptoms.

Interfering Factors
A poorly cleansed bowel is the most common interfering factor. Unless fecal matter is satisfactorily cleansed from the colon, small polyps or a source of blockage will not show up well on the x-ray film.

Patient Preparation
Preparation requires a three-step process over a 1- to 2-day period: (1) diet restrictions; (2) physiologic cleansing of large bowel with oral laxatives; and (3) mechanical cleansing with enema. Twelve- and 18-hour protocols are common. Check with the examining department for specifics.

1. Explain the purpose and procedure of the test.
2. Give a written reminder of the following instructions:
   (a) A clear liquid diet before testing
   (b) Stool softeners, laxatives, and enemas will be given in order to obtain the clearest possible x-ray films. Giving agents such as X-Prep, citrate of magnesia, and bisacodyl will result in emptying of the ascending and right-to-mid-transverse colon (proximal large bowel). Administering enemas cleanses the left transverse descending and sigmoid colon and rectum of stool. Suppositories may also be used to empty the rectum.
   (c) No food is to be eaten after the evening meal, and no liquids are to be taken from midnight until the examination is completed. Oral medications are not permitted.

Patient Aftercare
1. Provide food, fluids, and rest after the examination is completed. This examination is the most fatigue-producing of all x-ray studies. Patients may be weak, thirsty, or tired after the test is finished.
2. A laxative should be given for at least 2 days following the x-ray studies or until stools are normal in consistency and color.
3. Stools must be checked and recorded for color and consistency for at least 2 days in order to determine whether all the barium has been evacuated. Stools will be light in color until all barium has been expelled. Outpatients should be given a written reminder to inspect stools for 2 days.

Clinical Alert

1. See page 631 for clinical considerations for barium.
2. The use of multiple enemas prior to a diagnostic procedure, especially on a person at risk for electrolyte imbalances, could induce a rather rapid hypokalemia. Enema fluid, if not expelled from the body, can be absorbed through the bowel wall, thereby diluting it in the interstitial space and ultimately in all extracellular space.
3. A judgment should be made about the administration of cathartics or enemas in the presence of acute abdominal pain, ulcerative colitis, or obstruction. Consult the physician or radiology department and consider the following points:
   (a) When giving enemas, remember that introducing large quantities of water into the bowel should be avoided in patients with megacolon because of the danger of water intoxication. In general, patients with toxic megacolon should *not* be given enemas.
   (b) If any obstruction is suspected in the colon, the water from large enemas may be reabsorbed and impaction can occur.
   (c) If there is an obstruction in the rectum, it will be difficult or impossible to give the cleansing enemas, for the fluid will not flow into the colon. Consult the physician or radiology department in these matters.
4. Strong cathartics in the presence of obstructive lesions and acute ulcerative colitis can be hazardous or life-threatening.
5. The danger of introducing barium into the colon and the preparation for the procedure should always be considered. Be prepared for complications when barium sulfate or a similar contrast medium is introduced into the GI tract.
6. Barium may aggravate acute ulcerative colitis or cause a partial to complete obstruction.
7. The NPO order also includes oral medications.
8. Preparations for the test will vary from one x-ray department to another.
9. Barium should not be used as a contrast for intestinal studies when a bowel perforation is suspected. Leakage of barium through a perforation may cause peritonitis. Iodinated contrasts should be used when perforation is suspected.

Special Considerations for Barium Enemas on Children and the Elderly

1. Because the success of examination of the large intestines is dependent upon the bowel remaining filled with contrast during filming, special techniques are used for infants and young children and the infirm or uncooperative adult patient.
2. After insertion of a small enema tip, the buttocks of the infant are gently taped together in order to prevent leakage during the study.
3. For the older patient, a special retention enema tip may be employed. This device resembles a regular enema tip, but it has a segment that is capable of being inflated after insertion. Following the completion of the examination, the retention balloon is deflated and can be comfortably extracted.

Special Considerations for Barium Enema with Colostomy

1. See pages 631 and 632 for assessment criteria.
2. Laxatives can be taken.
3. Suppositories are useless.
4. Usually a suggested diet can be followed.
5. If irrigation is needed, use a preassembled colostomy irrigation kit or use a soft 28 Foley catheter attached to a disposable enema bag.
6. In those persons with a double-barreled colostomy, the irrigation solution may be expelled through the rectum as well as the stoma.
7. Advise the patient that a Foley catheter is used to introduce the barium into the stoma.
8. Recommend that the patient bring supplemental colostomy supplies to the testing department for post-test care.

Aftercare of Patients with Stomas

Persons with descending or sigmoid colostomies may need a normal saline or tap water irrigation to wash out the barium.

Advise those who normally irrigate the colostomy to wear a disposable pouch for several days until all the barium has passed.

Cholecystography (Gallbladder Radiography)

Normal Values
Normal functioning gallbladder and ducts without stones

Explanation of Test
This x-ray study involving the use of an oral iodine contrast substance such as Telepaque (iopanoic acid), Oragrafin (sodium spodate), and Priodax (iodoalphionic acid) is done to evaluate the functioning of the gallbladder (filling, concentration, contraction, and emptying) and to determine the presence of disease or gallstones. Because gallstones are

not usually radiopaque, it is necessary to fill the gallbladder with a radiopaque substance that permits stones to show up as shadows. After administration of the iodinated substance, it takes about 13 hours for it to reach the liver and to be excreted into the bile, where it is stored in the gallbladder. This test is effective only if the liver cells are functioning normally and are capable of excreting the radiopaque dye into the bile.

Procedure
Ultrasound studies of the gallbladder are commonly used alone or in conjunction with oral cholecystography, because of a high degree of accuracy and ease of performance. Calculi or diseases that are suggested but not positively identified by one type of imaging procedure are often verified by the other type of study.

1. A series of up to three x-ray examinations is made with the patient assuming the following positions: lying on the abdomen, lying with the right side of the body elevated away from the table, sitting, or standing. Total examining time is 1 hour.
2. In some instances, a high-fat drink may be given to make the gallbladder contract, and after 20 to 60 minutes another x-ray examination is conducted. Sincalide, when injected intravenously, also causes contraction of the gallbladder in 5 to 15 minutes and subsequent evacuation of bile.

Clinical Implications
Abnormal results reveal

1. Cholelithiasis (gallstones)
2. No evidence of gallbladder

>   **Note:** If the gallbladder is chronically inflamed or contains stones, it may not show up at all. This will provide presumptive evidence of disease if on two different occasions the gallbladder cannot be demonstrated.

3. Presence of gas within the gallbladder or ducts, which is always abnormal
4. Papillomatous or adenomatous tumors of the gallbladder
5. Congenital anomalies
6. Obstruction of cystic duct

Scheduling of Test
1. Thyroid scans, ^{131}I uptake, and protein-bound iodine (PBI) must be performed before a gallbladder examination.
2. Barium studies should be performed after gallbladder studies are completed, because barium may interfere with the results.
3. When a series of GI x-ray studies is made in a single day, the usual

order of examination is (1) gallbladder, (2) barium enema, and (3) upper GI x-ray film.

Patient Preparation
1. Explain the purpose and procedure of the test.
2. Tell the patient that this test often has to be repeated, so if it is requested again, there is no need to be alarmed.
3. Emphasize the importance of drinking a large amount of water with the contrast capsules. Give a written reminder.
4. Be familiar with the procedures of your medical facility. Prepare the patient with the following information:
   (a) A low-fat meal is eaten the evening before the x-ray examination.
   (b) An oral laxative or stool softener is given after the meal.
   (c) The iodine contrast is given orally, usually in the form of tasteless capsules. Some departments prefer two doses of oral contrast given on consecutive days before x-ray filming, others prefer a single dose followed by a second dose only if the first is unsuccessful.
   (d) Some x-ray departments require the patient to have an enema.
   (e) No food is permitted from the time the contrast is given until the examination is completed. Usually, water and coffee or tea without cream and sugar are permitted if the examination is not done in conjunction with intestinal studies.

Patient Aftercare
1. Provide fluids, food, and rest after the examination is completed.
2. Observe the patient for allergic reaction to the iodine contrast substance.

Clinical Alert

These tablets may act as a laxative in some patients with right-sided colostomies or ileostomies. If this happens, the patient needs extra oral fluids at once.

1. This examination is contraindicated in
   (a) Jaundiced patients who will be unable to metabolize and concentrate the iodine in the gallbladder because of liver disease
   (b) Patients sensitive to iodine
   (c) Vomiting patients
   (d) Patients with diarrhea
2. Observe for reactions to iodine. See pages 628–630 for additional assessment criteria.

T-Tube Cholangiography;
Intravenous Cholangiography

Normal Values
Patent common duct

Explanation of Test
The intravenous cholangiogram is an examination done to study the biliary ducts. It is usually performed after nonvisualization of the gallbladder following an oral choledochogram. A contrast is injected intravenously and followed by radiographic and tomographic evaluation. With intravenous injection of contrast there can be visualization of the gallbladder in persons unable to take oral contrast media or unable to absorb them from the GI tract.

The T-tube cholangiogram is done after gallbladder surgery to evaluate the patency of the common bile duct before removal of the T-tube (a T-tube is a self-retaining drainage tube that is attached to the common bile duct during surgery). An iodine contrast dye is injected into the T-tube; then a fluoroscopic examination is made. This test is usually done about 10 days after the operation.

Procedure
For T-tube cholangiogram

1. The patient lies on the x-ray table while a contrast medium such as Hypaque is injected into the T-tube.
2. Normally no pain or discomfort is experienced. Some persons may feel pressure upon injection.
3. The procedure takes at least 15 minutes. On leaving the x-ray department, the T-tube should be unclamped and draining freely unless otherwise ordered. This avoids prolonged, often irritating, contact of the residual dye with the bile duct.

For intravenous cholangiogram

1. A "scout film" of the right upper quadrant is made.
2. The patient lies on the x-ray table while a contrast agent, usually Cholografin, is injected. This process takes about 15 minutes.
3. Films are taken every 15 to 30 minutes until the common bile duct visualizes.
4. Following visualization of the biliary ducts, tomographic studies are performed.
5. If the patient's gallbladder has not been removed, the examination may include fluoroscopy of the gallbladder with the patient standing.

Clinical Implications
Results will reveal whether the lower end of the duct is clear.

Patient Preparation

1. Explain the purpose and procedure of the test.
2. The meal before the x-ray study is omitted. If the examination is in the morning, hold breakfast; if the examination is in the afternoon, hold lunch. Decrease the patient's fluid intake as well. A laxative may be administered the afternoon before the examination, and after midnight nothing can be eaten. Fluids are usually allowed upon completion of infusion.
3. The intravenous cholangiogram is a lengthy procedure requiring 2 to 4 hours and, in some instances, longer.

Patient Aftercare

1. After the test, nausea, vomiting, and transient elevated temperature may occur as a reaction to the iodine contrast.
2. Record observations and notify the physician.

Clinical Alert

1. Persistent fever, especially with chills, may signify inflammation of the bile duct.
2. Follow-up care to monitor for hemorrhage, pneumothorax, and/or peritonitis is essential after percutaneous transhepatic cholangiography.

Other Tests Used in the Examination of the Biliary System

Intravenous cholangiography—Radiographic visualization of the large hepatic ducts and the common ducts after intravenous injection of a contrast medium

Operative cholangiography—Performed by cannulation of the exposed cystic duct or common bile duct at laparotomy and subsequent injection of a contrast agent.

Percutaneous transhepatic cholangiography—A needle or catheter is introduced percutaneously into the liver and bile duct. The contrast agent is then injected, and opacification of the hepatic and common ducts occurs. The dilated biliary tree is opacified up to the point of obstruction, usually in the common duct. It is done on the jaundiced patient whose liver cells are unable to transport contrast when administered by oral or intravenous routes.

T-tube (or postoperative) cholangiography—The hepatic and common ducts can be opacified by injecting a contrast agent through the external opening of a drainage T-tube that has been placed in the common duct during surgery.

Intravenous cholecystography—Radiographic visualization of the gallbladder after intravenous injection of a contrast agent

Oral cholangiography—Radiographic visualization of the biliary ducts after oral administration of a contrast agent

Oral cholecystography—Radiographic visualization of the gallbladder after ingestion of an opaque medium

Endoscopic retrograde cholangiopancreatography (ERCP)—This endoscopic procedure uses a contrast substance to evaluate the patency of pancreatic and common bile ducts, the duodenal papilla, and the normalcy of the gallbladder (see p. 738).

Esophageal Radiography

Normal Values
Normal size, contour, swallowing, movement of material through the esophagus; peristalsis of esophagus

Explanation of Test
Usually, the esophagus is examined together with the stomach, duodenum, and upper part of the jejunum. By common usage, this examination is referred to as an upper GI series. In addition, the esophagus may be examined separately because of specific complaints pertaining to this region of the GI tract.

This x-ray and fluoroscopic examination is done to visualize the position, patency, and contour of the esophagus. The technique of examination will vary, depending on such factors as the presence or absence of a lesion and the amount of obstruction. Preliminary films without contrast media are made to identify opaque foreign bodies in the neck and thorax, displacement of trachea, or air or fluid in mediastinal tissues or pleural cavities.

The use of an oral contrast medium, barium sulfate or diatrizoate meglumine, will permit visualization of the lumen of the esophagus. Many laboratories employ a very viscous barium preparation that resembles toothpaste in order to fully coat the esophageal walls. Swallowing small pledgets of cotton soaked in barium is useful when the esophagus is being examined for the presence of small or sharp foreign bodies such as fish bones. Congenital abnormalities of the esophagus can be detected by this method as well as esophageal involvement in scleroderma, diverticulae, cancer, stricture with inflammation, and spasms. It is difficult to identify esophageal varices, but if present, they are an indication of cirrhosis of the liver.

Procedure
1. The patient lies on the examining table in the x-ray department while a preliminary plain-film study is made.
2. Barium sulfate or diatrizoate meglumine is swallowed while the

patient is in a standing position in front of the fluoroscope. All of the chalky substance must be swallowed.
3. The barium swallow is followed by x-ray studies. In some instances, delayed films may also be done.
4. Examining time is 45 minutes.

Clinical Implications
1. Abnormal results indicate
   (a) Congenital abnormalities
   (b) Esophageal involvement in scleroderma
   (c) Diverticulae
   (d) Cancer
   (e) Stricture with inflammation and spasm
   (f) Acute ulcerative esophagitis
   (g) Chronic fibrosing esophagitis
   (h) Peptic ulcer of the esophagus
   (i) Achalasia (cardiospasm)
   (j) Chalasia (cardioesophageal relaxation)
   (k) Polyps
   (l) Foreign bodies
   (m)Rupture
   (n) Paralysis
2. Esophageal varices may be difficult to identify but, if present, they are an indication of cirrhosis of the liver.

Patient Preparation
1. Explain the purpose and procedure of the test. Give a written reminder. Because barium has a chalky taste, it is often flavored.
2. No food or liquids are permitted from midnight until the examination is completed.

Patient Aftercare
1. Provide food and fluids after the test is completed.
2. If barium is used during the examination, a laxative should be given after the examination is completed.
3. Check stool for barium (color and consistency) to determine that all the barium has been evacuated.

Intravenous Urography (IVU) (Excretory Urography or IV Pyelography [IVP])

Normal Values
1. Normal size, shape, and position of the kidneys, ureters, and bladder. Normal kidneys are approximately as long as three and one-

half vertebral bodies. Size of kidneys is estimated in relation to the shadows cast against the vertebra on the x-ray film.
2. Normal renal function
    (a) Two to 5 minutes after the injection of the contrast material, the kidney outline will appear. Threadlike strands of the contrast material will be seen in the calyces.
    (b) When the second film is taken 5 to 7 minutes after the injection, the renal pelvis can be noted.
    (c) In the last stages of film-taking, the ureters and bladder can be visualized as the contrast material makes its way down the lower urinary tract.
3. No signs of residual urine should be found on the postvoid film.

Explanation of Test
An IVU is one of the most frequently ordered tests in instances of suspected renal disease or urinary tract dysfunction. A radiopaque iodine contrast substance, such as sodium diatrizoate (Hypaque) or n-methylglucamine iothalamate (Conray), is injected intravenously, concentrating the contrast substance in the urine. Then a series of x-ray films is made at set intervals over a 20- to 30-minute period. A final postvoid film is taken after the patient has been asked to empty his or her bladder.

The result allows for visualization of the size, shape, and structure of the kidneys, ureters, and bladder, and the ability of the bladder to empty sufficiently. Renal function is reflected by the length of time it takes the contrast material to appear and be excreted in each kidney. Kidney disease, ureteral or bladder stones, and tumors can be detected with this test.

An IVU is indicated in the initial investigation of any suspected urologic problem, especially in the diagnosis of lesions of the kidney and ureters and in the determination of renal function. The term *intravenous urogram* is preferred to IVP because urogram implies visualization of the entire urinary tract, whereas pyelogram refers specifically to the kidneys.

Tomography of the kidney may also be done at this time to obtain better visualization of renal pathology and tumors. This will increase the examination time, for more films will be taken. If kidney tomography or nephrotomogram is ordered separately, the procedure and preparation are the same as for IVU.

Procedure
1. A preliminary x-ray film is taken with the patient in a supine position in order to assure that the bowel has been properly emptied and that kidney placement can be visualized.
2. The contrast material is injected intravenously, usually in the antecubital vein.

3. During and following the intravenous injection, the patient should be forewarned that he or she may experience the following sensations: warmth, flushing of the face, salty taste, and nausea.
   (a) Should these sensations occur, the patient should be instructed to take slow, deep breaths.
   (b) As a precaution, an emesis basin should be handy.
   (c) Assess for other untoward signs such as respiratory difficulty, heavy sweating, numbness, and palpitations, and urticaria.
4. Following injection of the contrast material, at least three x-ray films are taken at set intervals.
5. The patient is then asked to go to the bathroom to void, after which another film is taken to determine bladder emptying.
6. Total examination time is about 45 minutes.

Clinical Implications
1. Abnormal IVU findings reveal
   (a) Altered size, form, and position of the kidneys, ureters, and bladder
   (b) Duplication of the pelvis or ureter
   (c) The presence of only one kidney
   (d) Hydronephrosis
   (e) A supernumerary kidney
   (f) Renal or ureteral calculi (stones)
   (g) Tuberculosis of the urinary tract
   (h) Cystic disease
   (i) Tumors
   (j) The extent of renal injury following trauma
   (k) Prostate enlargement (male)
   (l) Very large kidneys suggesting obstruction or polycystic disease
   (m) Evidence of renal failure with kidneys of normal size, suggesting an acute rather than a chronic process
   (n) Irregular scarring of the renal outlines, suggesting chronic pyelonephritis
2. A delay in the appearance time of the radiopaque contrast indicates renal dysfunction. No contrast may indicate very poor function or no function at all.

Interfering Factors
1. Feces or gas not cleared from the intestinal tract will obscure the view of the urinary tract.
2. Retained barium and the resulting gaseous distention from a previous barium examination can obscure the kidneys. (For this reason, barium tests should be scheduled to follow an IVU when possible.)

Patient Preparation
1. Explain the purpose and procedure of the test. Give a written reminder.
2. Because dehydration is necessary for the contrast material to be concentrated in the urinary tract, instruct the patient that no food, liquid, or medication is to be taken 12 hours before the examination. This usually means NPO after the evening meal.

   Note: Elderly or debilitated patients with poor renal reserves may not tolerate dehydration procedures (NPO, laxatives, enemas). In such instances, consult with the radiologist or the patient's physician to see if these procedures are contraindicated and if the patient should be given fluids during the normal NPO period.
   For infants and small children, the NPO time will usually vary from 6 to 8 hours preceding the test. However, be sure to obtain specific orders, because each child will require different limits.

3. Usually, a laxative is prescribed for the evening before the examination and an enema the day of the examination.
   (a) Patients with intestinal disorders such as ulcerated colitis probably should not be given a cathartic. Special orders should be obtained in such instances.
   (b) Elderly patients need special attention for possible assistance to the bathroom.
4. Children under 7 years should not be given cathartics or enemas before the examination. Should the preliminary x-ray film show gas obscuring the kidneys, a few ounces of formula or carbonated drink may help push the gas aside.
5. Check stool and abdomen for distention to assure that barium from a previous enema has been eliminated and that the bowel evacuation efforts have been successful.
6. See pages 628–630 for assessment criteria.

Patient Aftercare
1. Provide fluid and food immediately after the examination.
2. Inform the patient about the importance of drinking fluids to overcome dehydration and feelings of weakness.
3. Encourage bed rest following the examination, up to 8 hours for elderly and debilitated patients.
4. Observe and record any of the following mild reactions to the iodine material: hives, skin rashes, nausea, swelling of the parotid glands (iodinism).
   (a) Consult with the physician if the signs and symptoms persist.
   (b) Administration of oral antihistamines may relieve the more severe symptoms.

Clinical Alert

1. Contraindications to an IVU include
   (a) Hypersensitivity to iodine preparation
   (b) The presence of combined renal and hepatic disease
   (c) Oliguria
   (d) A BUN of more than 40 mg/100 ml (40 mg/dl)
   (e) Multiple myeloma, unless the patient can be kept well hydrated during and after the study
   (f) Advanced pulmonary tuberculosis
   (g) Patients receiving drug therapy for chronic bronchitis, emphysema or asthma
2. Whenever a radiopaque iodine substance is injected, some physiologic changes can be expected. Hypertension, hypotension, tachycardia, arrhythmia, or other electrocardiographic (ECG) changes are the types of conditions expected to occur.
3. Radiopaque contrast media containing iodine are given with caution to patients with hyperthyroidism or a history of asthma, hay fever, or other allergies.
4. Patients should be observed for any anaphylactic or severe reaction to iodine as evidenced by signs of shock, respiratory distress, a precipitous drop in blood pressure, fainting, or convulsions.
5. In all cases except emergencies, the contrast media should not be injected sooner than 90 minutes after eating.
6. Intravenously injected iodine can be highly irritating to the intima of the veins and may cause a painful vascular spasm.
   (a) Intravenous injection of 1% procaine solution may help relieve vascular spasm and pain.
   (b) Sometimes local vascular irritation is severe enough to induce thrombophlebitis. The area may be treated with warm compresses to relieve pain. The attending physician should be notified. In some cases, anticoagulant therapy is prescribed.
7. Patients should be observed for local reaction to iodine as evidenced by extensive redness, swelling, and pain at the injection site. A leakage of even a small amount of iodine contrast into the subcutaneous tissues can ultimately cause sloughing of the area, which may require skin grafting.
   (a) When extravasation is recognized, the local injection of hyaluronidase may hasten reabsorption of the iodine and resolution of the reaction.
   (b) The use of local applications of warm saline packs may alleviate discomfort, but it does not prevent sloughing.

Retrograde Pyelography

Normal Values
Normal contour and size of ureters and kidneys

Explanation of Test
This test is generally used to confirm findings suspected on the IVU. This test is also indicated when the IVU yields insufficient results because of nonvisualization of kidney (congenital absence of the kidney), decreased renal blood flow that restricts renal function and obstruction, when the IVU shows that one kidney is not working properly or provides evidence of a stone, or when the patient is allergic to intravenous contrast material. This x-ray examination of the upper urinary tract uses cystoscopy to introduce catheters into the ureters to the level of the renal pelvis. An iodine contrast dye is injected into the catheter and films are taken. The chief advantage of retrograde pyelography is that a dense contrast substance can be injected directly under controlled pressure so that visualization is good. The extent of impairment of renal function that may be present does not influence the degree of visualization.

Procedure
1. The examination is usually done in the surgical department in conjunction with cystoscopy.
2. The examination is preceded by sedation and analgesia and insertion of a local anesthetic into the urethra (see section on *cystoscopy*). General anesthesia may be used.
3. Total examination time is less than 1.5 hours.

Clinical Implications
Abnormal results reveal

1. Intrinsic disease of ureters and pelvis of the kidney
2. Extrinsic disease of the ureters such as obstructive tumor or stones

Interfering Factors
Because of the tendency of barium to interfere with the test results, these studies must be done before barium x-rays.

Patient Preparation
1. Explain the purpose and procedure of the test.
2. A legal consent form must be signed before examination.
3. The patient is allowed no foods or liquids after midnight before the test.
4. Cathartics, suppositories, or enemas are usually ordered before the examination.

Patient Aftercare
1. Observe for allergic reaction to iodine contrast dye.
2. Following the examination, check vital signs for at least 24 hours (every 15 minutes times 4, then every hour times 4, then every 4 hours times 4). If general anesthetic was used, care is the same.
3. Record accurate urine output and appearance for 24 hours. Hematuria and dysuria are common for several days after the examination.
4. Administer analgesics if necessary. Pain is common the first few days following the examination and may require something stronger than aspirin (*e.g.*, codeine).

> **Clinical Alert**
>
> If ordered, renal function tests of blood and urine must be completed before this examination is done.

Other Tests Used in Examination of the Urinary System
Excretion urography or intravenous pyelography (*IVP*)—After intravenous injection of a contrast agent, the collecting system (calyces, pelvis, and ureter) of each kidney is progressively opacified. Radiographs are made at intervals of 5 to 15 minutes until the urinary bladder is opacified.

Drip infusion pyelography—A modification of conventional pyelography. Increased volume of a contrast agent is administered by continuous intravenous infusion.

Cystography—The urinary bladder is opacified by introduction of a contrast agent through a urethral catheter. After the patient has voided, air may be introduced to obtain a double contrast study.

Retrograde cystourethrography—After catheterization, the bladder is filled to capacity with a contrast agent; radiographic techniques then visualize the bladder and urethra.

Voiding cystourethrography—After contrast material has been instilled into the urinary bladder, films are made of the bladder and urethra during the act of voiding.

Lymphangiography

Normal Values
Normal lymphatic vessels and nodes

Explanation of Test

This x-ray examination of the lymphatic channels and lymph nodes uses a radiopaque iodine contrast oil, such as Ethiodol, injected into the small lymphatics of the foot. The test is commonly ordered for patients with Hodgkin's disease and cancer of the prostate to check for nodal involvement. Lymphography is also indicated in diagnosing edema of an extremity with an unknown cause, in evaluating the extent of adenopathy and the staging of lymphomas, and in localizing affected nodes for treatment planning, either surgery or radiotherapy.

Procedure

1. The patient is asked to lie on the examining table in the x-ray department.
2. A blue dye is injected intradermally between each of the first three toes of each foot in order to stain the lymphatic vessels.
3. Under local anesthesia, a 1- to 2-inch incision is made in the dorsum of each foot about 15 to 30 minutes later.
4. The lymphatic vessel is identified and a cannula attached for an extremely *low* pressure injection of the iodine contrast medium.
5. When the contrast medium reaches the level of the third and fourth lumbar vertebra (as seen in fluoroscopy), the injection is discontinued.
6. Films taken of the abdomen, pelvis, and upper body demonstrate the filling of the lymphatic vessels.
7. A second set of films is obtained in 12 to 24 hours to demonstrate filling of the lymph nodes.
8. The nodes in the equinal, external iliac, common iliac, and paraaortic areas, as well as the thoracic duct and supraclavicular nodes, can be visualized.
9. When the injection is made in a lymphatic of the hand, the axillary and supraclavicular nodes are demonstrated.
10. Because the dye persists in the nodes for 6 months to a year, repeat studies can be used to confirm disease activity and follow the results of treatment without injection of dye.
11. The total examination time may take up to 3 hours, which can be very tiring.
12. The patient returns to the x-ray department for additional films in 24 hours.

Clinical Implications

Abnormal results indicate

1. Retroperitoneal lymphomas in patients with Hodgkin's disease
2. Metastasis to lymph nodes
3. Abnormal lymphatic vessels

Patient Preparation
1. Explain the purpose and procedure of the test. A legal permit must be signed.
2. No fasting is necessary; the patient can eat and drink during the procedure if he or she desires.
3. There may be some discomfort when the local anesthetic is injected into the feet.
4. An oral antihistamine is administered to any patient the physician suspects may be allergic to the iodized oil used as a contrast medium.

Patient Aftercare
1. Check the patient's temperature every 4 hours for 48 hours after the examination.
2. Allow the patient to rest after the test.
3. If ordered, elevate the legs to prevent swelling.
4. Be aware of complications such as delayed wound healing or infection at site of incision, edema of legs, allergic dermatitis, headache, sore mouth and throat, skin rashes, transient fever, lymphangitis, and oil embolism.

Clinical Alert

1. The test is usually contraindicated in
   (a) Known iodine hypersensitivity
   (b) Severe pulmonary insufficiency
   (c) Cardiac disease
   (d) Advanced renal or hepatic disease
2. The major complication of the procedure is related to embolization of the contrast media into the lungs. This will diminish pulmonary function temporarily and, in some patients, may produce lipid pneumonia.

Mammography

Normal Values
Essentially normal breasts. If calcification is present, it is evenly distributed—normal duct contrast with gradual narrowing of branches of the ductal system.

Explanation of Test
Soft-tissue mammography is the securing of an x-ray image of the breast on photographic film or on paper using the technology of the

Xerox office copier. Its primary use is to discover cancers that escape detection by all other means. Cancers of less than 1 cm in size cannot be regularly detected by routine clinical examination. Because the average cancer has probably been present in a woman's breast for 10 to 12 years before it reaches the clinically palpable size of 1 cm, the prognosis for cure is excellent if breast cancer is detected in this preclinical or presymptomatic phase. Breast cancer can be detected as early as 2 to 3 years before clinical appearance.

Mammography (x-ray diagnosis of breast disease) is based on gross characteristics. A low-energy x-ray beam is required to delineate the breast structures on mammograms. This radiation dose is quite acceptable for use in frequent reexamination, particularly when one considers that only a relatively small volume of tissue is in the low-energy x-ray beam and that the radiation to the eyes and gonads of the patient is too small for measurement.

Benign lesions push breast tissue aside as they expand while malignant lesions may invade the surrounding breast tissues. The x-ray criteria for diagnosing lesions of the breast are 85% accurate in identifying carcinomas and give less than 10% false-positive diagnoses.

Background
1. Most breast lumps are not malignant. Eight out of 10 are benign.
2. For women over age 40, the benefits of using low-dose mammography to find early, curable cancers outweigh a possible risk from radiation.

Indications for Mammography
1. To detect clinically nonpalpable cancers in women over age 40
2. When signs and symptoms of breast cancer are present
   (a) Skin changes
   (b) Nipple or skin retraction
   (c) Nipple discharge or erosion
3. Breast pain
4. "Lumpy" breast; multiple masses or nodules
5. Pendulous breasts that are difficult to examine
6. Survey of opposite breast after mastectomy
7. Patients at risk for having breast cancer (*e.g.*, having family history of breast cancer)
8. Adenocarcinoma of undetermined site
9. Previous breast biopsy
10. Examination of tissue biopsied from breast

Note: The American Cancer Society recommends a baseline mammogram for all women between 35 and 40 years of age, an annual or biannual mammogram for ages 40 to 49, and a yearly mammogram after 50 years of age.

Procedure
1. The patient is asked to identify the area of lumps or thickening, if any.
2. The breasts are exposed and held in position on the film holder to reduce air pockets, skin folds, and wrinkles in order to get the clearest films.
3. Two views are usually taken of each breast.
4. Following x-ray examination, the radiologist or technologist will often palpate the breasts.
5. Total examining time is about one half hour.

Clinical Implications
1. Abnormal findings reveal
   (a) Benign breast mass. On mammogram it appears as a round, smooth mass with definable edges. If there are calcifications in the mass, they are usually coarse.
   (b) Cancerous mass. On mammogram it appears as an irregular shape with extensions into the adjacent tissue. An increased number of blood vessels are present. Primary and secondary signs of breast cancer are apparent.
2. Speculated mass, on occasion, may be smooth and regular.
3. Calcification in malignant mass (duct carcinoma) or in adjacent tissue (lobular carcinoma) is described as innumerable punctate calcifications resembling fine grains of salt or rodlike calcifications when thin, branching, and curvilinear.
4. The likelihood of malignancy increases with the number of calcifications in a cluster. However, a cluster with as few as three calcifications, particularly if they are irregular, can occur in cancer.
5. Typical parenchymal patterns:
   N_1: Normal
   P_1: Mild duct prominence or less than one quarter of the breast
   P_2: Marked duct prominence
   DY: Dysplasia. Some diagnosticians believe that the dysplasia group is 22 times more likely to develop breast cancer than those with normal results
6. Findings of breast cancer when contrast is injected is associated with extravasation of contrast, filling defects, obstruction, an irregular narrowing of ducts.
   (a) Intraductal papilloma. Contrast mammography (ductograms, galactograms) is a most valuable aid in diagnosing intraductal papillomas. Mammary duct injection is used when cytologic examination of breast fluid is abnormal and in cases of breast discharge. In contrast mammography, about 1 ml of a radiopaque substance such as 50% sodium diatrizoate is injected after careful cannulation of a discharging duct in the breast with a blunt 25-gauge needle.

7. Difficult diagnoses
    (a) Colloid (gelatinous or mucinous) and medullary (circum-scribed) carcinomas are difficult to diagnose by mammography.
    (b) Soft-tissue mammography is notoriously poor in the localizing of nonpalpable intraductal papillomas. Sometimes the calcifi-cations of cancer and sclerosing adenosis may be indistinguish-able, particularly if the adenosis is not bilateral.

Patient Preparation
1. Explain the purpose, procedure, benefits, and risks of the test. Mammography is the single best method for detecting breast can-cer in a curable stage. Some discomfort is experienced when the breast is compressed.
2. Instruct the patient not to use any deodorant, perfume, powders, or ointment in the underarm area of the breasts on the day of the examination. Residue on the skin from these preparations can ob-scure the mammograms.
3. Advise the patient to wear a blouse with a skirt or slacks rather than a dress, since it is necessary to remove the clothing from the upper half of the body.
4. Suggest that patients who have painful breasts refrain from coffee, tea, cola, and chocolate 5 to 7 days before testing.

Transillumination Light Scan of Breast; Diaphanography

Normal Values
Normal tissue light absorption patterns

Explanation of the Test
This study projects red and infrared light through the breasts to differ-entiate benign and malignant tumors. It is known that light in the red and near-infrared spectrum varies in its absorbency and scattering characteristics as it passes through tissue. The basic premise of light scanning is that a soft-tissue organ such as the breast acts as a light filter. The manner in which the breast filters light differs from a very dense glandular breast to a fatty breast. The process is similar to shin-ing a flashlight beam through a person's hand and it does not include x-ray filming. A computerized television camera, focused on the breast, converts the light into images. The test is most useful in young women, women with dense breasts, and women with fibrocystic breasts in which benign tumors occur with the breast connective tissue. The tech-nique is also valuable in the evaluation of women with nipple dis-charge, for those who are afraid of the radiation risk of mammography

and refuse x-rays, silicone-injected and silicone-augmented breasts, and patients requiring frequent follow-up. It is particularly helpful in the evaluation of patients with mammary dysplasia, a disease difficult to assess by mammography. The scar tissue of mastectomy patients can also be examined for recurrence of carcinoma.

Procedure
1. The test is performed in a darkened room with the patient leaning far forward so that lesions near the chest wall are not missed.
2. The examiner moves a hand-held emitter similar to a flashlight over each breast.
3. Total examining time is 15 to 20 minutes.

Clinical Implications
1. Tissue variations are shown in computer-enhanced hues of blue and red. Malignancies often show as deep purple.
2. Areas of malignancy will absorb more light than benign tissues and appear to transilluminate to a lesser degree.

Interfering Factors
False positives are associated with hematoma, mastitis, sclerosing adenosis, fibroadenoma, and papillomatosis.

Patient Preparation
Explain the purpose and procedure of the test, its benefits, and the fact that it has no known risk factors. There is no discomfort involved.

> **Clinical Alert**
>
> This test is not a substitute for mammography.

Computed Tomography (CT) of the Brain/Head
(Computerized Axial Tomography [CAT])

Normal Values
No evidence of tumor or pathologic activity
Typically low electron and tissue density areas appear black, and high electron and tissue density areas appear as shades of gray. The whiter the shading, the higher the density.

Explanation of Test
Computed tomography of the head is a simple, routine x-ray examination that uses a special machine with a scanner system to evaluate suspected intracranial pathology. A narrow beam of attenuated x-rays

that allows little internal scatter of radiation is transmitted through the body part being evaluated and measured by special detectors. A computer provides rapid, complex calculations and determines the degree of multiple x-ray beams that are not absorbed by all the tissue in their path. The result is a three-dimensional picture of the anatomic structure of the head that includes the internal structure of the cranium, brain tissue, and surrounding cerebrospinal fluid (CSF). This transverse image of the head is similar to a view of the head looking down from the top.

The basic parameter measured by CT method is the attenuation coefficient of tissue. This reflects the electron density as well as the elemental composition of tissue. When there is more phosphorus in gray matter than in white matter (a change in elemental composition), the result is a difference in attenuation coefficient for low-energy x-rays, even though the densities of these tissues are the same. Because clotted blood, cystic fluid, bone, CSF, and air have somewhat different coefficients, it is possible to demonstrate the anatomic distribution in these tissues.

By rotation of the x-ray source around the head, several attenuation readings are obtained and computer-processed. These detailed cross-sectional, three-dimensional pictures of the head are free of blurred images, are displayed on a screen, photographed, and are stored in an x-ray film. In the procedure, the patient's head is placed in the scanner and is then scanned in successive "slices." Destructive, atrophic, space-occupancy intracranial pathology, and such congenital abnormalities as hydrocephalus may be diagnosed. A CT scan can demonstrate minor differences in density and composition of different structures. For this reason, it is helpful in differentiating tumors from soft tissues, air spaces from CSF, and normal blood from clotted blood. If there is a disruption in permeability, such as a break in the blood–brain barrier, the accumulation of contrast after intravenous administrations can also be demonstrated by the basal increase in attenuation coefficients.

Computed tomography scanning is a noninvasive diagnostic technique that has virtually eliminated the use of pneumoencephalography and sometimes eliminated angiography. The scope of the information afforded by CT scanning is such that a large number of patients requiring investigation for neurologic complaints need be subjected only to plain skull x-ray, a radioisotope brain scan, or a computerized head scan. In neurologic practice, the common lesions that require identification are cerebral neoplasms, inflammation, hematomas, infarctions, infections, and cerebral edema that often accompanies these lesions. The CT scan is the best screening test for this purpose.

In interpreting the scan, the radiologist identifies structures by appearance: their shape, size, symmetry, and position. On a typical CT brain scan, CSF appears black, bones appear white, and the brain appears to be various shades of gray. The radiologist then looks for changes in the tissue density. Usually, a space-occupying lesion will produce a characteristic displacement or deformity of some part of the ventricular system, and the extent of tissue change is defined. Scans for specific indications can be done in different planes, using thinner slices when the examination is one for the evaluation of small, intracranial structures such as the pituitary gland, optic nerves, and ossicles in the middle ear. These studies require a good deal of cooperation from the patient.

Procedure

1. Each examination takes 20 to 40 minutes to complete (10 scans per examination). During this time, the patient must lie perfectly still, but there is no other discomfort involved.
2. The patient lies on a motorized couch with his or her head resting in a head holder set in a movable frame (gantry) that revolves around the head. The face is not covered. No movement is experienced by the patient. A monotonous sound is heard that some people compare to a dulled sound of a broken washing machine. The head is enclosed and braced as if the patient were sitting under a hair dryer in a beauty salon.
3. If tissue density enhancement is desired (a questionable area that needs further clarification), an iodinated radiopaque substance may be injected intravenously. This contrast material can induce vomiting in some patients.
4. More pictures are taken after a short waiting period.
5. During and following the intravenous injection, the patient may experience the following sensations: warmth, flushing of the face, salty taste, and nausea.
   (a) If these sensations occur, instruct the patient to take slow, deep breaths.
   (b) Have an emesis basin ready as a precaution.
   (c) Watch for other untoward signs, such as respiratory difficulty, heavy sweating, numbness, and palpitations.

Clinical Implications
Tissues With Increased Density

Tissue abnormalities can be identified by the tissue-density alterations they exhibit in the scan pictures. Calcium is an important factor contributing to the increased density of a lesion. Meningiomas and low-grade astrocytomas are neoplasms that may show up as white areas because of their high tissue density. Calcium also collects in angiomas, aneurysms, and degenerative and infected tissue. Any hematoma can be distinguished easily. In intracranial hemorrhage, once clotting has occurred, serum is absorbed and tissue density is much higher than in the normal brain. Hemoglobin and calcium ions play an important part in this increase of average density. From a surgical point of view, the demonstration of a hematoma, its size, relationship to ventricles, or the extent of surrounding edema may be valuable. In subarachnoid hemorrhage, scans may be used to locate a small hematoma. Where aneurysms are multiple, this may be a valuable means of identifying or confirming which aneurysm has, in fact, ruptured. In craniocerebral trauma, computerized scanning provides an easy method of distinguishing between extradural, subdural, or intracerebral hematoma and cerebral edema resulting from brain damage.

Tissues With Decreased Density
Diminished tissue density on scanning is caused by many pathologic conditions. The breakdown of cell structure in infarctions, infections, necrosis in malignant tumors, cyst formation, degenerative processes, benign cysts, and edema are the main changes that will reduce tissue density and are observed as darker areas on the scan pictures.

Tissues Requiring Contrast Media
Lesions having tissue densities that are the same as those of the surrounding normal brain are difficult to identify in the routine scan. The basis for use of this contrast enhancement is that the breakdown of the blood–brain barrier permits small amounts of administered contrast substances to pass into the abnormal brain. Contrast enhancement is indicated when there is evidence of a tumor, multiple sclerosis, aneurysm, or vascular abnormality. Contrast enhancement is used in 80% to 85% of patients with a history of headache and seizures. A quantity of 300 ml of a radiopaque sodium-iodine solution is given by an intravenous infusion, and scans must be repeated. By administering venous contrast, abnormal areas can be enhanced, thus helping to detect underlying processes.

Interfering Factors
1. A false-negative CT result may occur in identifying areas of hemorrhage. One of the limitations of the test is that, as hematomas age, their appearance on CT scans changes from a high intensity to a low intensity level. This is partly due to the fact that older hematomas become more transparent to x-rays.
2. Movement will result in inaccurate pictures.
3. Because it is basically an anatomic technique, it is not useful for measurement of tissue perfusion, metabolism or vessel blood flow. For this reason it is not the best technique for evaluating small arteriovenous malformations, early ischemic disease of the brain, or subdural hematomas.

Patient Preparation
1. Explain the purpose and procedure of the test. Provide written explanation and reminders. The patient should be aware of risks that

include possible adverse effects such as radiation exposure and possible allergic reactions to iodine contrast media. The x-ray dose per examination is essentially the same as in a routine skull x-ray.

2. Generally, the patient should not eat or drink 2 to 3 hours prior to the test if contrast study is planned. Prescribed medications can be taken prior to CT studies. Diabetics should take their insulin and be allowed to eat. CT scanning time can be adjusted so that the examination does not interfere with the patient's medications.

3. Reassure the patient that scanning results in no more radiation than in conventional x-ray studies.

4. Check for allergy in food or drugs that contain iodine. If a contrast iodine intravenous substance is administered during the test (indications may not be present before testing), nausea and vomiting, warmth, and flushing of the face may occur. See pages 628–630 for additional assessment criteria.

5. Reassure the patient that claustrophobic fears of being in the machine are common. Show a picture of the scanner.

6. Administer analgesics and sedatives to patients with painful neck stiffness or injuries to the back of the head, and to those who are unable to cooperate by lying still. Any movement by the patient will give poor results.

Patient Aftercare

1. Determine whether or not an iodine contrast substance was used during the test. If the contrast material was used, observe and record any of the following mild reactions to the iodine material: hives, skin rashes, nausea, swelling of parotid glands (iodism).

2. Consult with the physician if the signs and symptoms persist.

3. Administer oral antihistamines to possibly relieve the more severe symptoms.

4. Documentation should include assessment of need for information, patient instruction given, time examination was completed, how the patient tolerated the procedure, and any signs or symptoms of reaction to contrast.

Computed Tomography (CT) of the Body (Computerized Axial Tomography [CAT] Body Scan; Computerized Transaxial Tomography [CTT] Body Scan)

Normal Values

No tumor or pathologic activity is evident. Air appears black on CT scans, bone appears white, soft tissue appears in shades of gray. The pattern of shades and their correlation to different densities in the body, with the added dimensions of depth, assist in identifying normal body structures and organs.

Explanation of Test

The body scanner is used primarily to give a clear, computerized image of the chest, abdomen, and pelvis and as an important diagnostic aid in the identification of neoplastic and inflammatory diseases. CT scanning of the neck, spine, and extremities can also be done. CT examination of the lumbar spine is also a reliable test for the evaluation of disk herniation or stenosis. Rapid scanning at a certain level can be done to determine changes in blood flow as in instances of aortic dissection and in determining vascularity of a mass (simple level dynamic scan technique).

The body scanner is 100 times more sensitive than the traditional x-ray machine in critical areas. Ordinary machines take a flat picture, with organs in the front of the body appearing to be superimposed over organs in the back of the body. The result is a two-dimensional picture of a three-dimensional object. The scanner also produces a two-dimensional picture, but by taking many cross-sectional views of organs of the body and displaying the pictures in turn on an x-ray film, a three-dimensional appearance is created. Typical x-rays show only major contrasts between body densities such as bones, soft tissue, and air. Fine density differences, as between structures within the liver, do not usually register on an x-ray film but will appear on a body scan. CT scanning of the abdomen, chest, or pelvis will, in most cases, require administration of iodinated contrast material before and during the examination.

Procedure

1. In most laboratories, CT examination of the abdomen is preceded by having the patient drink a special contrast preparation several minutes prior to the commencement of the study. This contrast material will outline the bowel so it can be differentiated more readily from other structures.
2. The patient lies on his or her back in a comfortable position in the scanner. The head remains outside of the scanning unit.
3. The patient should be still and follow breathing instructions.
4. No movement is felt by the patient as the x-ray beam makes a 180-degree scan of the body, one degree at a time, in three or four different planes.
5. A television picture of the inside of the living body is seen almost immediately.
6. If there is a questionable area that needs further clarification, such as unusual tissue densities, a contrast iodine substance is injected intravenously and more pictures are taken after a short waiting period. In addition, all patients having CT scans of the pelvis will be

given a barium contrast enema. Furthermore, all female patients undergoing pelvic testing will require the insertion of a vaginal tampon.

7. During and following the intravenous infusion or injection, the patient may experience warmth, flushing of the face, salty taste, and nausea.
   (a) If these sensations occur, instruct the patient to take slow, deep breaths.
   (b) Have an emesis basin available as a precaution.
   (c) Watch for other untoward signs, such as respiratory difficulty, heavy sweating, numbness, and palpitations.
8. The total examination time is 40 to 60 minutes.

Clinical Implications
Abnormal CT scan findings reveal

1. Tumors, nodules, and cysts of the whole body
2. Ascites
3. Abscessed or fatty liver
4. Aneurysm of abdominal aorta
5. Lymphoma
6. Enlarged lymph nodes
7. Pleural effusion
8. Radioactive iodine used in previous testing
9. Cancer of pancreas
10. Liver metastasis
11. Retroperitoneal lymphadenopathy
12. Collection of blood, fluid, or abnormal fat
13. Skeletal metastasis
14. Cirrhosis of liver

Interfering Factors
1. Retained barium can obscure organs in the upper and lower abdomen. (Barium tests should be scheduled to *follow* a CT scan when possible.)
2. Inability of the patient to lie quietly. Movement will result in inaccurate pictures.

Patient Preparation
1. Explain the purpose and procedure of the test. Provide written explanation and reminders. The patient should be aware of the benefits and risks, which are the same as for CT scanning of head.
2. Prescribed medications can be taken prior to CT studies. Diabetics should take their insulin and be allowed to eat. The CT scanning time can be adjusted so that the examination does not interfere with a patient's medication.
3. Inform the patient that an iodine contrast substance may be administered before and during the examination. Elicit any history of allergy to iodine. See pages 628–630 for additional assessment cri-

teria. Pelvic CT examinations usually require both intravenous and rectal contrast administration.

4. Abdominal cramping and diarrhea may occur in some patients. For this reason, drugs such as glucagon, Lipomul, or Donnatal will be ordered to decrease side effects.

5. Caution the patient not to eat solid foods on the day of the examination. Clear liquids are usually permitted up to 2 hours before examination. Check with the diagnostic department for specific protocols, because instructions concerning eating will vary. For CT of the abdomen, the patient is usually NPO.

6. Warn the patient that if a contrast iodine intravenous substance is administered during the test (indications are usually not present before testing), he or she may experience warmth, flushing of the face, salty, metallic taste, and nausea or vomiting.

7. Reassure the patient that claustrophobic fears of being in the machine are common. Show a picture of the scanner.

8. Sedation and analgesics may be ordered if it is difficult for the patient to lie quietly for a long period of time.

Patient Aftercare
If an iodine contrast material was used, observe the patient and record any of the following mild reactions to the iodine material: hives, skin rashes, nausea, swelling of parotid glands (iodism).

1. Consult with the physician if the signs and symptoms persist.

2. Administer oral antihistamines to relieve the more severe symptoms.

3. Document the preparation and instruction of the patient or significant others, the time the procedure was completed, and how the patient tolerated the procedure. Record the use of a control substance and the presence or absence of reaction to iodine contrast material.

Digital Subtraction Angiography (DSA)
(Transvenous Digital Subtraction)

Normal Values
Normal carotid and vertebral arteries, normal abdominal aorta and branches, normal renal arteries, normal peripheral vessels.

Explanation of Test
Digital angiography is a computer-based imaging method of vascular study that uses venous or arterial catheterization to examine the arteries of the body, especially the carotids. However, the intracranial vessels, aortic arch, and abdominal and renal arteries are also examined

for patency and flow using this method. Digital subtraction angiography was first used as an intravenous technique, but because of its limitations, other methods of iodine contrast administration have been investigated. For this reason, intra-arterial injection may be needed for evaluation of viscera and detailed vascular anatomy. The presence of the contrast blocks the path of x-rays and makes the blood vessels visible on x-ray film. Basically, what happens is that an image taken just before contrast injection is subtracted from that taken when the contrast material is in the vascular system. The resulting image shows only the distribution of the contrast substance. Digital subtraction is used to isolate a clinically relevant subset of information; this technique is particularly useful in preoperative and postoperative evaluations for vascular and tumor surgery.

In addition to reducing the risk associated with arterial puncture, the procedure precludes the potential trauma and emboli complications associated with arterial catheterization techniques. Because arterial punctures are not always necessary, this test may be routinely performed on an outpatient basis with considerably less risk and at lower cost than conventional angiography.

Visualization of the extra- and intracranial carotid and vertebral vasculature is possible in patients with a history of stroke, transient ischemic attacks, bruit, or subarachnoid hemorrhage. In the latter indication, the procedure may be used as an adjunct to CT scanning and may be performed just before the CT scan in cases where there is evidence of an aneurysm, vascular malformation, or hypervascular tumor.

Procedure

1. A local anesthetic is administered following careful cleansing of the antecubital area in the right arm. The basilic vein is easier to cannulate than the cephalic. For some studies, the femoral vein is used.
2. The catheter is usually advanced over a guide wire into the superior vena cava. The catheter is connected to a 250-ml bottle of normal saline that is administered slowly. Also connected to the catheter is a power injector that administers an iodine substance very rapidly after a variable delay to allow the contrast substance to clear the pulmonary circulation (depending on vessels being studied). Pictures are taken and stored on magnetic tapes or videodiscs.
3. As soon as the vessels being studied have been defined, the procedure is terminated and the catheter is removed.
4. A bandage is placed over the venous insertion site. Pressure is applied to the puncture site for about 5 minutes.
5. Total examining time is 30 to 45 minutes.

Clinical Implications

Abnormal results reveal the following:

1. Stenosis of arteries
2. Large aneurysms
3. Large jugular tumors and masses
4. Total occlusion of arteries
5. Thoracic outlet syndrome
6. Large or central pulmonary emboli
7. Vascular parathyroid adenoma
8. Pheochromocytoma
9. Ulcerative plaque
10. Tumor circulation
11. Abnormalities that can be identified with 65% accuracy are as follows:
    (a) Total occlusion of internal carotid arteries
    (b) Ulcers without web stenosis or thrombosis
    (c) Aortic arch occlusion
    (d) Subclavian steal
    (e) Meningiomas

Interfering Factors

1. All examinations, especially intracranial, are very sensitive to minimal amounts of patient motion such as respiration. Motion artifacts result in poor images. For this reason, uncooperative or agitated patients cannot be studied. Swallowing in the cooperative person also results in unsatisfactory images. Measures to reduce swallowing, such as having the patient hold his breath, bite on a block, or exhale through a straw, do not yield consistent results.
2. Vessel overlap of external and internal carotid arteries makes it almost impossible to obtain a select view of an individual artery. This is because contrast fills both arteries almost simultaneously. Incidence of uninterpretable studies ranges from 6% to 16%.
3. The examination is not totally reliable in ruling out small aneurysms, severe stenoses of intracranial arteries, and arteriovenous malformations.

Clinical Alert

Tests should be used cautiously in renal insufficiency and unstable cardiac disease. Assess for contraindications to the iodinated contrasts listed on pages 628–630.

Patient Preparation

1. Explain the purpose and procedure of the test and document any instructions given. Explain the benefits and risks (see number 5, below). The patient must be able to hold his or her breath when so instructed and to be very still during the test. A legal permit must be signed.

2. Determine whether or not allergy exists to iodine or contrast medium. See pages 628–630 for additional assessment criteria.
3. In many instances, glucagon is administered intravenously just before any abdominal examinations. This will reduce motion artifacts by stopping peristalsis.
4. No food or fluids should be taken within 2 hours of the study in order to prevent possible vomiting if there is a reaction to the iodine contrast.
5. The patient needs to be aware of the risk and benefits. This method of testing is decidedly less risky than conventional arteriography: There is less radiation than conventional x-ray, and there have been no known fatalities and no known strokes. However, risks will vary from one testing center to the next. Risks include rare complications such as thrombosis of a vein or infection. Overall, the risks are less than in routine angiography, especially when the lower pressure venous circulation is catheterized. By the venous route, the arteries, which are already under high pressure, are able to clear contrast through normal circulation and at their own rate. For this reason, there is less risk of loosening plaque. Another benefit to the patient is that all of the arteries in a specific area are visualized in one series of exposures. This overview gives the radiologist the advantage of being able to evaluate the entire blood supply to an area of interest at one time. In routine angiography, one specific artery at a time is visualized.

Patient Aftercare
1. Check vital signs for stability.
2. Observe the site of venous insertion for signs of infection, hemorrhage, or hematoma, and use infection control measures for site care.
3. Observe for signs of allergic reaction to iodine. Mild side effects of iodine that may occur are nausea, vomiting, dizziness, or urticaria. Watch for complications that can include abdominal pain, hypertension, congestive heart failure, angina, and myocardial infarctions. The possibility of renal failure in susceptible persons exists because there is a higher contrast level given than in conventional arteriograms.
4. Instruct the patient to increase fluid intake up to 2000 ml over the next 24 hours to facilitate excretion of the iodine contrast.

Arthrography

Normal Values
Normal filling of structures of encapsulated joint: joint space, bursae, menisci, ligaments, and articular cartilage

Explanation of Test
Multiple x-ray examinations in specific positions of the soft-tissue structures of encapsulated joints are made following the injection of a contrast agent or agents into the capsular space. The knee is the most frequent site of study for the evaluation of menisci and ligaments. This test is indicated in the investigation of persistent unexplained joint discomfort and is done using sterile technique. However, the shoulder, hip, elbow, wrist, and temporomandibular joints may also be examined using this method. These examinations are performed using local anesthetics and under careful aseptic conditions.

Procedure
1. The patient is asked to lie on his or her back on the examining table.
2. Skin over the joint is cleansed using sterile technique.
3. A local anesthetic is injected around the puncture site. It is usually not necessary to anesthetize the joint space itself.
4. Any effusion in the joint is aspirated by the examining physician. Then a contrast agent or agents (gas, water, or soluble iodine) is injected. After the needle is removed, the joint is manipulated to ensure distribution of the contrast material. In some cases, the patient may be asked to walk around the room and exercise the joint for a few minutes.
5. During the examination, other positions will be assumed by the patient to obtain multiple x-ray views of the joint.
6. A special frame may be attached to widen the joint space under investigation. Cotton pillows and sandbags are also used for this purpose.
7. Actual examining time is 30 to 40 minutes.

Clinical Implications
Abnormal results reveal

1. Arthritis
2. Dislocation
3. Tears of ligaments
4. Rupture of rotator cuff
5. Synovial abnormalities

Patient Preparation
1. Explain the purpose and procedure of the test.
2. Determine whether or not the patient has any known allergies to iodine or contrast substance.

Patient Aftercare
1. The joint should be at rest for 12 hours.
2. An elastic bandage is applied to the knee joint for several days.
3. Ice can be applied for swelling if it occurs. Some persons will experience pain requiring a mild analgesic.
4. Cracking or clicking noises may be heard in the joint for 1 or 2 days

following the test. This is normal. Notify the physician if crepitant noises persist.

Myelography

Normal Values
Normal lumbar or cervical myelogram

Explanation of Test
Myelography is a radiographic study in which iodine contrast material is introduced into the spinal subarachnoid space so that the spinal cord and nerve roots may be outlined and any distortion of the dura mater may be detected.

The test is done to detect neoplasms, ruptured intravertebral disks, or extraspinal pathology such as arthritic lumbar stenosis and cervical ankylosing spondyloses. This examination is indicated when compression of spinal or posterior fossa neural structure or nerve roots is suspected. The test is usually requested when surgical treatment for a ruptured vertebral disk or release of stenosis is considered. Persons who are candidates for testing are those with unrelieved back pain, pain radiating down the leg, those with absent ankle and knee reflexes, claudication of neurospinal origin, and persons with past history of cancer who lose leg and bladder control.

Three types of myelograms are done: positive contrasts using water-soluble iodine, iodized oil, and negative air contrast. The water-soluble contrast is the commonly used substance for myelograms. Both water-soluble and air contrast are followed by CT scanning, which improves visualization. In low-dose myelograms, a very small amount of water-soluble contrast is injected, followed immediately by scanning. An air myelogram is often a last resort examination and is also the test of choice for persons who are too large for the conventional CT myelogram and for those in traction, because of unstable spinal fractures.

Procedure
1. The test is usually done in the x-ray department.
2. The puncture area is shaved if necessary.
3. The patient is positioned lying on his or her abdomen during the procedure.
4. The procedure is the same as for lumbar puncture (see p. 248), except for the added procedure of injection of the contrast substance and fluoroscopic x-ray films; with water-soluble contrast, a narrow-bone needle (22 gauge) may be used. A lumbar puncture is done when lumbar pathology is suspected, and a cervical puncture

for cervical pathology is done so that there will be a higher concentration of contrast in the area of interest. In children, the lumbar puncture level is much lower than in adults to avoid the risk of puncturing the spinal cord. Depending on the specific contrast used, the substance may be removed (oil) or left to be absorbed by the body (water or air).
5. The table is tilted during the procedure. A shoulder and foot brace help to maintain correct position.
6. Total examining time is 30 to 90 minutes.

Clinical Implications
Abnormal results will reveal distortion of the outline of the subarachnoid space, indicating

1. Ruptured intervertebral disk
2. Compression and stenosis of spinal cord
3. Exact level of intravertebral tumors
4. Obstruction of spinal canal
5. Avulsion of nerve roots

Patient Preparation
1. Explain the purpose, procedure, benefits, and risks of the test. Disadvantages of water and air contrast include poor visualization, and, in air contrast, painful headache because of difficulty in controlling gas as it is introduced. Disadvantages of oil contrast studies are irritation of tissues and poor absorption of the oil on subarachnoid space. This oily substance is still visible in x-ray examination up to one year following the original examination. About 1 in 20 examinations uses oil; air is rarely used.
2. A legal consent form must be signed by the patient before the test may be administered.
3. Explain that the examination table may be tilted during the test, but that the patient is securely fastened and will not fall off the table.
4. Advise the patient that clear liquid intake is encouraged to lower any incidence of headache after the test. If the test is scheduled close to a meal time, there may be a food restriction.
5. Minimal discomfort is usually associated with the myelogram itself. However, if the patient has trouble moving, a pain reliever may be ordered to make it easier for positioning and movement during the test.

Patient Aftercare
1. Bed rest is necessary for several hours after the test. If water-soluble contrast is used, the head of the bed is kept elevated at 45 degrees for 8 to 24 hours and the patient is advised to lie quietly. This position will reduce the rate of upward dispersion of the me-

dium and keep contrast out of the head where it can cause headache. If oil contrast is used, the patient will usually be prone for 2 to 4 hours, then on his or her back for 2 to 4 hours. If all the oil contrast has not been withdrawn, the head will be elevated to prevent the substance from flowing into the brain.

2. Fluid intake is encouraged to hasten absorption of any retained contrast media, to replace CSF, and to reduce chance of headache.
3. Check for bladder distention and the ability to void adequately, especially if metrizamide has been used.
4. Check vital signs every 4 hours for at least 24 hours after the examination.

Clinical Alert

1. Observe the patient for possible complications, including nausea, headache, fever, seizure, paralysis, arachnoiditis (inflammation of the coverings of the spinal cord), drowsiness, stupor, stiffness of the neck, sterile meningitis reaction (severe headache and symptoms of arachnoiditis, slow wave patterns on electroencephalogram).
2. Manipulation of CSF pressure may cause an acute exacerbation of symptoms, which may require immediate surgical intervention. No lumbar punctures should be done unless really needed.
3. This test is to be avoided unless there is strong and sufficient reason to suspect a lesion. Multiple sclerosis, for example, may be worsened by the procedure.
4. Be certain to determine whether water-soluble oil or air contrast is used in the procedure, because aftercare interventions will differ.
5. If nausea or vomiting occurs after a water-soluble contrast has been used, do not administer phenothiazine antinauseants such as Compazine.

BIBLIOGRAPHY

Abrams HL (ed): The Little Brown Library of Radiology. Boston, Little, Brown, 1983

Alterescu KB: What about special procedures. Am J Nurs 86(12):1363–1367, December 1985

Ballinger PW: Merrill's Atlas of Roentgenographic Positions and Standard Radiologic Procedures, 6th ed. St. Louis, CV Mosby, 1985

Council on Scientific Affairs: Mammographic screening in asymptomatic women aged 40 years and older. JAMA 261 (17):1989

Douglas E et al: Digital subtraction angiography of the heart and lungs. Orlando, Grune & Stratton, 1986

Federle M: Computed Tomography in the Evaluation of Trauma, 2nd ed. Baltimore, Williams & Wilkins, 1986

Felson B: The chest roentgenologic workup: What and why? Respir Care 25(9):955–959, 1980

Greenfield GB: Radiology of Bone Diseases, 4th ed. Philadelphia, JB Lippincott, 1986

Grossman ZD, et al: The Clinician's Guide to Diagnostic Imaging. 2nd ed. New York, Raven Press, 1987

Gyll C, Black NS: Pediatric Diagnostic Imaging. New York, John Wiley & Sons, 1986

Hahn K: Clinical do's and don'ts—when a patient is scheduled for GI studies. Nursing '89 19(3):88, March, 1989

Heiken JP: Manual of Clinical Magnetic Resonance. New York, Raven Press, 1986

Hjelm-Karlsson K: Effects of information to patients undergoing intravenous pyelography: An intervention study. J Adv Nurs 14(10):853–862, October, 1989

Hoffman DA, et al: Effects of imaging radiation on the developing embryo and fetus: A review. HHS Publication No. FDA 81-8170. Washington, DC, U.S. Government Printing Office, 1981

Kereiackes JB, Rosenstein M: Handbook of radiation doses in nuclear medicine and diagnostic x-ray. Boca Raton, FL, CRC Press, 1980

Meschan I, Ott DJ: Introduction to Diagnostic Imaging. Philadelphia, WB Saunders, 1984

Monroe D: Patient teaching for x-ray and other diagnostics (upper GI, small bowel series and barium enema). RN S2(12):36–40, December, 1989

Monroe D: Patient teaching for x-ray and other diagnostics (CT scan, myelogram, cerebral arteriogram). RN S2(9):50–56, September, 1989

Monroe D: Patient teaching for x-ray and other diagnostics (cardiac cath). RN 54(2):44–46, February, 1991

Monroe D: Patient teaching for x-ray and other diagnostics (IVP). RN 53(9):42–44, September, 1990

Monroe D: Patient teaching for x-ray and other diagnostics (ERCP and Oral Cholecytogram). RN 53(4):52–56, April, 1990

Peters ME, et al: Handbook of Breast Imaging. New York, Churchill-Livingstone, 1989

Pinnar J: Patient teaching for x-ray and other diagnostics (thallium and stress tests). RN 54(3):32–36, March, 1991

Sanchez F: Fundamentals of chest x-ray integrations. Crit Care Nurse 6(5):41–54, September/October, 1986

Seeram E: Computers in diagnostic radiology. Springfield, IL, Charles C Thomas, 1989

Skucas J (ed): Radiographic Contrast Agents, 2nd ed. Rockville, MD, Aspen, 1989

Van Breda A, Katzen B: Digital Subtraction Angiography: Practical Aspects. Thorofare, NJ, Charles B. Slack, 1986

Weinreb R: Magnetic Resonance Imaging of the Body. Philadelphia, WB Saunders, 1987

CYTOLOGY AND GENETIC STUDIES

CYTOLOGY STUDIES

Introduction

Cytologic Study

Exfoliated cells in body tissues and fluid are studied to (1) count the cells, (2) determine the type of cells present, and (3) detect and diagnose malignant and premalignant conditions. The staining technique developed by Dr. George N. Papanicolaou has been especially useful in diagnosis of malignancy and is now routinely used in the cytologic study of the female genital tract, as well as in many types of nongynecologic specimens.

Some cytologic specimens (*e.g.*, smears of the mouth, genital tract, and nipple discharge) are relatively easy to obtain for study. Other samples are from less accessible sources (*e.g.*, amniotic fluid, pleural effusions, and cerebrospinal fluid), and special techniques such as fine-needle aspiration (see p. 689), are required for collection. Tissue samples obtained in surgery are also examined, and skin biopsies for fibroblast culture are done. In all studies, the source of the sample and its method of collection must be noted so that the evaluation can be based on complete information.

Specimens for cytologic study are usually composed of many different cells. Some are normally present, whereas others indicate pathologic conditions. Under certain conditions, cells normally observed in one sample may be indicative of an abnormal state when observed elsewhere. All specimens are examined for the number of cells, cell distribution, surface modification, size, shape, appearance and staining properties, functional adaptations, and inclusions. The cell nucleus is also examined. Any increases or decreases from normal values are noted.

Gynecologic specimens are smeared and fixed in 95% alcohol. (Some types of spray fixative are also available.) Nongynecologic specimens are generally collected without preservative, and they must be handled carefully to prevent drying or degeneration. Check with your individual laboratory for collection requirements. It is important for all cytology specimens to be sent to the laboratory as soon as they are obtained to prevent disintegration of cells or any other process that could cause alteration of the material for study.

Clinical Alert

1. The test is only as good as the specimen received.
2. Specimens collected from patients in isolation should be clearly labeled on the specimen container and requisition

form with appropriate warning stickers. The specimen container should then be placed in two protective bags before transporting it to the laboratory.

In practice, cytologic studies will be commonly reported as

1. Inflammatory
2. Benign
3. Atypical
4. Suspicious for malignancy
5. Positive for malignancy (*in situ* versus invasive)

Histology

Material submitted for tissue examination may be classified according to the histologic or cellular characteristics. A basic method for classifying cancer according to the histologic or cellular characteristics of the tumor is Broder's classification of malignancy.

Grade I   Tumors showing a marked tendency to differentiate; 75% or more of cells differentiated

Grade II   75%–50% of cells differentiated, slight to moderate dysplasia and metaplasia

Grade III   50%–25% of cells differentiated, marked dysplasia, marked atypical, and cancer *in situ*

Grade IV   25%–0% of cells differentiated

The TNM system is a method of identifying tumor stages according to spread of the disease. This system evolved from the work of the International Union Against Cancer and the American Joint Committee on Cancer. In addition, the TNM system further defines each specific type of cancer, such as breast, head, or neck. This staging system (on pp. 690 and 691) is employed for previously untreated and treated cancers and classifies the primary site of cancer and its extent and involvement, such as lymphatic and venous invasion.

Cytologic Study of Fine-Needle Aspiration

Normal Values

Negative. No abnormal cells present.

Explanation of Test

Fine-needle aspiration is a method of obtaining diagnostic material for cytologic study that causes a minimal amount of trauma to the patient. Bacteriologic studies may also be done on material obtained during fine-needle aspiration. Unfixed material, either left in the syringe or on

(*text continues on page 692*)

TNM System

Three capital letters are used to describe the extent of the cancer:

T   Primary tumor
N   Regional lymph nodes
M   Distant metastasis

Chronology of Classification

c   Clinical-diagnostic
p   Postsurgical treatment—pathologic
s   Surgical-evaluative
r   Retreatment
a   Autopsy

This classification is extended by the following designations:

T Subclasses (Extent of Primary Tumor)

	TX	Tumor cannot be adequately assessed
	T0	No evidence of primary tumor
	Tis	Carcinoma *in situ*
T1, T2, T3, T4		Progressive increase in tumor size and involvement

N Subclasses (Involvement of Regional Lymph Nodes)

	NX	Regional lymph nodes cannot be assessed clinically
	N0	Regional lymph nodes demonstrably abnormal
N1, N2, N3, N4		Increasing degrees of demonstrable abnormality of regional lymph nodes

Histopathology

	GX	Grade cannot be assessed
	G1	Well-differentiated grade
	G2	Moderately well-differentiated grade
G3, G4		Poorly to very poorly differentiated grade

Metastasis

MX	The minimum requirements to assess the presence of distant metastasis cannot be met
M0	No evidence of distant metastasis
M1	Distant metastasis present
	Specify sites of metastasis_____

(Continued)

TNM System (*Continued*)

The category M1 may be subdivided according to the following notations:

Pulmonary	PUL		Bone marrow	MAR
Osseous	OSS		Pleura	PLE
Hepatic	HEP		Skin	SKI
Brain	BRA		Peritoneum	PER
Lymph nodes	LYM		Other	OTH

In certain sites further information regarding the primary tumor may be recorded under the following headings:

Lymphatic Invasion (L)

LX   Lymphatic invasion cannot be assessed
L0   No evidence of lymphatic invasion
L1   Evidence of invasion of superficial lymphatics
L2   Evidence of invasion of deep lymphatics

Venous Invasion (V)

VX   Venous invasion cannot be assessed
V0   Veins do not contain tumor
V1   Efferent veins contain tumor
V2   Distant veins contain tumor

Residual Tumor (R)

This information does not enter into establishing the stage of the tumor but should be recorded for use in considering additive therapy. When the cancer is treated by definitive surgical procedures, residual cancer, if any, is recorded.

Residual Tumor Following Surgical Treatment

RX   Residual tumor at primary site cannot be assessed
R0   No residual tumor
R1   Microscopic residual tumor
R2   Macroscopic residual tumor

M   Symbol—in parentheses indicates multiple tumors
Y   Symbol—Y prefix indicates classification occurring with intense multimodality therapy
r   Symbol—r prefix indicates recurrent tumors after a disease-free interval

(Adapted from Beahrs OH, Myers MH [eds]: Manual for Staging of Cancer, 3rd ed. Philadelphia, JB Lippincott, 1988) a needle rinsed in sterile saline, may be taken to the microbiology department for study.

Procedure
1. Superficial or palpable lesions may be aspirated without radiologic aid, but nonpalpable lesions are aspirated with radiographic aid in placement of the needle.
2. After the needle is properly positioned, the plunger of the syringe is retracted to create negative pressure. The needle is moved up and down, and sometimes at several different angles. The plunger of the syringe is released and the needle is removed.
3. The material obtained is expressed onto slides that are then smeared together and fixed immediately. The needle may be rinsed in sterile saline or 50% alcohol for further studies.

Clinical Implications
Abnormal results are helpful in identifying

1. Infectious processes. The infectious agent may be seen or characteristic cellular changes may indicate the infectious agent that is present.
2. Benign conditions. Some characteristic cellular changes may be present, indicating the presence of a benign process.
3. Malignant conditions, either primary or metastatic. If the disease is metastatic, the findings may be reported as consistent with the primary malignancy.

Patient Preparation
Explain the purpose and procedure, benefits, and risks.

Patient Aftercare
Assess the patient for signs of inflammation and use site care infection control measures. Pain may be common in sensitive areas such as the breast, nipple, and scrotum.

Clinical Alert

1. Traumatic complications are rare. Fine-needle aspiration of the lung infrequently results in pneumothorax. Local extension of the malignancy is a consideration, but studies have shown this to be an extremely rare occurrence.
2. A negative finding on a fine-needle aspirate does not rule out the possibility that a malignancy is present. The cells aspirated may have been from a necrotic area of the tumor or a benign area adjacent to the tumor.

Cytologic Study of Liver Biopsies

Normal Values
Negative for malignant or other abnormal cells and tissue

Explanation of test
Cellular material from the liver may be useful in evaluating the status of the liver in diffuse disorders of the parenchyma and the diagnosis of space-occupying lesions. Liver biopsy is especially useful when the clinical findings and laboratory test portions are not diagnostic (when the AST level is 10 to 20 times less than the upper defined limit and the ALP level is less than 3 times the limit), and when the diagnosis or etiology cannot be established by other means (enlarged liver of unknown origin and systemic disease affecting the liver, such as miliary tuberculosis) (Ravel, 1989).

Procedure
1. See section on fine-needle biopsy on page 689.
2. The test is done at the bedside under local anesthesia. Specimens may be obtained using ultrasound radiologic guidance and a tissue core biopsy needle, such as the Menghini needle, which will provide histologic and cytologic material, or one may use a fine-needle aspirate needle, which will obtain cytologic material only.
3. Tissue specimens should be placed in 10% formalin for fixation.
4. Touch prints on glass slides may be made prior to fixation to be submitted for cytologic evaluation. Needle rinses in 50% alcohol or saline may provide helpful diagnostic material as well.
5. Direct slides from needle aspirates may be made, with the slides being fixed immediately in 95% alcohol. See Chapter 12 on endoscopic examination and liver biopsy on page 751.

Interfering Factors
The reported effectiveness of liver aspirates or biopsies varies in the limited published information. Because a very small fragment of tissue, often partially destroyed, is taken in a random manner from a large organ, localized disease is easily missed.
1. False negatives may be due to
   (a) Sampling error. Detection rate of liver metastases is approximately 50% to 70% with blind biopsy and about 85% (range 67%–96%) using ultrasound guidance. Also, many *diseases* produce nonspecific changes that may be spotty, healing, or minimal (Ravel, 1989).
   (b) Degeneration or distortion caused by faulty preparation of specimen
2. False positives may be due to misinterpretation of markedly reactive hepatocytes.

Patient Preparation
The patient should be told the purpose of the test, the nature of the procedure, and the benefits and risks. The procedure usually causes minimal discomfort. There is a small but definite risk of intra-abdominal bleeding and bile peritonitis.

Patient Aftercare
1. See section on fine-needle aspirations.
2. Bed rest with 24 hours of observation after biopsy is usually ordered.

Clinical Implications
Abnormalities in test results of liver biopsies may be helpful in detecting the following:

1. Benign disorders such as
    (a) Metabolic disorders
        (1) Fatty metamorphosis
        (2) Hemosiderosis
        (3) Accumulation of bile (may be due to hepatitis, obstructive jaundice, or malignancy)
        (4) Diabetes
    (b) Hepatic cirrhosis
    (c) Abscess
    (d) Hepatic cysts (congenital or hydatid)
2. Malignant processes such as
    (a) Primary tumors of the liver
        (1) Hepatocellular carcinoma
        (2) Cholangiocarcinoma
    (b) Metastatic tumors

Clinical Alert

Contraindications to percutaneous liver biopsy include

1. A prothrombin time in the anticoagulant range (2–3 seconds over control values)
2. Other bleeding disorders
3. A platelet count of less than 50,000 mm^3
4. Marked ascites
5. Suspected vascular tumor of the liver
6. Infection of the biliary tract or subdiaphragmatic or right hemothoracic infection.
7. Inability of the patient to cooperate during the procedure
8. See section on fine-needle aspirations on page 689.

Cytologic Study of the Respiratory Tract

(See also Chap. 7, under "Respiratory Tract Cultures.")

Normal Values

Negative

Background

The lungs and the passages that conduct air to and from the lungs form the respiratory tract, which is divided into the upper and lower respiratory tracts. The upper respiratory tract consists of the nasal cavities, the nasopharynx, and the larynx; the lower respiratory tract consists of the trachea and the lungs. Cytologic studies of sputum and bronchial specimens are quite important as diagnostic aids because of the frequency of cancer of the lung and the relative inaccessibility of this organ. Also detectable are cell changes that may be related to the future development of malignant conditions and to inflammatory conditions.

Sputum is composed of mucus and cells. It is the secretion of the bronchi, lungs, and trachea and is therefore obtained from the lower respiratory tract (bronchi and lungs). Sputum is ejected through the mouth but originates in the lower respiratory tract. Saliva produced by the salivary glands in the mouth is *not* sputum. A specimen can be correctly identified as sputum in microscopic examination by the presence of dust cells (carbon dust-laden macrophages). Although the glands and secretory cells in the mucous lining of the lower respiratory tract produce up to 100 ml of fluid daily, the healthy person does not cough up sputum.

Procedure

For Obtaining Sputum

1. The preferred material is an early morning specimen. Three specimens are usually collected on three separate days.
2. The patient must inhale air to the full capacity of the lungs and then exhale the air with an expulsive deep cough.
3. The specimen should be coughed directly into a wide-mouthed clean container containing 50% alcohol. (Some cytology laboratories prefer the specimen to be fresh if it will be delivered to the laboratory immediately.)
4. The specimen should be covered with a tight-fitting clean lid.
5. The specimen should be labeled with the patient's name, age, date, diagnosis, and number of specimens (1, 2, or 3) and sent immediately to the laboratory.

For Obtaining Bronchial Secretions

Bronchial secretions are obtained during bronchoscopy (see Chap. 12). Diagnostic bronchoscopy involves removal of bronchial secretions and tissue for cytologic and microbiologic studies. Secretions obtained are collected in a clean container and taken to the cytology laboratory. If microbiologic studies are ordered, the container *must* be sterile.

For Obtaining Bronchial Brushings
Bronchial brushings are obtained during bronchoscopy. The material collected can be smeared directly on all-frosted slides and immediately fixed, or the actual brush may be placed in a container of 50% ethyl alcohol or saline (check with the laboratory for their preference) and delivered to the cytology laboratory.

Bronchopulmonary Lavage
Bronchopulmonary lavage may be used to evaluate patients with interstitial lung disease. Saline is injected into the distal portions of the lung and aspirated back through the bronchoscope into a specimen container. This essentially "washes out" the alveoli. The fresh specimen should be brought directly to the laboratory. A total cell count and a differential cell count are performed to determine the relative numbers of macrophages, neutrophils, and lymphocytes.

Patient Preparation
1. Explain the purpose and procedure of the test.
2. Emphasize that sputum is not saliva.
3. Advise the patient to brush his or her teeth and rinse his or her mouth well before obtaining the specimen to avoid introduction of saliva into the specimen.

Clinical Implications
Abnormalities in sputum and bronchial specimens may sometimes be helpful in detecting the following:

1. Benign atypical changes in sputum as in
   (a) Inflammatory diseases
   (b) Asthma (Creola bodies, Curschmann's spirals, and eosinophils may be found, but they are not diagnostic of the disease.)
   (c) Lipid pneumonia. (Lipophages may be found, but they are not diagnostic of the disease.)
   (d) Asbestosis (ferruginous or asbestos bodies)
   (e) Viral diseases
   (f) Benign diseases of lung such as bronchiectasis, atelectasis, emphysema, and pulmonary infarcts
2. Metaplasia, which is the substitution of one adult cell type for another. Severe metaplastic changes are found in patients with
   (a) History of chronic cigarette smoking
   (b) Pneumonitis
   (c) Pulmonary infarcts

(d) Bronchiectasis
(e) Healing abscess
(f) Tuberculosis
(g) Emphysema
(Metaplasia often adjoins a carcinoma or a carcinoma *in situ*.)
3. Viral changes and the presence of virocytes (viral inclusions may be seen), as in
(a) Viral pneumonia
(b) Acute respiratory disease caused by adenovirus
(c) Herpes simplex
(d) Measles
(e) Cytomegalic inclusion disease
(f) Varicella
4. Degenerative changes, as seen in viral diseases of the lung
5. Fungal and parasitic diseases (in parasitic diseases, ova or parasite may be seen)
6. Tumor (benign and malignant)

Interfering Factors
False negatives may be due to

1. Delays in preparation of the specimen, causing a deterioration of tumor cells
2. Sampling error. (Diagnostic cells may not have exfoliated into the material examined.)

   Note: Incidence of false negatives is about 15%, in contrast to about 1% in studies for cervical cancer. This high incidence occurs even with careful examination of multiple deep cough specimens.

Cytologic Study of the Gastrointestinal Tract

Normal Values
Negative. Squamous epithelial cells of the esophagus may be present.

Explanation of Test
Exfoliative cytology of the gastrointestinal tract is useful in diagnosis of benign and malignant diseases. However, it is not a specific test for these diseases. Many benign diseases, such as leukoplakia of the esophagus, esophagitis, gastritis, pernicious anemia, and granulomatous diseases, may be recognized because of their characteristic cellular changes. Response to radiation may also be noted from cytologic studies.

Procedure
1. For esophageal studies, a nasogastric Levin tube is passed approximately 40 cm (to the cardioesophageal junction) with the patient in a sitting position.
2. For stomach studies, a Levin tube is passed into the stomach (approximately 60 cm) with the patient in a sitting position.
3. For pancreatic and gallbladder drainage, a special double-lumen gastric tube is passed orally to 45 cm, with the patient in a sitting position. Then the patient is placed on his or her right side and the tube is passed slowly to 85 cm. It takes about 20 minutes for the tube to reach this distance. Tube location is confirmed by biopsy. Lavage with physiologic salt solution is done during all upper gastrointestinal cytology procedures.
4. Specimens can also be obtained during endoscopy procedures.
5. During endoscopy, cytologic brushings may be taken of suspicious areas. The material obtained may be smeared on a slide and immediately fixed, or the brush may be placed in a specimen cup containing 50% alcohol or saline (check with the cytology laboratory for their preference) and taken to the laboratory for processing. (See Chap. 12 for endoscopic procedures.)

Patient Preparation
1. The patient should be told the purpose of the test, the nature of the procedure, and to anticipate some discomfort from the procedure.
2. A liquid diet is usually ordered 24 hours before testing. The patient is encouraged to take fluids throughout the night and in the morning before the test.
3. No oral barium should be administered for the preceding 24 hours.
4. Laxatives and enemas are ordered for colon cytology studies.
5. Because insertion of the nasogastric tube can cause considerable discomfort, the patient and clinician should devise a system (*e.g.*, raising a hand) to indicate discomfort.
6. The patient should be informed that panting, mouth-breathing, or swallowing can help to ease the insertion of the tube.
7. Sucking on ice chips or sipping through a straw also makes insertion of the tube easier.

Clinical Alert

Immediately remove the tube if the patient shows signs of distress: coughing, gasping, or cyanosis.

Patient Aftercare
1. The patient should be given food, fluids, and rest after the tests are completed.
2. Provide rest. Patients having colon studies will be feeling quite tired.

Clinical Implications
1. The characteristics of benign and malignant cells of the gastrointestinal tract are the same as for cells of the rest of the body.
2. Abnormal results in cytologic studies of the esophagus may be a nonspecific aid in the diagnosis of
    (a) Acute esophagitis, characterized by increased exfoliation of basal cells with inflammatory cells and polymorphonuclear leukocytes in the cytoplasm of the benign squamous cells
    (b) Vitamin B_{12} and folic acid deficiencies, characterized by giant epithelial cells
    (c) Malignant diseases, characterized by typical cells of esophageal malignancy
3. Abnormal results in studies of the stomach may be a nonspecific aid in the diagnosis of
    (a) Pernicious anemia, characterized by giant epithelial cells. An injection of vitamin B_{12} will cause these cells to disappear within 24 hours.
    (b) Granulomatous inflammations seen in chronic gastritis and sarcoid of the stomach, which are characterized by granulomatous cells
    (c) Gastritis, characterized by degenerative changes and an increase in the exfoliation of clusters of surface epithelial cells
    (d) Malignant diseases, most of which are gastric adenocarcinomas. Lymphoma cells can be differentiated from adenocarcinoma. The Reed–Sternberg cell, a multinucleated giant cell, is the characteristic cell found along with abnormal lymphocytes in Hodgkin's disease.
4. Abnormal results in studies of the pancreas, gallbladder, and duodenum may reveal malignant cells (usually adenocarcinoma), but it is sometimes difficult to determine the exact site of the tumor.
5. Abnormal results in examination of the colon may reveal
    (a) Ileitis, characterized by large multinucleated histocytes (bovine tuberculosis commonly manifests itself in this area)
    (b) Ulcerative colitis, characterized by a hyperchromatic nuclei surrounded by a thin cytoplasmic rim
    (c) Malignant cells (usually adenocarcinoma)

Interfering Factors

The barium and lubricant used in Levin tubes will interfere with good results, because their presence will distort the cells and prevent accurate evaluation.

Cytologic Study of the Female Genital Tract
(Papanicolaou Smear)

Normal Values

Normal: no abnormal cells
Maturation Index (MI): The MI is a ratio of parabasal to intermediate
to superficial cells. The following are representative ratios:

Normal child	80/20/0
Preovulatory adult	0/40/60
Premenstrual adult	0/70/30
Pregnant adult (2nd mo.)	0/90/10
Postmenopausal adult (age 60)	65/30/5

Explanation of Test

The Papanicolaou (Pap) smear is used principally for diagnosis of precancerous and cancerous conditions of the genital tract, which includes the vagina, cervix, and endometrium. This test is also used for hormonal assessment and for diagnosis of inflammatory diseases. Because the Pap smear is of great importance in the early detection of cervical cancer, it is recommended that all women over the age of 20 have the test at least once a year.

The value of the Pap smear depends on the fact that cells readily exfoliate (or can be easily stripped) from genital cancers. Cytologic study can also be used for assessing response to the effect of administered sex hormones. It should be noted that the microbiologic examination on cytology samples is not as accurate as bacterial culture, but it can provide valuable information.

Specimens for cytologic examination of the genital tract are usually obtained by vaginal speculum examination or by colposcopy with biopsy. Material from the cervix, endocervix, and posterior fornix is obtained for most smears. Smears for hormonal evaluation are obtained from the vagina.

All Pap smears are usually reported on a five-point scale. The meaning of the classes varies, however, and is not universally agreed upon. The following is the scale:

1. Absence of atypical or abnormal cells, negative
2. Atypical cytology, dysplastic, borderline but not neoplastic

3. Cytology suggestive of but not inclusive of malignancy (*suspect* is term often used)
4. Cytology strongly suggestive of malignancy or strongly suspect
5. Cytology conclusive of malignancy, cancer cells present

Clinical Alert

It is important to remember that cytologic findings alone do not form the basis of a diagnosis of cancer or other diseases. Often they are used to justify further procedures, such as biopsy.

Cells are also examined for hormonal effect and organisms. Cells examined for hormonal effect may be reported on a six-point scale.

1. Marked estrogen effect
2. Moderate estrogen effect
3. Slight estrogen effect
4. Atrophic
5. Compatible with pregnancy
6. No evaluation—specimen too bloody or inflamed or scanty

Cells can also be examined for microorganisms using routine staining techniques. These cells may be reported on a five-point scale.

1. Normal flora
2. Scanty or absent
3. *Trichomonas*
4. *Monilia*
5. Other (cocci, coccobacilli, mixed bacteria)

In an effort to standardize reporting of cervical/vaginal cytology specimens, the Division of Cancer Prevention and Control, National Cancer Institute (NCI), organized a workshop in December of 1988. The Besthesda System of reporting was developed as a result of that workshop, and this reporting system is being adopted by numerous laboratories nation-wide. The terminology of this reporting system appears in Table 11–1.

Background

Characteristic physiologic cellular changes occur in the genital tract from birth through the postmenopausal years. Hormonal evaluation by cytologic examination should be performed only on vaginal smears taken from the lateral vaginal wall or from the vaginal fornix. Smears from the ectocervix or endocervix cannot be used for hormonal evaluation because certain conditions, such as metaplasia and cervicitis, in-

(*text continues on page 704*)

TABLE 11–1.
The 1988 Bethesda System for Reporting Cervical/Vaginal Cytological Diagnoses

Statement on Specimen Adequacy
Satisfactory for interpretation
Less than optimal
Unsatisfactory
Explanation for less than optimal/unsatisfactory specimen:
  Scant cellularity
  Poor fixation or preservation
  Presence of foreign material (e.g. lubricant)
  Partially or completely obscuring blood
  Excessive cytolysis or autolysis
  No endocervical component in a premenopausal women who
    has a cervix
  Not representative of the anatomic site
  Other

General Categorization
Within normal limits
Other:
  See descriptive diagnosis.
  Further action recommended

Descriptive Diagnoses
Infection
Fungal
  Fungal organisms morphologically consistent with *Candida*
    species
  Other

Effects of mechanical devices (*e.g.*, intrauterine contraceptive
  device)
Effects of nonsteroidal estrogen exposure (*e.g.*,
  diethystilbestrol)
Other
Epithelial Cell Abnormalities
Squamous Cell
• Atypical squamous cells of undetermined significance
  (recommended follow-up and/or type of further
  investigation: specify)
• Squamous intraepithelial lesion (SIL) (comment on
  presence of cellular changes associated with HPV if
  applicable)
Low-grade squamous intraepithelial lesion, encompassing:
  Cellular changes associated with HPV
  Mild (slight) dysplasia/cervical intraepithelial neoplasia
    grade 1 (CIN 1)
High-grade squamous intraepithelial lesions,
  encompassing:
    Moderate dysplasia/CIN 2
    Severe dysplasia/CIN 3
    Carcinoma in situ/CIN 3
• Squamous cell carcinoma
Glandular Cell
• Presence of endometrial cells in one of the following
  circumstances:
    Out of phase in a menstruating women

Bacterial
Microorganisms morphologically consistent with *Gardnerella* species
Microorganisms morphologically consistent with *Actinomyces* species
Cellular changes suggestive of *Chlamydia* species infection, subject to confirmatory studies
Other
Protozoan
Trichomonas vaginalis
Other
Viral
Cellular changes associated with cytomegalovirus
Cellular changes associated with herpesvirus simplex
Other
(Note: for human papillomavirus [HPV], refer to "Epithelial Cell Abnormalities, Squamous Cell")
Other
Reactive and Reparative Changes
Inflammation
Associated cellular changes
Follicular cervicitis
Miscellaneous (as related to patient history)
Effects of therapy
Ionizing radiation
Chemotherapy

In a postmenopausal woman
No menstrual history available
• Atypical glandular cells of undetermined significance (recommended follow-up and/or type of further investigation: specify)
Endometrial
Endocervical
Not otherwise specified
• Adenocarcinoma
Specify probable site of origin: endocervical, endometrial, extrauterine
Not otherwise specified
• Other epithelial malignant neoplasm: specify
Nonepithelial Malignant Neoplasm: Specify
Hormonal Evaluation (Applies To Vaginal Smears Only)
• Hormonal pattern compatible with age and history
• Hormonal pattern incompatible with age and history: specify
• Hormonal evaluation not possible
Cervical specimen
Inflammation
Insufficient patient history
Other

terfere with a correct assessment. There are three major cell types occurring in a characteristic pattern in vaginal smears.

1. Superficial squamous cells (mature squamous, usually polygonal, containing a pyknotic nucleus)
2. Intermediate squamous cells (mature squamous, usually polygonal, containing a clearly structured vesicular nucleus, which may be either well preserved or peptolytically changed as a result of bacterial cytolysis)
3. Parabasal cells (immature squamous, usually round or oval, containing one or, rarely, more than one relatively large nucleus). These cells occur either well preserved or in proteolytic clusters as a result of degeneration or necrosis.

> **Note:** Deviation from physiologic cell patterns may be indicative of pathologic conditions.

Hormonal cytology is valuable in the assessment of many endocrine-related conditions, especially ovarian function.

Procedure
1. The patient is usually asked to remove clothing from the waist down.
2. The patient is placed in a lithotomy position on an examining table.
3. A speculum lubricated only with water is inserted into the vagina to expose the cervix.
4. The posterior fornix and external os of the cervix are scraped with a wooden spatula and obtained material is spread on slides and placed in preservative or fixative.
5. Label the specimen with name, date, woman's age, reason for examination, last menstrual period, and area from which specimen is obtained.
6. Examination takes only about 5 minutes.

> **Note:** The best time to take a Pap smear is 5 to 6 days after the end of the menstrual period.

Procedure for Hormonal Smears, "Maturation Index"
Obtain a specimen by scraping the proximal portion of the lateral wall of the vagina, avoiding the cervical area. Otherwise the same as above.

Clinical Implications
1. Abnormal cytology responses can be classified as protective, destructive, reparative (regenerative), or neoplastic.
2. Inflammatory reactions and microbes can be identified to help in the diagnosis of vaginal diseases.

3. Precancerous and cancerous lesions of the cervix can be identified. The stages of neoplastic disease can be arbitrarily classified as dysplasia (mild, moderate, and severe), carcinoma *in situ* (preinvasive carcinoma), microinvasive carcinoma, and invasive carcinoma.
4. Hormonal cytology reports will include several factors:
   (a) Hormonal cell pattern: The report will state that the pattern is, or is not, compatible with the age and menstrual history of the patient. The reason for noncompatibility is given.
   (b) Maturation index: Maturation index is a proportion of the major cell types (parabasal, intermediate, and superficial) in each 100 cells counted. The MI will be expressed as a ratio (*e.g.*, MI = 100/0/0). See "Normal Values" for representative MIs.
5. The following facts should be kept in mind when hormonal cytology reports are reviewed (see Table 11–2).
   (a) The degree of maturity of the epithelium cannot be expressed in degrees of estrogenic effects or estrogen deficiencies, because more than one hormonal stimulus is involved (estrogen, progesterone, and adrenal hormones).
   (b) Surgical removal of the ovaries does not necessarily result in epithelial atrophy.
   (c) Only two cell types can be identified with accuracy if the age and menstrual history of the patient are not known.
      (1) Abundant superficial squamous cells, indicative of unequivocal estrogenic effect
      (2) Parabasal cells, indicative of lack of cell maturation due to lack of hormone stimulation
   (d) From a single specimen, it is impossible to predict whether ovulation will occur, whether it has recently occurred, or what stage of menstrual cycle the patient is in. Serial specimens must be examined to obtain the above results.
   (e) An intermediate cell type is always intermediate, regardless of its size.
   (f) No hormonal assessment should be made without knowing the age of the patient, her menstrual history, and her history of hormone administrations.

Interfering Factors
1. Medications such as tetracycline and digitalis, which affect the squamous epithelium, will alter test results.
2. The use of lubricating jelly in the vagina and recent douching will interfere with test results by distorting the cells and preventing accurate evaluation.
3. The presence of infection will interfere with hormonal cytology.
4. Heavy menstrual flow may make the interpretation of the results difficult and may obscure atypical cells.

TABLE 11–2.
Vaginal Cytologic Smear Findings in Gynecologic
and Related Endocrinopathies

Condition	Usual Smear Types
Adrenal hyperplasia, congenital	Atrophic to atypical intermediate proliferation
Adrenogenital syndrome (hyperplasia)	Atrophic to atypical intermediate proliferation
Adrenal tumor (masculinizing)	Usually atrophic; sometimes "multihormonal" with cells from all layers
Chiari–Frommel syndrome	Markedly atrophic
Cushing's syndrome	Intermediate proliferation or atypical regressive types
Eunuchoidism, ovarian	Atrophic
Feminizing testicular syndrome	Proliferative; nuclear sex chromatin negative
Follicular cytosis	Persistently high estrogen index (EI) and karyopyknotic index (KI)
Gonadal dysgenesis	Atrophic; nuclear sex chromatin negative in 80%
Hirsutism, genetic	Normal cycling
Hypothalamic (psychogenic) amenorrhea	Most often atrophic to slight proliferation but great variation from atrophic to highly proliferative
Menopausal syndrome	At first highly proliferative, some with cycling; later, intermediate proliferation or atrophic
Ovarian tumors, feminizing	Proliferative, some with high EI and KI, occasionally regressive
Ovarian tumors, masculinizing	Variation, many atrophic, some with atypical proliferation or "multihormonal"
Precocious puberty, constitutional	Proliferative, some with high EI and KI, some with cycling
Pituitary hypogonadism	Atrophic to slight proliferation
Pseudocyesis	"Progestational" types with varying regression
Stein–Leventhal syndrome	Variation; most with intermediate proliferation, occasionally highly proliferative
Uterine defect (congenital absence or irresponsiveness)	Normal cycling

(Adapted from Rakoff AI: Hormonal cytology in gynecology. Clin Obstet Gynecol 4:1045–1061, 1961). In Keebler CM, Reagan JW (eds): Manual of Cytotechnology, 6th ed. Chicago, American Society of Clinical Pathologists, 1983)

Patient Preparation
1. Explain the test purpose and procedure.
2. Instruct the patient not to douche for 2 to 3 days before the test because this may remove the exfoliated cells.
3. Have the patient empty her bladder and rectum prior to examination.
4. Ask the patient to give the following information:
   (a) First day of last menstrual period
   (b) Use of hormone therapy or birth control pills
   (c) All medications taken
   (d) Any radiation therapy
   This information must be sent to the laboratory along with specimens for cytology.

Cytologic Study of Aspirated Breast Cysts and Nipple Discharge

Normal Values
Negative for neoplasia

Background
Nipple discharge is normal usually only during the lactation period. Any other nipple discharge is abnormal and when it occurs, breasts should be examined for mastitis, duct papilloma, or intraductal cancer. (However, certain situations increase the possibility of finding a normal nipple discharge, such as pregnancy, perimenopause, and use of birth control pills.) About 3% of breast cancers and 10% of benign lesions of the breast are associated with abnormal nipple discharge.

The contents of all breast cysts obtained by needle biopsy are examined to detect malignant cells.

Procedure
1. Breast cyst
   The contents of the identified breast cyst are obtained by percutaneous aspiration.
2. Nipple discharge

   Note: This procedure should be confined to patients who have no palpable masses in the breast or other evidence of breast cancer.

   (a) The nipple should be washed with a cotton pledget and patted dry.
   (b) The nipple is gently stripped, or milked, to obtain a discharge.
   (c) Fluid should be expressed until a pea-sized drop appears.
   (d) The patient may assist by holding a bottle of fixative beneath the breast so that the slide may be dropped in immediately.

    (e) The discharge is spread immediately on a slide and then dropped into the fixative bottle containing 95% alcohol.

    (f) The specimen is identified with pertinent data, including from which breast it was obtained.

    (g) The specimen is sent without delay to the laboratory.

Clinical Implications
Abnormal results are helpful in identifying

1. Benign breast conditions, such as mastitis and intraductal papilloma
2. Malignant breast conditions, such as papilloma intraductal cancer or intracystic infiltrating cancer

---

Clinical Alert

Any discharge, regardless of color, should be examined. A bloody or blood-tinged discharge is especially significant.

Interfering Factors
Use of drugs that alter hormone balance, such as phenothiazines, digitalis, diuretics, and steroids, often results in a clear nipple discharge.

Cytologic Study of Urine

Normal Values
Negative. Epithelial and squamous cells are normally present in urine. (See also Chap. 3, especially "Microscopic Examination of Sediment.")

Explanation of Test
Cells from the epithelial lining of the urinary tract exfoliate readily into the urine. Urine cytology is most useful in the diagnosis of cancer and inflammatory diseases of the bladder, the renal pelvis, the ureters, and the urethra. This study is also valuable in detecting cytomegalic inclusion disease and other viral diseases and in detecting bladder cancer in high-risk populations, such as workers exposed to aniline dyes, smokers, and patients previously treated for bladder cancer. A Papanicolaou stain of smears prepared from the urinary sediment, filter preparations, or cytocentrifuged smears is useful to identify abnormalities.

Procedure
1. Obtain a clean voided urine specimen of at least 180 ml (adults) and 10 ml (children).

2. Obtain a catheterized specimen, if possible, if cancer is suspected.
3. Deliver the specimen immediately to the cytology laboratory. Urine should be as fresh as possible when it is examined. If a delay is expected, an equal volume of 50% alcohol may be added as a preservative.

Clinical Implications

1. Findings possibly indicative of *inflammatory conditions* of the *lower urinary tract*
   (a) Epithelial hyperplasia
   (b) Atypical cells
   (c) Abundance of red blood cells
   (d) Leukocytes

   > **Note:** Inflammatory conditions could be due to any of the following:
   >
   > (a) Benign prostatic hyperplasia
   > (b) Adenocarcinoma of the prostate
   > (c) Kidney stones
   > (d) Diverticula of bladder
   > (e) Strictures
   > (f) Malformations

2. Findings indicative of viral diseases
   (a) Cytomegalic inclusion disease: large intranuclear inclusions

   > **Note:** Cytomegalic inclusion disease is a viral infection that usually occurs in childhood but is also seen in cancer patients treated with chemotherapy and in transplant patients treated with immunosuppressives. The renal tubular epithelium is usually involved
   >
   > (1) Cytomegaloviruses or salivary gland viruses are related to the herpes varicella agents.
   > (2) Infected people may excrete virus in the urine or saliva for months.
   > (3) About 60% to 90% of adults have experienced infection.
   > (4) In closed populations such as the mentally retarded or households, high infection rates may occur at an early age.

   (b) Measles: Characteristic cytoplasmic inclusion bodies may be found in the urine preceding the appearance of Koplik's spots.

3. Findings possibly indicative of malacoplakia and granulomatous disease of the bladder or upper urinary tract
   (a) Histiocytes with multiple granules in an abundant, foamy cytoplasm
   (b) Michaelis–Gutmann bodies in malacoplakia

4. Cytologic findings possibly indicative of malignancy
   If the specimen shows evidence of any of the changes associated with malignancy, cancer of the bladder, renal pelvis, ureters, kidney, and urethra may be suspected. Metastatic tumor should be ruled out as well.

Cytologic Study of Cerebrospinal Fluid (CSF)

Normal Values
1. Total cell count
   Adult: 0–10/mm^3 (all mononuclear cells)
   Infant: 0–20/mm^3
2. Negative for neoplasia
3. A variety of normal cells may be seen. Large lymphocytes are most common. Small lymphocytes are also seen, as are elements of the monocyte–macrophage series.
4. The CSF of a healthy person should be free of all pathogens.

Explanation of Test
Spinal fluid obtained by lumbar puncture is examined for the presence of abnormal cells and for an increase or decrease in the normally present cell population. Most of the usual laboratory procedures for study of CSF involve an examination of the white cells and a white blood cell count; chemical and microbiologic studies are also done. In recent years, cell studies of the CSF have been used to identify neoplastic cells. These studies have been especially helpful in the diagnosis and treatment of the different phases of leukemia disorders. The nature of neoplasia is such that for tumor cells to exfoliate, they must actually invade the CSF circulation and enter such areas as the ventricle wall, the choroid plexus, or the subarachnoid space.

Procedure
1. Usually, three specimens of at least 1 to 3 ml are obtained by lumbar puncture (see Chap. 5, p. 248).
2. Generally, only one specimen of 1 to 3 ml goes to the cytology laboratory. Other tubes are sent to different laboratories for examination.
3. The specimen is labeled with the patient's name, date, and type of specimen.
4. The sample is sent immediately to the cytology laboratory for processing.

Clinical Alert

The laboratory should be given adequate warning that a CSF specimen will be delivered. Time is a critical factor; cells begin to disintegrate if the sample is kept at room temperature for more than 1 hour.

Clinical Implications

1. Cerebrospinal fluid abnormalities may be helpful in the detection of
    (a) Malignant gliomas that have invaded the ventricles or cortex of the brain. White blood cells (WBC) $\leq$ 150/mm^3 (The sample may be normal in 75% of patients.)
    (b) Ependymoma (neoplasm of differentiated ependymal cells) and medulloblastoma (a cerebellar tumor) in children
    (c) Seminoma and pineoblastoma (tumors of the pineal gland)
    (d) Secondary carcinomas
        (1) Secondary carcinomas metastasizing to the central nervous system have multiple avenues to the subarachnoid space through the bloodstream.
        (2) The breast and lung are common sources of metastatic cells exfoliated in the CSF. Infiltration of acute leukemia is also quite common.
    (e) Central nervous system leukemia
    (f) Fungal forms
        (1) Congenital toxoplasmosis
            WBC: 50–500/mm^3 (mostly monocytes present)
        (2) Coccidioidomycosis
            WBC: 200/mm^3
    (g) Various forms of meningitis
        (1) Cryptococcal meningitis
            WBC: 800/mm^3 (lymphocytes are more abundant than polynuclear neutrophilic leukocytes)
        (2) Tuberculous meningitis
            WBC: 25–1000/mm^3 (mostly lymphocytes present)
        (3) Acute pyogenic meningitis
            WBC: 25–10,000/mm^3 (mostly polynuclear neutrophilic leukocytes present)
    (h) Meningoencephalitis (primary amebic meningoencephalitis)
        (1) WBC: 400–21,000/mm^3
        (2) Red blood cells are also found.
        (3) Wright's stain may reveal amebas.

   (i) Hemosiderin-laden macrophages, as in subarachnoid hemorrhage

   (j) Lipophages from central nervous system destructive processes

2. Characteristics of neoplastic cells

   (a) Sometimes marked increase in size, most likely sarcoma and carcinomas

   (b) Exfoliated cells tend to be more polymorphic as the neoplasm becomes increasingly malignant.

Interfering Factors

The lumbar puncture can occasionally cause contamination of the specimen with squamous epithelial cells or spindly fibroblasts.

Cytologic Studies of Effusions

Normal Values

Negative for abnormal cells

Background

Effusions are accumulations of fluids. They may be exudates, which generally accumulate as a result of inflammation, or transudates, which are fluids not associated with inflammation. Below is a comparison of these two effusions.

Exudate

1. Accumulates in body cavities and tissues because of malignancy or inflammation
2. Associated with an inflammatory process
3. Viscous
4. High content of protein, cells, and solid materials derived from cells
5. May have high WBC content
6. Clots spontaneously (because of high concentration of fibrinogen)
7. Malignant cells as well as bacteria may be detected
8. Specific gravity >1.015

Transudate

1. Accumulates in body cavities from impaired circulation
2. Not associated with an inflammatory process
3. Highly fluid
4. Low content of protein, cells, or solid materials derived from cells
5. Has low WBC content
6. Will not clot
7. Malignant cells may be present
8. Specific gravity <1.015

Fluid contained in the pleural, pericardial, and peritoneal or abdominal cavities is a serous fluid. Accumulation of fluid in the peritoneal cavity is called *ascites*.

Explanation of Test

Cytologic studies of effusions—either exudates or transudates—are sometimes helpful in determining the cause of these abnormal collections of fluids. The effusions are found in the pericardial sac, the pleural cavities, and the abdominal cavities. *The chief problem in diagnosis is in differentiating malignant cells from reactive mesothelial cells.*

Procedure

Material for cytologic examination of effusions is obtained by either thoracentesis or paracentesis. Both of these procedures involve surgical puncture of a cavity for aspiration of a fluid.

Thoracentesis

1. Chest roentgenograms should be available at the patient's bedside so that the location of fluid may be determined.
2. The patient may be administered a sedative.
3. The chest is exposed. The physician inserts a long thoracentesis needle with a syringe attached.
4. At least 40 ml of fluid is withdrawn. It is preferable to withdraw 300 ml to 1000 ml of fluid.
5. The specimen is collected in a clean container and heparin may be added, particularly if the specimen is very bloody (5–10 units heparin per 1 ml of fluid). Alcohol should *not* be added.
6. The specimen should be labeled with the patient's name, date, source of the fluid, and diagnosis.
7. The covered specimen should be sent immediately to the laboratory. (If the specimen cannot be sent at once, it may be refrigerated.)

Paracentesis (Abdominal)

1. The patient should be asked to void.
2. The patient is placed in the Fowler's position.
3. A local anesthetic is given.
4. A no. 20 needle is introduced into the patient's abdomen and the fluid is withdrawn, 50 ml at a time, until 300 ml to 1000 ml is withdrawn.
5. Follow the same procedure as in numbers 5, 6, and 7 of *Thoracentesis*, above.

Clinical Alert

Paracentesis may precipitate hepatic coma in a patient with chronic liver disease. The patient must be watched constantly for indications of shock: pallor, cyanosis, or dizziness. Emergency stimulants should be ready.

Clinical Implications

1. All effusions contain some mesothelial cells. (Mesothelial cells comprise the squamous layer of the epithelium covering the surface of all serous membranes.) The more chronic and irritating the condition, the more numerous and atypical are the mesothelial cells. Histiocytes and lymphocytes are common.

2. Evidence of abnormalities in serous fluids is characterized by

    (a) Degenerating red blood cells, granular red cell fragments, and histiocytes containing blood. Presence of these structures means that injury to a vessel or vessels is part of the condition causing fluid to accumulate.

    (b) Mucin, which is suggestive of adenocarcinoma

    (c) Large numbers of polymorphonuclear leukocytes, which is indicative of an acute inflammatory process such as peritonitis

    (d) Prevalence of plasma cells, which suggests the possibility of antibody formation

    (e) Numerous eosinophils, which suggest parasitic infestation, Hodgkin's disease, or a hypersensitive state

    (f) Presence of many reactive mesothelial cells together with hemosiderin histiocytes, which may indicate

    (1) Leaking aneurysm

    (2) Rheumatoid arthritis

    (3) Lupus erythematosus

    (g) Malignant cells

3. Abnormal cells may be indicative of

    (a) Malignancy. The most important criterion of cancer is the arrangement of chromatin within the nuclei.

    (b) Inflammatory conditions

Interfering Factors

Vigorous shaking and stirring of specimens will cause altered results.

Patient Preparation

Explain the purpose of the test and procedure.

Cutaneous Immunofluorescence Biopsy

Normal Values

A descriptive interpretative report is made.

Explanation of Test

Biopsy of the skin for direct epidermal fluorescent studies is indicated in the investigation of certain disorders such as lupus erythematosus, blistering disease, and vasculitis. Skin biopsies are also used to confirm the histopathology of skin lesions to rule out other diagnoses and to follow the results of treatment.

Procedure
A 4-mm punch biopsy specimen of involved or uninvolved skin is obtained.

Clinical Implications
Biopsy of skin will show

1. The lesions of discoid lupus erythematosus as a bandlike immunofluorescence of immunoglobulins and complement components. Similar findings in a biopsy of the normal skin are consistent with systemic lupus erythematosus and may be used to follow the results of treatment.
2. In blistering diseases such as pemphigus and pemphigoid, where circulating antibodies may not be present, a lesion may show intercellular epidermal antibody of pemphigus or basement membrane antibody of pemphigoid.

Estradiol Receptor and Progesterone Receptor in Breast Cancer (ERA, PRA)

Normal Values
Estradiol: Negative; ≤3 femtomoles/mg of protein
Progesterone: Negative; ≤5 femtomoles/mg of protein

Explanation of Test
Estrogen and progesterone receptors in the cells of breast cancer tissues are measured to determine whether or not a tumor is likely to respond to endocrine therapy or to the removal of the ovaries.

Procedure
A 1-g specimen of quickly frozen tumor is examined for saturation and expressed in a Scatchard plot.

Clinical Implications
1. Positive test for estrogen occurs at levels greater than 3 femtomoles and for progesterone binding at levels of 5 femtomoles and above.
2. Approximately 55% of estrogen receptor–*positive* tumors will respond to endocrine therapy.
3. Estrogen receptor–*negative* tumors rarely respond to endocrine therapy.
4. The finding of positive progesterone increases the predictive value of selecting patients for hormonal therapy. There is some incidence to suggest that progesterone receptor synthesis is estrogen dependent.

STUDIES OF INHERITED DISORDERS

Introduction

Many disease states can reflect hereditary components. However, general clinical studies usually focus upon the disorder itself rather than upon its heredity. Therefore, this section addresses conditions that require information about genetic backgrounds in order to be diagnosed properly. Chromosomal and linkage studies are two methods used for the diagnosis of inherited disorders. (Related disorders are discussed in the hematology section, Chap. 2, and the prenatal section, Chap. 16.)

Indications for Testing

1. *Genetic Counseling.* Specific diagnostic studies of biologically related family members may be necessary to determine the risk of disease recurrence or occurrence for the children, the parents, and other family members, especially if reproduction is an option.
2. *Prenatal Care.* (See Chap. 16.) In some instances, psychological and medical management of a potential problem pregnancy may greatly improve outcomes. On the other hand, serious fetal abnormalities may sometimes cause the parents to opt for termination of the pregnancy. Others will choose to sustain pregnancy in spite of uncertain or negative outcomes.
3. *Diagnosis.* Diagnosis of certain diseases is related to chromosome or DNA studies.

Overview of Chromosomes and Genes

Genetic information is coded in deoxyribonucleic acid (DNA), which is found in the chromosomes. Chromosomes are physical structures in the cell and nucleus that can be directly, although not easily, observed. Each chromosome consists of many thousands of genes, which are considered to be smaller segments of DNA responsible for specific genetic traits. (Single genes cannot be directly seen.)

Chromosomes (and the genes that comprise them) are found in pairs. There are 23 pairs. One of each pair comes from the father and the other comes from the mother. Twenty-two of these pairs (the autosomes) are essentially identical. The twenty-third pair consists of the sex chromosomes. Women have two X chromosomes. Men have an X and a Y chromosome. The Y chromosome has very few genes. These determine the development of the man.

Single abnormal genes can generate a wide range of problems that manifest themselves in a few basic ways.

1. *Dominant Inheritance.* A single copy of an abnormal gene is enough to produce a disorder. An affected parent has a 50% chance of transmitting this specific abnormal gene to any child. Of course, when the disorder is seen for the first time, it may be presumed that a new mutation has occurred in the egg or the sperm. For some conditions, expression of the disorder may be variable. This leads to the possibility that one of the parents may have the abnormal gene in question. Examples of dominant inherited disorders include Huntington's chorea and neurofibromatosis.
2. *Recessive Inheritance.* Both copies of the gene must be abnormal for the problem to be apparent. If both parents carry the same recessive gene, there is a 25% chance that their child will inherit two copies of the abnormal gene and will develop a problem. Cystic fibrosis and sickle cell disease are examples of recessive gene disorders.
3. *X-linked (Sex-linked) Inheritance.* Because men have only a single copy of X chromosome genes, abnormalities of these genes will not be "covered up" by a second normal copy (as happens in women). When the female is a carrier, a 50% chance exists for any son to be affected by the disease or for any daughter to be a carrier of the disease. Examples of sex-linked disorders include hemophilia and Duchenne muscular dystrophy.
4. *Multifactorial Inheritance.* This causes some defects through the interactions of many genes with each other. Often these interactions are associated with environmental factors. Risks vary according to the disorder. Examples of multifactorial disorders are congenital dislocation of the hip and pyloric stenosis.

Chromosome Analysis

Normal Values
Women: 44 autosomes + 2 X chromosomes; karyotype: 46, XX
Men: 44 autosomes, 1 X, 1Y chromosome; karyotype; 46, XY

Background
The karyotype is a study of the chromosome constitution of an individual. It involves determination of chromosome number and chromosome structure. Alterations in either can produce a wide range of problems. The standard karyotype can be useful for determining diagnosis and for providing genetic counseling. Extra or missing pieces of most chromosomal material cause developmental problems. Despite much speculation, we generally do not know how the abnormality translates into structural or functional anomalies. Predictions related to expecta-

tions from specific findings almost always depend upon comparisons with clinical findings of other cases that present the same abnormality.

Explanation of Test

Standard chromosome studies can be helpful in evaluation of the following clinical situations:

1. Multiple malformations
2. Failure to thrive
3. Mental retardation
4. Ambiguous genitalia or hypogonadism
5. Recurrent miscarriages
6. Infertility
7. Primary amenorrhea or oligomenorrhea
8. Delayed puberty
9. Analysis of products of conception that result from stillbirths or miscarriages (particularly with malformations)
10. Prenatal diagnosis of abnormalities related to chromosome disorders (*e.g.*, Down syndrome in mothers over 35 years of age)
11. Detection of parents with chromosomal mosaicism or translocations who may be at high risk for transmitting genetic abnormalities to their children
12. Sex determination prior to delivery
13. With certain cancers and leukemias, abnormalities of the chromosomes may help determine prognosis and/or stage of the disease. Interpretation of such studies is complex and subject to change as new information becomes available.

Procedure

Specimens for chromosome analyses are generally obtained from the following sources:

1. Leukocytes from peripheral blood are used most frequently because they are the most easily obtained. At least 3 days are necessary to prepare the cells. Interpretation may take additional time, directly proportional to the complexity of the analytical process.
2. Bone marrow biopsies can sometimes be completed within 24 hours. However, the detailed results are rarely as satisfactory as those obtained from leukocyte analysis. Bone marrow analysis is often done to diagnosis certain leukemias.
3. Fibroblasts from skin or surgical specimens can be grown and preserved in long-term culture mediums for future studies. A sufficient amount of the specimen for studies usually requires at least a week for growth. These specimens are especially helpful in the detection of mosaicism (different chromosome constitutions in different tissues).

4. Amniotic fluid obtained through amniocentesis requires more than a week to produce a sufficient amount of specimen for analysis. These studies are often done for prenatal detection of chromosomal abnormalities.
5. Chorionic villus sampling, or CVS, can be done at an earlier stage of pregnancy (about 9 weeks) than amniocentesis. In fact, some initial CVS studies can be done almost immediately after conception. Occasional false positives represent mosaicism of the placenta (the presence of several cell lines, some of which may not be found in the fetus). These studies need confirmation through long-term culture.
6. Cells may be grown from fetal tissue or from early products of conception in order to determine the reason for the loss of the pregnancy. Cells from the fetal side of the placenta may be the easiest to grow. However, these studies are frequently not successful.

   Note: The buccal smear for sex chromosome detection taken from a cheek cell specimen is rarely useful. In fact, it is often inaccurate, especially in the newborn period. However, it may occasionally be helpful for determining the presence or absence of the Y chromosome.

Definition of Karyotype

The karyotype is an arrangement of the chromosomes of a cell into a specific order from the largest to the smallest so that their number and structure can be analyzed. Today, this is routinely done with banding, a technique that permits the appreciation of differences in structure between the different pairs. Prior to the institution of banding, it was often impossible to group the correct pairs of chromosomes, so they were arranged in groups according to size and structure and labeled A through G. The X chromosomes were part of group C and the Y chromosomes belonged to group E. Now, they are usually placed with each other, apart from the other groups.

The different pairs of chromosomes are distinguished by several of the following characteristics:

1. Length
2. The location of the centromere (the constriction that divides chromosomes into long [q] arms and short [p] arms)
3. Ratio of the long and short arms to each other
4. Secondary constrictions
5. Satellites, which are small variable pieces of DNA seen at the ends of arms of some of the chromosomes

6. Staining or banding patterns. A variety of different stains and techniques can be used. The most common is Giemsa banding. Most of the other methods, such as centromeric or fluorescent staining, are used only for select situations.

Nomenclature of the Karyotype
The following is the standard convention:

1. The first number is the total number of chromosomes.
2. The sex chromosome complement follows (usually XX for normal women or XY for normal men).
3. Missing, extra, or abnormal chromosomes are then identified.
4. "p" refers to the short arm; "q" to the long arm.
5. Bands are numbered from the centromere out. As techniques have improved, these have been subdivided. For example, in the two-digit number 32, the first number (3) is the band and the second number (2) is the subdivision of that band (band 32). Decimal points indicate further division under the same system; for example, 32.41 is the first subdivision (1) of the fourth subdivision (4) of band 32.
6. A three-letter code at the end designates the banding technique. The first letter is the type of banding; the second letter denotes the general technique; and the third letter indicates the stain. Probably the most common is GTG; G bands by trypsin using Giemsa. Special or unusual techniques are normally used only in very select circumstances.

More than 80 other abbreviations can be used to label other structural findings. Some of the more common ones are mentioned in clinical implications of chromosome analyses on page 721.

Occasionally, it is possible to associate a chromosomal finding with specific genes and to understand the clinical picture from these results. However, for the most part, the link between a specific chromosomal abnormality and a specific set of findings is not well understood. Implications that result from karyotype studies usually come from correlations with previous cases rather than from any theoretical considerations. Well-known chromosomal syndromes can present many variables. Therefore, predictions must be made cautiously.

Clinical Alert

Most laboratories provide explanations of results. However, it may be necessary to talk directly with laboratory personnel to understand fully a difficult karyotype.

Clinical Implications

Some chromosomal abnormalities include the following:

1. Abnormalities of number
   (a) Autosomes
       Trisomy 21 (Down's syndrome)
       Trisomy 18
       Trisomy 13
   (b) Sex chromosomes
       Turner syndrome (single X)
       Klinefelter syndrome (XXY)
       XYY
       XXX
2. Abnormalities of structure
   (a) Deletions
       Cat cry syndrome (5p-)
       18 p- (missing short arm of chromosome 18)
       Prader–Willi syndrome (15q- in some cases)
   (b) Duplications
       3q2 trisomy (extra material from the second band in the long arm of the third chromosome—Cornelia de Lange resemblance)
   (c) Translocations
       t(11;22) (translocation of chromosomes 11 and 22)
   (d) Isochromosomes
       i(Xq) (a single chromosome with duplication of the long arms of the X chromosome; a variant of Turner syndrome)
   (e) Ring chromosomes
       r(13) (a chromosome 13 with the ends of the long and short arms joined together, giving a ring)
   (f) Mosaicism
       46,XX/45,X (two cell lines, one normal female and the other for Turner syndrome)

Patient Preparation

1. Some states will require an informed, signed, and witnessed consent.
2. Explain purpose, procedure, and any known risks of tests.
3. Provide appropriate parental counseling regarding implications of test outcome.

Patient Aftercare

1. If amniotic fluid specimen is obtained for analysis, follow same precautions as listed in Chapter 16.
2. Provide timely and compassionate information, support and guidance for parents and child (and/or other family members) dependent upon test outcome (*e.g.*, risk of disease occurrence or recurrence).

Special Chromosome Studies

The fragile X syndrome is one of the most common genetic causes of mental retardation. An X-linked trait, it is most common in men. Women can carry the gene without exhibiting any of the characteristics. However, some women are as severely affected as men. This syndrome takes its name from the finding of a small area on the long arm of the X chromosome that looks like a break in the arm (although it actually is not). It is necessary to grow the cells in a special media to see this finding. A regular karyotype will miss it. Even with the special media, not all cells will show the finding. In women who are carriers, the syndrome becomes harder to detect as the woman ages.

In rare conditions, special areas such as excess chromosome breakage (as for Fanconi anemia) or abnormalities of the centromeres (Roberts syndrome) are examined. These require special requests.

Direct Detection of Abnormal Genes

In the past, abnormal genes were detected through the effects they produced. These effects typically presented themselves as biochemical or physical manifestations. Now, it is possible to detect directly the specific sequence of DNA that causes an abnormality. This technology relies upon the ability to synthesize probes (pieces of DNA with specific sequences). Such probes hybridize with (attach to) specific complementary sequences and can be labeled for easy detection. Probes manufactured for this purpose are called Allele Specific Oligonucleotides, or ASOs.

Sometimes detection relies upon the presence of restriction sites. In this case, DNA can be "chopped" into pieces by enzymes that attack specific sequences. The pieces that result depend upon the presence of restriction sites (areas that have the requisite sequences). If only a few of these are present, the pieces will usually be large. If there are only a few for a particular enzyme, they will be small.

Genes can contain several different DNA abnormalities. The bases that make up the genetic sequence may be changed. In some cases, they may be missing entirely or in part or may be partially duplicated. Any of these abnormalities can change the sequence at a restriction site. This means that sometimes a fragment will change in size because of a change in the DNA. When this happens, it provides a method for the detection of a change in a gene. Of course, many changes do not involve restriction sites and so are not detectable by this method.

Linkage Studies

Specific genes have specific locations or loci (singular: locus) on chromosomes. It is sometimes possible to track an abnormal gene that is undetectably by standard methods by detecting something located nearby that is transmitted along with the abnormal gene. Chromosomes can show harmless variations (polymorphisms) of their structure. These polymorphisms sometimes help to locate the site of a gene when appropriate family studies are done. Similarly, other genes may be easily detected through their biochemical products, through physical findings, or by specific molecular probes.

Because chromosomes are specific physical structures, all genes on any specific one should be transmitted as a single unit. Actually, because of the process of crossing over during formation of egg and sperm cells, there is some recombination between the two members of any chromosome pair—a switching of material from one to another. Still, the more physically close any two genes are, the more likely it is that they will stay together, or be linked in transmission. Linkage studies are based on this fact. It means that even if a gene cannot be identified directly, it may be possible to test for another gene nearby and to use that as a marker.

This is like trying to trace a package on a train going from coast to coast. All the baggage cars on one line may look alike, but if it is known that there is a distinctive caboose, this caboose can be tracked and linked to the car with the package. Of course, at each layover the cars may be switched onto other trains. If the cars right in front and right in back of the one with the package can be identified, it is unlikely that the package car would have been switched out by itself.

Basically, then, flanking markers, one on each side of the gene, reduce the likelihood of undetected crossovers that might destroy the linkage. The closer the flankers are, and the more of them, the better the identification process. Calculations may be complex, but they can express a percentage chance that the gene in question has been passed on.

Again, it needs to be emphasized it is usually not enough to know that gene A is linked to gene B. Which form of gene A is linked to which form of gene B in the family at risk is the crucial question. Typically, this can only be done by studies on that particular family.

Such studies, which may need extended families to clarify linkage, can be laborious and time consuming. Therefore, if possible, the family should discuss the situation with a medical geneticist or genetic counselor as early in the pregnancy as possible.

Linkage studies are becoming more common as molecular techniques evolve. Traditionally, these studies involved specific genes that were highly variable, such as the blood groups, or the immune response (HLA) genes. At times, chromosome studies were also helpful. This process has been greatly enhanced by the discovery of *restriction fragment length polymorphisms* (RFLP), a term often found in linkage reports. It has been found that certain areas of the DNA that comprise the chromosomes are highly variable (polymorphic) within human populations. These variations affect the process whereby that portion of DNA is separated into pieces by different types of enzymes. The length of the DNA fragments that result (longer or shorter) depends upon the sensitivity to different enzymes at different positions. These can give DNA "fingerprints" that become markers at a large number of sites. Although the technical work involved often differs from classical linkage studies, the end result is hopefully the same.

Ideally, related techniques can be used specifically to detect gene disorders (*e.g.*, sickle cell anemia). These studies are more specific than linkage and can be done on one person.

Bibliography

American Society for Cytotechnology: The 1988 Bethesda System for Reporting Cervical/Vaginal Cytological Diagnoses. JAMA 267(7): August 18, 1989

Antonarakis A: Diagnosis of genetic disorders. N Engl J Med 320:155, 1989

Beahrs OH, Myers MH (eds): Manual for Staging of Cancer, 3nd ed. Philadelphia, JB Lippincott, 1988

Cann HM, et al: Diagnosis of genetic disease by linkage analyses. Birth Defects 23:33, 1987

Clodak GW, et al: The role of fine needle aspiration biopsy in early diagnosis of prostate cancer. *In* Karr J, Caffey D, Gardner W Jr (eds): Prognostic Cytometry and Cytopathology of Prostate Cancer. New York, Elsevier Science Publishing, 1989

Fiesor G et al: Enhancing cervical cancer detection using nucleic acid hybridization and acetic acid tests. Nurse Pract 7(26):29–30, July 1990

Galpard H: Biochemical diagnosis of genetic disease. Experientia 42:1075, 1986

Henry JB (ed): Clinical Diagnoses and Management of Laboratory Methods, 18th ed. Philadelphia, WB Saunders, 1984, p 299

Kaiser LR: Diagnostic and therapeutic uses of pleuroscopy (thorascopy) in lung cancer. Surg Clin North Am, 67:1081–1086, October, 1987

Kallacky MA, MacMillan W, Sheets EE: Should you be doing colposcopy? Patient Care: June 15, 1988

Keebler CM, Reagan JW (eds): Manual of Cytotechnology, 6th ed. Chicago, American Society of Clinical Pathologists, 1984

Keebler CM, Reagan JW (eds): Manual of Cytotechnology, 3rd ed. Chicago, American Society of Clinical Pathologists, 1979

Kiang D, Kollenda R: Breast cancers negative for estrogen receptor but positive for progesterone receptor, a true entity. J Clin Oncol 5:662–666, 1987

Koss LG: Diagnostic Cytology and Its Histological Bases, 3rd ed. Philadelphia, JB Lippincott, 1979

Leavelle DE (ed): Mayo Medical Laboratories Interpretive Handbook. Rochester, MN, Mayo Medical Laboratories, 1990

McCauly KM, Oi RH: Evaluating the Papanicolaou smear: Four possible colposcopic findings and corresponding management strategies, Part 2. Consultant, 29(1): 36–42, January, 1989

Muench KH: The Genetic Basis for Human Disease. New York, Elsevier–Dalton, 1979

Newborn screening fact sheets. Pediatrics 83(3):449–464, March, 1989

Raufman JP, et al: Endoscopic procedures in the AIDs patients: Risks, precautions, indications, and allegations. Gastroenterol Clin North Am 17(3):495–506, September, 1988

Ravel R: Clinical Laboratory Medicine: Clinical Application of Laboratory Data, 5th ed. Chicago, Year Book Medical Pub, 1989

Rivera ML: Pelviscoscopy: Broadening the scope of laparoscopy. Today's OR Nurse 11:16–20, November 1989

Soloway HB, et al: Operational considerations in maternal serum AFP screening. MLO 20(12):37–40, 1988

Sugarbaker PH: Endoscopy in cancer diagnosis and management. Hosp Pract:111–112, November, 1984

Watson A, Griffiths M: Cervicography: The nurse's role. Nurs Times 185(29): July 9, 1989

Wolberg WH, Tanner MA, Loh WL: Fine needle aspiration for breast mass diagnoses. Arch Surg 124:814–888, 1989

COMMON ENDOSCOPIC STUDIES

12

Introduction

Endoscopy is the examination and inspection of body organs or cavities by endoscopes. These instruments can also provide access for certain kinds of surgical procedures and/or treatments. Endoscopes, known generally as *fiberoptic instruments*, are used for direct visual examination of certain internal body structures. These instruments have lighted lens systems attached to either a rigid or flexible tube. Flexible scopes are the state of the art. Light travels through an optic fiber by means of multiple reflections. Fiberoptic instruments, composed of these fiber bundle systems, redirect and transmit light around twists and bends in cavities and hollow organs of the body. An image fiber and a light fiber allow for visualization at the distal tip of the scope. A suction port allows instillation of drugs, lavage, suction, and insertion of brushes, forceps, or other instruments for suction. The fiberoptic scope can be inserted into orifices or other areas of the body not easily accessible or directly visualized by other means. Procedures can be done for diagnosis of pathologic conditions or for therapy, such as removal of tissue or foreign objects. These examinations are done under local or general anesthetics. Biopsied tissue is submitted to the laboratory for histologic examination.

This chapter includes discussions of the following procedures:

1. *Arthroscopy*, which is examination of joints
2. *Bronchoscopy*, which is visualization and examination of the trachea and bronchi
3. *Cervicography*, which is not an actual endoscopic examination but involves photography of the cervix; often done in conjunction with colposcopy
4. *Colonoscopy*, which is examination of the large intestine
5. *Colposcopy*, which is direct visualization of the vagina and cervix
6. *Cytoscopy*, which involves inspection of the bladder, urethra, utereral orifices, or prostate (in men)
7. *Endoscopic retrograde cholangiopancreatography (ERCP)*, which entails visualization of pancreatic and bile ducts
8. *Esophageal manometry*, which is not an actual endoscopic examination but is often done for patients who need esophagogastroduodenoscopy; pressure readings evaluate esophageal muscle contraction
9. *Esophagogastroduodenoscopy (EGD)*, or gastroscopy, which allows visual examination of the upper gastrointestinal tract (UGI)
10. *Mediastinoscopy*, which involves examination and biopsy of mediastinal lymph nodes
11. *Medical laparoscopy*, which entails visualization of tissue of different abdominal organs, such as the liver and stomach

12. *Peritonoscopy*, which is visualization of uterus, fallopian tubes, and ovaries
13. *Proctoscopy*, *sigmoidoscopy*, *proctosigmoidoscopy*, which allow visualization of the rectum and sigmoid colon
14. *Thoracoscopy*, which involves examination of pleura, pleural spaces, mediastinum, and pericardium
15. *Urodynamic studies*, although not an actual endoscopic examination, are often done in conjunction with cytoscopy. They are performed to study voiding patterns and to identify possible causes of incontinence

Mediastinoscopy

Normal Values
No evidence of disease; normal lymph glands

Explanation of Test
This examination, performed under general anesthesia, requires insertion of a lighted mirror-lens instrument, similar to a bronchoscope, through an incision at the base of the neck. It is done to biopsy mediastinal lymph nodes. Because these nodes receive lymphatic drainage from the lungs, biopsies may identify such diseases as carcinoma, granulomatous infection, sarcoidosis, coccidiodomycosis, or histoplasmosis. Mediastinoscopy has virtually replaced scalene fat pad biopsy for suspected nodes on the right side of the mediastinum. It is the routine method of establishing tissue diagnosis and staging of lung cancer and for evaluating the extent of lung tumor metastasis. Nodes on the left side of the chest are usually biopsied through left anterior thoracotomy (mediastinotomy) or, occasionally, by scalene fat pad biopsy.

Procedure
1. Mediastinoscopy is considered a surgical procedure and is normally performed under general anesthesia.
2. The biopsy is done through a suprasternal incision.
3. The total procedure time is approximately 1.5 hours.

Clinical Implications
1. Abnormal findings may include
   - (a) Sarcoidosis
   - (b) Tuberculosis
   - (c) Histoplasmosis
   - (d) Hodgkin's disease
   - (e) Granulomatous infections/inflammatory processes
   - (f) Carcinomatous lesions
   - (g) Coccidiodomycosis
   - (h) *Pneumocystis carinii*
2. Assists in defining extent of metastatic process

Patient Preparation
1. Explain the purpose of this examination and the process the patient can expect to experience.
2. A legal surgical consent form must be appropriately signed and witnessed before the procedure begins (see p. 2 and p. 8, Chap. 1).
3. Preoperative care is the same as that for any patient having general anesthesia and surgery.
4. The patient must be NPO for 8 or more hours before the test.

Patient Aftercare
Following the examination, care is the same as for any patient who has had surgery and a general anesthetic.

1. Evaluate breathing and lung sounds.
2. Check wound for bleeding and hematoma.

Clinical Alert

1. Previous mediastinoscopy is a contraindication to a repeat examination because adhesions make satisfactory dissection of nodes extremely difficult or sometimes impossible.
2. Complications can result from the risks associated with general anesthesia or from pre-existing diseases and conditions.

Bronchoscopy

Normal Values
Normal trachea, bronchi, nasopharynx, pharynx, and select peripheral airways (conventional bronchoscopy cannot visualize alveolar structures)

Explanation of Test
This test permits visualization of the trachea, bronchi, and select bronchioles with a flexible or, less frequently, a rigid bronchoscope. It is done to diagnose tumors, coin lesions, or granulomatous lesions; to find the site of hemorrhage; to evaluate trauma or nerve paralysis; to biopsy; to take brushings for cytologic examinations; to improve drainage of secretions; to identify inflammatory infiltrates; and to lavage and remove foreign bodies. Bronchoscopy can determine resectability of a lesion as well as provide the means to diagnose bronchogenic carcinoma.

The examination is usually done under local anesthesia combined with some form of sedation in an outpatient department, diagnostic center, or operating room. It can also be done in a critical care unit when the patient is unresponsive or his or her breathing is assisted by a ventilator.

Procedure

1. A local anesthetic is sprayed and swabbed to the back of the nose, the tongue, the pharynx, and the epiglottis. If the patient has a history of bronchospasms, steroids and aminophylline are frequently administered prior to the procedure.
2. The flexible bronchoscope is inserted carefully through the mouth or nose into the pharynx and the trachea. It can also be inserted through an endotracheal tube or through a tracheostomy. Suctioning, oxygen delivery, and biopsies are accomplished through the ports designed for these purposes.
3. Because of sedation with Valium, Versed, or Demerol, the patient is not usually uncomfortable. However, when the bronchoscope is passed, some patients may feel they cannot breathe or that they are suffocating.
4. Examining time is usually 30 to 45 minutes, depending upon techniques. Endotracheal intubation takes longer than nasal intubation.
5. An arterial blood gas measurement performed after bronchoscopy is desirable. Arterial blood oxygen may remain altered for several hours after the procedure. In addition, sputum specimens taken after bronchoscopy may be ordered for cytology or culture and sensitivity. These must be handled and preserved according to institutional protocols.
6. Continuous pulse oximetry readings indicate levels of oxygen saturation before, during, and after the procedure.

Clinical Implications

Abnormalities revealed through bronchoscopy include

1. Abscesses
2. Bronchitis
3. Carcinoma (right lung more than left)
4. Tumors (usually appear more often in larger bronchii)
5. Tuberculosis
6. Alveolitis
7. Signs of nonresectability by surgery (*e.g.*, involvement of tracheal wall by tumor growth, immobility of a main-stem bronchus, widening and fixation of the carina)
8. *Pneumocystis carinii*
9. Inflammatory process
10. Cytomegalic inclusion virus infection
11. Aspergillosis
12. Idiopathic nonspecific pulmonary fibrosis
13. Cryptococcus neoformans
14. Coccidioidomycosis
15. Histoplasmosis
16. Blastomycosis
17. Phycomycosis

Clinical Considerations

These data must be available prior to the procedure: history and physical examination, chest x-ray (recent), recent arterial blood gases, and electrocardiogram (ECG) if the patient is over age 40 or has heart disease. Appropriate blood work, urinalysis, pulmonary function tests, and sputum studies (especially for acid-fast bacilli must be done as well). It is often an outpatient/day surgery procedure.

Patient Preparation

1. Reinforce information related to the purpose, procedure, benefits, and risks of the test.
2. Emphasize that no pain is expected because lungs do not have pain fibers.
3. Explain that the local anesthetic has a bitter taste and that numbness occurs in a few minutes. Feelings of a thickened tongue and the sensation of something in the back of the throat that cannot be coughed out or swallowed are not unusual. These sensations will pass within a few hours following the procedure.
4. An informed consent must be properly signed and witnessed (see p. 2 and p. 8, Chap. 1).
5. The patient must be NPO for at least 6 hours before the procedure to reduce the risk of aspiration. Gag, cough, and swallowing reflexes are blocked.
6. Wigs, nailpolish, makeup, dentures, jewelry, and contact lenses must be removed prior to the examination.

   Note: Morphine sulfate is contraindicated in patients who have bronchospasm or asthma because it can cause bronchospasm. Analgesics, barbiturates, tranquilizers/sedatives, and atropine may be ordered and administered one-half to 1 hour before bronchoscopy. The patient should be as relaxed as possible before and during the procedure. The patient also needs to know that anxiety is normal. In spite of these measures, the patient may need additional intravenous sedatives administered during the procedure.

7. Use of relaxation techniques may help the patient to relax and to breath normally during the procedure. The more relaxed the patient is, the easier it is to complete the procedure.
8. The right lung, by convention, is normally examined before the left lung.

Patient Aftercare

1. Usually the patient is NPO for at least 2 hours. Be certain that swallow, gag, and cough reflexes are present before allowing food or liquids to be ingested orally.
2. Provide gargles to relieve mild pharyngitis. Monitor ECG, blood

pressure, pulse/oximeter readings, color, lung sounds, and respiratory patterns, according to institution protocols.
3. Monitor temperature, pulse, and respiratory rate.
4. Oxygen per mask or nasal cannula may be ordered following the procedure.
5. Sometimes a chest x-ray may be ordered to check for pneumothorax or to evaluate lungs following the procedure.
6. Sputum specimens may be ordered. One must preserve these in the proper medium/solution.
7. Head of bed may be elevated.

Contraindications to Bronchoscopy

The following are contraindications to bronchoscopy:

1. Severe hypoxemia
2. Severe hypocapnia (carbon dioxide retention)
3. Certain cardiac arrhythmias, cardiac states
4. History of being hepatitis B carrier
5. Bleeding/coagulation disorders
6. Severe tracheal stenosis

Clinical Alert

Observe for possible complications, which may include

1. Shock
2. Cardiac arrhythmias
3. Hypoxemia
4. Laryngospasm (inspiratory stridor, a "crowing" sound)
5. Bronchospasm (pallor and increasing dyspnea are signs)
6. Infection and/or gram-negative bacterial sepsis/empyema
7. Pneumothorax
8. Respiratory failure
9. Bleeding following biopsy (rare, but can occur if there is excessive friability of airway or massive lesions, or if patient is uremic or has hematologic disorders)
10. Anaphylactic reactions to drugs
11. Seizures
12. Febrile state
13. Hypoxia, respiratory distress

Special Pediatric Considerations

Bronchoscopy instruments can decrease a small airway lumen even more by causing inflammation and edema. Consequently, a child can rapidly become hypoxic. Resuscitation and oxygen administration equipment and drugs must be readily accessible. Close monitoring of respiratory and cardiac status is imperative after the procedure should complications develop and require treatment.

Thoracoscopy

Normal Values
Thoracic cavity normal and free of disease

Explanation of the Test
Thoracoscopy is the examination of the thoracic cavity by means of an endoscope. This procedure is making somewhat of a comeback because it can be used as a diagnostic device when other methods of diagnosis fail to present adequate and accurate findings. Moreover, some of the risks associated with traditional diagnostic thoracotomy procedures are reduced. Thoracoscopy provides the means to visualize parietal and visceral pleura, pleural spaces, thoracic walls, the mediastinum and the pericardium without the need for more extensive procedures. It can be used to perform biopsies, to perform laser procedures, and to assess tumor growth, pleural effusion, emphysema, inflammatory processes, and conditions predisposing to pneumothorax.

Procedure
1. Thoracoscopy is considered an operative procedure. The patient's state of health, the particular positioning needed, and the procedure itself determine the need for either local or general anesthesia.
2. Admission is frequently scheduled the morning of the procedure. Many patients are discharged the following day, provided the lung has re-expanded properly and chest tubes have been removed.

Clinical Implications
Abnormal findings can include

1. Carcinoma/extent of metastasis
2. Empyema
3. Pleural effusion
4. Conditions predisposing to pneumothorax
5. Inflammatory processes

Patient Preparation
1. Reinforce and explain the purpose of the examination and the process the patient can expect to experience.
2. The surgical consent form must be appropriately signed and witnessed before the procedure begins (see p. 2 and p. 8, Chap. 1).
3. Required blood tests, urinalysis, recent chest x-ray, and ECG (for certain individuals) must be completed and available for review prior to the procedure.
4. The patient must be fasting for 8 hours before the procedure.

5. An intravenous line needs to be inserted for the administration of intraoperative intravenous fluids and intravenous medication.
6. Skin preps and correct positioning need to be done in the operating room.
7. After the actual thoracoscopy is completed, a chest tube is placed and connected to negative suction.

Patient Aftercare
1. A postoperative chest x-ray is taken to check for abnormal air or fluid in the lung space.
2. Monitor vital signs, amount and color of chest tube drainage, fluctuation of fluid in the chest tube, bubbling in the chest bottle, and respiratory status, including arterial blood gases. Report abnormalities to the physician promptly.
3. Administer pain medication as necessary. Encourage relaxation exercises as a means to lessen the perception of pain.
4. Encourage coughing and deep breathing frequently. Assist the patient to splint the incision to lessen discomfort. Promote leg exercises while in bed and encourage frequent ambulation.
5. Use open-ended questions in an effort to provide the patient with the opportunity to express concerns.

Clinical Alert

Possible complications include

1. Respiratory distress/hypoxia   3. Hemorrhage
2. Infection   4. Emyema

Esophagogastroduodenoscopy (EGD)
(Endoscopy, Gastroscopy)

Normal Values
Upper gastrointestinal tract within normal limits

Explanation of Test
This test allows the physician to visualize the lumen of the upper gastrointestinal tract with a fiberoptic instrument designed for that purpose. Esophagogastroduodenoscopy is indicated for patients with dysphagia and weight loss, especially those with moderate to heavy alcohol and tobacco consumption. This method is useful to determine the cause of upper gastrointestinal tract bleeding, to confirm suspi-

cious findings on x-rays, to establish a diagnosis for a symptomatic patient with negative x-ray reports, to biopsy upper gastrointestinal tract lesions, and to diagnose hiatal hernia or esophagitis. It can also be used to determine whether a gastric ulcer is benign or malignant or to perform a follow-up exam for gastrectomy.

Endoscopy is a general term that denotes visual inspection of any body cavity with an endoscope. Endoscopic examination of the upper gastrointestinal tract (mouth to upper jejunum), therefore, may be referred to when the following examinations are ordered: panendoscopy, esophagoscopy, gastroscopy, duodenoscopy, esophagogastroscopy, or esophagogastroduodenoscopy.

Procedure

1. This examination is usually performed in a gastrointestinal laboratory, in surgery, or in critical care settings.
2. A spray is used to anesthetize the patient's throat.
3. An intravenous tranquilizer is often given prior to initiation of the procedure. The patient becomes relaxed and somewhat sleepy.
4. The endoscope is then gently inserted into the esophagus and is advanced slowly into the stomach and duodenum. Air is insufflated through the scope to distend the area being examined so that good visualization of the mucosa may take place. Biopsies and brushings for cytology may be obtained during the examination. Photos may also be taken.
5. Feelings of pressure or bloating are normal, but there should be no pain.
6. Immediately after the examination is completed, the patient will be asked to relax and to remain lying on his or her side.
7. The EGD takes about 10 to 20 minutes.

Clinical Implications

Abnormal results may indicate

1. The location of the hemorrhage site
2. Hiatal hernia
3. Esophagitis
4. Neoplastic tissue
5. Gastric ulcers, both benign or malignant

Patient Preparation

1. Explain the purpose of the procedure, what the patient can expect of the experience, and the benefits and risks of the test. Reassure the patient that the endoscope is thinner than most food swallowed. Remind the patient that they may be quite sleepy during the EGD.
2. Instruct the patient to be NPO for 8 hours before the examination. In the hospital, this restriction usually begins at midnight prior to the examination. Give the patient written instructions about fast-

ing. A legal permit must be signed and properly witnessed (see p. 2 and p. 8, Chap. 1).

3. Oral hygiene needs to be done before coming to the gastrointestinal laboratory. Assist with oral care as necessary.
4. Encourage the patient to urinate and to defecate before the examination.

Patient Aftercare
1. After the test is completed, no food or liquids are permitted for 2 hours (or longer if the patient cannot swallow).
2. Be certain the patient can swallow properly before offering liquids or food.
3. Check blood pressure, pulse, and respirations every 30 minutes times four.
4. A side-lying position in bed, with the side rails up, should be maintained until the sedative has worn off (usually about 2 hours). This position usually prevents aspiration in case of emesis.
5. Encourage the patient to belch so that air inserted into the stomach during the examination is expelled.
6. The patient should not experience discomfort or side effects once the sedative has worn off. Occasionally, a patient may complain of a slight sore throat.

Clinical Alert
Complications are rare. However, the following can occur:

1. Perforation
2. Bleeding
3. Local irritation of blood vessels
4. Drug reactions
5. Complications from unrelated diseases such as myocardial infarction or cerebrovascular accident
6. Death is an extremely rare occurrence.

Esophageal Manometry

Normal Values
Normal esophageal and stomach pressure readings
Normal contraction and no acid reflux

Explanation of Test
This procedure tests the esophagus for normal contractile activity by means of pressure readings.

Indications for Testing

1. Abnormal esophageal muscle function
2. Difficulty in swallowing
3. Heartburn
4. Chest pain of unknown cause
5. Regurgitation
6. Vomiting

Other tests often done in conjunction with manometry include acid reflux tests and the Bernstein test (see below). These measurements are useful for evaluating heartburn, esophagalitis, and chest pain of undetermined cause.

Procedure

1. A local anesthetic is applied to the nasal passage with a cotton swab.
2. A small tube is passed through the nose while the patient is in a sitting position. Tiny holes in the sides of this tube allow for the measurement of pressure within the esophagus and stomach.
3. After the tube is passed, the patient lies supine for the remainder of the test.
4. Small amounts of water are placed in the mouth. The patient is then asked to swallow the water.
5. This part of the test takes approximately 40 minutes.
6. *Acid reflux testing*
   A second small tube is passed alongside the one already in place. This tube is actually a probe that is sensitive to acid. When the valve at the bottom of the esophagus is not functioning, acid from the stomach comes back up the esophagus and the probe in the esophagus senses the acid.
7. *Bernstein testing*
   Hydrochloric acid (0.1 N HCl) is infused for 10 minutes into the esophagus to reproduce symptoms of heartburn or chest discomfort. In the first 5 minutes of testing, normal saline is infused as a control. Testing takes approximately 15 minutes. The patient may be either lying down or sitting up.

Clinical Implications

Abnormal results reveal

1. Achalasia (failure of muscles such as sphincters to relax)
2. Esophageal spasm
3. Acid reflux

Patient Preparation

1. Explain the purpose, procedure, and benefits of the test. State that serious complications are unknown.
2. The patient should be kept NPO for 6 hours prior to testing.
3. If the patient is diabetic, notify the testing department.

Patient Aftercare
1. Advise the patient that a sore throat and nasal passage irritation is common within the first 24 hours after the examination.
2. Observe for nasal bleeding.

Endoscopic Retrograde Cholangiopancreatography (ERCP)

Normal Values
Patent pancreatic ducts, hepatic ducts, common bile ducts, duodenal papilla (Ampulla of Vater), and normal gallbladder (if present)

Explanation of Test
This examination of the biliary system is done through a side-viewing flexible fiberoptic endoscope by instillation of contrast medium into the duodenal papilla or ampulla of Vater. It is used to evaluate jaundice, pancreatitis, persistent abdominal pain, pancreatic tumors, retained common duct stones, or extra- and intrahepatic biliary tract disease as well as malformations and strictures, and as a follow-up study in confirmed or suspected cases of pancreatic disease.

The ERCP manometry can be done to obtain pressure readings in the bile duct, pancreatic duct, and sphincter of Oddi at the papilla. Measurement is obtained by a catheter that is inserted into the endoscope and placed within the sphincter zone.

Procedure
1. If the patient has had barium x-rays prior to ERCP, a flat plate of the abdomen (KUB) should be done to be certain that no barium is present to obscure the view. Screen for chest pain, shortness of breath, myocardial infarct, epigastric pain with bleeding, acute infections (including active hepatitis *or* pancreatitis). Older debilitated people may be more prone to complications. The presence of fever or flu-like symptoms may necessitate cancellation of the procedure.
2. The patient gargles or has the throat sprayed with a topical anesthetic.
3. An intravenous line is started and drugs such as meperidine, diazepam, or midazolam are administered before and during the procedure as needed for sedation. The very ill patient often needs only a small dose of sedation. Resuscitation equipment needs to be available.
4. The patient assumes the left lateral position while the endoscope is inserted via a mouthpiece through the esophagus to the duodenum.

At this point, a prone position is assumed with the left arm positioned behind the patient.

5. Simethicone may be instilled to reduce bubbles from bile secretions. Glucagon or atropine may be given intravenously during the procedure to relax the duodenum so that the papilla can be cannulated. Anticholinergics also are often administered during the procedure. (Atropine can increase heart rate.)

6. A catheter is passed into the ampulla of Vater and an x-ray contrast substance is instilled through the cannula to outline the pancreatic and common bile ducts. Fluoroscopy and x-rays are done at this time.

7. Biopsies or cytology brushings may also be taken before the endoscope is removed.

8. The procedure can last up to 2 hours. The patient's vital signs, ECG, and oxygen saturation (pulse oximetry) should be monitored throughout the procedure.

9. Side effects and drug allergy reactions (diaphoresis, pallor, restlessness, hypotension) need to be watched for.

Clinical Implications

Abnormal results will reveal the presence of stones, stenosis, and other abnormalities that are indicative of

1. Biliary cirrhosis
2. Primary sclerosing cholangitis
3. Cancer of bile ducts
4. Pancreatic cysts
5. Pseudocysts
6. Pancreatic tumor
7. Cancer of head of pancreas
8. Chronic pancreatitis
9. Pancreatic fibrosis
10. Cancer of duodenal papilla
11. Papillary stenosis

Patient Preparation

1. Explain the purpose, procedure, benefits, and risks of the test. If this is an outpatient procedure, the patient should arrange for a ride home and should leave all valuables at home. Results of appropriate blood work, urinalysis, x-rays, and scans should be on the chart. Vital signs need to be recorded.

2. A legal permit must be signed and properly witnessed (see p. 2 and p. 8, Chap. 1).

3. Nothing by mouth is permitted for 12 hours before the ERCP.

4. Inform the patient that she or he
   (a) Should swallow when requested to do so (prevents damage to the oral pharynx)
   (b) May experience a choking sensation
   (c) Will have to lie quietly during the time x-rays are taken
   (d) Should breathe deeply to relieve gagging
   (e) Will be suctioned for the purpose of secretion clearance

Patient Aftercare

1. Check vital signs, including temperature, according to protocols.
2. Do not give food or fluids for at least 2 hours after the procedure or until the gag reflex returns. Make sure the patient can swallow before offering liquids or food.
3. Urinary retention may be a complication.
4. Observe the patient for signs of complications such as cholangitis or pancreatitis. Check for elevation in temperature (may be the first sign of inflammation).
5. Monitor for respiratory or central nervous system depression from narcotics. (Except for diazepam, naloxone may be used to counter these narcotic effects.)
6. Explain that some abdominal discomfort may be present for several hours after the procedure.
7. Drowsiness from the medication may last up to 24 hours. The patient should not perform any tasks that require mental alertness for this period of time.
8. A sore throat can be relieved by gargles and ice chips or fluids.
9. Notify physician of the following
   (a) Prolonged, sharp abdominal pain
   (b) Fever
   (c) Nausea or vomiting

Colposcopy

Normal Values
Normal vagina and cervix

Explanation of Test
Colposcopy is the examination of the vagina and cervix with a colposcope. This instrument with a magnifying lens visualizes the vagina and the endocervix. Indications for this procedure include an abnormal Papanicolaou (Pap) smear and/or any cervical lesion. This examination aids the diagnosis of benign, preclinical, and other cancerous lesions. Patients with abnormal Pap smears commonly undergo colposcopy. Biopsies and scrapings of cells are done under direct visualization. Colposcopy is also valuable for assessing women with a history of exposure to diethylstilbestrol.

Advantages of colposcopy include

1. Lesions can be localized and their extent can be determined.
2. Inflammatory processes can be differentiated from neoplasia.
3. Invasive or noninvasive disease processes can be differentiated.

Colposcopy *cannot* readily detect endocervical lesions. Cervicitis and other changes can produce abnormal findings. When combined with findings from Pap smears, colposcopy can be a means of enhancing diagnostic accuracy. (See Tables 12–1 and 12–2 regarding correlation of findings and advantages and disadvantages of Pap smears and colposcopy. See Chap. 11, p. 700 for Pap smear procedure.)

Whitish areas of epithelium (leukoplakia), mosaic staining patterns, irregular blood vasculature, hyperkeratosis, and other abnor-

TABLE 12–1.
Correlation of Colposcopic and Histologic Findings

Colposcopic Term	Colposcopic Appearance	Histologic Correlate
Original squamous epithelium	Smooth, pink; indefinitely outlined vessels; no change after application of acetic acid	Squamous epithelium
Columnar epithelium	Grapelike structures after application of acetic acid	Columnar epithelium
Transformation zone	Tongues of squamous metaplasia; gland openings; nabothian cysts	Metaplastic squamous epithelium
White epithelium	White, sharp-bordered lesion visible only after application of acetic acid; no vessels visible	From minimal dysplasia to carcinoma in situ
Punctation	Sharp-bordered lesion; red stippling; epithelium whiter after application of acetic acid	From minimal dysplasia to carcinoma in situ
Mosaic	Sharp-bordered lesion, mosaic pattern; epithelium whiter after application of acetic acid	From minimal dysplasia to carcinoma in situ
Hyperkeratosis	White patch; rough surface; already visible before application of acetic acid	Usually hyperkeratosis or parakeratosis; seldom carcinoma in situ or invasive disease
Atypical vessel	Horizontal vessels running parallel to surface; constrictions and dilatations of vessels; atypical branching, winding course	From carcinoma in situ to invasive carcinoma

(Staff A: Colposcopy. In Danforth DN, Scott JR (eds): Obstetrics and Gynecology, 5th ed. Philadelphia, JB Lippincott, 1986, pp 1057–1067)

TABLE 12–2.
Pros and Cons of Colposcopy and Cytology

Advantages	Disadvantages
Colposcopy	
Localizes lesion	Inadequate for detection of endocervical lesions
Evaluates extent of lesion	More intensive training is necessary
Differentiates between inflammatory atypia and neoplasia	Cervicitis and regenerative changes may produce abnormal findings
Differentiates between invasive and noninvasive cervical lesions	
Enables follow-up	
Cytology	
Ideal for mass screening	Cannot localize lesion
Economical	Inflammation, atrophic changes, or folic acid deficiency may produce suspicious changes
Specimen can be obtained by most medical personnel	Many steps between patient and cytopathologist allow misdiagnosis
Detects lesion in endocervical canal	Value of single smear is limited
Detects endocervical and endometrial carcinoma	False-negative rate is 5%–10%
High correlation with biopsy material (>90%)	

(Killachey MA, MacMillan R, Shuts EE: Should you be doing colposcopy? Patient Care: 240, June 15, 1988)

mal-appearing tissues show up on colposcopy. Leukoplakia vulvae is a precancerous condition characterized by white to grayish infiltrated patches on the vulvar mucosa. The colposcope has a definite advantage for detecting atypical epithelium, designated in the literature as *basal cell activity*. Atypical epithelium cannot be called benign and, yet, does not fulfill all criteria for carcinoma in situ. Its early detection promotes cancer prophylaxis.

Patients receiving colposcopy may often be spared having to undergo surgical conization (the removal of a cone of tissue from the cervix). More recently, colposcopy is being used for evaluation of male genitals for sexual transmitted diseases, condylomata, and human papilloma virus.

Procedure

1. With the patient in a lithotomy position, the vagina and cervix are exposed with a speculum after the internal and external genitalia have been carefully examined. A Pap smear is obtained at this time. No part of the colposcope is inserted into the vagina (see Fig. 12–1).

FIGURE 12–1.
The colposcope. (Courtesy of Carl Zeiss, Inc., New York)

2. The cervix and vagina are then swabbed with 3% acetic acid as needed during the procedure to improve visibility of epithelial tissues by apparent precipitation of nuclear proteins within the cells. The cervical mucus must be completely removed. Do not use cotton-wool swabs because fibers left on the cervix may interfere with proper visualization.
3. Actual visualization with the colposcope begins with white light and lower magnification. An attempt is made to focus upon sites of

white epithelium or irregular cervical contours. The light is then switched to a green filter for magnification of vascular changes.

(a) Suspicious lesions are diagramed, and photographs are taken for the permanent health care record.

(b) The transformation zone and squamocolumnar junction (where squamous epithelium meets columnar epithelium of the cervix) are areas where many women exhibit atypical cells. It is imperative that these zones be visualized completely, especially in older women, because of changes associated with aging.

4. Biopsies of the lesions are done with a fine biopsy forceps. Some patients note discomfort at this time.

(a) Endocervical curettage must be performed prior to colposcope-directed biopsy so that detached epithelial fragments during colposcopy do not cause false-positive results in the endocervical curettage. Endocervical curettage biopsy samples should be placed in formalin.

(b) Sterile saline or cotton balls soaked in sterile water should be used to rinse acetic acid from the vaginal area to prevent burning or irritation. Bleeding can be stopped by applying toughened silver nitrate cautery sticks or using ferric subsulfate (Monsel's solution).

5. Total examining time is 10 to 15 minutes.

6. A small amount of vaginal bleeding for a few hours is not abnormal.

7. A paracervical block may be necessary for those patients who are extremely anxious.

Clinical Implications

Abnormal lesions or unusual epithelial patterns include the following:

1. Leukoplakia
2. Abnormal blood vessels
3. Slight-to-moderate-to-marked dysplasia
4. Punctation (sharp borders, red stippling, epithelium whiter with acetic acid)
5. Mosaic (sharp borders, mosaic pattern, epithelium whiter after acetic acid)
6. Hyperkeratosis (white, rough, visible without acetic acid)

Clinical Alert

1. Patients may have a vasovagal response. Have the patient sit for a short while before standing.
2. Cramping may be relieved by anti-inflammatory agents such as ibuprofen.

3. Cervical scars from previous events may prevent satisfactory visualization.
4. Complications may include heavy bleeding, infection, or pelvic inflammatory disease.
5. Development of cervical changes and potential cervical carcinoma is of greater risk for these patients. An annual Pap smear is mandatory for them.

Patient Aftercare
1. Instruct the patient to abstain from sexual intercourse and not to insert anything into the vagina for 2 to 7 days after the procedure.
2. Excessive bleeding, pain, fever, or abnormal vaginal discharge should be reported immediately.

Cervicography

Cervicography is done in conjunction with colposcopy or by itself. It is a photographic method that records an image of the entire cervix. The patient assumes a lithotomy position and the cervix is exposed by means of a speculum. Mucus needs to be wiped away. Then 5% acetic acid is applied to the area and swabbed for a few minutes. Photographs of the cervix are then taken with a specially designed 35-mm camera. Following this, aqueous iodine is applied to the cervix in the same way and another picture is taken. Finally, an endocervical smear is taken and transferred onto a slide for later evaluation. The patient should be told that brown vaginal discharge (from the iodine) for a few days is not unusual.

The photographs are processed into slides (cervigrams). This procedure allows the entire cervix to be visible on one slide. It can provide evidence for colposcopic consultations. Moreover, the cervigram can be done in conjunction with a routine gynecologic examination. It has been shown to be more sensitive to the early detection of cervical intraepithelial neoplasia and invasive cervical cancer than the Pap smear has been.

Flexible Proctoscopy; Sigmoidoscopy; Proctosigmoidoscopy

Normal Values
Normal rectum and sigmoid colon mucosa

Explanation of Test

These tests involve the examination of a 25-cm area of the rectum and sigmoid with a proctosigmoidoscope. Flexible proctosigmoidoscopes are commonly used. These instruments are tubes usually measuring 60 cm in length. They incorporate a lighted lens system for illuminating the rectum and sigmoid. Their main use is the detection and diagnosis of cancers in these areas of the gastrointestinal tract. These examinations should be routine in cancer screening for those individuals over the age of 40.

Note: Men over 45 years of age are at high-risk for adenocarcinoma of the rectum.

These tests can also evaluate hemorrhoids, blood in the stool, bowel symptoms, and unexplained anemia.

Procedure

1. For rigid proctoscopy, the patient assumes a knee-to-chest position. The proctoscope or sigmoidoscope is then carefully inserted into the rectum. When the flexible proctoscope is used, the patient must be in the left lateral position for this examination.
2. The examination can be done with the patient in bed or on a special tilt table.
3. Usually, the procedure takes 3 to 5 minutes. If the longer, flexible instrument is used, examining time may take 5 to 10 minutes.
4. The patient may feel a very strong urge to defecate and may experience a feeling of bloating. These sensations are normal.

Clinical Implications

Findings may reveal the following: edematous, red, or denuded mucosa; granularity; friability; ulcers; cysts; thickened areas; changes in vascular pattern; pseudomembranes; spontaneous bleeding; or normal mucosa. They may help to confirm or to rule out the following conditions:

1. Inflammatory bowel disease
   (a) Chronic ulcerative colitis
   (b) Crohn's disease
   (c) Proctitis (acute and chronic)
   (d) Pseudomembranous colitis
2. Polyps
   (a) Adenomatous
   (b) Familial
   (c) Diminutive
3. Cancer and tumors
   (a) Adenocarcinoma
   (b) Carcinoids
   (c) Other tumors such as lipomas

4. Anal and perianal conditions
   (a) Hemorrhoids
   (b) Abscesses and fistulas
   (c) Strictures and stenoses
   (d) Rectal prolapse
   (e) Fissures
   (f) Contractures

Patient Preparation
1. Explain the purpose of the test and the process the patient may expect to experience.
2. The patient does not need to fast. However, a light diet the evening before the test may be necessary.
3. Laxatives and an enema may be given the night before the examination, or one or more enemas or a rectal laxative suppository may be administered 1 hour before the procedure. (For all ages, a small enema or possibly two, 1 hour before the scheduled examination is considered ample preparation by many endoscopy departments.)

Clinical Alert

1. Patients with acute symptoms, particularly those individuals with suspected ulcerative or granulomatous colitis, should be examined *without* any preparation (without enemas, laxatives, or suppositories).
2. Perforation of the intestinal wall is an infrequent complication of these tests.
3. Notify the patient's physician prior to administering laxatives or enemas to a pregnant women.

Colonoscopy

Normal Values
Normal large intestine mucosa

Explanation of Test
Colonoscopy is the visualization and examination of the large intestine with a fiberoptic colonoscope that has been inserted through the anus to the ileocecal valve. Air passed through an accessory channel of the colonoscope distends the intestinal walls. This technique can differentiate inflammatory disease from neoplastic disease or can evaluate polypoid lesions beyond the reach of the sigmoidoscope. Suture lines after bowel resection, anastomoses, or surveillance of those individuals at

high risk for colon cancer, polyps, foreign bodies, and specimens can be removed via the colonoscope. Photographs can also be taken. Before colonoscopy was available, major abdominal surgery was the only way to remove colon polyps to determine if they were benign or malignant. Periodic colonoscopy is a valuable adjunct to the follow-up of persons with previous polyps, colon cancer, or family history of colon cancer.

Clinical Implications

1. Polyps
2. Tumors
3. Areas of ulceration
4. Inflammation
5. Colitis, diverticula
6. Bleeding sites
7. Strictures
8. Discovery or removal of foreign bodies

Procedure

1. A clear liquid diet is usually ordered for 48 to 72 hours before the examination. The patient must fast for 8 hours before the procedure. Laxatives may be ordered for 1 to 3 days before the test, and enemas are sometimes ordered to be given the night before. To be effective, a purgative must produce fluid diarrhea. This shows that unaltered small intestinal contents are emerging and colonic residue has been cleared. Enemas must be repeated until solid matter is no longer expelled.
2. Another common form of preparing the patient involves the administration of an oral saline iso-osmotic and isotonic (with respect to bowel contents) laxative. This washout solution may contain a number of salts such as potassium chloride, sodium chloride, bicarbonate, an additive such as polyethylene glycol, and distilled or deionized water. The glycol acts as an osmotic agent, so there is no net ion absorption or loss; water and electrolyte balances should not change significantly. The patient is asked to drink 3 to 6 L of the prescribed solution over a 2- to 3.5-hour period. The typical dosage is 1 gallon. It can be administered by nasogastric tube if necessary. This laxative acts quickly. First results can be expected in 30 minutes to 1 hour. Ingestion is continued until defecation is clear liquid. However, the physician should be notified prior to administering more than 6 L of this solution. No special diet, laxative, or enemas are required with this method. However, patients with congestive heart failure or renal failure may be at great risk for fluid volume overload if this preparation is used.
3. The colonoscopy is done under analgesia by using combinations of medications such as Demerol (meperidine hydrochloride), Valium (diazepam), or Versed (midazolam). The patient should be alert enough to inform the doctor of any untoward reactions during the examination.
4. Occasionally, intravenous anticholinergics and glucagon may be used to relax local bowel spasms.
5. The patient assumes the left side or Sim's position. A well-lubri-

cated colonoscope is inserted approximately 12 cm into the bowel. The patient should take deep breaths through the mouth during this time. Air is then introduced into the bowel to aid viewing. As the colonoscope advances, the patient may need to be repositioned several times to aid in the visualization of the colon. Feelings of pressure or mild pain are not unusual.

6. The examination may take from 30 minutes to 1.5 hours. Better views are obtained during withdrawal of the colonscope than during insertion. Therefore, a more careful examination is usually performed during withdrawal.

Clinical Considerations

1. Keep colon electrolyte lavage preparations refrigerated. However, the patient may drink the solution at room temperature. Use within 48 hours. Discard any unused portions.
2. Prior to testing, a complete blood count, current protime, platelet count, and thromboplastin times results should be known or available.
3. Preparation for those patients with a colostomy or paralyzed patients is the same. They will usually receive at least 4 L of oral prep solution.
4. Persons with known heart disease should receive prescribed antibiotics before testing.
5. Patients should not mix or drink anything with the liquid bowel preparation. Do not add ice or glucose to the solution.

Patient Preparation

1. Explain the purpose, procedure, benefits, and risks of the test. If used, one 12-ounce glass of liquid prep is to be taken every 10 minutes. (Each gallon holds 10.7 twelve-ounce glasses.) The entire gallon should be taken in 2 hours, if possible. Timing is important. Slower drinking does not clean the colon properly.
2. Some patients will be on a clear liquid diet for 72 hours before the test and NPO, except for medications, after a clear liquid supper the evening before the test.
3. Administer purgatives and cleaning enemas as ordered. Preparation is complete when fecal discharge is clear. If returns are not clear after 4 L of solution have been ingested, continue until returns are clear (up to *6 L total*). (See previous note, p. 748, number 2.)
4. A legal consent form must be signed, preferably by the patient, and properly witnessed (see Chap. 1).
5. Iron preparations should be discontinued 3 or 4 days before the examination because iron residues produce an inky black stool that interferes with inspection. Also, the stool can be viscous and difficult to clear. Aspirin and aspirin-containing products should also be discontinued 1 week before the examination because of the bleeding problems or localized hemorrhages they may cause.

6. Some protocols call for a patent or capped intravenous line to be in place.
7. Persons with heart valve disease need antibiotics before the test.

Patient Aftercare

1. The patient should be NPO for 2 hours after the examination.
2. Stools should be observed for visible bleeding. The patient should be instructed to report abdominal pain, because perforation and hemorrhage are possible complications.
3. Vital signs should be checked frequently for 2 hours after the procedure.
4. Most frequent adverse reactions to oral purgatives include nausea, vomiting, bloating, and rectal irritation, and chills.

Clinical Alert

1. Solid food should never be given less than 2 hours before the oral cleansing regimen.
2. Orally administered colon lavage is contraindicated in
   (a) Actual or suspected ulcers
   (b) Gastric outlet obstruction
   (c) Weight less than 20 kg
   (d) Toxic colitis
   (e) Megacolon
3. Relative contraindications for colonoscopy include
   (a) Perforating disease of the colon
   (b) Peritonitis
   (c) Radiation enteritis
   (d) Recent abdominal or bowel surgery
   (e) Acute conditions of the anus and rectum
   (f) Serious cardiac or respiratory problems (such as recent myocardial infarction)
   (g) Situations in which the bowel cannot be adequately prepared for the procedure.
4. Observe for possible complications, including
   (a) Perforations
   (b) Hypotensive episodes
   (c) Cardiac or respiratory arrest, which can be provoked by the combination of oversedation and intense vagal stimulus from instrumentation
   (d) Hemorrhage, especially if polypectomy has been performed
   (e) Death, which is extremely rare but possible

5. If colon preparations are administered by lavage to the unconscious patients or to those with impaired gag reflexes, observe for aspiration or regurgitation, especially if a nasogastric tube is in place. Keep the head of the bed elevated. Have continuous suction equipment readily available.
6. No barium studies are to be done during the preparation period.

Peritoneoscopy, Laparoscopy, Pelviscopy

Normal Values
Gynecologic examination: normal size shape and appearance of uterus, fallopian tubes, and ovaries
Medical examination: normal liver, gallbladder, spleen, and greater curvature of the stomach

Explanation of Test
These examinations of the intra-abdominal and pelvic cavities are done using a laparoscope or pelviscope inserted through the anterior abdominal wall. The pelvic organs as well as abdominal organs, such as the greater curvature of the stomach or the liver, can be viewed. The separate types of examinations done are peritoneoscopy (medical laparoscopy), laparoscopy (gynecologic), and pelviscopy (gynecologic). These procedures are frequently performed under general anesthesia in a surgical setting; however, many are also done by means of local anesthesia.

Peritoneoscopy is most commonly used to evaluate liver disease and to obtain biopsies. This procedure is done when the liver is too small, when previous liver biopsy proves inadequate, when contraindications to percutaneous liver biopsy exist (ascites), when there is unexplained portal hypertension or unexplained liver function abnormalities, and when the liver cannot be properly palpated for doing a conventional liver biopsy. It does away with the need to do a blind liver biopsy. Other indications for peritoneoscopy include unexplained ascites, staging of lymphomas, staging and follow-up of ovarian cancer, or abdominal masses. Sometimes patients with advanced chest, gastric, pancreatic, endometrial, and rectal tumors are evaluated by peritoneoscopy before attempting surgical intervention.

Gynecologic laparoscopy and pelviscopy are used to diagnose cysts, adhesions, fibroids, malignancies, inflammatory processes, or infections in persons with pelvic and abdominal pain. Evaluation of the fallopian tubes can be done for infertile patients. These procedures provide a means to remove adhesions, to obtain biopsies, to do select operative procedures, or to do tubal ligations. Gynecologic laparoscopy or pelviscopy is commonly performed under general anesthetia as a same-day surgical procedure.

These techniques replace laparotomy because they are less stressful to the patient, use small incisions, can be done in shorter periods of time, may be done under local, spinal, or general anesthetics, reduce potential for formation of adhesions, and hasten healing and recovery time.

Pelviscopy differs from laparoscopy in two major respects—*endocoagulation* as a method for controlling bleeding and *endoligation* as a technique that permits suturing using extracorporeal (outside the body) or intracorporeal (inside the body) ligating and suturing methods with special instruments.

The pelviscope is also angled at 30 degrees for better visualization. A video-camera attachment offers the physician a choice of viewing the process on a video screen instead of the scope. Printouts and videotapes of the pelviscopy can be produced. Thus, pelviscopy is both a diagnostic and an operative modality.

Procedure Using Local Anesthetic

1. The patient is supine during all procedures except gynecologic laparoscopy, in which case the patient is placed in a lithotomy position.
2. The skin is cleansed and a local anesthetic is injected into the area where the scope will be introduced. A sterile field is maintained.
3. An intravenous line is placed so that medications may be given intravenously as needed.
4. An indwelling catheter is placed into the bladder to reduce the risk of bladder perforation.
5. A small incision is made near the umbilicus through which a trocar is introduced, followed by passage of the pelviscope or laparoscope. Sometimes, more than one puncture site will be made so that accessory instruments can be used during the procedure. Carbon dioxide introduced into the peritoneal cavity causes the omentum to rise away from the organs and allows for better visualization. A few stitches or steri-strips are usually needed to close the incisions. Band-Aid type bandages are applied as dressings. Total examining time averages 30 minutes to 1 hour.

Clinical Implications

Abnormal findings can reveal

1. Endometriosis
2. Ovarian cysts
3. Pelvic inflammatory disease
4. Metastasis stage of cancer
5. Uterine fibroids
6. Abscesses

7. Enlarged fallopian tubes (hydrosalpinx)
8. Ectopic pregnancy
9. Infection
10. Adhesions
11. Ascites
12. Cirrhosis
13. Liver nodules (often an indication of cancer)
14. Engorged peritoneal vasculature (correlates with portal hypertension)

Clinical Alert

These procedures may be contraindicated in persons known to have

1. Advanced abdominal wall cancer
2. Severe respiratory or cardiovascular disease
3. Intestinal obstruction
4. Palpable abdominal mass
5. Large abdominal hernia
6. Chronic tuberculosis
7. History of peritonitis

The procedure should be interrupted and a laparotomy instituted in the event of uncontrolled bleeding or suspected malignancy.

Patient Preparation
1. Laboratory tests and other appropriate diagnostic modalities need to be completed prior to these procedures.
2. Bowel prep may include an enema or suppository.
3. Explain the purpose and procedure of the test and the type of anesthesia chosen (general, spinal, or local) as well as postoperative expectations such as activity, deep breathing, and shoulder pain.
4. A legal permit must be signed (see Chap. 1, p. 2 and p. 8).

Patient Aftercare
1. Check blood pressure frequently after the procedure (institutional practice dictates frequency.)
2. Observe for infection, hemorrhage, and bowel or bladder perforation.
3. Advise the patient that shoulder and abdominal discomfort may be present for 1 to 2 days because of carbon dioxide gas remaining in the abdominal cavity. This can be controlled with mild oral analgesics. Sitting or resting in a semi-Fowler's position can also alleviate discomfort.
4. If the patient has a general or spinal anesthetic, follow the usual cautions and procedures for the care of any person having those types of anesthesia.

Cystoscopy (Cystourethroscopy)

Normal Values
Normal structure and function of the bladder, urethra, ureteral orifices, and male prostate

Explanation of Test
These examinations are used to diagnose and to treat disorders of the lower urinary tract. They provide views of the interior bladder, the urethra, the prostatic urethra, and the ureteral orifices through tubular, lighted, telescopic lens instruments called cystoscopes or cystourethroscopes. Urethroscopy is an important part of this examination because it allows visualization of the male prostate gland. (Kidney function may be studied separately through ureteral catheterization and collection of urine specimens from each kidney.)

Cystoscopy is the most common of all urologic diagnostic methods. It may be indicated when the following conditions exist:

1. Unexplained hematuria (gross or microscopic)
2. Recurrent or chronic urinary tract infection
3. Infection resistant to medical treatment
4. Unexplained urinary symptoms such as dysuria, frequency, urgency, hesitancy, intermittency, straining, incontinence, enuresis, or retention
5. Bladder tumors (benign and malignant)

Intravenous pyelogram (IVP) does not allow proper visualization of the area from the neck of the bladder to the end of the urethra. Cystoscopy makes it possible to diagnose and to treat abnormalities in this area.

Cystoscopy may be used to perform meatotomy and to retrieve small stones and other foreign bodies from the urethra, ureter, and bladder. Biopsy specimens can be obtained, bladder stones can be crushed, bladder tumors can be fulgurated, and strictures can be dilated through the cystoscope. In conjunction with cystoscopy, ureteroscopy can be done to determine the cause of hematuria, to detect tumors and stones, and to manipulate stones. The instruments used come in many sizes and variations, including flexible fiberoptic cystoscopes.

Procedure
1. The examination can be performed in an operating room designed for that purpose or in the urologist's office. Patient's age, state of health, and extent of surgical procedure determine setting.
2. The external genitalia are scrubbed and sprayed with an antiseptic solution such as Betadine (povidone-iodine) after the patient is placed in the lithotomy position with legs in stirrups. Proper grounding, padding, and draping follow.

3. A local anesthetic jelly is instilled into the urethra. For the male patient, the anesthetic is held in the urethra by a clamp applied near the end of the penis. For best results, the local anesthetic is applied 5 to 10 minutes before passage of the cystoscope.
4. The scope is connected to an irrigation system with solutions that are nonconductive and retain clarity during the procedure (*e.g.,* glycone or sterile water). This solution also distends the bladder for better visualization.

   Note: During transurethral resection procedures, venous sinuses may be opened and irrigation fluid may enter the circulatory system. Therefore, isotonic solutions such as sorbitol, mannitol, or glycine must be used.

5. The actual examination takes 15 minutes; however, the patient's time in the examining room may be about 1 hour.
6. Should blood or other matter be present in the bladder, the fiberoptic cystoscope will not provide as clear a view as a rigid cystoscope because it is more difficult to flush.
7. Institutional policies dictate specifics related to perioperative care and procedures.

Clinical Implications
Abnormal conditions revealed by cystoscopy include

1. Prostatic hyperplasia/hypertrophy
2. Cancer of the bladder
3. Bladder stones
4. Urethral strictures or abnormalities
5. Prostatitis
6. Ureteral reflux (shown on cystogram)
7. Vesical neck stenosis
8. Urinary fistulas
9. Ureterocele
10. Diverticula
11. Abnormally small or large capacity bladder
12. Polyps

Patient Preparation
1. Explain the purpose and procedure of the test. Care and tact are paramount in dealing with these patients. Cultural, social, and modesty issues are an important part of psychological support. Advise the patient that there is little pain or discomfort from cystoscopy. However, a strong desire to void may be expected.
2. Bowel prep and other laboratory and diagnostic tests may be necessary if more extensive procedures are planned in conjunction with the cystoscopy.

3. If cystoscopy is performed in the hospital, the patient must sign a legal consent form (see Chap. 1, p. 2 and p. 8).
4. The patient may take a full liquid breakfast, and liquids may be encouraged until the time of the examination to promote urine formation if the procedure is a simple cystoscopy done under local anesthesia. NPO guidelines are followed when spinal or general anesthesia is planned.
5. Sometimes an intravenous line may be started for the administration of intravenous medications such as diazepam (Valium) and midazolam (Versed) to relax the patient. Amnesia may be a side effect. Younger men may experience more pain and discomfort than older men. Women usually require less sedation because the female urethra is shorter. The patient should be instructed to relax the abdominal muscles to lessen discomfort.

Patient Aftercare

1. After cystoscopy, the patient should be monitored (or be instructed to self-monitor) for voiding patterns as well as bladder emptying. Check vital signs frequently in the immediate postcystoscopy period.
2. Fluids should be encouraged.
3. Sometimes clots will form. This may cause the patient difficulty in voiding.
4. Report heavy bleeding or difficult urination to the urologist promptly.
5. Urinary frequency, dysuria, pink to light red wine color, or urethral burning is common after cystoscopy.
6. Antibiotics are usually prescribed 1 day before and 3 days after cystoscopy to prevent infection.
7. The potential for gram-negative shock is present with urologic procedures because the urethra is such a vascular organ that any break in the tissues may allow bacteria to enter the bloodstream directly. Observe for and promptly report chills, fever, increasing tachycardia, hypotension, and back gain to the physician.
8. Ureteral catheters may be left in place to facilitate urinary drainage.
9. Routine catheter care is necessary for retention or ureteral catheters that are placed.

Clinical Alert

1. If urethral dilatation has been part of the procedure, the patient is advised to rest and to increase fluid intake.

2. Edema may cause urinary retention, hesitancy, small urinary stream, or urinary dribbling anytime within hours to a week after surgery. Warm sitz baths and mild analgesics may be helpful until the edema subsides. However, an indwelling catheter may be necessary to relieve retention.

Urodynamic Studies, Cystometrogram (CMG), Urethra Pressure Profile, Rectal Electromyogram, and Cystourethrogram

Normal Values
Normal bladder sensation of fullness, heat, and cold. Normal adult capacity is 400 to 500 ml, and residual urine is less than 30 ml. First desire to void is at 175 to 250 ml. Fullness is felt at 350 to 450 ml. Stream is strong and uninterrupted.

Patients will have low voiding pressure without dyssynergia (failure of muscular coordination) and with detrusor muscle reflex contraction that can be suppressed upon command. Rectal electromyographic readings will be normal. Urethra pressure profile reveals normal urethral closing mechanism.

Explanation of Test
These techniques are used to identify abnormal voiding patterns in incontinent persons by determining if a detrusor muscle and external sphincter reflex exists. The cystometrogram reflects intactness of the neuroanatomic connections between the spinal cord, the brain, and the bladder. These studies are indicated when there is evidence of neurologic disease such as spina bifida, myelomeningocele, spinal cord injury, tumors, extensive pelvic dissection, cordotomy, neurectomy, cerebrovascular aneurysm, or specific neuropathies such as multiple sclerosis, diabetes, and tabes dorsalis. This examination can also be used to evaluate patients with symptoms of dysuria, scant or weak urinary stream, frequency, enuresis, overflow or stress incontinence, residual urine, or recurrent infection. Cystometrogram is often done in conjunction with cystoscopy. Neurogenic bladder dysfunctions are grouped into five classes according to the bladder responses: autonomic, reflex, uninhibited, sensory paralytic, and motor paralytic. Frequently, crossover between categories exists.

Procedure
Cystometrogram Procedure
1. The patient is asked to void and the urine flow rate, voiding pressure, and amount of urine voided are recorded.
2. An indwelling catheter is inserted into the bladder and residual urine is noted. The catheter is then connected to the cystometer. (A cystometer is a device for studying the neuromuscular mechanism of the bladder by measuring bladder capacity and pressure.) The bladder is gradually filled with sterile saline or water or carbon dioxide gas in predetermined increments, and pressure readings are taken at these increments.
3. During the cystometric examination, observations are recorded about the patient's perception of heat and cold, bladder fullness, urge to void, and ability to inhibit voiding when bladder contractions occur.
4. After fluid or gas instillation and measurements are completed, the catheter may be either removed or left in place. Incontinence, voiding patterns, and voided amounts are recorded if the catheter is removed. Gas is removed prior to other studies or to catheter removal.
5. The patient should be instructed to report the following sensations:
   (a) Flushing   (d) Nausea
   (b) Sweating   (e) Bladder fullness
   (c) Pain   (f) Strong urge to void
6. After the cystometric examination, cholinergic and/or anticholinergic drugs (*e.g.,* Banthine [methantheline bromide], atropine, or Urecholine [bethanechol chloride]) may be injected to determine their effects upon bladder function. Answers to the following questions are sought:
   (a) Is an atonic bladder capable of being stimulated by cholinergic parasympathomimetic drugs such as Urecholine, *or* are detrusor muscle fibers so decompensated that no response can be elicited?
   (b) Can overactive motor stimuli be altered sufficiently with cholinergic blocking parasympatholytic drugs, such as atropine, to allow a near-normal bladder volume that will produce an acceptable voiding pattern?

   To determine the effect of these drugs, the cystometric study may be performed as a control, followed by repeat study 20 to 30 minutes after injection of the drugs.
7. A change in posture from supine to standing or walking may be required during the examination.
8. *Sleep examination* studies may be performed in conjunction with an electroencephalogram to evaluate persons having nocturnal incontinence. (See Chap. 15 for EEG study.)

Rectal Electromyographic Procedure

1. Electrodes are applied close to the anus, and a ground is attached to the thigh.
2. A needle electrode may be introduced into the periurethral striated muscle.
3. These electrodes record electromyographic activity during voiding and produce a simultaneous recording of urine flow rate. (See Chap. 15 for EMG study.)

Urethral Pressure Profile Procedure

A special catheter, connected to a transducer, is slowly withdrawn and the pressures along the urethra are recorded.

Cystourethrogram Procedure

1. This study evaluates stress incontinence (in women), and bladder wall and urethral abnormalities, and tumors. It can be used to assess reflux and to identify urine extravasation following trauma.
2. An x-ray contrast medium is instilled into the bladder through a catheter until the bladder is filled. The catheter is clamped and x-rays are done with the patient assuming several different positions.
3. After the catheter is removed, more x-rays are taken as the patient voids and the contrast passes through the urethra (voiding cysto-urethrogram).

Clinical Implications

Abnormal results reveal motor and sensory defects and abnormal patterns that point to inappropriate or absent contractions of the pelvic floor muscle and internal sphincter during voiding.

1. The most common cause of incontinence is a vesical-sphincter dyssynergia. This is a disturbance of muscular coordination between the external urethral sphincter/pelvic floor musculature and the detrusor muscle. The dyssynergia is thought to be responsible for incomplete emptying of the bladder, inappropriate voiding, perineal dampness, and predisposition to urinary tract infections.
2. Detrusor hyperreflexia is a detrusor muscle reflex that the patient cannot suppress on command due to upper or lower motor neuron lesions, as in
   (a) Cerebrovascular aneurysm
   (b) Parkinson's
   (c) Multiple sclerosis
   (d) Cervical spondylosis
   (e) Spinal cord injury above conus medullaris
3. Urethrovesical causes of hyperreflexia are benign prostatic hypertrophy and stress urge incontinence.
4. Detrusor areflexia, in which the detrusor reflex cannot be evoked because the peripheral innervation of the detrusor muscle has been interrupted, results in difficulty in initiating voiding without a residual volume. If it is due to interrupted peripheral innervation of

the detrusor muscle, the cause may be associated with trauma to cauda equina or conus medullaris, spinal arachnoiditis, spinal cord birth defects, diabetic neuropathy, or anticholinergic effects of phenothiazides. In postmenopausal women, the urethral pressure profile may be altered because the mucosal sphincter is deprived of estrogen.

Patient Preparation
1. Explain the purpose and procedure of the test. Be sensitive to the patient's potential anxiety and embarrassment. Tell the patient that he or she may experience slight discomfort and the urge to void.
2. No sedation is given because patient participation is necessary to verify sensations and perceptions. However, the patient must avoid movement during the examination.

Patient Aftercare
1. Encourage the patient to increase oral fluid intake to dilute the urine and to minimize bladder sensitivity.
2. Explain that some minor discomfort or burning may be noted soon after the procedure is completed, especially if carbon dioxide is used.

Clinical Alerts

1. Use of sterile technique can reduce the incidence of urinary tract infections. Preprocedural urinary tract infections can lead to sepsis as a result of bacterial spread.
2. Certain patients with cervical cord lesions may sustain an autonomic reflex that produces an elevated blood pressure, severe headache, lower pulse rate, flushing, and diaphoresis. Propantheline bromide (Pro-Banthine) alleviates these symptoms.

Arthroscopy

Normal Values
Normal joint: normal vasculature and color of the synovium, capsule, menisci, ligaments, and articular cartilage. This is a surgical procedure normally done under general anesthesia.

Explanation of Test

It is a visual examination of the joint using an arthroscope. It is used most commonly for the diagnosis of athletic injuries and in the differential diagnosis of acute or chronic joint disorders. For example, degenerative processes and injuries can be accurately differentiated. Wound irrigation as well as some actual surgical procedures can be performed at the same time. Postoperative rehabilitation programs can be initiated to shorten recovery periods. Arthroscopy may also be done to assess response to treatment or to identify whether other corrective procedures are indicated.

Although the knee joint is the site most frequently examined, the shoulder, ankle, hip, elbow, wrist and metacarpophalangeal joints can also be explored. Calcium deposits, biopsy specimens, bone spurs, torn meniscus or cartilage, and scar tissue can be removed during the procedure. Currently, many of these procedures are performed on a "same-day surgery" basis.

Clinical Implications

Abnormal results reveal the following:

1. Torn or displaced meniscus or cartilage. These persons complain of clicking, locking, and/or swelling of the joint.
2. Trapped synovium
3. Loose fragments of joint contents
4. Torn/ruptured ligaments
5. Necrosis
6. Nerve entrapment
7. Fractures/nonunion of fractures
8. Ganglions
9. Infections
10. Osteochondritis dissecans—inflammation of bone/cartilage—occurs when cartilage fragment and underlying bone detach from the articular surface (common in the knee).
11. Chronic inflammatory arthritis
12. Secondary osteoarthritis caused by injury, metabolic disorders, and use of weight-bearing joints
13. Chondromalacia of femoral condyle—wearing down of back of kneecap in persons who complain of grinding

Procedures

1. The examination is usually performed under general anesthesia for the following reasons:
   (a) The joint is very painful.
   (b) If a lesion is found, definitive treatment or surgical intervention can be done at the same time.
   (c) The patient is not subjected to the discomfort from an inflated tourniquet.

(d) Complete muscle relaxation permits a thorough examination and eliminates risk of inadvertent patient movement while the instrument is in the joint.

2. The surgical site is draped and prepped according to institutional protocols. Proper monitoring equipment is attached to the patient.

3. A tourniquet is applied to the appropriate area of the extremity after it is exsanguinated by the use of an elastic bandage or elevation. Some surgeons will choose not to inflate the tourniquet unless bleeding cannot be cleared by irrigation.

4. The joint is aspirated with a 15- or 16-gauge needle. (A specimen may be sent to the laboratory.) The joint is then injected with 75 to 100 ml of normal saline or lactated Ringer's solution to distend the joint before inserting the arthroscope. Additional puncture sites allow for use of accessory instruments. The wound is irrigated throughout the procedure.

5. Joint washings are collected and examined for loose bodies or cartilage fragments.

6. All parts of the joint are carefully examined. Photographs or videotapes of the procedure may be taken. Surgical interventions may be chosen for those problems able to be corrected in this manner.

7. As the arthroscope, accessory pieces, and irrigating needles are slowly withdrawn, the joint is compressed to squeeze out excess fluid.

8. Steroids or local anesthetics may be injected into the joint for postoperative pain control and reduction of inflammation. The wound is closed with sutures or adhesive strips and small dressings. Compressive dressings and splints or immobilizers may be applied.

9. Total examining time varies from 45 minutes to 1.5 hours or longer if actual surgery is done.

Patient Preparation

1. History and physical examination, requisite laboratory work, x-rays, and other preoperative requirements should be completed and documented on the patient's record.

2. Explain the purpose and procedure of the test. The patient should be NPO from midnight before the examination unless otherwise ordered (e.g., scheduled late in the day).

3. A legal permit must be signed by the patient and properly witnessed.

4. Pedal pulses are checked. Surgical site is prepped, positioned, and draped according to institutional protocols. An intravenous line is started.

5. Crutch walking should be taught prior to the procedure if this is anticipated postoperatively.

Patient Aftercare

1. Assess vital signs, bleeding, and neurologic and circulatory status of the affected extremity (color, pulse, temperature, capillary refill times, and sensation).
2. Apply ice immediately and elevate (if ordered) to minimize swelling and pain. Dressing changes and suture removal are at the physician's discretion. Dressing is kept clean and dry.
3. Appropriate pain medication should be administered.
4. The patient can usually be up and about after recovery from the anesthetic. Crutches may be used. Degree of weight-bearing and motion of the area is at the discretion of the physician.
5. Exercises and physical therapy may be ordered postoperatively. These are designed to strengthen and maximize use of the joint.
6. If discharged the same day, arrangements for transportation to home by another person needs to be arranged preoperatively.
7. Patient should consume no alcohol for 24 hours after the procedure. Progress diet from fluid to regular as tolerated.
8. Instruct patient to report loss of sensation, numbness, tingling, coldness, duskiness (bluish color), swelling, or abnormal pain to the physician immediately.

Clinical Alert

1. Arthroscopy is usually contraindicated if ankylosis or fibrosis is present because it is almost impossible to maneuver the examining instrument in this type of joint.
2. For knee arthroscopy, the posterior approach is not used because of the neurovascular structures present in that area.
3. Do not place pillows under the knee because flexion contractures can occur as a result. If the patient's *entire* leg is ordered to be elevated, make sure the knee is not flexed.
4. If there is risk of sepsis or if sepsis is present in any part of the body, the procedure should not be done.
5. Arthroscopy is usually not done less than 7 to 10 days after arthrography because chemical synovitis caused by a contrast medium can adversely affect the visual examination. However, it may be necessary to perform arthroscopy if the patient is experiencing severe pain. In this case, the joint will be thoroughly irrigated to remove contrast medium.
6. Be alert for signs of thrombophlebitis postoperatively. Instruct patient to watch for calf tenderness, pain, and heat and to report these symptoms to the physician immediately. Warn the patient not to massage the affected area.

7. Other complications may include hemarthrosis, adhesions, neurovascular injury, pulmonary embolus, effusion, scarring, and compartmental syndrome as a result of swelling. Compartmental syndrome is a musculoskeletal complication that occurs most commonly in the forearm or leg. The compartment of fascia surrounding muscles does not expand when edema occurs. Assess the neurovascular status of an affected extremity at least every hour for 24 hours after the procedure.

BIBLIOGRAPHY

Barnie DC: Care planning in the endoscopy unit: Master care plan for the pre-endoscopy patient. SGA J 11(2):97–99, Fall, 1988

Barnie DC: Care planning for the endoscopy unit: Master care plan for the post-procedure patient. Gastroenterol Nurs 11(4):266–267, Spring, 1989

Barsevick AM, Louver D: Women's informational needs about colposcopy. Image. 22(1):23–26, Spring, 1990

Beck ML: Guiding your patient a step at a time through a colonoscopy. Nursing 11(6):28–31, 1981

Beck ML: Preparing your patient psychologically for an esophagogastro-duodenoscopy. Part I. Nursing 11(1):28–31; Part II, 11(2):88–91, 1981

Bennett JR et al: Therapeutic Endoscopy and Radiology of the Gut, 2nd ed. Baltimore, Williams & Wilkins, 1990

Bora WF, et al: The role of orthoscopy in treatment of disorders of the wrist. Contemp Orthop 12:28–36, April, 1986

Brunner LS, Suddarth DS: The Lippincott Manual of Nursing Practice, 4th ed. Philadelphia, JB Lippincott, 1986

Bushing J: An introduction to cystoscopy. Nurs Times: 17–32, October 6, 1985

Cunningham JT: Peritoneoscopy: Indications, technique, and diagnostic yield. Hosp Med: 128–144, August, 1985

Friedman EA (ed): Atlas of Colposcopy. Philadelphia, WB Saunders, 1981

Golanamski M: Thoracoscopy. AORN J 50(1):80–85, July, 1989

Grundemann BJ, Meeker MH (eds): Alexander's Care of the Patient in Surgery, 7th ed. St. Louis, CV Mosby, 1983

Grundemann BJ, Meeker MH (eds): Questions and Answers About Orthoscopy Patient Care. Darien, CT, Patient Care Communications, 1984

Hollen EM, Toomley IV, Given S: Bronchoscopy. Nursing 12(6):120–122, 1982

Isselbacher KJ, et al (eds): Harrison's Principles of Medicine, 9th ed. New York, McGraw-Hill, 1980

Kaiser LR: Diagnostic and therapeutic uses of pleuroscopy (thorascopy) in lung cancer. Surg Clin North Am 67:1081–1086, October, 1987

Kallacky MA, MacMillan W, Sheets EE: Should you be doing colposcopy? Patient Care: June 15, 1988

McCauly KM, Oi RH: Evaluating the Papanicolaou smear: Four possible colposcopic findings and corresponding management strategies, Part 2. Consultant 29(1): 36–42, January, 1989

Nichols CD: Wrist orthoscopy. AORN J 49(3):759–771, March, 1989

Raufman JP, et al: Endoscopic procedures in the AIDs patient: Risks, precautions, indications, and allegations. Gastroenterol Clin North Am 17(3):495–506, September, 1988

Rivera ML: Pelviscoscopy: Broadening the scope of laparoscopy. Today's OR Nurse 11:16–20, November, 1989

Sugarbaker PH: Endoscopy in cancer diagnosis and management. Hosp Pract: 111–112, November, 1984

Thawley SE: Endoscopic sinus surgery: A functional approach. MO Med 84:237–241, May, 1987

Watson A, Griffiths M: Cervicography: The nurse's role. Nurs Times 185(29), July 9, 1989

ULTRASOUND STUDIES

Introduction

Overview
Ultrasonography is a noninvasive procedure for visualizing soft-tissue structures of the body by recording the reflection of ultrasonic waves directed into the tissues. This diagnostic procedure, which requires very little patient preparation, is now being used in many branches of medicine for accurate diagnosis of certain pathologic conditions. It may be used diagnostically with the obstetric and gynecologic patient, the cardiac patient, and in patients with abnormal conditions of the kidney, pancreas, gallbladder, lymph nodes, liver, spleen, thyroid, and peripheral blood vessels. Frequently, it is used in conjunction with radiography or nuclear medicine scans. The procedure is relatively quick (often requiring only a few minutes to an hour) and causes little discomfort. At this time, no harmful effects have been established at the low intensities that are used (under 100 mW/cm^2). However, the ultrasound technique is a relatively new procedure, and long-term effects have not been documented. As with any diagnostic procedure, ultrasound must be weighed by its benefit and risk and should not be used frivolously.

Principles of the Technique
Ultrasound employs high-frequency sound waves to examine the position, form, and function of anatomic structures (*e.g.*, the heart) and beautifully demonstrates fetal movements. Using principles first employed in sonar, ultrasound involves transmission of a sound frequency higher than that detectable by the human ear. Sonar stands for *sound visualization and ranging* and is akin to radar. Ultrasonograms are really echo-reflection maps. The visualization of even a very early fetus in utero is simply a scaled down version of submarine detection and copies the miniaturization technique of metal flaw detection in modern engineering practice.

The two basic parameters measured by ultrasound are differences in tissue acoustic impedance and sound-frequency shifts due to motion.

The ways in which these basic parameters are obtained are as follows:

1. An ultrasound beam is directed into the patient's body.
2. By vibration, the beam is propagated through body tissue.
3. The body tissue, being composed of structures of different acoustic impedances, reflects the sound waves in various ways. Flow through the carotid arteries is manifested by a frequency shift in the echoes reflected from moving blood cells.
4. Reflected sound waves are electronically processed and shown on imaging displays.

5. Recordings of the reflected sound waves may be made on Polaroid film, x-ray film, chart paper, slides, videotape, or digital recording media. The record may be called a scan.

Evidences of pathology are detectable because lesions are of a different density and elasticity than the surrounding normal tissue. However, ultrasound cannot be used diagnostically with the air-filled lung or the gas-filled intestine because the ultrasound beam is almost totally reflected by air-containing organs. For this reason, the ultrasound beam cannot be employed where air-filled lung, gas-filled intestine, or bone will come between the beam and the part of the body being studied.

Display Techniques
The complexities of the ultrasonic equipment used in ultrasound studies as well as the physical principles involved are beyond the scope of this text. However, it is helpful to have a general understanding of the types of equipment used and the techniques for displaying the image.

In the past, several different methods of displaying the echoes were used (A-mode, B-mode). Modern equipment typically uses a real-time display that is shown on a cathode ray tube (CRT) or high-resolution television monitor. With this method, images are generated rapidly and repetitively through the same section of tissue, allowing the motion of interfaces to be observed. Real-time scanning allows for visualization of moving structures such as the living fetus, heart, and blood vessels. Motion of abdominal organs due to breathing and peristalsis may be observed.

Recording Display Images
Some laboratories videotape a portion or all of the real-time ultrasound exam. However, permanent "hard copy" images are generally required for further investigation and for legal reasons. To obtain this hard copy format, a frame from the real-time study is "frozen" and then photographed or recorded digitally.

Doppler Method
A phenomenon known as the Doppler effect can be used to detect the motion of a reflector, such as a pulsating structure or moving cells within a blood vessel. Doppler can also be used to measure and characterize blood flow (*e.g.*, velocity). Color flow Doppler is a recent advance that provides a colored image rather than a grey-scale image. Color Doppler depicts the direction of flow and the velocity of blood flow in varying shades of blue and red.

Doppler and color flow Doppler examinations can be used to establish the patency of a given blood vessel. It is useful for studying the cerebrovascular system, abdominal vessels, fetal blood vessels, and peripheral blood vessels. Further discussion of these tests may be found in Chapter 15.

Uses of Ultrasound

1. Obstetrical use of ultrasound is the most common application of this diagnostic modality. This is because the fluid-filled uterus is an ideal environment from which to gain information with diagnostic ultrasound. It is used in the perinatal as well as the prenatal and neonatal periods.

2. Ultrasound has been used frequently in diagnosis of brain disorders to determine shifts in the intracranial midline structures; however, this technique is used less often since the advent of computed tomography (CT) of the head. Ultrasound studies are still useful when CT and radionuclide studies are not available. Real-time study may also be used in following young children with hydrocephalus and in the evaluation of intracranial hemorrhage.

3. Other uses of ultrasound include studies of the genitourinary system, with promising results identified in the examination of the urinary bladder, scrotum, prostate, and in the diagnosis of renal masses.

4. A 98.8% accuracy rate has been reported in use of ultrasound to detect aortic aneurysms.

5. Diagnostic ultrasound also permits direct visualization of the pancreas. As with the procedures already mentioned, it has both advantages and disadvantages. Major advantages are that the pancreas can be seen in its normal state and that ultrasound gives information different from x-rays, because it is dealing with acoustic properties. Tissue echogenicity is an important aid in scanning; generally, thinner patients yield the highest quality scans. The major disadvantage of ultrasound is related to its high reflectivity at bone and air interfaces. Adequate visualization of the pancreas is often obscured by ribs, stomach, and colon. Even with its inherent drawbacks, diagnostic ultrasound has found an important role in the workup of a patient with suspected pancreatic pathology. Its noninvasive aspect makes serial examination possible, and this allows us to follow the progress of pathologic states. Information about tissue character can also narrow the diagnostic possibilities.

6. Echograms of the neck include thyroid, parathyroid, lymph nodes, and carotids. Echograms of the thyroid have their greatest value when used in conjunction with palpation of the gland by an experienced clinician. It is useful in differentiating cysts from tumors. Real time Doppler ultrasound is commonly used in the evaluation of carotid vascular disease.

7. Echograms of the eye aid ophthalmologists in removal of foreign bodies and allow the ophthalmologist to study the posterior parts of

the eye, especially when the lens is opaque (as in cataracts or in vitreous hemorrhage). It is also helpful in evaluating retinal detachment.

8. Ultrasound studies of the gallbladder will detect disease as well as gallstones. The overall accuracy of gallbladder ultrasound is approximately 90%. Diseases of the gallbladder often are not detected when conventional x-ray techniques are used because the organ cannot concentrate the contrast used in testing. Ultrasonography does not depend on organ function and, thus, can be used even in the presence of significant jaundice, which would interfere with radiologic techniques dependent on organ function. Liver and spleen ultrasound studies are also done.

9. Well-circumscribed, solitary breast masses greater than 1 cm in diameter can be evaluated. Under certain circumstances, it is possible to make a determination of the nature of mass as either cystic or solid.

10. Gallium scanning combined with ultrasound is a very useful method of evaluating suspected abscesses, and aspiration of pus collections can also be aided by ultrasound.

11. Ultrasound can also be used in evaluating persons with increasing abdominal girth and suspected ascites.

Procedure (General)

1. A gel or lubricant such as mineral oil is applied to the skin over the area to be examined. The oil or gel as a conductor of the sound waves.

2. In certain cases, water is used as the conductor. The patient is then either immersed in a water bath or a water bath is hung over the area to be scanned.

3. A transducer is held by an examiner who watches the display on a CRT while moving this device over a specific area of the body.

4. Sonography of structures in the abdominal region will most often require the patient to control breathing patterns. Deep inspiration and/or exhalation techniques may be used.

5. The examination is performed by a technician called a *sonographer*.

6. Scan pictures of the recorded images are made.

7. The examination causes no physical discomfort. However, if the examining time is long, the patient could become very tired.

8. Tests usually take at least 35 to 45 minutes. This test time refers to the actual time the patient is in the examining department.

9. Some examinations require fasting and enemas.

10. Certain tests are best performed with a full urinary bladder.

11. Each individual examining department will determine its own guidelines.

Contact Technique versus Water Bath Technique

Because air provides a poor medium for transmission of ultrasound beams, another medium must be used to couple the ultrasonic energy from the probe into the patient. Two major kinds of coupling agents have been used: water and various kinds of oils and gels.

1. *Water bath.* Early scanning devices relied heavily on the immersion of the patient in a water bath. This method provided good detail of internal structure and good sound beam control, but it was cumbersome, and the condition of the patient often made immersion inadvisable. Several newer ultrasound devices have returned to the water bath as a coupling agent. This is especially true when visualizing small organs such as the eye, the thyroid, and breast.
2. *Contact method.* This technique uses oils, glycerin, and water-soluble gels that are applied directly to the patient's skin. The transducer is swept across the skin with the probe always moving along a layer of the coupling material. Advantages of this technique are that it is easy to use and the device is portable.

Rectal and vaginal transducers have recently been introduced for the evaluation of prostate, uterine, and adnexal regions. The advantage is that these devices can often supply information in organs that were otherwise difficult to visualize sonographically because of overlying intestinal gas.

Benefits and Risks of Ultrasound Studies

1. Noninvasive procedure (with no radiation risk)
2. Requires little, if any, patient preparation
3. Procedure is safe for both patient and examiner. (To date, the procedure has been shown to be safe even for the developing fetus.)
4. As far as we know, examination can be repeated as many times as necessary without being injurious to patient. There is no harmful cumulative effect prove to date.
5. Studies can obviate the need for extended hospitalization.
6. Because ultrasound studies demonstrate structure rather than function, they may be useful with patients whose organ function is impaired.
7. Useful in detection and examination of moving parts, such as the heart
8. Does not require the injection of contrast materials, isotopes, or ingestion of opaque materials
9. Fasting is not required in many instances

Disadvantages of Ultrasound Studies

1. An extremely skilled technician is required to operate the transducer. The scans must be read immediately and interpreted for

adequacy. If the scans are not satisfactory, the examination must be repeated.

2. Air-filled structures (*e.g.*, lungs) cannot be studied by ultrasonography.
3. Certain patients (*e.g.*, restless children, extremely obese patients) cannot be studied adequately unless they are specially prepared.

Patients Difficult to Study

The following general categories of patients may provide some difficulties in ultrasound studies:

1. Postoperative patients. If possible, dressings should be removed and a sterile coupling agent and probe should be applied gently to the skin.
2. Patients with abdominal scars. The scar tissue causes attenuation of the ultrasound.
3. Children. Because the procedure requires the patient to remain very still, some children may need to be sedated so that their movements do not cause artifacts. However, the technologist remains with the child during the entire procedure so in most cases, there is little apprehension and little need for sedation.
4. Obese patients. Certain patients cannot be studied adequately in any case. For example, it may be very difficult to obtain an accurate scan on a very obese patient due to the alteration of the sound beam. There is no prep that would help in this case.

Interfering Factors

1. Barium has an adverse effect on the quality of abdominal studies, so echograms should be scheduled before barium studies are done.
2. If a patient has a large amount of gas in the bowel, the examination will be rescheduled because air (bowel gas) is a very strong reflector of sound and will not permit visualization.
3. Because gel or lubricant on the skin is used as a conductor, the examination cannot be performed over an area of open wounds or dressings.

Inadequate contact between the skin and the probe may be one of the causes of unsatisfactory scans. Sufficient quantities of the coupling agent, such as oil, must be applied to the skin and frequently reapplied.

Obstetric Sonogram

Normal Values

Normal image of placental position, size, and structure
Normal fetal position and size with evidence of fetal movement, and cardiac and breathing activity
Adequate amniotic fluid volumes.

Accuracy of Obstetric Measurements

Crown–rump length measured prior to 12 weeks has predictive value of ±5 days.

Biparietal diameter measured at 17 to 26 weeks has predictive value of ±11 days.

Biparietal diameter measured in third trimester has predictive value of ±3 weeks.

Gestational age is also estimated by measuring fetal extremities, particularly the femur, head, and abdominal circumferences, orbits, and numerous other anatomic structures.

Explanation of Test

Ultrasound studies of the obstetric patient are valuable in (1) confirming pregnancy, (2) facilitating amniocentesis by locating a suitable pool of amniotic fluid, (3) determining fetal age, (4) confirming multiple pregnancy, (5) ascertaining whether fetal development is normal, through sequential studies, (6) determining fetal viability, (7) localizing the placenta, (8) confirming masses associated with pregnancy, and (9) postmature pregnancy (evaluation of amount of amniotic fluid and degree of placental calcification). A pregnancy can be dated with considerable accuracy if one sonogram is done at 20 weeks and a follow-up is done at 32 weeks. There is a good reliability between those two points in fetal growth. This validation is most important when early delivery is anticipated and prematurity is to be avoided. Conditions in which determination of pregnancy duration are useful are maternal diabetes, Rh immunization, preterm labor, and any medical condition that is worsening with the progress of labor (Table 13-1).

The pregnant uterus is ideal for echographic evaluation because the amniotic fluid-filled uterus provides strong transmitting interfaces between the fluid, placenta, and fetus. Ultrasonography has become the method of choice in evaluating the fetus, thus eliminating the need for potentially injurious x-ray studies that were used previously. Because ultrasonography as used in obstetrics is about 98% accurate in detecting placental site, radionuclide studies of the pregnant patient have been abandoned.

Procedure

1. The pregnant woman lies on her back with her abdomen exposed during the test. This may cause some shortness of breath and supine hypotensive syndrome and can be relieved by elevating the upper body or by turning the patient onto her side.

2. In the second trimester, the patient is usually scanned with a full bladder. Exceptions to this requirement are made when ultrasound is used to locate the placenta prior to amniocentesis, in the evaluation of an incompetent cervix, or in labor and delivery. A full bladder allows the examiner to assess the true position of the placenta, repositions the uterus and cervix for better visibility,

TABLE 13–1.
Major Uses of Obstetric Sonography

First Trimester
Confirm pregnancy
Confirm viability
Rule out ectopic pregnancy
Confirm gestational age*
  Birth control pill use
  Irregular menses
  No dates
  Postpartum pregnancy
Previous complicated pregnancy
  Caesarean delivery
  Rh incompatibility
  Diabetes mellitus
  Fetal growth retardation
Clarify dates/size discrepancy
  Large for dates—rule out
    Leiomyomata
    Bicornuate uterus
    Adnexal mass
    Multiple gestation
    Poor dates
    Missed abortion
    Blighted ovum

Second Trimester
Establish or confirm dates†
If no fetal heart tones
Clarify dates/size discrepancy
  Large for dates—rule out
    Poor estimate of dates
    Molar pregnancy
    Multiple gestation
    Leiomyomata
    Polyhydramnios
    Congenital anomalies
  Small for dates—rule out
    Poor estimate of dates
    Fetal growth retardation
    Congenital anomalies
    Oligohydramnios
If history of bleeding—rule out total
  placenta previa
If Rh incompatibility—rule out fetal
  hydrops

Third Trimester
If no fetal heart tones
Clarify dates/size discrepancy
  Large for dates—rule out
    Macrosomia (diabetes mellitus)
    Multiple gestation
    Polyhydramnios
    Congenital anomalies
    Poor estimate of dates‡
  Small for dates—rule out
    Fetal growth retardation
    Oligohydramnios
    Congenital anomalies
    Poor estimate of dates‡
Determine fetal position—rule out
  Breech
  Transverse lie
If history of bleeding—rule out
  Placenta previa
  Abruptio placentae
Determine fetal lung maturity
  Amniocentesis for lecithin/sphingo-
    myelin ratio
  Placental maturity (grade 0–3)
If Rh incompatibility—rule out fetal
  hydrops

* *Accuracy ±3 days*
† *Accuracy ±1 to 1½ weeks*
‡ *Accuracy only ±3 weeks*
(*Athey PA, Hadlock FP: Ultrasound in Obstetrics and Gynecology, 2nd ed. St Louis, CV Mosby,*
1985)

serves as a reference point, and acts as a sonic window to the pelvic organs.

3. During the first trimester, some laboratories utilize a *transvaginal* approach when performing obstetrical sonograms. This method does *not* require a full bladder. A slim transducer, properly covered and lubricated, is gently introduced into the vagina. Because the sound waves do not have to transverse abdominal tissue, exquisite image detail is produced. Check with the individual laboratory to determine the approach to be used.

4. A coupling agent (*e.g.*, special transmission gel, mineral oil, olive oil) is applied liberally to the skin to prevent air from absorbing sound waves. The sonographer slowly moves the transducer over the entire abdomen to obtain a picture of the uterine contents.

5. The examining time is about 30 to 60 minutes.

Clinical Implications

1. In the *first trimester*, the following information can be obtained:
   (a) Number, size, and location of gestational sacs
   (b) Presence or absence of fetal cardiac and body movement
   (c) Presence or absence of uterine abnormalities (*e.g.*, bicornuate uterus, fibroids) or adnexal masses (*e.g.*, ovarian cysts, ectopic pregnancy)
   (d) Pregnancy dating (*e.g.*, biparietal diameter, crown–rump length)
   (e) Coexistence and location of an intrauterine device

2. In the *second* and *third trimesters*, ultrasound can be performed to obtain the following information:
   (a) Fetal viability, number, position, gestational age, growth pattern, and structural abnormalities
   (b) Amniotic fluid volume
   (c) Placental location and maturity, abnormalities
   (d) Uterine fibroids and anomalies
   (e) Adnexal masses.

   Early diagnosis of fetal structural abnormalities makes the following choices possible: (1) intrauterine surgery or other therapy to fetus if possible; (2) discontinuation of pregnancy, and (3) preparation of family for care of child with a disorder, or plan or other options.

3. *Fetal viability*. Fetal heart activity can be demonstrated as early as 6 to 7 weeks by real-time scanners or 10 to 12 weeks by Doppler ultrasound. This information can be utilized in management of a woman who has vaginal bleeding. Incomplete, complete, and missed abortions can be differentiated. A molar pregnancy can be diagnosed but may be misdiagnosed by 9 to 10 weeks.

4. *Gestational age*. Indications for gestational age include uncertain dates for the last menstrual period or last normal menstrual period;

recent discontinuation of oral hormonal suppression of ovulation; bleeding episode during the first trimester; amenorrhea of at least 3 months' duration; uterine size that does not agree with dates; previous cesarean birth, and other high-risk conditions. The method of fetal age estimation utilized depends upon the stage of pregnancy: (1) determination of gestational sac size (about 4–5 weeks); (2) measurement of crown–rump length (between 6 and 12 weeks; (3) measurement of biparietal diameter (BPD) (starting at 12 weeks to term); (4) other parameters such as extremity length, especially femur, abdominal, and head circumferences (12 weeks to term). The crown–rump length method is the *most* accurate age estimator. Other age predictors such as BPD and femur length are most accurate during the second trimester. The accuracy of all other methods suffers as the pregnancy reaches term.

5. *Fetal growth.* Some of the conditions that serve as indicators for ultrasound assessment of fetal growth include the following: poor maternal weight gain or pattern of weight gain; previous intrauterine growth retardation (IUGR); chronic infections; ingestion of drugs such as anticonvulsants or heroin; maternal diabetes; pregnancy-induced or other hypertension; multiple pregnancy; and other medical or surgical complications. Serial evaluation of BPD and limb length can help differentiate between wrong dates and IUGR. *Doppler* evaluation of the umbilical artery, uterine artery, and fetal aorta can also assist in the detection of IUGR. Intrauterine growth retardation can be symmetric (the fetus is small in all diameters) or asymmetric (head and body growth vary). Symmetric IUGR may be due to low genetic growth potential, intrauterine infection, maternal undernutrition and/or heavy smoking, or chromosomal aberration. Asymmetric IUGR may reflect placental insufficiency secondary to hypertension, cardiovascular disease, or renal disease. Depending on the probable cause, the therapy varies.

6. *Fetal anatomy.* Depending on the gestational age, the following structures may be identified: head (including blood vessels and ventricles), neck, spine, heart, stomach, small bowel, liver, kidneys, bladder, and extremities. Structural defects may be identified prior to delivery. The following are examples of structural defects that may be diagnosed by ultrasound. Hydrocephaly, anencephaly, and myelomeningocele are often associated with polyhydramnios. Potter's syndrome (renal agenesis) is associated with oligohydramniosis. These can be diagnosed prior to 20 weeks, as can skeletal defects (dwarfism, achondroplasia, osteogenesis imperfecta) and fat disorders. Other structural anomalies that can be diagnosed by ultrasound are pleural effusion (after 20 weeks), intestinal atresias or obstructions (early to second trimester), hydronephrosis and bladder outlet obstruction (second trimester to term with fetal sur-

gery available). Two-dimensional studies of the heart, together with echocardiogram, allow diagnosis of congenital cardiac lesions and prenatal treatment of cardiac arrhythmias.

7. *Detection of fetal death.* Inability to visualize the fetal heart beating and the separation of bones in the fetal head are signs of death. With real-time scanning, the absence of cardiac motion for three minutes is diagnostic of fetal demise.

8. *Placental position and function.* The site of implantation, such as anterior, posterior, under, or in lower segment, can be described, as well as the location of the placenta on the other side of midline. The pattern of uterine and placental growth and the bladder fullness influence the apparent location of the placenta. For example, in approximately 15% to 20% of all pregnancies when ultrasound scanning is done in the second trimester, the placenta seems to be overlying the os. At term, the evidence of placenta previa is only 0.5%; therefore, the diagnosis of placenta previa can seldom be confirmed until the third trimester. Placenta abruptia (premature separation of placenta) can also be identified.

9. *Fetal well-being.* The following physiologic measurements can be accomplished with ultrasound: heart monitor, beat-to-beat variability, fetal breathing movements (FBM), urine production (following serial measurements of bladder volume), fetal limb and head movements, and analysis of vascular wave forms from fetal circulation. Fetal breathing movements are decreased with maternal smoking and alcohol use, and increased with hyperglycemia. Fetal limb and head movements serve as an index of neurologic development. Identification of amniotic fluid pockets is also used to evaluate fetal status. A pocket of amniotic fluid measuring at least 1 cm is associated with normal fetal status. The presence of one pocket measuring less than 1 cm or the absence of a pocket is abnormal. It is associated with increased risk of perinatal death.

10. *Assessment of multiple pregnancy.* Two or more gestational sacs, each containing an embryo may be seen after 6 to 7 weeks. Of those diagnosed in the first trimester, only approximately 30% will deliver secondary to loss or absorption of one. Of value is the assessment of the relative fetal growth of twins, where IUGR or twin-to-twin transfusion is suspected. One cannot unequivocally diagnose whether they are monozygotes or heterozygotes with ultrasound alone. Routine ultrasound cannot be totally relied upon to exclude the possibility of triplets or quadruplets, instead of only twins.

11. Male sex can be determined if fetal position is favorable; the genitalia of the male fetus may be identifiable. However, this is not the purpose of ultrasound. There is a low incidence of sex determination from the examination.

Interfering Factors

1. Artifacts can be produced when the transducer is moved out of contact with the skin. This can be resolved by adding more coupling agent to the skin and repeating the scan.
2. Artifacts (reverberation) may be produced by echoes emanating from the same surface several times. This can be avoided by careful positioning of the transducer.
3. A posterior placental site may be difficult to identify because of the angulation of the reflecting surface or insufficient penetration of the sound beam due to the patient's size.
4. Schedule uterine examination before barium x-ray examination whenever possible because barium will deflect the ultrasound beam.

Patient Preparation

1. A brief explanation of procedure to be performed is given, emphasizing that it is not uncomfortable or painful, or that it does not involve ionizing radiation that may be harmful to the mother and fetus. The studies can be repeated without harm, but the procedure is being studied carefully to determine whether there are any long-term adverse side effects. Benefits of the procedure should be explained.
2. Most studies are performed using a transabdominal approach with a full bladder. The patient is asked to drink five or six glasses of fluid (coffee, tea, water, juice, soda) approximately 1 to 2 hours before the examination. If she is unable to do so, intravenous fluids may be administered. She is asked to refrain from voiding until the examination is completed. Tell the patient the examination will be done when she has a strong urge to void. Discomfort due to pressure applied over a full bladder may be experienced. If the bladder is not sufficiently filled, three to four 8-ounce glasses of water should be ingested, and rescanning is done 30 to 45 minutes later. The examination will not be conducted if the bladder is empty.
3. Some laboratories use a transvaginal (endovaginal) approach during the first trimester of pregnancy. No patient preparation is required for this method. Contact the laboratory performing the study to determine method to be used.
4. Explain that a liberal coating of coupling agent must be applied to the skin so that there is no air between the skin and the transducer, and so that the transducer will pass easily across the skin. A sensation of warmth may be felt. The woman should be advised not to wear good wearing apparel.
5. The woman may face the screen, and the sonographer can explain and interpret the picture. The father of the baby is encouraged to observe the testing. Some institutions provide a photograph or videotape for the family to keep.

Clinical Alert

1. A full bladder may not be needed or desired in patients in the late stages of pregnancy or active labor. However, if a full bladder is required, and the woman has not been instructed to report with a full bladder, at least another hour of waiting time may be required before the examination can begin.
2. A transvaginal (endovaginal) scan does *not* require the patient to have a full bladder. Contact the laboratory to determine method to be utilized.
3. Fetal age determinations are most accurate during the crown–rump stage in the first trimester. The next most accurate time for age estimation is during the second trimester. Sonographic dating during the third trimester has a large margin of error (up to ±3 weeks).

Gynecologic Sonogram; Pelvic and Uterine Mass Diagnosis

Normal Values

Normal pattern image of bladder, uterus, ovaries, fallopian tubes, and vagina, and the prostate in men

Explanation of Test

Pelvic ultrasound examines the area from the umbilicus to the pubic bone in both men and women. Ultrasound studies may be used in the evaluation of pelvic masses, postmenopausal bleeding, and to aid in the diagnosis of cysts and tumors. Information can be provided on the size, location, and structure of the masses. These examinations cannot give definitive diagnoses of pathology, but they can be used as an adjunct procedure when the diagnosis is not readily apparent. These studied are also used in treatment planning and follow-up radiation therapy of gynecologic cancer.

This test may be performed using a transvaginal (endovaginal) *or* transabdominal approach. With the transvaginal method, a slim, covered, and lubricated transducer is gently introduced into the vagina. A full bladder is *not* required. Because the sound waves do not have to traverse through abdominal tissue, exquisite image detail is produced. This approach is most advantageous for examining the obese patient, the patient with a retroverted uterus or those who have difficulty maintaining bladder distention. The transvaginal method is the approach of choice in monitoring follicular size during fertility workups and during the aspiration of follicles for *in vitro* fertilization.

For pelvic sonograms using the transabdominal approach, a full bladder is necessary. The distended bladder serves four purposes: (1) It acts as a "window" for transmission of the ultrasound beam; (2) it pushes the uterus away from the pubic symphysis, thus providing a less obstructed view; (3) it pushes the bowel out of the pelvis; and (4) it may be used as a comparison in evaluating the internal characteristics of a mass under study.

Procedure (Transabdominal Method)
1. The patient lies on the back on the examining table during the test.
2. A coupling agent is applied to the area under study.
3. The active face of the transducer is placed in contact with patient's skin and swept across the area being studied.
4. Examination time is about 30 minutes.

Procedure (Transvaginal [Endovaginal] Method)
1. The patient lies on an examining table with hips slightly elevated in a modified lithotomy position. The patient is draped.
2. A vaginal transducer, protected by a sterile sheath, is lubricated and introduced into the vagina. Some laboratories prefer that the patient insert the transducer herself. A depth of less than 8 cm is all that is usually required.
3. Scans are performed by using a slight rotation or "planning" movement of the transducer handle.
4. Examination time is about 15 to 30 minutes.

Interfering Factors
1. Results may be only fair, may vary with the patient's habitus and preparation (see "Clinical Implications"), and can only be used in conjunction with other studies. However, masses 1 cm and smaller can be seen with high-resolution equipment.
2. The success of a transabdominal scan is dependent upon full bladder distention.

Clinical Implications
1. Ultrasound studies may raise the suspicion that a uterine fibroid exists; such studies, however, cannot confirm this diagnosis. It may be difficult to differentiate a uterine fibroid from a solid adnexal tumor.
2. Very small adnexal masses may not be demonstrated by ultrasound studies. Masses identified on ultrasound may be evaluated in terms of size and consistency.
3. *Cysts*
   (a) Ovarian cysts (the most common ovarian mass detected by ultrasound) will appear as smoothly outlined, well-defined masses. Cysts cannot be confirmed as either malignant or be-

nign, but ultrasound studies can increase the suspicion that a particular mass is malignant.

(b) A corpus luteum cyst is a single simple cyst commonly visualized in early pregnancy.

(c) Theca-lutein cysts are associated with hydatidiform mole, choriocarcinoma, or multiple pregnancy.

(d) Parovarian cysts are thin-walled cystic masses that can become quite large. When the urinary bladder is not distended, these large cysts are often situated low in the pelvis and confused with the urinary bladder.

(e) Because normal ovaries often have numerous visible small cysts, the diagnosis of polycystic ovaries is difficult on the basis of ultrasound alone.

(f) Dermoid cysts or benign ovarian teratomas are found in the young adult woman and have an extremely variable appearance. Because of their echogenicity, they are often missed on ultrasound. The only initial clue may be an indentation of the urinary bladder. When a dermoid is suspected on ultrasound, a pelvic x-ray should be obtained.

4. Solid ovarian tumors such as fibromas, fibrosarcomas, Brenner tumors, dysgerminomas, and malignant teratomas are not distinguishable by diagnostic ultrasound. Ultrasound will document the presence of a solid lesion but can go no further in narrowing the diagnosis.

5. Metastatic tumors of the ovary are common and may be solid or cystic in ultrasonic appearance. They are quite variable in size and may be bilateral. Because ascites is often present, the pelvis and remainder of the abdomen should be scanned for fluid.

6. Pelvic inflammatory disease: Ultrasound differentiation between pelvic inflammatory disease and endometriosis is difficult. Evaluation of laboratory results plus clinical history leads to correct diagnosis. Other entities may have similar ultrasonic presentations and include (1) appendicitis with rupture into the pelvis, (2) chronic ectopic pregnancy, (3) post-trauma with hemorrhage into the pelvis, and (4) pelvic abscesses from various causes such as Crohn's disease or diverticulitis.

7. Bladder distortion: Any distortion of the bladder raises the possibility of an adjacent mass. Tumor, infection, and hemorrhage are the major causes of increased thickness to the urinary bladder wall. Masses such as calculi and catheters may be seen within the bladder lumen. Urinary bladder calculi are highly echogenic. A urinary bladder diverticulum appears as a cystic mass adjacent to the urinary bladder. It may be mistaken for a cystic mass arising from some other pelvic structure, so attempts are made to demonstrate its communication to the bladder.

8. Ultrasound studies can help to determine whether a pelvic mass is mobile.
9. Solid pelvic masses such as fibroids and malignant tumors may be differentiated from cystic masses, which will show sound patterns similar to the bladder.
10. Lesions may be shown to have metastasized.
11. Studies may aid in the planning of tumor radiation therapy.
12. Position of an intrauterine contraceptive device may be determined.

Patient Preparation
1. Explain the purpose and procedure of the test. Fasting is not required.
2. For transabdominal scans, have patient drink four glasses of water or liquid 1 hour before the examination. Advise the patient not to void until the test is over.
3. If a transvaginal (endovaginal) approach is to be used, no patient preparation is required. Contact the laboratory performing the study to determine method to be used.
4. Reassure the patient that there is no pain or discomfort involved.

Clinical Alert

If the patient is NPO or in certain emergency situations, the patient may be catheterized and the bladder filled via the catheter.

Kidney Sonogram

Normal Values
Normal pattern image indicating normal size and position of kidney

Explanation of Test
This noninvasive test, often done to differentiate renal masses, has become an accepted clinical procedure following intravenous pyelography (IVP). It is of value in monitoring the status of the transplanted kidney. Using IVP, the exact location of a renal mass can be located before ultrasonic examinations are performed. However, in the case of impaired renal function and iodine allergies that preclude the use of IVP, renal echograms are fairly reliable and easy to do. They can be used alone or with a nuclear scan to establish a diagnosis. The size of the kidneys can be determined without the need for contrast agents. The location of the kidneys can also be determined. This is particularly useful information in planning radiation therapy for a renal tumor.

Procedure
1. The patient lies quietly in a prone or lateral position on an examining table. However, the right kidney may also be examined with the patient supine, employing the liver as an acoustic window.
2. Warm oil or gel is applied to the patient's skin.
3. For visualization of the upper poles of the kidney, the patient must inspire as deeply as possible.
4. The total study time varies from 30 to 45 minutes.

Clinical Implications
1. Abnormal pattern readings reveal
   (a) Cysts
   (b) Solid masses
   (c) Hydronephrosis
   (d) Obstruction of ureters
   (e) Nonopaque calculi
2. Studies can provide information on the size, site, and internal structure of a nonfunctioning kidney.
3. Studies can differentiate between bilateral hydronephrosis, polycystic kidneys, and the small, end-stage kidneys of glomerulonephritis or pyelonephritis.
4. Ultrasound may be used to follow the kidney development in children with congenital hydronephrosis. This approach is safer than repeated IVP studies.
5. Perirenal hematomas or abscesses may be discovered.
6. Solid lesions may be differentiated from cystic lesions.

Interfering Factors
Retained barium from x-rays will cause poor results.

Patient Preparation
1. Explain the purpose and procedure of the test.
2. Assure the patient that there is no pain involved; the only discomfort is that caused by lying quietly for a long period of time.
3. Explain that fasting is usually necessary. Check with your ultrasound department for guidelines.

Clinical Alert
1. Scans cannot be done over open wounds or dressings.
2. This examination must be performed before barium x-ray. If such scheduling is not possible, at least 24 hours must elapse between barium procedure and renal echogram.
3. Biopsies are often done using ultrasound as a guideline. If a biopsy is done, a surgical permit must be signed by the patient.

Pancreas Sonogram

Normal Values
Normal pattern image indicating normal size and position of pancreas. The normal gland is an echo-producing structure and will be more echogenic than the normal liver.

Background
The pancreas is an extremely inaccessible abdominal organ; various diagnostic procedures have been attempted to ascertain pathologic conditions of this organ. Ultrasound studies are probably the safest and most accurate procedures available. With gray-scale ultrasound equipment, the normal pancreas can be visualized 75% to 95% of the time. A sonogram of the pancreas in combination with a pancreas nuclear scan will increase the percentage greatly.

Explanation of Test
Ultrasound studies are done to establish a diagnosis of chronic pancreatitis, pseudocysts, and carcinoma. This is the method of choice in screening suspected pancreatic disease and in monitoring the response of pancreatic tumors to therapy. The results of these studies are used as a guide for percutaneous aspiration and biopsy. Liver and pancreatic ultrasound studies may be done at the same time. The pancreas may be visualized more easily and precisely by echogram than by any other method.

Although sonography is helpful in evaluation of patients who develop complications of acute pancreatitis, it is of little help in evaluation of patients who present with acute pancreatitis. This is primarily due to the associated ileus and gas-filled bowel that prohibit adequate visualization of the pancreas in patients presenting in an acute phase of pancreatitis.

Procedure
1. The patient lies on his or her back on the examining table.
2. The skin is covered with a layer of mineral oil or scan gel.
3. The patient will be asked to regulate breathing patterns as instructed during the exam.
4. Occasional position changes may be required during the exam.
5. In some cases, the patient is asked to drink water in order to outline the stomach and duodenum, thereby affording better visualization of the pancreas.
6. Total time of the examination is about 30 minutes.

Patient Preparation
1. Explain the purpose and procedure of the test.
2. Check with the individual laboratory to determine whether or not fasting is required.

Clinical Implications
1. Abnormal image patterns can identify the following conditions:
   (a) Acute and chronic pancreatitis
   (b) Possible sequelae of pancreatitis
   (c) Pseudocysts
   (d) Carcinoma of pancreas
2. In the patient with pancreatitis, the borders of the pancreas are more distinct, and the fibrous tissue septae inside the gland become more apparent.

Clinical Alert

If the patient with pancreatitis has an unusual amount of bowel gas, the scan will need to be repeated or a CT scan done.

---

3. In ultrasound studies, pseudocysts appear as well-defined masses and usually have echo-free interiors. Pancreatic pseudocysts may not always be echo-free. Debris secondary to necrosis and enzymatic action on surrounding tissue presents as echogenic regions within a pseudocyst. (A pseudocyst occurs when a portion of the pancreas is deprived of its normal route of drainage through the pancreatic duct. Enzymes continue to be secreted from walled-off cysts with no mucosal lining.)
4. Pancreatic carcinoma may be identified as an irregular mass with scattered internal echoes and poorly defined borders. This condition may easily be confused with lymph node enlargement secondary to lymphoma.

Interfering Factors
1. Air, gas, or bone near the pancreas could interfere with visualization of the organ.
2. If the stomach, costal cartilage, or fat overlies the pancreas, visualization is impeded.
3. The obese patient presents an impediment to visualization because of the difficulty of ultrasound waves passing through layers of fat.
4. Movement of the organ can cause difficulties, but this is less of a problem if real-time imaging techniques are used.
5. Barium from recent radiographic studies will cause problems in visualization.

Gallbladder and Biliary System Sonogram

Normal Values
Normal pattern image indicating normal size and position of the gall-
bladder and bile ducts
Normal adult gallbladder is 3 cm wide and 7.5–10 cm long.

Explanation of Test
This test is used to differentiate hepatic disease from biliary obstruction. The gallbladder and sometimes the common bile and cystic duct
can be identified using echography. This method is the procedure of
choice when a patient with poor liver function has an elevated serum
bilirubin and contrast x-rays cannot be performed. The test is very
helpful in evaluation of a patient with suspected gallstones whose gallbladder fails to opacify during oral or intravenous gallbladder x-rays.
   Sonography is an excellent examination in the determination of
stones or chronic cholecystitis. A normal study will very likely rule out
these conditions. It is a worthwhile initial study in persons with
chronic right upper quadrant pain because the common duct, head of
pancreas, intrahepatic ducts, liver parenchyma, and porta hepatis can
also be seen during gallbladder study.

Procedure
1. The patient lies on his or her back on the examining table.
2. Generally, scans are performed in supine, decubitus (lateral), or
   upright positions.

Clinical Implications
1. Abnormal pattern images indicate
   (a) Enlarged gallbladder
   (b) Obstruction of common bile duct
   (c) Thickened gallbladder wall, sometimes a sign of chronic chole-
       cystitis
   (d) Dilatation of biliary tree
   (e) Stones (calculi) in gallbladder and common bile duct

   Note: Gallstones smaller than 2 to 3 mm in diameter often can be
      visualized with the new high-resolution equipment. These
      stones are often the most dangerous because they can obstruct
      the flow of bile by entering the bile ducts. Stones usually cause
      dense echoes in the gallbladder area.

2. Inflammation of the gallbladder (cholecystitis) will be indicated by
   a slightly enlarged sonolucent structure with thickened walls.
3. Carcinoma of gallbladder
4. Polyps within gallbladder

Patient Preparation
1. Explain the purpose, procedure, and benefits of the test. No ionizing radiation is involved.
2. Instruct the patient not to eat solid food for 12 hours before the examination to allow the greatest dilatation of the gallbladder.
3. Water is permitted.
4. In some instances, enemas will be ordered before testing.

Clinical Alert

When it is difficult to differentiate between an abnormal gallbladder and a normal gallbladder with good contractility, the patient will be given a fatty substance such as Lipomul and another scan will be done to check contractility.

Lymph Node and Retroperitoneal Sonogram

Normal Values
Normal lymph nodes, which are smaller than a fingertip (about 1.5 cm), are not visible with ultrasound. Only when the lymph nodes enlarge, as with tumor, infection, or in a nodal group, are they visible.

Explanation of Test
Ultrasound has made the investigation of the retroperitoneum much easier. Generally, the retroperitoneum is a somewhat inaccessible area for conventional x-ray examination. This test is ordered for patients with aortic or iliac lymph node enlargement when lymphoma is suspected. Lymph node enlargement can be evaluated using ultrasound without the use of contrast agents. Also, retroperitoneal tumor response to therapy can be monitored without lymphangiography. Localization of lymph node masses by this method before radiotherapy is very useful in planning treatment and may be used as a follow-up study to assess shrinkage of the mass. These studies are easy to do and fairly reliable with a 28% chance of error. Ultrasound studies of the lymph nodes are often done in conjunction with lymphangiography.

Procedure
1. The patient lies on his or her back during the test.
2. Scans in two planes—longitudinal and transverse—must be taken.
3. If scans are taken below the umbilicus, the patient should have a full bladder to push the bowel out of the pelvis.

Clinical Implications
1. Abnormal pattern readings indicate
    (a) Retroperitoneal adenopathy
    (b) Retroperitoneal tumors
2. Lymph nodes that have enlarged will be more homogeneous than surrounding structures. However, echoes from enlarged nodes are not always a reliable indicator of their cause.

Patient Preparation
1. Explain the purpose and procedure of the test.
2. A 12-hour fast from solid food before the test is usually required.
3. Water is permitted.

Interfering Factors
With scans taken below the umbilicus, a gas- or feces-filled bowel may cause difficulty in differentiating lymph nodes.

Liver Sonogram

Normal Values
Normal pattern image indicating normal size, shape, and position of liver and normal relationship to adjacent anatomic structures

Explanation of Test
This noninvasive diagnostic technique is used to determine the cystic, solid, or complex nature of a liver defect. Pleural effusion can be seen and the intrahepatic ducts and veins can also be visualized. This examination is an excellent guide in evaluating ascites and is used before biopsy. Liver echograms are also used with good results mainly to differentiate cysts and abscesses from tumors. Liver sonograms are extremely useful in conjunction with hepatic radioisotope studies. Unfortunately, liver echograms are not reliable in detecting metastasis, especially in persons whose liver is high and largely under the rib cage.

Procedure
1. The patient lies on his or her back on the examining table.
2. It is important to have the patient take a deep breath and hold it. Deep inspiration places the liver as caudal as possible and costal margins and ribs are avoided.
3. Scans in several different planes are taken: supine longitudinal, supine transverse, and supine oblique.

Clinical Implications
1. Abnormal pattern readings reveal
    (a) Biliary duct obstruction
    (b) Cirrhosis

(c) Necrotic tumors

(d) Liver masses (intrahepatic, extrahepatic, subhepatic)

(e) Metastasis to liver

(f) Cause of jaundice

2. Cystic masses, solid masses, and abscesses may be distinguished from one another (cystic lesions have an echo-free nature, whereas abscesses may contain internal echoes). Solid masses will have internal echoes and will alternate the sound beam more than cystic lesions or abscesses.

3. A cirrhotic liver is more echogenic (contains more echoes) than the normal liver.

4. Serial scans can be used to determine the volume of the liver.

5. Adenocarcinoma and other primary liver tumors will have a dense central echo pattern surrounded by a less echo-producing halo. The image pattern is thus called the *bull's-eye*.

Patient Preparation

1. Explain the purpose and procedure of the test.

2. Check with the laboratory for fasting requirements.

Interfering Factors

Images of the right lobe may be somewhat obscured by rib artifacts.

Spleen Sonogram

Normal Values

Normal pattern image; diffuse, homogeneous, low-level echo pattern

Explanation of Test

This test is useful when the spleen is enlarged, because it is then easily detectable. Ultrasound is often used when a splenectomy is contemplated, such as with thrombocytopenic purpura. This study can be used to estimate spleen size and volume and may spare the patient discomfort from other kinds of diagnostic procedures. It can help to demonstrate the presence of hemostasis or fluid collections in or around the spleen in persons who have had a left upper quadrant injury. Following splenectomy, this test is used to search for a subphrenic abscess. Ultrasound is often used in conjunction with a radioisotope scan, except with pregnant women.

Procedure

1. The patient lies on his or her back or abdomen on the examining table during the test.

2. The examining time is about 30 minutes.

Clinical Implications
1. Abnormal pattern readings will reveal filling defects associated with an enlarged spleen, splenic metastasis, and cysts.
2. Although splenic metastases are rare, they will produce stronger than normal echoes.
3. Cysts within the spleen are identified because they give off no echoes.
4. In pregnant women who have experienced trauma to the spleen, a splenic hematoma may develop, causing distortion of the border of the spleen; hemorrhagic areas may be separated by a band of echoes.
5. The spleen is often large and echo-free in early sickle cell disease, but it shrinks in size and produces echoes in later stages of the disease.

Patient Preparation
1. Explain the purpose and procedure of the test.
2. Fasting from food for 12 hours before the examination is usually necessary.
3. Water is permitted.

Thyroid Sonogram

Normal Values
Normal pattern image of thyroid; echoes are uniformly reflected throughout the gland; boundaries are unevenly displayed. (The normal thyroid is moderately echogenic; on a transverse scan, the trachea is posterior to the thyroid gland.)

Explanation of Test
This ultrasound study is used to determine the size of the thyroid, to differentiate cysts from tumors, and to reveal the depth and dimension of thyroid goiters and nodules. The response of a mass in the thyroid to suppressive therapy can be monitored by successive examinations. Theoretically, this technique offers the possibility of a good estimation of thyroid weight—information that is important in radioiodine therapy for Graves' disease.

The examination is easy to do, is done before surgery, and gives 85% accuracy. Often, these studies are done in conjunction with radioactive iodine uptake tests. With pregnant patients, ultrasound studies are the method of choice; radioactive iodine is harmful to the developing fetus.

Procedure
1. The patient lies on his or her back on the examining table, with the neck hyperextended.

2. Oil is applied to the patient's neck.
3. A pillow is placed under the shoulder for comfort and to bring the transducer into better contact with the thyroid.
4. An alternate procedure involves separation of the neck surface from the transducer by a plastic bag filled with water. The water-filled bag is clipped on a stand and hung over the patient's neck. This water bath device allows for proper transmission of the ultrasound waves through the thyroid.
5. Examining time is about 30 minutes.

Clinical Implications
1. An abnormal pattern reading will present a cystic, complex, or solid echo pattern.
2. Solitary "cold" nodules 1 to 3 cm in size identified on radioisotope scans can be described as cystic or solid nodules by means of the ultrasound studies. Approximately 20% of these cold nodules prove to be cysts, the great majority of which are benign. Sixty percent are solid benign tumors, and the remaining 20% are solid malignant tumors.
3. Cysts, which are generally benign, are usually echo-free, with many echoes occurring distal to the posterior wall.
4. Solid tumors generally represent benign adenomas.
5. Thyroid adenoma will be demonstrated by a core of high-amplitude echoes with a halo of low-amplitude echoes.
6. Thyroid carcinomas appear to be lesions that are echo poor with an irregular display or peripheral echoes.

Interfering Factors
1. Nodules less than 1 cm in diameter may escape detection.
2. Cysts not originating in the thyroid may show the same ultrasound characteristics as thyroid cysts.
3. Lesions of more than 4 cm in diameter frequently contain areas of cystic or hemorrhagic degeneration and give a mixed echogram that is difficult to correlate with specific disease.

Patient Preparation
Explain the purpose and procedure of the test.

Abdominal and Aorta Sonogram

Normal Values
Normal pattern image showing regular contour and diameter of the aorta. The walls strongly reflect echoes, whereas the blood-filled lumen is echo-free.

Normal pattern image of upper abdominal organs indicating no discernible pathology

Explanation of Test

Abdominal ultrasound includes all the upper abdominal organs from the xiphoid to the umbilicus and includes the gallbladder, liver, pancreas, kidneys, aorta, and spleen. Sonograms may be organ-specific, such as pancreas sonogram. They are commonly ordered by region, such as upper abdomen. The greatest value of the aortic echogram is in the assessment of abdominal aortic aneurysms. Ultrasound is the least invasive diagnostic procedure available. The aorta is one of the easiest abdominal structures to visualize ultrasonically because of the marked change in acoustic impedance produced by the elasticity of its walls and its blood-filled internal structure. Echograms can evaluate the body tissues from below the xyphoid process to the aortic bifurcation. Ultrasound is an ideal method for serial examinations before and after surgery and in patients with small aneurysms. Clots within the aorta are evaluated by using ultrasound and Doppler in combination. For the pregnant patient, ultrasound studies are the only abdominal diagnostic method used.

Procedure

1. The patient lies on his or her back or side on the examining table and may also be asked to sit up during the test.
2. The skin surface in the testing area is lubricated with a gel to permit maximum contact between transducer and body surface.
3. The length of examination is usually 30 to 45 minutes.

Clinical Implications

The typical abnormal pattern readings reveal aortic aneurysms with or without thrombus. See individual organ tests for abnormal results.

Interfering Factors

Retained barium from x-ray procedures will give poor results.

Patient Preparation

1. Explain the purpose and procedure of the test.
2. Explain that there is no pain or discomfort involved.
3. Instruct the patient not to eat solid food for 12 hours before testing.
4. Water is permitted.

Clinical Alert

This examination must be scheduled before barium x-ray procedures. If this cannot be arranged, at least 24 hours must elapse between barium tests and aortic and abdominal echogram.

Heart Sonogram
(Echocardiogram; Doppler Echocardiography)

Normal Values
Normal position, size, and movement of heart valves and chamber walls are recorded in three modes: unidimensional, two-dimensional, and Doppler. The following values may vary from physician to physician:

Diagnostic Movements and Dimensions	Expected Values
Left ventricular (LV) dimensions $\begin{cases} \text{diastolic} \\ \text{systolic} \end{cases}$	3.7–5.6 cm
Ejection fraction $\begin{cases} \text{thickness} \\ \text{motion} \end{cases}$	0.6–1.1 cm
Interventricular septum (IVS)	⅔ LVPW motion
LV posterior wall thickness	0.6–1.1 cm
Ratio: $\dfrac{\text{IVS}}{\text{LVPW}}$	<1.3
LV outflow tract width (early systolic)	2–3.5 cm
Right ventricular dimensions	0.7–2.3 cm
Change	0–0.6 cm
Aortic root dimension	2–3.7 cm
Left atrial size	1.9–4 cm
Mitral valves: amplitude	1.5–2.5 cm
Diastolic closing velocity (EF slope)	50–150 mm/sec
Aortic cusp separation	1.6–2.6 cm
Pre-ejection period	Q wave to aortic opening
Ejection time	Period of aortic opening
Mean V_{cf} (left ventricular velocity of fiber shortening)	1.22–1.73 circm/sec
Peak V_{cf}	1.15–2.10 circm/sec

(*Feigenbaum H:* Echocardiography, *4th ed. Philadelphia, Lea & Febiger, 1986.*

Explanation of Test
This noninvasive technique for examining the heart can provide information about the position, size, movements of the valves and chambers, and velocity of blood flow by means of reflected ultrasound. Echoes from pulsed high-frequency sound waves are used to locate and study the movements and dimensions of cardiac structures such as the valves and chamber walls. Because the heart is a blood-filled organ, sound can be transmitted through it readily to the opposite wall and to the heart–lung interface. This test is commonly used to determine biologic and prosthetic valve dysfunction, and pericardial effusion, to evaluate velocity/direction of blood flow, to furnish direction for further diagnostic study, and to follow cardiac patients over an extended period. One of the advantages of this diagnostic technique is that it is a noninvasive procedure that can be performed at the patient's bedside using mobile equipment, or it can be done in the laboratory.

The three types of echocardiograms provide different diagnostic parameters. Unidimensional echocardiograms consist of A mode, B mode, and M mode. The A and B modes record the amplitude of the ultrasound signal as spikes or dots of varying intensity. The M mode, the most common unidirectional echocardiogram, measures both amplitude and motion, thus permitting the evaluation of the movement of cardiac structures.

Two-dimensional echocardiograms utilize a transducer that emits more than one ultrasonic beam. Despite the fact that it is unable to record a complete chamber or valve as a whole, it permits viewing structures with a spatial orientation.

Doppler echocardiograms record the velocity of moving objects, including the movement of blood through the heart, providing information on dynamics of blood flow through shunts and regurgitant valves. Newer techniques use color monitors to enhance information obtained.

In order to provide information relative to the function of heart structures during high cardiac output states, stress echocardiograms are used. Increased rate and contraction velocity can be achieved through the use of Persantine, ergometers, and pacing via an esophageal electrode.

Procedure
1. A specific diagnosis should accompany the request for the test (*e.g.*, "rule out pericardial effusion" or "determine severity of mitral stenosis").
2. The patient lies on his or her back and may be asked to turn on left side and sit up, leaning slightly forward. The skin surface is lubricated with a gel. The transducer is held over the left fourth intercostal space, apex, and subcostally for scanning.
3. There is no pain or discomfort involved. Electrocardiogram (ECG) leads are attached for a simultaneous ECG and ultrasonic record (see Chap. 15).
4. Examination time is 30 to 45 minutes.

Clinical Implications
Abnormal values help to diagnose the following:

1. Valvular stenosis
2. Valve prolapse
3. Pericardial effusion/tamponade
4. Subaortic stenosis
5. Free wall/septal rupture
6. Other valvular diseases
7. Congenital heart disease
8. Chamber size variations
9. Wall motion dysfunction

10. Cardiac thrombi
11. Endocarditis
12. Myocardial aneurysm
13. Prosthetic valve function

Patient Preparation
Explain the purpose and procedure of the test.

Interfering Factors
1. Dysrhythmias
2. The hyperinflation of the lungs with mechanical ventilation, especially with PEEP of greater than 10 mm, precludes adequate ultrasound imaging of the heart.
3. False-negative and false-positive diagnoses have been identified (especially in M-mode echocardiograms), including pleural effusion, dilated descending aorta, pericardial fat pad, tumors encasing the heart, clotted blood, and loculated effusions.
4. Doppler study results can vary greatly if the transducer position does not provide satisfactory angles for the beam.

Eye and Orbit Sonograms

Normal Values
Pattern image indicating normal soft tissue of eye and retrobulbar orbital areas, retina, choroid, and orbital fat

Explanation of Test
Ultrasound can be used to describe both normal and abnormal tissues of the eye when no alternative visualization is possible because of opacities. This information is of invaluable assistance in the management of eyes with large corneal leukomas or conjunctival flaps and in the evaluation of eyes for keratoprosthesis. Orbital lesions can be detected and distinguished from inflammatory and congestive causes of exophthalmus with a high degree of reliability. An extensive preoperative evaluation before vitrectomy surgery or for vitreous hemorrhages is also done. In this case, the vitreous cavity is examined to rule out retinal and choroidal detachments and to detect and localize vitroretinal adhesions and intraocular foreign bodies. Also, persons who are to have intraocular lens implants after removal of cataracts must be measured for exact length of the eye. These exact measurements must be to the nearest tenth of a millimeter.

Procedure
Two techniques are used: immersion and contact. The immersion technique gives a more sophisticated evaluation because the transducer is placed away from the eye in a water bath.

1. The eye area is anesthetized by instilling eye drops.
2. If the immersion technique is used, the probe is immersed within the fluid, and sound waves are directed along the visual axis.
3. In the contact method, the probe gently touches the corneal surface.
4. If a lesion in the eye is detected, as much as 30 minutes may be required to accurately differentiate pathology.
5. Orbital examination can be done in 8 to 10 minutes

Clinical Implications
1. Abnormal patterns are seen in
   (a) Alkali burns with corneal flattening and loss of anterior chamber
   (b) Detached retina
   (c) Keratoprosthesis
   (d) Extraocular thickening in thyroid eye disease
   (e) Pupillary membranes
   (f) Cyclitic membranes
   (g) Vitreous opacities
   (h) Orbital mass lesions
   (i) Inflammatory conditions
   (j) Vascular malformations
   (k) Foreign bodies
2. Abnormal patterns are also seen in tumors of various types based on specific ultrasonic patterns.
   (a) Solid, such as meningioma, glioma, and neurofibroma
   (b) Cystic, such as mucocele, dermoid, and cavernous hemangioma
   (c) Angiomatous, such as diffuse hemangioma
   (d) Lymphangioma
   (e) Infiltrative, such as metastatic lymphoma and pseudotumor

Interfering Factors
If at some time the vitreous humor in a particular patient has been replaced by a gas, no result can be obtained.

Patient Preparation
1. Explain the purpose and procedure of the test.
2. Topical anesthetic drops are instilled into the eyes before examination. This is usually done in the examining department.

Patient Aftercare
1. Instruct the patient to refrain from rubbing the eyes until the effects of anesthetic have disappeared. This type of friction could cause corneal abrasions.
2. Advise the patient that minor discomfort and blurred vision may be experienced for a short time.

Urinary Bladder Sonogram

Normal Values
Normal pattern image of the exact dimensions and contour of the bladder and little residual volume

Explanation of Test
This examination is done in the investigation of possible bladder tumor and provides a simple method of estimating postvoid residual urine volume. This test reduces the need for urinary catheterization and risk of subsequent urinary tract infection.

Procedure
1. The patient is placed in a supine position.
2. A gel is applied to the lower abdomen.
3. Total examining time is 20 to 30 minutes.

Clinical Implications
Abnormal results reveal the following:

1. Tumors of bladder
2. Ovarian carcinoma extension to bladder
3. Thickening of bladder wall
4. Masses posterior to bladder
5. Obstruction of lower urinary tract showing residual urine

Interfering Factors
1. Poor technique
2. Overlying gas or fat tissue

Patient Preparation
1. Explain the purpose and procedure of the test.
2. The bladder should be full to start, then emptied to complete the examination.

Patient Aftercare
Return to normal routine of nursing unit.

Intrauterine Contraceptive Device (IUCD, IUD) Localization

Normal Values
An intrauterine device (IUD) can be visualized ultrasonically if it has not perforated the uterus.

Explanation of Test

Ultrasonography has been found useful for confirming the presence and exact location of an IUD and for identifying the type of contraceptive device within the endometrial cavity. X-ray studies will only indicate that the device is in the pelvis. Most of these devices are sufficiently different in acoustic impedance from the normal uterus, so they are easily detected. The precise appearance depends on the type of device used, the position of the device within the uterus, and the position of the device relative to the transducer.

Procedure

1. The patient lies on her back on the examining table. A full bladder is necessary.
2. A coupling gel is applied to the entire abdomen.
3. The transducer is moved across the area being studied.
4. Total examining time is about 30 minutes.

Clinical Implications

1. A typical pattern will identify the presence of an IUD.
2. If the device has perforated the uterus, it is seldom possible to visualize it ultrasonically because it blends with the surrounding bowel echoes.

Interfering Factors

Overlying gas or obesity interferes with obtaining a satisfactory result.

Patient Preparation

1. Explain the purpose and procedure of the test.
2. Fasting is not required.
3. Instruct the patient to drink three to four glasses of liquid, preferably water, 1 hour before examination. Advise the patient not to void until the test is completed.
4. The only discomfort involved is the feeling of a full bladder.

Breast Sonogram

Normal Values

Symmetric echo pattern in both breasts, including subcutaneous, mammary, and retromammary layers

Explanation of Test

Ultrasound mammography is useful for differentiating cystic, solid, and complex lesions, in diagnosing disease in women with very dense breasts, and in the follow-up of women with fibrocystic disease. It is recommended as the initial method of examination in young women with palpable masses and pregnant women with a newly palpable mass. The pregnant patient presents a dilemma because malignancies in pregnancy grow rapidly, and the increased glandular tissue causes difficulties in mammography. Ultrasound may now be used to evaluate women who have silicone-prosthesis (as opposed to silicone-injected) augmented breasts. The prosthesis is readily penetrated by the ultrasound beam. Such prostheses are known to obscure masses on physical examination, and x-ray beams are absorbed by the prosthesis, thus obscuring portions of the breast parenchyma.

When ultrasound is used in combination with x-ray mammography, diagnostic accuracy is improved. In addition, ultrasound mammography is an alternative for women who absolutely refuse to have an x-ray mammogram or those who should not be exposed to diagnostic radiation.

Procedure
1. The patient is asked to lie down on the examining table, which contains a machine with a tank that holds chlorinated, chemically treated, heated water. Visible at the bottom of the tank is a transducer that produces the ultrasound waves and detects their echoes. The patient will hear the sounds of the machine in operation as it records the echoes. (Water is a very good conductor of the ultrasound waves.) One breast at a time is immersed in the water.
2. Total examining time is 15 minutes.
3. Some laboratories will evaluate a suspicious area identified on a mammogram by utilizing a hand-held transducer that is applied to the overlying skin of the breast. Total examining time for this technique is approximately 10 minutes.

Clinical Implications
Unusual and distinctive echo patterns will indicate the presence of

1. Cysts
2. Benign solids
3. Malignant tumors
4. Tumor metastasis to muscles and lymph nodes

Interfering Factors
1. Women with back problems or those with limited flexibility may have difficulty maintaining the positions necessary for the procedure.
2. Although the tank is built to accommodate breasts of most sizes, 1% of breasts are too large to examine by this method.

Patient Preparation
1. Explain the purpose and procedure of the examination. There is no discomfort involved. Many diagnostic departments will show the patient a videotape that explains the test.

2. On the day of examination, the patient should wear a two-piece outfit because the garments on the torso will be removed prior to examination.
3. No powders, lotions, or other cosmetics should be applied to the upper body on the day of examination.

Patient Aftercare
The breasts are dried, and the patient is advised to contact her referring physician for outcomes.

Scrotal Sonogram

Normal Values
Normal scrotal structure

Explanation of Test
This study is useful in diagnosing scrotal abscess, "missed torsion," hydrocele, and spermatocele. Sonography is ideal for evaluating chronic scrotal swelling when the possibility of a testicular tumor exists and is valuable in clarifying the ambiguous nuclear studies. It is also the best means of evaluating the clinically normal scrotum when screening for occult disease. Because sonography cannot assess perfusion, it is not the initial examination in an "acute scrotum."

Procedure
1. The patient lies on his back and the penis is gently taped back to the lower abdominal wall.
2. After an acoustical gel is applied to the skin, the transducer is repeatedly passed over the scrotum. Sonographic images are generated.
3. Total examining time is 30 to 60 minutes.

Clinical Implications
Abnormal results are associated with

1. Abscess (cystic and solid pattern)
2. Infarcted testes of missed torsion (solid pattern)
3. Tumor
4. Hydrocele
5. Spermatocele
6. Adherent scrotal hernia
7. Missed torsion
8. Chronic epididymitis

Prostate Sonogram (Transrectal)

Normal Values
Normal sizes, contour, and consistency of prostate tissue

Explanation of Test
This diagnostic technique is valuable in the diagnosis of prostatic cancer when used in association with rectal examination and laboratory testing of blood samples for levels of prostate-specific antigen (see p. 333).

Carcinoma of the prostate is the second most common cause of cancer-related deaths in American men. Sonography can be used to evaluate prostate tissue, the seminal vesicles, and surrounding tissue. Small, subclinical tumors may be identified using this method. It is also useful in evaluating palpable nodules and as a guide for biopsy. Sonography may be used to stage a known carcinoma and to assist in radiation "seed" placement. The volume of the prostate can be determined, and transrectal sonography may also be used in the evaluation of micturition disorders.

Procedure
1. Approximately 1 hour before the study, a self-administered enema is used to eliminate fecal material from the rectum.
2. The patient lies on his left side with knees bent toward the chest.
3. A digital rectal exam usually precedes insertion of the rectal transducer.
4. A draped and lubricated rectal probe is inserted. Water may be introduced into the sheath surrounding the transducer. The patient may feel slight pressure at this time.
5. Scans are performed in various planes by using a slight rotational movement of the transducer.
6. Total exam time is approximately 30 minutes.

Clinical Implications
Abnormal results are associated with

1. Prostatitis
2. Benign prostatic hypertrophy
3. Carcinoma of the prostate

Interfering Factors
Fecal material in the rectum will interfere with exam results.

Patient Preparation
1. Explain the purpose and procedure of the examination.
2. Approximately 1 hour before the study, a self-administered enema is used to eliminate fecal material from the rectum.

Patient Aftercare
Return to normal routine at home or in the nursing unit.

BIBLIOGRAPHY

Athey PA, Hadlock FP: Ultrasound in Obstetrics and Gynecology, 2nd ed. St. Louis, CV Mosby, 1985

Babcock DS, Hand BK: Cranial Ultrasound of Infants. Baltimore, Williams & Wilkins, 1981

Callen PW: Ultrasonography in Obstetrics and Gynecology, 2nd ed. Philadelphia, WB Saunders, 1988

Dakin R et al: Transrectal ultrasound of the prostate. Journal of Diagnostic Medical Sonography 1:1–5, January, 1989

Feigenbaum H: Echocardiography, 4th ed. Philadelphia, Lea & Febiger, 1986

Fleischer AC, James AE: Diagnostic Sonography. Philadelphia, WB Saunders, 1989

Goldberg BB: Measurements in Ultrasound: A Reference Manual. Chicago, Year Book Medical Pub, 1988

Hackeloer BJ et al: Ultrasound Mammography. New York, Springer–Verlag, 1988

Hagen–Ansert SL: Textbook of Diagnostic Ultrasonography, 3rd ed. St. Louis, CV Mosby, 1989

Jensen MD, Bobak I: Maternity and Gynecologic Care: The Nurse and the Family, 4th ed. St. Louis, CV Mosby, 1988

Kremkau FW: Diagnostic Ultrasound: Physical Principles and Exercises, 3rd ed. Philadelphia, WB Saunders, 1989

Martin JP: Prep talks–transrectal ultrasound: A new screening tool for prostate cancer. Am J Nurs 91(2):69, February, 1991

Mendelson EB et al: Gynecologic imaging: Comparison of transabdominal and transvaginal sonography. Radiology 166:321–324, 1988

Peters BE, Kocherl GP: Diagnostic Medical Ultrasound Examination Review, 2nd ed. New Hyde Park, NY, Medical Examination Publishing, 1989

Sabbagha RE et al: Diagnostic Ultrasound Applied to Obstetrics and Gynecology, 2nd ed. Philadelphia, JB Lippincott, 1987

Sarti DA: Diagnostic Ultrasound: Text and Cases. Chicago, Year Book Medical Pub, 1987

Taylor K: Atlas of Ultrasonography. New York, Churchill Livingstone, 1985

Thijsson JM et al: Ultrasonography in Ophthamology. New York, Kluwer Academic, 1988

Weill FS et al: Renal Sonography, 2nd ed. New York, Springer–Verlag, 1986

PULMONARY FUNCTION STUDIES; BLOOD GAS ANALYSES

Introduction

Pulmonary Physiology
There are three aspects of pulmonary function: perfusion, diffusion, and ventilation. *Perfusion* consists of the passage of blood through pulmonary vessels; *diffusion* consists of the movement of oxygen and carbon dioxide across alveolar capillary membranes; *ventilation* consists of exchanging air between alveolar spaces and the atmosphere.

During breathing, the lung–thorax system acts as a bellows that provides fresh air to the alveoli for adequate gas exchange. Like springs, the lung tissue possesses the property of elasticity. When the inspiratory muscles contract, the thorax and lungs expand, and when the muscles relax and the force is removed, the thorax and lungs recoil to their resting position. In addition, when the thorax and lungs expand, the alveolar pressure is lowered below atmospheric pressure and air flows into the trachea, bronchi, bronchioles, and finally the alveoli. Expiration is mainly passive and is brought about by the recoil of the thorax and lungs to their resting position; alveolar pressure is increased above atmospheric pressure, and air flows out. The primary purpose of the pulmonary blood flow is to conduct mixed venous blood through the capillaries of the alveoli so that oxygen (O_2) can be added and carbon dioxide (CO_2) removed.

Use of Tests
Pulmonary function tests are designed to determine the presence, nature, and extent of pulmonary dysfunction caused by obstruction or restriction, or a combination of both.

When ventilation is disturbed by an increase in airway resistance, the ventilatory defect is called an *obstructive* defect. When ventilation is disturbed by a limitation in chest wall excursion, the defect is called a *restrictive* defect. When ventilation is disturbed by both increased airway resistance and limitation of chest wall excursion, the defect is called a combined or *mixed* defect. See Table 14–1 for conditions that affect ventilation.

The results of pulmonary function studies may reveal abnormalities in the airways, alveoli, and pulmonary vascular bed early in the course of disease when physical examinations and x-ray tests are still normal. In addition, the location of an airway abnormality can be determined—for example, upper airway, large airway, or small airway.

Indications for Tests
1. Early detection of pulmonary or cardiac pulmonary disease
2. Differential diagnosis of all patients with dyspnea

TABLE 14–1.
Conditions That Affect Ventilation

Diagnosis	Basic Disturbance in Ventilation	Underlying Pathology
Obstructive Defects		
Asthma	Increased airway resistance	Bronchial edema, bronchospasm, and obstructive mucus
Bronchitis	Increased airway resistance	Same as above
Emphysema	Increased airway resistance	Loss in radial traction or respiratory airway due to destruction of alveolar septa
Restrictive Defects		
Kyphoscoliosis	Limitation on chest cavity expansion	Increase in elastic resistance of chest wall due to abnormal curvature of spine
Obesity	Same as above	Increase in elastic resistance of chest wall due to increase in adipose tissue, especially of abdomen
Muscular dystrophy	Same as above	Weakness of inspiratory muscles
Pneumoconiosis	Same as above	Increase in elastic resistance of lung due to fibroses of pulmonary tissue
Mixed Defect		
Pulmonary congestion	Increases in both airway resistance and limitation in expansion of chest cavity	Obstructive due to bronchial edema and compression of respiratory airway due to increased interstitial and intravenous fluid pressure. Restrictive due to increase in elastic resistance of lung due to increased interstitial and intravenous fluid pressure

3. Assessment of patient's ability to tolerate anesthetics during surgery, particularly if the removal of lung tissue is contemplated
4. Determination of the risk of using certain diagnostic procedures
5. Detection of early respiratory failure
6. To follow course of disease in patients known to have bronchopulmonary disease
7. Periodic examination of workers in industries in which a lung hazard exists
8. Epidemiologic study of populations to provide clues to the causes of pulmonary diseases

Classification of Pulmonary Diseases

1. Restrictive diseases
   Characterized by interference with elastic behavior of lungs, causing them to be stiff; actual reduction in the volume of air that can be inspired

Examples of Restrictive Diseases	*Caused by*
Chest wall disease	Injury, kyphoscoliosis, spondylitis, muscular dystrophy, and other neuromuscular diseases
Extrathoracic conditions	Obesity, peritonitis, ascites, and pregnancy
Interstitial lung disease	Interstitial pneumonitis, fibrosis, pneumoniosis, granulomatosis, and edema
Pleural disease	Pneumothorax, hemothorax, pleural expansion, and fibrothorax
Space-occupying lesions	Tumors and cysts

2. Obstructive diseases
   Characterized by need for unusual effort to produce air-flow; respiratory muscles must work with difficulty to overcome resistive forces during breathing. Patient experiences prolongation and impairment of airflow during expiration.

Examples of Obstructive Diseases	*Caused by*
Peripheral airway disease	Bronchitis, bronchiecstasis, bronchiolites, bronchial asthma
Pulmonary parenchymal disease	Emphysema
Upper airway disease	Pharyngeal and laryngeal tumors, edema, infections, foreign bodies, tracheal tumors, collapse or stenosis of airway.

3. Combined or mixed (a component of both) obstruction and restriction caused by pulmonary congestion.

Classification of Tests

Most pulmonary function tests evaluate the status of the airways, vascular system, and alveoli in an indirect, overlapping way. The patient's age, height, weight, and sex are recorded before testing because they are the basis for the determination of predicted values.

Pulmonary function tests are generally divided into three categories:

1. Airway flow rates typically include instantaneous and/or average airflow rates during a maximal forced exhalation to assess airway function.
2. Lung volumes/capacities typically include the various "air-containing compartments" of the lung to assess air trapping or hyperinflation.
3. Gas exchange typically includes the rate of gas transfer across the alveolar/capillary membranes to assess the diffusion process.

List of Symbols and Abbreviations*

Pulmonary function studies and blood gas analyses measure quantities of gas mixtures and their components, blood and its constituents, and various factors affecting these quantities. The symbolic expression of these quantities was standardized at a conference held in 1950 by American physiologists. The list of symbols and abbreviations given here is based on those standards.

Once you have mastered the meaning of the major and secondary symbols, you should be able to interpret any combination of these symbols. This list will introduce you to general principles and will then apply them to measurements included in the chapter.

General Principles
Gas Volumes
Large capital letters denote primary symbols for gases.

V = Gas volume
$\dot{V}$ = Gas volume per unit time (the dot over the symbol indicates the factor per unit time)
P = Gas pressure or partial pressure of a gas in a gas mixture or in blood
F = Fractional concentration in gas

Small capital letters indicate the type of gas measured.

A = Alveolar gas
D = Dead space gas
E = Expired gas
I = Inspired gas
T = Tidal gas

* Adapted from Pulmonary terms and symbols: A report of the ACCP-ATS Joint Committee on Pulmonary Nomenclatures. Chest 67: 583, 1975

Chemical symbols for gases may be placed after the small capital letters listed above.

O_2 = Oxygen
CO = Carbon monoxide
CO_2 = Carbon dioxide
N_2 = Nitrogen

Combinations of Symbols

The following are some of the ways these symbols may be combined in the measurement of gases:

V_T = Tidal volume
V_E = Volume of expired gas
P_ACO_2 = Partial pressure of carbon dioxide in alveolar gas

Blood Gas Symbols

Large capital letters are used in primary symbols for blood.

C = Concentration of a gas in blood
S = Percent saturation of hemoglobin with CO or CO_2
Q = Volume of blood
$\dot{Q}$ = Volume of blood per unit time (blood flow)

To indicate whether blood is capillary, venous, or arterial, *lower case letters* are used as subscripts.

v = Venous blood
a = Arterial blood
c = Capillary blood
s = Shunted blood

Combinations of Symbols

Blood gas symbols may be combined in the following ways:

PO_2 = Oxygen tension or partial pressure of oxygen
$PvCO_2$ = Venous oxygen tension or partial pressure of oxygen in venous blood
PaO_2 = Arterial oxygen tension or partial pressure of oxygen in arterial blood
P_AO_2 = Alveolar oxygen tension or partial pressure of oxygen in the alveoli
PCO_2 = Partial pressure of carbon dioxide
$PaCO_2$ = Partial pressure of carbon dioxide in arterial blood
$PvCO_2$ = Partial pressure of carbon dioxide in venous blood
SO_2 = Oxygen saturation

SaO_2 = Percent saturation of oxygen in arterial blood
SvO_2 = Percent saturation of oxygen in venous blood
TCO_2 = Total carbon dioxide content

Lung Volume Symbols

The following list indicates symbols used in measuring lung volumes as well as the units used in expressing these measurements:

FVC = Forced Vital Capacity—maximal amount of air that can be exhaled forcibly and completely following a maximal inspiration (units : liters)

FEV_1 = Forced Expiratory Volume in 1 second—volume of air expired during the first second of the FVC maneuver (units : liters)

FEV_3 = Forced Expiratory Volume in 3 seconds—volume of air expired during the first 3 seconds of the FVC maneuver (units : liters)

$FEF_{200-1200}$ = Forced Expiratory Flow between 200 ml and 1200 ml—flow of expired air measured after the first 200 ml and during the next 1000 ml of the FVC maneuver (units : liters/sec)

FEF_{25-75} = Forced Expiratory Flow between 25% and 75%—flow of expired air measured between 25% and 75% of the FVC maneuver (units : liters/sec)

PEFR = Peak Expiratory Flow Rate—maximum flow of expired air attained during an FVC maneuver (units : liters/sec or liters/min)

PIFR = Peak Inspiratory Flow Rate—maximum flow of inspired air achieved during a forced maximal inspiration (units : liters/sec or liters/min)

FEF_{25} = Instantaneous flow rate at 25% of lung volume achieved during an FVC maneuver (units : liters/sec or liters/min)

FEF_{50} = Instantaneous flow rate at 50% of lung volume achieved during an FVC maneuver (units : liters/sec or liters/min)

FEF_{75} = Instantaneous flow rate of 75% of lung volume achieved during an FVC maneuver (units : liters/sec or liters/min)

FIVC = Forced Inspiratory Vital Capacity—maximal amount of air that can be inhaled forcibly and completely following a maximal expiration (units : liters)

FRC = Functional Residual Capacity—volume of gas contained in the lung at the end of a normal expiration (units : liters)

IC = Inspiratory Capacity—maximal amount of air that can be inspired from end tidal expiration (unit : liters)

ERV = Expiratory Reserve Volume—maximal amount of air that can be expired from end tidal expiration (units : liters)

RV = Residual Volume—volume of gas left in the lung following a maximal expiration (units : liters)

VC = Vital Capacity—maximal volume of air that can be expired following a maximal inspiration (units : liters)

TLC = *T*otal *L*ung *C*apacity—volume of gas contained in the lungs following a maximal inspiration (units : liters)

D_LCO = Carbon monoxide diffusing capacity of the lung—rate of diffusion of carbon monoxide across the alveolar/capillary membrane (*i.e.*, rate of gas transfer across the alveolar/capillary membrane (units : ml/min/torr)

CV = *C*losing *V*olume—volume at which the lower lung zones cease to ventilate, presumably as a result of airway closure (units : percent of VC)

MVV = *M*aximal *V*oluntary *V*entilation—maximal number of liters of air a patient can breathe per minute by a voluntary effort (units : liters/min)

$V_{ISO}\dot{V}$ = Volume of isoflow—volume in which flow was the same with air and with helium during an FVC maneuver

Miscellaneous Symbols

The following is an assortment of symbols you may encounter throughout the chapter:

A = Age in years
W = Weight in pounds
H = Height in inches
torr = A unit of pressure equal to 1/760 of normal atmospheric pressure or to the pressure necessary to support a column of mercury 1 mm high at 0°C and standard gravity
f = Frequency of breathing
C = Compliance
He = Helium
Hg = Mercury
D = Diffusing capacity
CO = Carbon monoxide
D_LCO_2 = Oxygen diffusing capacity of the lung (ml/min/torr)
$A\text{-}aDO_2$ = Alveolar-to-arterial oxygen gradient
BSA = Body surface area (unit : m²)
H_2CO_3 = Carbonic acid
HCO_3 = Bicarbonate
TGV = *T*horacic *G*as *V*olume (also expressed as V_{TG})
R_{aw} = Airway resistance
F-V = Flow volume
V-T = Volume time
*p*H = Negative logarithm of the hydrogen ion concentration, used as a positive number to indicate acidity or alkalinity
V-T = Volume time
BE = Base excess/deficit

PULMONARY FUNCTION TESTS

Spirometry

Lung capacities, volumes, and flow rates are clinically measured by a spirometer. The spirometer has a breathing system that allows gas to be breathed in and out and allows for the addition or removal of accurate amounts of gas. The electrical recording of the amounts of gas breathed in and out forms a spirogram. Spirometers can be grouped into two major categories: the mechanical (volume displacement) types, such as water-filled, sliding wedge, and bellows, and the electronic (flow sensing) types, such as Fleisch pneumotach and hot-wire anemometer.

The water-seal spirometer has been the basic tool for many years. This spirometer consists of a bell suspended in a container of water (Fig. 14–1). The bell rises and falls in response to the breathing of the patient, who inhales and exhales into a tube connected to the spirometer. The proportional movements of the bell are recorded, either on a

FIGURE 14–1.
The Collins Stead–Wells spirometer. (Courtesy of Warren E. Collins, Inc, Braintree, MA)

kymograph (a rotating drum on which a tracing is made with a stylus) or by an electrical potentiometer. Measured or actual values are then compared with the predicted values by means of regression equations using age, height, weight, and sex and are expressed as a percent of predicted. Typically a percent of predicted greater than 80% is considered to be within normal limits.

Spirometry is designed to determine the effectiveness of the various forces involved in the movement of the lungs and chest wall. The values obtained will provide quantitative information about the degree of obstruction to air flow and/or the restriction of the amount of air that can be inspired.

Spirometry can be recorded as either a volume–time tracing or a flow–volume tracing from which the following measurements can be made:

1. Forced vital capacity (FVC): Maximum amount of air exhaled forcefully and rapidly following a maximal inspiration (measured in liters and reported at body temperature pressure saturated [BTPs])
2. Forced expiratory volumes (*e.g.*, FEV_1, FEV_2, FEV_3): The volume of air exhaled at the first, second, and third seconds of the FVC, respectively (measured in liters and reported at BTPs), the volumes exhaled during the first and third seconds of forced vital capacity.
3. Air-flow rates (*e.g.*, FEF 200–1200; FEF 25–75; FEF 75–85)

Procedure for Spirometry
1. The patient is fitted with a mouthpiece that is connected to the spirometer.
2. A noseclip is used so that only mouth breathing is possible.
3. The patient is either sitting down or standing up.
4. The patient is asked to inhale maximally, hold his or her breath momentarily, and then exhale forcibly and completely.
5. The patient is allowed to rest, and the preceding step is repeated twice. (A minimum of three tracings are obtained and the two best should compare within 5% of one another.)
6. The procedure takes approximately 15 to 20 minutes to perform.
7. The best tracing is used to provide the spirometric measurements of FVC, FEV_1, $FEF_{200-1200}$, FEF_{25-75}, and so forth.

AIRWAY FLOW RATES

Airway flow rates provide information about the severity of airway obstruction in terms of air trapping and serve as an index of dynamic function. The lung volume at which the flow rates are measured is a most important value.

Forced Vital Capacity (FVC); Forced Expiratory Volume (FEV); Timed (FEV$_t$)

Normal Values

Forced vital capacity is approximately 3000 to 5000 ml. The total FVC should be exhaled in approximately 6 seconds. The FEV$_t$ is expressed in liters.

81%–83% exhaled in 1 second = FEV$_1$
90%–94% exhaled in 2 seconds = FEV$_2$
95%–97% exhaled in 3 seconds = FEV$_3$

Predicted values for a patient of a specific age and height may be determined by use of a nomogram (Fig. 14–2).

Explanation of Test

The FEV$_t$ is valuable in quantifying the amount and severity of airway obstruction. The maximum amount of air that can be exhaled rapidly after a maximum deep inspiration is recorded. Three separate exhalations are measured and the highest volume is recorded as the FVC. The recording is given in liters or as the FVC : VC ratio.

The volumes exhaled within 1, 2, and 3 seconds are referred to as FEV$_1$, FEV$_2$, and FEV$_3$ or timed VCs. These measurements are useful in the evaluation of a patient's response to bronchodilators. If the FEV$_1$ and/or the FEF$_{25-75}$ is below 80% of the predicted, a bronchodilator such as metaproterenol or isoetharine is administered with a mini-nebulizer and the spirometry is repeated. An increase in the FEV$_1$ and/or the FEF$_{25-75}$ of 20% or more above the prebronchodilator level receives a significant response to the bronchodilator consistent with a reversible obstructive airway disease such as asthma. The person with emphysema typically does not demonstrate a response to bronchodilators because of the nature of the disease state.

Clinical Implications

1. Obstructive lung disease is a cause of reduced volume and flow rates.
2. Decreased values occur in chronic lung diseases that cause trapping of air, such as emphysema, pulmonary fibrosis, and asthma.
3. In restrictive lung disease, the FVC is reduced; however, the flow rates can be normal or elevated.

Patient Preparation

Explain the purpose and procedure of the test.

FIGURE 14–2.
This is an example of a typical nomogram for determining various expiratory flow rates in normal males (*A*) and normal females (*B*). The values are determined by laying a ruler across the height scale and age scale (corresponding to the patient's height and age) and then reading the values where the ruler crosses the other scales. When the test site has computer equipment, the values are computed electronically. (Burton GG, Gee GN, Hodgkin JE: Respiratory Care: A Guide to Chemical Practice. Philadelphia, JB Lippincott, 1977)

Flow-Volume Loops (F-V Loops)

Normal Values
Normal curves or loops are characteristic of absence of lung disease.

Explanation of Test
This test is designed to provide both a graphic analysis and a quantitative measurement of flow rates at any lung volume. It is used to evaluate the dynamics of both large and medium size (central) airways and is quite helpful in ruling out peripheral or small airway obstruction.

FVC

FIGURE 14–2. (Continued)

Values obtained in this determination include the FVC, FEV, FEF_{25-75}, PEFR, PIFR, FEF_{25}, FEF_{50}, and FEF_{75}. See Figure 14–3 for an example of a flow-volume loop.

Procedure
The procedure is the same as for spirometry except for the addition of a maximal forced inspiration at the end of the forced expiratory maneuver.

Clinical Implications
Abnormal flow volume loops are indicative of

1. Obstructive lung disease
   (a) Small airway obstructive disease, as in emphysema and asthma
   (b) Large airway obstructive disease, such as tumors of trachea and bronchioles
2. Restrictive diseases when the disease is far advanced.

Patient Preparation
Explain the purpose and procedure of the test.

FIGURE 14–3.
Flow-volume loop. $FEV_{0.5, 1.0}$, and $_{3.0}$ = forced expiratory volumes at 0.5 second, 1 second and 3 seconds respectively. $FEF_{25, 50}$, and $_{75}$ = forced expiratory flows at 25%, 50%, and 75% of lung volume, respectively.

Peak Inspiratory Flow Rate (PIFR)

Normal Values
An average value of at least 300 L/min
Predicted values are based on age, sex, and height.

Explanation of Test

This measurement of flow rate is used to identify reduced breathing on inspiration and is totally dependent on the effort the patient makes in inspiration. The PIFR is the maximum flow of air achieved during a forced maximal inspiration.

Procedure

1. The PIFR is obtained from the flow-volume loop procedure using the spirometer with an X–Y recorder.
2. The patient is asked to inspire maximally, exhale forcibly and completely, and then inspire forcibly and completely (Fig. 14–3).

Clinical Implications

1. The value is reduced in neuromuscular disorders, weakness, poor effort, and extrathoracic airway obstruction (*i.e.*, substernal thyroid, tracheal stenosis, and laryngeal paralysis).
2. The PIFR will be altered by upper airway obstruction.

Interfering Factors

Poor patient effort

Patient Preparation

Explain the purpose and procedure of the test.

Peak Expiratory Flow Rate (PEFR)

Normal Values

An average of at least 450 L/min
Predicted values are based on age, sex, and height.

Explanation of Test

This measurement of lung volume flow rate is used as an index of large airway function. It is the maximum flow of expired air attained during an FVC maneuver.

Procedure

1. The PEFR is obtained from the flow-volume loop procedure using the spirometer with an X–Y recorder (see Fig. 14–3).
2. The patient is asked to inspire maximally, exhale forcibly and completely, and then inspire forcibly and completely.

Clinical Implications

1. The value is normally decreased in obstructive disease such as emphysema when air is trapped.
2. The value is usually normal in restrictive lung disease, except in severe restriction, when it is reduced.

Interfering Factors
Poor patient effort

Patient Preparation
Explain the purpose and procedure of the test.

LUNG VOLUMES AND CAPACITIES

Lung volumes can be considered as basic subdivisions of the lung (not anatomic subdivisions) and may be subdivided as follows:

1. Total lung capacity (TLC)
2. Tidal volume (VT)
3. Inspiratory capacity (IC)
4. Functional residual capacity (FRC)
5. Expiratory reserve volume (ERV)
6. Vital capacity (VC)
7. Residual volume (RV)

Combinations of two or more volumes are termed *capacities*. These volumes and capacities are shown graphically in Figure 14–4. Also shown are values found in normal adult men. Measurement of these values with devices such as the spirometer with the appropriate requi-

FIGURE 14–4.
Subdivisions of lung volume in the normal adult. (Geschickter CF: The Lung in Health and Disease. Philadelphia, JB Lippincott, 1973)

site instrumentation can provide information about the severity of airway obstruction and can serve as an index of dynamic function. There are two basic methods for the determination of lung volumes:

1. The multiple-breath nitrogen washout technique (open circuit)
2. The helium dilution technique (closed circuit)

Both methods employ the use of a gas (oxygen or helium, respectively) to either wash out or dilute the air left in the lung at end tidal expiration.

Functional Residual Capacity (FRC)

Normal Values
Approximately 2400–3000 ml
Predicted values are based on age, height, weight, and sex.
The observed value should be 75% to 125% of the predicted value.

Explanation of Test
This test is used to evaluate both restrictive and obstructive defects of the lung. Changes in the elastic properties of the lungs are reflected in the FRC and residual volume (RV). This test measures the volume of gas contained in the lungs at the end of a normal quiet expiration (*i.e.,* FRC). The residual volume is expressed mathematically as the difference between the FRC and expiratory reserve volume (ERV) (RV = FRC − ERV) (see below).

Procedure
1. The patient is fitted with nose clips and asked to breathe through the mouthpiece on the lung volume apparatus.
2. Depending on the instrument, the patient either
   (a) Breathes 100% oxygen (O_2) until the alveolar nitrogen (A_{N_2}) reaches 1% or 7 minutes elapses (whichever comes first). Calculation of the FRC is based on the fact that 81% of the air in the lung is N_2. The N_2 is "washed" out of the lungs by having the patient breathe 100% O_2 and then measuring the volume of N_2 collected

   or

   (b) Rebreathes a 10% to 12% helium (He) and room-air concentration until equilibrium is reached
3. Results are recorded by either an X–Y recorder on semilog paper (Fig. 14–5) or by a respirometer on a kymograph drum.

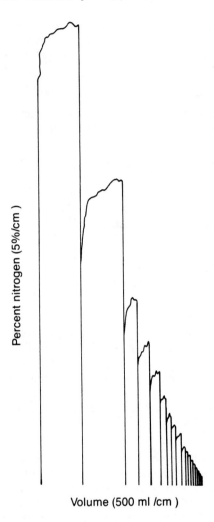

Volume (500 ml /cm)

FIGURE 14–5.
Typical tracing of a multiple breath nitrogen workout curve for determining FRC. The patient breathes 100% oxygen until alveolar nitrogen reaches 1%.

4. At the end of the test, the following values are computed. The choice of the formula depends on the method being used.

$$FRC = \frac{\% \, N_2 \text{ final} \times V_E}{\% \, A_{N_2}}$$

(nitrogen washout or open circuit technique)

or

$$FRC = \frac{\% \text{ He initial} - \% \text{ He final}}{\% \text{ He final}} \times \text{initial volume}$$

(helium dilution or closed circuit technique)

5. The test should be repeated a second time, and results between the FRCs should not vary by more than 5% to 10%.

Clinical Implications

1. A value less than 75% is indicative of restrictive disease.
2. A value of greater than 125% demonstrates air trapping, which is consistent with obstructive airway disease. An increase in the FRC represents hyperinflation, which may result from emphysematous changes, asthmatic or fibrotic obstruction of the bronchioles, compensation for surgical removal of lung tissue, or a thoracic cage deformity.

Patient Preparation

1. Explain the purpose and procedure of the test.
2. Obtain the patient's age, sex, weight, and height, and record this information before doing the test.

Residual Volume (RV)

Normal Values

Approximately 1200–1500 ml
Predicted values are based on age, sex, and height.

Explanation of Test

This test can be helpful in differentiating between either a restrictive or obstructive ventilatory defect. It is a measurement of the volume of gas remaining in the lungs after a maximal exhalation. Because the lungs cannot be completely emptied and because all the gas cannot be expelled by maximal expiratory effort, it is the only volume that cannot be measured directly from the spirometer. This value is calculated mathematically: Residual volume equals the functional residual capacity minus the expiratory reserve volume ($RV = FRC - ERV$) (see Fig. 14–4).

Procedure

The RV is determined indirectly from other tests. There is no procedure.

Clinical Implications

1. An increase in the RV indicates that in spite of a maximal expiratory effort, the lungs still contain an abnormally large amount of

gas. This type of change occurs in young asthmatics and is usually reversible. An increase in RV of greater than 125% of the predicted value is typically referred to as air trapping.
2. Increases of the RV are also characteristic of emphysema, chronic air trapping, and chronic bronchial obstruction.
3. The RV and the FRC usually increase together, although this is not always true.
4. The RV sometimes decreases in diseases that occlude many alveoli.
5. A RV of less than 75% of predicted value is consistent with restriction.

Interfering Factors
Residual volume normally increases with age.

Patient Preparation
Explain the purpose and procedure of the test.

Expiratory Reserve Volume (ERV)

Normal Values
Approximately 1200–1500 ml
Predicted values are based on age and height.

Explanation of Test
This test measures the largest volume of gas that can be exhaled following normal resting expiration. This measurement is used to identify lung or chest wall restriction. The ERV can be estimated mathematically by subtracting the inspiratory capacity (IC) from the vital capacity (VC). The ERV comprises approximately 25% of the VC and can vary greatly in subjects of comparable age and height.

Procedure
1. Record the patient's age and height.
2. Have the patient breathe normally for several breaths and then exhale maximally into a spirometer from the end tidal expiratory level.
3. Results are recorded on a spirogram.

Clinical Implications
1. A decreased ERV implies a chest wall restriction due to non-pulmonary causes.
2. Decreased values are associated with elevated diaphragms as seen in massive obesity, ascites, or pregnancy. These decreased values also occur in conjunction with massive enlargement of the heart, pleural effusion, kyphoscoliosis, and thoracoplasty.

Patient Preparation
Explain the purpose and procedure of the test.

Inspiratory Capacity (IC)

Normal Values
Approximately 2500–3600 ml
Predicted values are based on age and height.

Explanation of Test
This test measures the largest volume of air that can be inhaled in one deep breath after a normal expiration or that can be inhaled from the end tidal expiratory level. This measurement is used to identify lung or chest wall restriction. This measurement mathematically equals the tidal volume plus the inspiratory reserve volume (V_T + IRV). This value is not commonly measured because many diseases do not affect inspiratory capacity.

Procedure
1. Record the age, sex, and height of the patient.
2. The patient is asked to breathe normally into a spirometer for several breaths and then to inhale deeply or maximally, expanding the lungs as much as possible from end tidal expiration. Normal breathing is then resumed.
3. Step 2 is usually repeated two or more times and the largest inspired volume is selected.

Clinical Implications
Changes in the IC usually parallel increases or decreases in the vital capacity.

Patient Preparation
Instruct the patient about the purpose and procedure of the test.

Vital Capacity (VC)

Normal Values
About 3000–5000 ml
Predicted values are based on age, sex, and height.

Explanation of Test
This measurement is used to identify defects that can be due to lung or chest wall restriction. It measures the largest volume of gas that can be expelled from the lungs after the lungs are first filled to the maximum

extent and then emptied to the maximum extent. The VC is the mathematical sum of the inspiratory capacity (IC) and the expiratory reserve volume (ERV; see Fig. 14–4).

Procedure

1. Have the patient inhale as deeply as possible and then exhale completely, with no forced or rapid effort.
2. The inhalation and exhalation are done into a spirometer and the results are recorded on a spirogram.
3. No time limit is set.
4. The procedure should be repeated at least twice, and the VCs should compare within 5% of each other.

Clinical Implications

1. A *reduced* VC is considered to be less than 80% of the predicted value.
2. The VC can be lower than expected in either a restrictive or an obstructive disorder.
3. Decreases of VCs can be related to depression of the respiratory center in the brain, neuromuscular diseases, pleural effusion, pneumothorax, pregnancy, ascites, limitations of thoracic movement due to pain, scleroderma, or kyphoscoliosis, and limitation of movement by tumors, ascites, or pregnancy.

Interfering Factors

1. The VC increases with physical fitness and height.
2. The VC decreases with age after about age 30.
3. The VC is generally less in women than in men of the same age and height.
4. The VC is decreased by approximately 15% in blacks and 20% to 25% in the oriental populations when compared to whites of the same age, height, and sex.
5. Inadequate patient effort is a cause of a VC that is lower than expected.

Patient Preparation

Explain the purpose and procedure of the test.

Total Lung Capacity (TLC)

Normal Values

Approximately 4000–6000 ml
Predicted values are based on age, height, and sex.

Explanation of Test

This test is used mainly to evaluate obstructive defects of the lungs as well as to delineate restrictive from obstructive pulmonary disease. It measures the volume of gas contained in the lungs at the end of a maximal inspiration. Mathematically, it is the sum of the VC and the RV or the sum of the primary lung volumes (see Fig. 14–4). This value is determined indirectly from other tests.

Procedure
1. The patient is instructed to breath normally into a spirometer and then inspire maximally and exhale maximally. The total amount of air exhaled is the VC (see above).
2. The total lung capacity is then derived by the following formula:

$$TLC = VC + RV$$

Clinical Implications
1. An obstructive defect is characterized by an *elevated* TLC. However, a normal or *increased* TLC does not mean that ventilation or the surface area for diffusion is normal.
2. The TLC may be normal or *increased* in bronchiolar obstruction with hyperinflation and in emphysema.
3. The TLC is *decreased* in edema, atelectasis, neoplasms, pulmonary congestion, pneumothorax, or thoracic restriction.

GAS EXCHANGE

Common measurements determine the rate of gas transfer across alveolar/capillary membranes to assess the diffusion process.

Carbon Monoxide Diffusing Capacity of the Lung (D$_L$CO)

Normal Values
Approximately 25 ml/min/torr
Predicted values are based on patient's height, age, weight, and sex
D$_L$CO (in men) = 15.5 (BSA) − 0.238 (A) + 6.8
D$_L$CO (in women) = 15.5 (BSA) − 0.117 (A) + 0.5
(A = age in years; BSA = body surface area in meters squared; factor 14.4 takes into account a normal hemoglobin)

Background
Carbon monoxide (CO) combines with hemoglobin about 210 times more readily than does oxygen (O$_2$). If there is a normal amount of hemoglobin in the blood, the only other significant limiting factor to CO uptake is the state of the alveolar capillary membranes. Normally, there is no CO in the blood to affect the test.

Two categories of factors determine the rate of gas (CO) transfer across the lung—physical and chemical. Physical determinants are CO driving pressure, surface area, thickness of capillary walls, and diffusion coefficient for CO. Chemical determinants are red cell volume + reaction rate with hemoglobin.

Explanation of Test
This test is used to diagnose pulmonary vascular disease, emphysema, and pulmonary fibrosis, and to evaluate the amount of functioning pulmonary capillary bed in contact with functioning alveoli. During the measurement of this value, alveolar volume (VA) is also determined. The D_L measures the diffusing capacity of the lungs for CO. The D_LO_2 is obtained by multiplying D_LCO by 1.23 ($D_LO_2 = D_LCO \times 1.23$).

Procedure
1. Record the patient's age, height, weight, and sex.
2. Two techniques are used by laboratories.
    (a) *Single-breath* or *breathing-holding technique.* With this method, the patient is asked to take a deep breath from a bag containing a mixture of 10% helium and 0.3% CO with the balance of room air. The patient holds his or her breath for 10 seconds and exhales (Fig. 14–6).

    $$D_LCO = \frac{V_A \times 60}{(BP\text{-}47)x_t} \ln \frac{F_ACO_o}{F_ACO_t}$$

    F_ACO_0 = initial alveolar CO concentrations
    F_ACO_t = alveolar CO concentration at breath-holding time
      VA = alveolar volume
      60 = conversion factor for seconds to one minute
        t = breath-holding time in seconds

    (b) *Steady-state technique.* The patient is asked to breathe from a bag containing 0.1% to 0.2% CO for several minutes. This method requires an arterial blood sample. During the last 2 minutes, the exhaled air is collected in a neoprine bag and analyzed for O_2, CO_2, and CO concentrations. An arterial blood gas is also drawn during the last 2 minutes.

    $$D_LCO = \frac{V_{CO}(STPD)}{PACO}$$

    VCO = ml of CO transferred/min
    PACO = partial pressure of CO in the alveoli

Clinical Implications
1. *Decreased values* are associated with
    (a) Multiple pulmonary emboli
    (b) Emphysema
    (c) Lung restriction

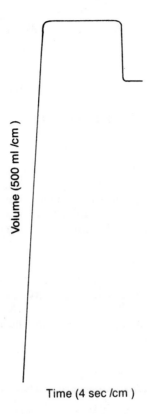

FIGURE 14–6.
Typical tracing for the single-breath carbon monoxide diffusing capacity maneuver. Patient inspires the diffusing gas test mixture maximally, holds breath for 10 to 12 seconds, and then exhales.

    (d) Pulmonary fibroses

(1) Sarcoidosis	(5) Anemia
(2) Scleroderma	(6) Pulmonary resection
(3) Systemic lupus erythematosus	(7) Pneumonia
(4) Asbestosis	

2. *Increased values* are observed in polycythemia, left-to-right shunts, and exercise.
3. The value is relatively normal in chronic bronchitis.

Interfering Factors
Exercise (with an increased cardiac output) and polycythemia will increase the value. Elevated levels of COHb (as seen in smokers) and anemia will decrease the value.

Maximum Voluntary Ventilation (MVV)

Normal Values
Approximately 170 L/min
Based on age, height, and sex; a healthy person may vary by as much as 25% to 35% of mean group values
MVV (in men) = 3.39 (H) − 1.26 (A) − 21.4
MVV (in women) = 138 − 0.77 (A)
(H = height in inches; A = age in years)

Explanation of Test
This test measures several physiologic phenomena occurring at the same time (*e.g.*, thoracic cage compliance, lung compliance, airway resistance, and muscle force available). It is a determination of the liters of air that a person can breathe per minute by a maximum voluntary effort.

Procedure
1. The patient breathes into a spirometer as deeply and rapidly as possible for 10 to 15 seconds. Generally, the frequency is 40 to 70 breaths per minute and tidal volume is 50% of VC (Fig. 14–7).
2. Actual value is then extrapolated from the 10- to 15-second time interval to a 1-minute time period.

Interfering Factors
Poor patient effort can be ruled out by using the following formula to predict the MVV of the patient:

$$\text{Predicted MVV} = 35 \times \text{FEV}_1$$

Time (2 sec /cm)

FIGURE 14–7.
Maximum voluntary ventilation. Patient breathes into a spirometer as deeply and rapidly as possible for 10 to 15 seconds.

This is a useful check to determine whether the recorded MVV is indicative of adequate patient effort.

Clinical Implications
1. Obstructive defects, chronic obstructive pulmonary disease (COPD), abnormal neuromuscular control, and poor patient effort are causes of reduced values.
2. In restrictive disease, the value will usually be normal.

Patient Preparation
1. Explain the purpose and procedure of the test.
2. Obtain and record the patient's age, height, and sex.

Closing Volume (CV)

Normal Values
Average is about 10% to 20% of vital capacity
Values derived from mathematical regression equations and based on age and sex
CV (in men) = 0.562 + 0.357 (A) + 4.15
CV (in women) = 2.812 + 0.293 (A) + 4.90
(A) = age in years

Explanation of Test
In the healthy person, the concentration of nitrogen diluted with 100% O_2 rapidly increases near the end of expiration. This rise is due to closure of the small airways in the lower alveoli. The point at which this closure occurs is termed *closing volume.*

This measurement is used as an index of pathologic changes occurring within the small airways (those airways less than 2 mm in diameter). The conventional pulmonary function tests are not sensitive enough to make this determination. The principle of the determination relies on the fact that the upper lung zones contain a proportionately larger residual volume of gas than the lower lung zones and that there is a gradient of intrapleural pressure from the top of the lung to the bottom of the lung. Additionally, the uniformity of gas distribution within the lungs can be measured.

Procedure
1. The patient is asked to exhale completely, inhale 100% oxygen, hold the breath for a few seconds, and then exhale completely at the rate of approximately ½ liter per second.
2. During the exhalation, both volume and percent of alveolar nitrogen are monitored simultaneously on an X–Y recorder. A sudden increase in nitrogen represents the closing volume (Fig. 14–8).

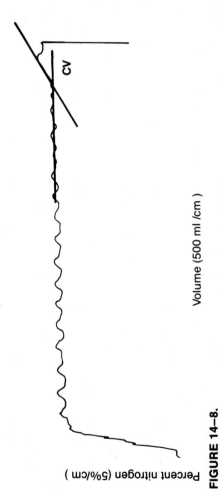

FIGURE 14–8.
Typical single-breath nitrogen washout curve for determination of closing volume (CV). The patient inspires 100% oxygen to total lung capacity and then exhales slowly (0.5 LPS) until the lung is empty.

Clinical Implications
1. The value is increased in diseases in which the airway is narrowed, such as bronchitis, and in chronic smokers and the elderly.
2. A change in the slope of the nitrogen curve by more than 2% is indicative of maldistribution of inspired air (*i.e.*, uneven alveolar ventilation).

Interfering Factors
Value increases with age.

Patient Preparation
Explain the purpose and procedure of the test.

Volume of Isoflow ($V_{ISO}\dot{V}$)

Normal Values
Values cover a wide range based on age (A).

$$V_{ISO}\dot{V} = 0.450 \text{ (A)} + 4.69$$

Explanation of Test
This test is designed to detect pathologic changes occurring in the small airways and may be more sensitive than conventional pulmonary function tests. Helium (He) has the unique property of lowering gas density. Therefore, after breathing a helium–oxygen gas mixture, the effects of convective acceleration and turbulence are negated. Any abnormality observed in the flow-volume loop is due then to an increase in resistance to laminar flow, which is indicative of small airway abnormalities or disease.

Procedure
1. The patient is fitted with nose clips and allowed to breathe into a mouthpiece connected to a spirometer that is interfaced with an X–Y recorder.
2. The patient is instructed to perform a flow-volume loop maneuver.
3. Next, the patient is asked to breathe an 80% He and 20% O_2 gas mix for several breaths and then perform another flow-volume loop maneuver.
4. From the tracings obtained in steps 2 and 3, the flow-volume loops are superimposed and the volume of isoflow is measured at the point in which the two loops intersect.

Clinical Implications
1. An *increased* volume of isoflow is consistent with the diagnosis of mild airway obstruction (*i.e.*, small airways disease).
2. A *decreased* volume of isoflow is normal.

Patient Preparation
Explain the purpose and procedure of the test.

Body Plethysmography

Normal Values
Based on height in inches (H) and weight in pounds (W)
TGV = approximately 2400 ml
TGV (in men) = 0.081 (H) − 2.94 (W)
TGV (in women) = 0.135 (H) − 0.008 (W) − 4.74
C = 0.2 L/cm H_2O
RAW = 0.6 cm−2.4 cm H_2O/L/sec

Explanation of Test
This test is designed to measure thoracic gas volume (TGV), compliance (C), and airway resistance (RAW). The TGV equals all the air contained within the thorax, whether or not it is in ventilatory communication with the rest of the lung. Compliance is an indication of the elasticity of the lung, and airway resistance is a measurement of resistance to air flow in the tracheobronchial tree.

The measurement of TGV via body plethysmography is an application of Boyle's law, that is, $PXV = PXV^1$ as long as T is constant.

P = pressure
V = volume
T = temperature

$$\text{Compliance (C)} = \frac{\text{change in volume}}{\text{change in pressure}} = \frac{V}{P}$$

Normal C = 0.2L/cm H_2O

$$\text{Airway resistance (RAW)} = \frac{\text{change in pressure}}{\text{change in flow}} = \frac{P}{F}$$

RAW = 0.2 − 2.5 cm H_2O/L/sec

Airway resistance increases with decreasing lung volume and decreases at higher lung volumes. Therefore, to provide a volume-standardized RAW measurement, airway conductance (GAW) and specific airway conductance (SGAW) are typically calculated.

$$\text{GAW} = \frac{1}{\text{RAW}} = 0.4 − 2.0 \text{ L/sec/cm } H_2O$$

$$\text{SGAW} = \frac{\text{GAW}}{\text{TGV}} = 0.112 − 0.400 \text{ L/sec/cm } H_2O\text{/liter}$$

Procedure
1. The patient is seated in the body box, fitted with nose clips, and asked to breathe through a mouthpiece connected to a transducer.
2. The box door is secured and the test is not begun for a few minutes, while the box pressure is allowed to stabilize.
3. The patient is instructed to perform a panting maneuver while holding his or her cheeks rigid and glottis open. The technician makes a recording of box pressure and mouth pressure on the oscilloscope. This recording provides the necessary data for mathematical derivation of TGV.
4. Next, the patient is instructed to breathe rapidly and shallowly. The technician makes a recording of box pressure changes versus flow on the oscilloscope, and this provides the necessary data for mathematical derivation of RAW.
5. For the C determination, a balloon catheter must be passed into the patient's esophagus through the nose. The balloon is then inflated with a few cubic centimeters of air, and the patient is instructed to breathe normally. The technician makes a recording of intraesophageal pressure changes during normal respiration (which mimics changes in intrapleural pressure), and this provides the necessary data for the mathematical derivation of C.

Clinical Implications
1. An *increased* TGV demonstrates air trapping, which is consistent with obstructive pulmonary disease.
2. An *increased* RAW demonstrates an increased resistance to air flow through the tracheobronchial tree, which is seen in asthma, emphysema, bronchitis, and other forms of obstruction. The RAW is useful in distinguishing between a restrictive ventilatory defect versus an obstructive ventilatory defect.
3. An *increase* in C (*i.e.*, lung is more distensible) is seen in obstructive diseases.
4. A *decrease* in C (*i.e.*, lung is more stiff) is seen in fibrotic diseases, restrictive diseases, pneumonia, congestion, and atelectasis.

Patient Preparation
1. The height, weight, and sex are recorded.
2. Explain the purpose and procedure of the test.

Patient Aftercare
Allow the patient to rest quietly after the test is completed.

Bronchial Provocation

Normal Values
Minimal to no change in airway dynamics (*i.e.*, FEV_1 and/or FEF_{25-75})
Positive response to inhaled antigen is equal to:
>20% decrease in FEV_1
and/or
>30% decrease in FEF_{25-75}

Explanation of Test
Occasionally, the diagnosis of asthma cannot be made with certainty from the history, physical examination, and conventional pulmonary function tests. This is a specific test for bronchial asthma. The asthmatic patient is more sensitive to the bronchoconstrictive effects of cholinergic agents (*e.g.*, methacholine chloride or histamine) than the normal person. Studies indicate that airway resistance tests are sensitive in monitoring the response to bronchoconstrictive agents.

Clinical Implications
A positive response to methacholine or histamine is consistent with bronchial hyperreactivity.

Procedure
1. The patient is instructed to perform an FVC maneuver, and the FEV_1 and FEF_{25-75} are measured.
2. The patient is now asked to take an inhalation of 1.25 mg of methacholine chloride/ml by means of a nebulizer, to wait 5 minutes, and then repeat the FVC maneuver. A 20% reduction in the FEV_1 or a 30% decrease in FEF_{25-75} is a positive response.
3. If there is no response, the dilution of methacholine chloride is progressively increased (2.50 mg/ml, 5.0 mg/ml, 10.0 mg/ml, and 25 mg/ml), and the patient repeats step 2. However, once a 20% reduction in the FEV_1 and/or a 30% decrease in FEF_{25-75} is observed at any dilution ratio, this represents a positive response, and the test is terminated. A bronchodilator is administered.
4. If a patient goes through all five dilution ratios without a 20% reduction in the FEV and/or 30% reduction in the FEF_{25-75}, this is a negative test.
5. If the methacholine causes no change, the patient can be tested with histamine at a later time. (Usually, the patient is tested first with methacholine, then with histamine.)

Patient Preparation
Explain the purpose and procedure of the test.

Carbon Dioxide (CO$_2$) **Response**

Normal Values
Breathing increasing concentrations of CO_2 should result in an increase in minute volume when compared to minute volume when breathing room air (0.03% CO_2).

Explanation of Test
This test is designed to evaluate the respiratory response to increasing levels of inspired CO_2 concentration. As levels of CO_2 increase in alveolar air, so does arterial CO_2. The central chemoreceptors respond by initiating impulses to the respiratory control centers, and this in turn causes an increase in the rate and depth of breathing in the healthy person.

Procedure
1. The patient's minute volume is determined while breathing room air. This is done by allowing the patient to breathe for several minutes into an instrument that records frequency (f) of breathing and tidal volume (V$_T$). The minute volume is then calculated for 1 minute by computing the value of f × V$_T$.
2. Next, the patient is instructed to breathe a gas mixture of 2% CO_2 and balance room air for 5 minutes. During the last 2 minutes, breathing (f) and V$_T$ are recorded.
3. Next, the patient breathes a gas mixture of 4% CO_2 and balance room air, and the above procedure is repeated. This is also done with 6% CO_2 and sometimes even 8% CO_2 and room air.
4. Finally, a graph is constructed that plots changes in minute volume against increasing inspired CO_2 concentrations.

Clinical Implications
Unresponsiveness to increasing inspired CO_2 concentrations suggests a disturbance in the normal physiologic pathway of ventilatory changes to hypercapnia.

EXERCISE PULMONARY FUNCTION TESTS

Normal Values
Normal exercise response:
No change in the electrocardiographic (ECG) complex
No systemic hypertension and normal arterial blood pressure
Normal air flow pattern during inspiration and expiration

Normal arterial blood gases and chemistry (CO_2, O_2, pH, HCO_2, lactate), based on an indwelling catheter
Normal pulmonary artery pressure

Background
Respiratory disease reduces the ability to perform exercise. Dynamic exercise employing large muscle groups is accompanied by increases in metabolic O_2 consumption and CO_2 production. The increase in metabolic demand leads to stresses on all the mechanisms taking part in O_2 and CO_2 transport. Exercise testing allows the measurement of the functional reserve in these mechanisms through the application of the engineering principles of testing under load. The analysis of bronchogenic and cardiovascular disorders includes procedures that measure respiratory outcomes and blood gas studies during exercise. The results of many pulmonary function tests and blood gas studies are normally altered during exercise in healthy persons. However, certain specific alterations will be noted when there is cardiovascular or respiratory impairment. In virtually all diseases affecting the lungs and circulation, exercise tests are of value in assessing severity and impairment due to an already diagnosed condition. Exercise testing may also allow the recognition of unsuspected abnormalities that are contributing to disability. The diagnosis of psychogenic dyspnea is considered if no expected abnormal response occurs indicative of disease. Listings of normal and abnormal changes in blood gas studies during exercise follow.

Normal Changes in Blood Gas Studies During Moderate Exercise

Value	Change
O_2 consumption	Increases
Respiratory quotient	Increases
Ventilation	Increases
Physiologic dead space	Increases
Cardiac output	Increases
Blood lactate	Increases
Arteriovenous O_2 content	Increases
V_D/V_T ratio	Decreases
Venous-admixturelike perfusion	Decreases
A-aDO_2	No change
Arterial blood gas tensions	No change

Abnormal Changes in Blood Gas Studies During Moderate Exercise

Value	Change	Disorders That Cause Increases or Decreases
Respiratory quotient	Increases	Acidemia develops if person is physically unfit or if cardiovascular system cannot cope with increased demands of the tissues during exercise
Lactate	Increases	
PaO_2	Decreases	Ventilatory impairment
$PaCO_2$	Increases	
P_AO_2	Decreases	Diffusion defect occurs when the area of alveolar surface available for diffusion is reduced. Conditions that cause such a structural change include pulmonary fibrosis, late stages of emphysema, and surgical removal of lung tissue

Explanation of Test

Exercise testing of pulmonary function is done to evaluate fitness, to identify work tolerance or intolerance in persons with obstructive and restrictive diseases. Efficiency of the cardiopulmonary system may be quite different during periods of exercise than at rest. For this reason, exercise testing is designed to assess ventilation, gas exchange, and cardiovascular function during increased demands. With such tests, dyspnea due to cardiovascular causes can be differentiated from that due to respiratory causes. Precise information about the mechanisms that influence O_2 and CO_2 transport during exercise can be obtained using a staged approach. This information is important because the ability to exercise or perform work represents an essential part of any definition of health. (Symptoms of limited exercise tolerance include onset of fatigue and shortness of breath.) Patients who require more than the normal amount of O_2 to perform work or exercise can be identified when they are exercised on a cycle ergometer or treadmill.

An exercise test can detect or exclude many conditions, even though the response may be nonspecific. For example, in a person complaining of severe shortness of breath in the presence of a normal exercise response, the likely cause is psychogenic. However, there are a few conditions in which a particular exercise response is strictly diagnostic: exercise-induced asthma and myocardial ischemia. Exercise tests are also of value in assessing the severity of impairment due to virtually all conditions affecting the lungs and circulation. In addition, exercise testing may uncover unsuspected abnormalities contributing to the person's disability.

The majority of clinical problems can be assessed during the simple procedures included in Stage 1. These procedures should always be done before more complex tests are undertaken. An abnormal result is an indication that more precise information is required, using either Stage 2 protocols, which are more complex but bloodless, or Stage 3 protocols, in which arterial blood is sampled. In 75% of cases, only Stage 1 need be performed. One hundred percent O_2 is often used during incremental exercise and is helpful in estimating the magnitude of a hypovolemic stimulus during air-breathing exercises to quantify the degree of any right-to-left shunt in known arterial hypoxemia and to determine the degree of O_2 supplementation needed to improve a person's exercise tolerance.

Clinical Alert

Absolute contraindications to exercise testing include

Acute febrile illness	Uncontrolled hypertension
Pulmonary edema	systolic >250 mm Mg
Uncontrolled asthma	diastolic >120 mm Mg
Unstable angina	

Relative contraindications to exercise testing include

Recent myocardial infarction	Epilepsy
(less than 4 weeks)	Respiratory failure
Resting tachycardia	Resting ECG abnormalities
>120 bpm	

Procedure

1. Stage 1

   (a) Assessments of blood pressure, ECG analysis, and spirometry measurments of expiratory air flow, tidal volume, and frequency of breathing are made using cycle ergometry and incremental exercise.

   (b) Measurements are made at the end of each minute; the test continues to a symtom-limited maximum. The O_2 intake and CO_2 output are measured if facilities are available.

   (c) Total examining time is 30 minutes.

2. Stage 2
   (a) More complex analytical methods are required.
   (b) Exercise is continued long enough to reach a steady state, usually 3 to 5 minutes.
   (c) Stage 1 measurements plus mixed venous CO_2 tension using a rebreathing technique are done.
   (d) Total examining time is 1 hour.
3. Stage 3
   (a) Blood gas sampling and analysis are required.
   (b) An indwelling catheter is inserted in the brachial artery. In some instances, capillary blood is substituted.
   (c) In addition to Stage 2 tests, measurements are obtained for cardiac output, alveolar ventilation, ratio of dead space to tidal volume, alveolar-arterial O_2 tension difference, venous admixture ratio, and lactate.
   (d) Total examining time is 90 to 120 minutes.

Clinical Implications
Altered values will reveal

1. Cardiac dysrhythmias
2. Cardiac ischemia as related to work rate
3. Degree of impairment in pulmonary restrictive diseases
4. Hypoventilation
5. Work rate at which metabolic acidosis appears
6. Cardiac output if pulmonary artery is catheterized during procedure
7. Decreased work tolerance in COPD

Interfering Factors
1. The exercise tolerance of any person is affected by the degree of impairment of
   (a) Mechanical factors
   (b) Ventilatory efficiency
   (c) Gas exchange factors
   (d) Cardiac status
   (e) Physical condition
   (f) Sensitivity of the respiratory control mechanism
2. Obese persons will have a higher than normal oxygen consumption at any given work rate, even though the muscular and work efficiency values are normal.

BLOOD GASES, ARTERIAL BLOOD GASES (ABGs)

Introduction

Reasons for obtaining arterial blood gases (ABGs)

1. Assessment of adequacy of oxygenation
2. Assessment of adequacy of ventilation
3. Assessment of the acid–base status by measuring the respiratory and nonrespiratory components

The ABGs are used to monitor critically ill patients, to establish baseline values, in the perioperative period, to follow up postoperative patients, in the detection and treatment of electrolyte imbalances, and in conjunction with pulmonary function testing.

Reasons for using *arterial* blood rather than *venous* blood to measure blood gases include the following:

1. Arterial blood is a good way to sample a mixture of blood that has come from various parts of the body.
   (a) Venous blood in an extremity gives information mostly about that extremity. The metabolism in the extremity can differ from the metabolism in the body as a whole. This difference is accentuated in the following instances:
      (1) In shock, when the extremity is cold or under-perfused
      (2) With local exercise of extremity, as opening and closing the fist
      (3) In local infection of the extremity
   (b) Blood from a central venous catheter usually is an incomplete mix of venous blood from various parts of the body. For a sample of completely mixed blood, a sample would have to be obtained from the right ventricle or pulmonary artery, and even then information is not obtained about how well the lungs are oxygenating the blood.
2. Arterial blood gives the added information of how well the lungs are oxygenating the blood.
   (a) If it is known that arterial oxygen (O_2) concentration is normal (indicating that the lungs are functioning normally), but that the mixed venous O_2 concentration is low, it can be inferred that the heart and circulation are failing.
   (b) Oxygen measurements of central venous catheter blood can tell if the tissues are getting oxygenated, but they do not separate the contribution of the heart from the lungs. If central venous catheter blood has a low O_2 concentration, it means either that
      (1) The lungs have not oxygenated the arterial blood well, so that venous blood has a low concentration.

(2) The heart is not circulating the blood well. In this case, the tissues of the body must take more than the usual amount of O_2 from each cardiac cycle because the blood is flowing slowly. This produces a low venous O_2 concentration.
3. Arterial samples provide information on the ability of the lungs to regulate acid–base balance through retention or release of CO_2 and the effectiveness of the kidneys in maintaining appropriate bicarbonate levels.

Note: The site of arterial puncture must satisfy the following three requirements:
1. Available collateral blood flow
2. Superficial or easily accessible
3. Periarterial tissues (should be nonsensitive)

The radial artery satisfies the criteria listed above, although the brachial and femoral are also arteries of choice.

Procedure for Obtaining Arterial Blood Sample
1. Place the patient in either a sitting or a supine position.
2. Perform the Allen's test to assess collateral circulation prior to performing the radial puncture. If collateral circulation in the ulnar artery is inadequate, another site should be chosen.
3. Elevate the wrist with a small pillow and ask the patient to extend the fingers downward (this will flex the wrist and move the radial artery closer to the surface).
4. Palpate the artery and rotate the patient's hand back and forth until a good strong pulse is felt.
5. Swab the area liberally with an antiseptic agent such as Betadine.
6. Optional: Anesthetize the area with a small amount of 1% Xylocaine (approximately 0.25 ml or less). This allows a second attempt without undue pain if the first attempt is a failure.
7. Using a 20- or 21-gauge needle and preheparinized self-filling syringe, puncture the artery and collect a 3- to 5-ml sample.
8. Withdraw the needle and place a 4″ × 4″ absorbent bandage over the puncture site and maintain pressure with two fingers for a minimum of 2 minutes.
9. Meanwhile, any air bubbles in the blood sample should be expelled as quickly as possible; the syringe should then be capped and gently rotated to mix heparin with blood.
10. Place the sample on ice and remove to the laboratory. This will prevent alterations in gas tensions because metabolic processes continue after blood is drawn.

Clinical Alert

1. Arterial gases will not indicate to what degree the patient is suffering from an abnormality. For this reason, the vital signs and mental function of the patient must be used as guides to determine adequacy of tissue oxygenation.
2. The arterial puncture site must have pressure applied and be watched carefully for bleeding.
3. Blood for electrolytes and gases must be drawn without trauma and must be protected from room to air at all times. Be aware that air bubbles in the syringe will also change gas values.
4. Include with information for the laboratory the fraction of inspired oxygen (F_IO_2) or room air. Note the time the sample is obtained. Do not use blood for ABGs after 3 hours.

Alveolar to Arterial Oxygen Gradient (A–aDO$_2$)

Normal Values
9 torr or less in a patient breathing room air

Explanation of Test
This test gives an approximation of the O_2 in the alveoli and arteries. It is used to identify the cause of hypoxemia and intrapulmonary shunting: (1) ventilated alveoli but no perfusion; (2) unventilated alveoli with perfusion; or (3) collapse of both alveoli and capillaries.

Procedure
An arterial blood sample is obtained, and the following mathematical formula is solved:

$$A–aDO_2 = P_AO_2–PaO_2$$
$$P_AO_2 = (BP-47)F_IO_2-PaCO_2 \times 1.25$$

$$\begin{aligned}
BP &= \text{barometric pressure} \\
47 &= \text{water vapor pressure} \\
F_IO_2 &= \text{fractional concentration of inspired oxygen (\textit{e.g.}, .21 for room air)} \\
PaCO_2 &= \text{partial pressure of arterial carbon dioxide} \\
1.25 &= \text{conversion factor for respiratory quotient} \\
PaO_2 &= \text{Arterial oxygen tension} \\
P_AO_2 &= \text{Alveolar oxygen tension} \\
D &= \text{difference}
\end{aligned}$$

Clinical Implications
1. *Increased* values may be due to
   (a) Mucus plugs
   (b) Bronchospasm
   (c) Airway collapse as seen in
      (1) Asthma
      (2) Bronchitis
      (3) Emphysema
2. Hypoxemia, due to an increased A-aDO$_2$ difference is also caused by
   (a) Atrial septal defects
   (b) Pneumothorax
   (c) Atelectasis
   (d) Emboli
   (e) Edema

Interfering Factors
Value increases with age and increasing O$_2$ concentration.

Arterial to Alveolar Oxygen Ratio (a/A Ratio)

Normal values
75% (regardless of age or F$_I$O$_2$)

$$a/A \text{ ratio} = \frac{PaO_2}{(BP-47)F_IO_2-(PaCO_2 \times 1.25)}$$

Partial Pressure of Carbon Dioxide (PCO$_2$)

Normal Values
PaCO$_2$ (arterial blood) 35–45 torr
PvCO$_2$ (venous blood) 41–51 torr
Carried in blood in two ways: 10% carried in plasma
                              90% carried in red blood cells

Explanation of Test
This test is a measurement of the pressure or tension exerted by dissolved CO$_2$ in the blood and is proportional to the partial pressure of CO$_2$ in the alveolar air. The test is commonly used to detect a respiratory abnormality and to determine the alkalinity or acidity of the blood. In order to maintain CO$_2$ within normal limits, the rate and depth of respiration vary automatically with changes in metabolism. The test is an index of the effectiveness of alveolar ventilation and is the

most physiologically reflective blood gas measurement. When taken as an arterial sample, it directly reflects how well air is exchanging with blood in the lungs.

The CO_2 tension in the blood and in cerebrospinal fluid (CSF) is the major chemical factor regulating alveolar ventilation. When the CO_2 of arterial blood rises from 40 torr to 45 torr, it causes a threefold increase in alveolar ventilation. A CO_2 of 63 torr in arterial blood increases alveolar ventilation tenfold. When the CO_2 concentration of breathed air exceeds 5%, the lungs can no longer be ventilated fast enough to prevent a dangerous rise of CO_2 concentration in tissue fluids. Any further increase in CO_2 begins to depress the respiratory center, causing a progressive decline in respiratory activity rather than an increase.

Procedure
1. Obtain an arterial blood sample.
2. Do not expose the sample to air.
3. A small amount of blood is then introduced into a blood gas analyzing machine (*e.g.*, Radiometer, Corning, IL) and the CO_2 tension is measured with a silver–silver chloride electrode (Severinghaus electrode).

Clinical Implications
1. A *rise* in PCO_2 is usually associated with hypoventilation; a *decrease*, with hyperventilation. Reduction in PCO_2 through its effect on plasma bicarbonate concentration decreases renal bicarbonate reabsorption. For each mEq/liter fall in HCO_3, the PCO_2 falls by 1 to 1.3 mm Hg. Because HCO_3 and PCO_2 bear this close mathematical relationship, and this ratio in turn defends the hydrogen ion concentration, the outcome is that the steady state PCO_2 in simple metabolic acidosis is equal to the last two digits of the *p*H. Also, addition of 15 to the bicarbonate level also equals the last two digits of the *p*H. Failure of the PCO_2 to achieve predicted levels defines the presence of superimposed respiratory acidosis on alkalosis.
2. The causes of *decreased* PCO_2 include
   (a) Hypoxia
   (b) Nervousness
   (c) Anxiety
   (d) Pulmonary emboli
   (e) Pregnancy
   (f) Pain
   (g) Other cause of hyperventilation
3. The causes of *increased* PCO_2 include
   (a) Obstructive lung disease
       (1) Chronic bronchitis
       (2) Emphysema

(b) Reduced function of respiratory center
  (1) Over-reaction
  (2) Head trauma
  (3) Anesthesia
(c) Other more rare causes of hypoventilation, such as Pickwickian syndrome

Clinical Alert

Increased PCO$_2$ may occur even with normal lungs if the respiratory center is depressed. Always check laboratory reports for abnormal values. When interpreting laboratory reports, remember that PCO$_2$ is a gas and is regulated by the lungs, not the kidneys.

Oxygen Saturation (SO$_2$)

Normal Values
Arterial blood saturation (SaO$_2$) = 95% or higher
Mixed venous blood saturation (SvO$_2$) = 75%

Explanation of Test
This measurement is a ratio of the actual oxygen (O$_2$) content of the hemoglobin compared to the potential maximum O$_2$-carrying capacity of the hemoglobin. The percentage of SO$_2$ is a measure of the relationship between O$_2$ and hemoglobin. The percentage of saturation does not indicate the O$_2$ content of arterial blood. The maximum amount of O$_2$ that can be combined with hemoglobin is called the O$_2$ capacity. The combined measurements of O$_2$ saturation, partial pressure of O$_2$, and of hemoglobin will indicate the amount of O$_2$ available to the tissue (tissue oxygenation). Pulse oximetry is a noninvasive technique that permits continuous real-time trending of SaO$_2$. Additional advantages over arterial samples are that equipment calibration is not necessary and no special preparation is needed for the sensor site.

Procedure
1. Arterial blood sample. Two methods for determining oxygen saturation are used.
  (a) The blood sample is introduced into the oximeter, which is a spectrophotometric device for determining the oxygen saturation of the blood. The value is measured directly with an oximeter.

(b) Oxygen saturation is calculated from the oxygen content and oxygen capacity determinations.

$$\text{Percentage saturation} = \frac{100 \times O_2 \text{ content volume \%}}{O_2 \text{ capacity volume \%}}$$

that is

$$\text{Percentage saturation} = 100 \times \frac{\text{volume of } O_2 \text{ actually combined with hemoglobin}}{\text{volume of } O_2 \text{ with which hemoglobin is capable of combination}}$$

The O_2 content of the blood sample is measured before and after exposure to the atmosphere.
2. Pulse oximetry. A small clip-like sensor is placed on a digit. The instrument, using transmitted light waves and sensors, determines oxygen saturation.

Limitations
1. Only measures percentage of oxygen being carried by hemoglobin. Therefore, it does not reveal the actual amount of oxygen available to the tissues.
2. Pulse oximetry equipment evaluates motion in the digit to localize pulsatile blood flow. Multiple factors, such as the following, can interfere with its ability to measure flow:
    (a) Digit motion
    (b) A decrease in flow to the digit (cool extremity and decreased peripheral pulses from hypotension, vasoconstrictive drugs, or localized obstruction).
    (c) Decrease in hemoglobin (anemia) or presence of abnormal hemoglobin (carboxyhemoglobin)

Oxygen (O_2) Content

Normal Values
Arterial blood: 15%–22 vol %
Venous blood: 11%–16 vol %
(Vol % = volume percentage = ml/100 ml of blood)

Explanation of Test
The actual amount of O_2 in the blood is termed the *oxygen content*. Blood can contain less O_2 than it is capable of carrying. About 98% of all O_2 delivered to the tissues is transported in chemical combination with hemoglobin. One gram of hemoglobin can carry or is capable of combining with 1.34 ml of O_2, whereas 100 ml of blood plasma can

carry only up to 0.3 ml of O$_2$. This measurement is determined mathematically by multiplying the number of grams of hemoglobin in 100 ml of blood by 1.34 times the saturation, plus the PaO$_2$ times .003.

Clinical Implications
Decreased arterial blood O$_2$ associated with increased arterial blood CO$_2$ can be due to

1. Chronic obstructive lung disease
2. Patients with respiratory complications postoperatively
3. Flail chest
4. Kyphoscoliosis
5. Neuromuscular impairment
6. Obesity hypoventilation

Procedure
1. An arterial or venous blood sample is obtained.
2. Mathematical formula:

$$O_2 \text{ content} = SaO_2 \times Hgb \times 1.34 + PaO_2 \times 0.003$$

Partial Pressure of Oxygen (PO$_2$)

Normal Values
PaO$_2$ 80 torr or greater: arterial sample
PvO$_2$ 30–40 torr: venous or peripheral blood sample

Background
Oxygen (O$_2$) is carried in the blood in two forms: dissolved and in combination with hemoglobin. Most of the O$_2$ in the blood is carried by hemoglobin. It is the partial pressure of a gas that determines the force it exerts in attempting to diffuse through the pulmonary membrane. The partial pressure reflects the amount of O$_2$ passing from the pulmonary alveoli into the blood and is directly influenced by the amount of O$_2$ being inhaled.

Explanation of Test
This is a measure of the pressure exerted by the amount of O$_2$ dissolved in the plasma. It is a test that measures the effectiveness of the lungs to oxygenate the blood, and is used to assess the effectiveness of oxygen therapy. The severity of impairment of the ability of the lungs to diffuse O$_2$ across the alveolar membrane into the circulating blood is indicated by the level of partial pressure of oxygen (PO$_2$).

Procedure
1. An arterial blood sample is obtained.
2. A small amount of blood is then introduced into a blood gas analyzing machine and the O$_2$ tension is measured.

Clinical Implications
1. *Increased levels* are associated with
    (a) Polycythemia
    (b) Increased F_LO_2
2. *Decreased levels* are associated with
    (a) Anemias
    (b) Cardiac decompensation
    (c) Insufficient atmospheric O_2
    (d) Intracardiac shunts
    (e) Chronic obstructive disease
    (f) Restrictive pulmonary disease
    (g) Hypoventilation due to neuromuscular disease
3. *Decreased* arterial PO_2 with normal or decreased arterial blood PCO_2 tension is associated with
    (a) Diffuse interstitial pulmonary infiltration
    (b) Pulmonary edema
    (c) Pulmonary embolism
    (d) Postoperative extracorporeal circulation

Carbon Dioxide (CO_2) Content or Total Carbon Dioxide (TCO_2)

Normal Values
23–30 mmol/L

Background
In normal blood plasma, more than 95% of the total CO_2 content is contributed by bicarbonate (HCO_3^-), *which is regulated by the kidneys.* The other 5% of CO_2 is contributed by the dissolved CO_2 gas and carbonic acid (H_2CO_3). Dissolved CO_2 gas, which is regulated by the lungs, therefore contributes little to the total CO_2 content. Total CO_2 content gives little information about the lungs.

HCO_3^- in the extracellular spaces exists first as CO_2, then as H_2CO_3, and, thereafter, much of it is changed to sodium bicarbonate ($NaHCO_3^-$) by the buffers of the plasma and red cells.

Explanation of Test
This test is a general measure of the alkalinity or acidity of the venous, arterial, or capillary blood. This test measures CO_2 from

1. Dissolved CO_2
2. Total H_2CO_3
3. HCO_3^-
4. Carbaminohemoglobin (CO_2HHb)

$$\text{Total carbon dioxide} = HCO_3^- + 0.03 \times PCO_2$$

Procedure
1. A venous or arterial blood sample of 6 ml is collected in a heparinized syringe.
2. If the collected blood sample cannot be studied immediately, the syringe should be placed in an iced container.

Clinical Implications
(See also Table 14-2)

1. *Elevated* CO_2 content levels occur in
   (a) Severe vomiting   (c) Aldosteronism
   (b) Emphysema   (d) Use of mercurial diuretics
2. *Decreased* CO_2 content levels occur in
   (a) Severe diarrhea   (e) Diabetic acidosis
   (b) Starvation   (f) Use of chlorothiazide diuretics
   (c) Acute renal failure
   (d) Salicylate toxicity

   Note: In diabetic acidosis the supply of ketoacids exceeds the demands of the cell. Blood plasma acids rise. Blood plasma HCO_3^- decreases because it is used in neutralizing these acids.

Clinical Alert

1. A double use of the term CO_2 is one of the main reasons why understanding acid–base problems may be difficult. Use the terms *CO_2 content* and *CO_2 gas* to avoid confusion. Remember the following:
   (a) *CO_2 content* is mainly bicarbonate and a base. It is a solution and is regulated by the kidneys.
   (b) *CO_2 gas* is mainly acid. It is regulated by the lungs.
2. Panic value is 6.0 or less and is usually associated with severe metabolic acidosis, with the pH often less than 7.1. This is a medical emergency.

Interfering Factors
A number of drugs may cause increased or decreased levels.

Blood pH

Normal Values
Arterial blood: 7.35–7.45
Venous blood: 7.31–7.41

Background

The pH is the negative logarithm of the hydrogen ion concentration in the blood. The sources of hydrogen ions are: (1) volatile acids, that can vary between a liquid and a gaseous state, and (2) nonvolatile acids that cannot be volatilized and are fixed (*e.g.*, dietary acids, lactic acids, and ketoacids).

Explanation of Test

This is a measurement of the chemical balance in the body and is a ratio of acids to bases. A determination of the blood pH is one of the best ways to tell if the body is too acid or too alkaline. Low pH numbers (<7.35) indicate an acid state, and higher pH numbers (>7.45) indicate an alkaline state. This balance is extremely intricate and must be kept within the very slight margin of 7.35 to 7.45 pH (alkaline) in the extracellular fluid. (Recall that 1–7 represents acidity; 7 is neutrality; and 7–14 represents alkalinity.) pH limits compatible with life are 6.9 to 7.8.

Procedure

1. An arterial blood sample is obtained.
2. Two methods of determining the pH are used: the direct method and the indirect method.
    (a) *Direct method:* A small amount of blood is introduced into a blood gas machine and the pH is measured.
    (b) *Indirect method:* The Henderson–Hasselbalch equation is solved.

$$pH = p\kappa' + \log \frac{(H_2CO_3) \text{ major blood base}}{(H_2CO_3) \text{ major blood acid}}$$

Clinical Implications

1. Generally speaking, the pH is *decreased* in acidemia because of increased formation of acids. pH is *increased* in alkalemia because of a loss of acids.
2. When attempting to interpret an acid–base abnormality, one must
    (a) Check the pH to see if there is an alkalemia or an acidemia.
    (b) Check PCO_2 to see if there is a respiratory abnormality. CO_2 is an acid: A CO_2 change that corresponds to the direction of pH change (*i.e.*, both are acidic) indicates that a CO_2 disturbance is causing the pH imbalance; an inverse change indicates a compensatory mechanism.
    (c) Check HCO_3^- or base excess to see if there is a metabolic abnormality. HCO_3^- is a base/alkali. An HCO_3 that deviates in the same direction as the altered pH (*i.e.*, both are alkaline) indicates HCO_3^- change is the primary etiology of pH change; an opposite change reflects compensation.

3. See Table 14–2 for a more complete explanation of the changes occurring in respiratory and metabolic acidemia and respiratory and metabolic alkalemia.
4. Metabolic acidemia (acidosis)
   (a) Renal failure
   (b) Ketoacidosis in diabetes and starvation
   (c) Lactic acidosis
   (d) Strenuous exercise
   (e) Severe diarrhea
5. Metabolic alkalemia (alkalosis)
   (a) Hypokalemia
   (b) Hypochoremia
   (c) Gastric suction or vomiting
   (d) Massive administration of steroids
   (e) Sodium bicarbonate administration
   (f) Aspirin intoxication
6. Respiratory alkalemia (alkalosis)
   (a) Acute pulmonary disease
   (b) Myocardial infarction
   (c) Chronic and acute heart failure
   (d) Adult cystic fibrosis
   (e) Third trimester of pregnancy and labor/delivery
   (f) Anxiety, neuroses, psychoses
   (g) Pain
   (h) Central nervous system diseases
   (i) Anemia
   (j) Carbon monoxide poisoning
   (k) Acute pulmonary embolus
   (l) Shock
7. Respiratory acidemia (acidosis)
   (a) Acute/chronic respiratory failure
   (b) Ventilatory failure
   (c) Neuromuscular depression
   (d) Obesity
   (e) Pulmonary edema
   (f) Cardiopulmonary arrest

Clinical Alert

1. Ventilation failure is a medical emergency. Aggressive and supportive measures must be taken immediately.
2. Observing the rate and depth of respiration may give a clue to blood *p*H.

(*text continues on page 854*)

TABLE 14–2.
Summary of Changes in Four Basic Forms of Acid–Base Imbalances

Form	pH	Bicarbonate (HCO$_3^-$)	pCO$_2$	Occurrence	Compensatory Mechanism
1. Respiratory acidosis due to decreased alveolar ventilation and retention of CO$_2$	↓	↑	↑	*Depression of respiratory centers* (a) Drug overdose (b) Barbiturate toxicity (c) Use of anesthetics *Interference with mechanical function of thoracic cage* (a) Deformity of thoracic cage (b) Kyphoscoliosis *Airway Obstruction* (a) Extrathoracic tumors (b) Asthma (c) Bronchitis (d) Emphysema *Circulatory Disorders* (a) Congestive heart failure (b) Shock	Renal reabsorption of the bicarbonate ion
2. Respiratory alkalosis due to increased alveolar ventilation and excessive blowing off of CO$_2$ and water	↑	↓	↓	*Hyperventilation* *Hysteria* *Lack of oxygen* *Toxic stimulation of the respiratory centers* (a) High fever (b) Cerebral hemorrhage (c) Excessive artificial respiration (d) Salicylates	Glomerular filtration of the bicarbonate ion

3. Metabolic acidosis due to accumulation of fixed body acids or loss of HCO_3^- (bicarbonate) from the extracellular fluid

3. *Acid addition*
   (a) Renal failure
   (b) Diabetic ketoacidosis
   (c) Lactic acidosis
   (d) Anaerobic metabolism
       Hypoxia
   Base subtraction
   (a) Diarrhea
   (b) Renal tubular acidosis

Hyperventilation through stimulation of central chemoreceptors

4. Metabolic alkalosis due to loss of fixed body acids or gain in bicarbonate (HCO_3^-) in the extracellular fluid

4. *Acid subtraction*
   (a) Loss of gastric juice
   (b) Vomiting
       Potassium or chloride depletion
   Base addition
   (a) Excessive bicarbonate or lactate administration

Hypoventilation

Heavier arrows indicate the primary abnormality

Note: *1. Although these four basic imbalances occur individually, a combination of two or more is observed more frequently. These disturbances may have an antagonistic or a synergistic effect upon each other.*
2. Compensation is most efficient in respiratory and nonrespiratory acidemia.
3. The degree of hypoventilation is precisely related to the degree of hypobicarbonatemia. For each mEq/L fall in bicarbonate, PCO_2 falls by 1 to 1.3 torr. A close mathematical relationship prevails between bicarbonate and PCO_2. Their ratio (HCO_3^- and PCO_2) defines the prevailing hydrogen ion concentration. For this reason, the steady-state PCO_2 in simple metabolic acidosis is equal to the last two digits of the pH. Failure of the PCO_2 to reach predicted levels defines the presence of superimposed respiratory acidosis or alkalosis.

(a) Acidosis usually *increases* respirations.
(b) Alkalosis usually *decreases* respirations.
3. Respiratory alkalemia may reflect hyperventilation due to hypoxemia. Correction of hypoxemia is essential to reverse alkalosis.
4. Metabolic alkalemia, which is compensated through hypoventilation, may produce hypoxemia.

Interfering Factors
A number of drugs may cause increased or decreased levels.

Base Excess/Deficit

Normal Values (±3 mEq/L)
Positive value indicates a base excess (*i.e.*, nonvolatile acid deficit).
Negative value indicates a base deficit (*i.e.*, nonvolatile acid excess).

Explanation of Test
This determination is an attempt to quantify the patient's total base excess or deficit so that clinical treatment of acid–base disturbances (specifically those that are nonrespiratory in nature) can be initiated. It is also referred to as the whole blood buffer base and is the sum of the concentration of buffer anions (in mEq/L) contained in whole blood. These buffer anions are the bicarbonate (HCO_3^-) ion in plasma and red blood cells, and the hemoglobin, plasma proteins, and phosphates in plasma and red blood cells.

Total quantity of buffer anions is 45 to 50 mEq/L or about twice that of HCO_3^-, which is 24 to 28 mEq/L. Thus, the quantity of HCO_3^- ions accounts for only about half of the total buffering capacity of the blood. Therefore, the base excess/deficit measurement provides a more complete picture of the buffering taking place and is a critical index of nonrespiratory changes in acid–base balance versus respiratory changes.

Procedure
Calculationi s made from the measurement of *p*H, $PaCO_2$, and hematocrit. These values are plated on a nomogram, and the base excess/deficit is read.

Clinical Implications
1. Negative value (below 3 mEq/L) reflects a nonrespiratory or metabolic disturbance. It indicates a true base deficit or a nonvolatile acid accumulation due to

(a) Dietary intake of organic and inorganic acids
(b) Lactic acid
(c) Ketoacidosis
2. Positive value (above 3 mEq/L) reflects a nonvolatile acid deficit or true base excess.

Anion Gap or R Factor

Normal Values
$<\pm12$ mEq/L
<16 mEq/L if potassium concentration is used to calculate the anion gap

Explanation of Test
This test is a measurement of the difference between sodium (Na^+) and potassium (K^+) ion concentrations (the measured cations) and the sum of chloride (Cl^-) and bicarbonate (HCO_3^-) (the measured anions). This difference reflects the concentration of anions that are present in the extracellular fluid. These components include phosphates, sulfates, ketone bodies, lactic acid, and proteins. Increased amounts of these unmeasured anions are produced in the acidotic state.

Primary hypocarbonatemia is brought about by any combination of these three mechanisms: (1) overproduction of acids, which causes replacement of $NaHCO_3^-$ by the Na salt of the offending acid (*e.g.*, Na lactate replaces HCO_3^- in lactic acidosis); (2) loss of $NaHCO_3^-$ through diarrhea along with renal retention of dietary NaCl, which causes hyperchloremic metabolic acidosis; (3) generalized renal failure or specific forms of renal tubular acidosis, which causes retention of acids that are normally produced by intermediary metabolism or by urinary excretion of alkali (Table 14–3).

Hyperbicarbonatemia with sustained increases of HCO_3^- levels is brought about by a source of *new* alkali and the presence of factors that stimulate renal retention of excess HCO_3^- (see Table 14–4). These mechanisms include excessive gastrointestinal loss of acid, exogenous alkali in persons whose kidneys avidly retain $NaHCO_3^-$, and renal synthesis of HCO_3^- in excess of daily consumption. Other pathophysiological factors that affect renal reabsorption of more than 25 mEq of HCO_3^- and contribute to sustained hyperbicarbonatemia include extracellular fluid volume contraction, hypercapnia, hypokalemia, hyperaldosteronemia, and hypoparathyroidism.

Procedure
This measurement is obtained by determining the difference between the sum of the serum cations and the sum of the serum anions.

TABLE 14–3.
Subclassification of Anion Gap Metabolic Acidosis
(Hypobicarbonatemia) into High- and Low-Potassium Forms*

Hyperkalemic Form	Hypokalemic Form
Acidifying agents	Diarrhea
Mineralocorticoid deficiency	Ureteral sigmoidostomy and mal-
Renal diseases such as systemic	functioning
lupus erythematosus, interstitial	Ileostomy
nephritis, amyloidosis, hydrone-	Renal tubular acidosis, both proxi-
phrosis, sickle cell nephropathy	mal and distal
Early nonspecific renal failure	

All metabolic acidoses can be classified on the basis of how they affect the anion gap. (After Narins RG et al: Diagnostic strategies in disorders of fluid, electrolyte, and acid-base homeostasis Am J Med 72[3]:510, 1982)

Clinical Implications

1. An anion gap occurs in acidosis due to excess metabolic acids and excess serum chloride levels. If there is no change in sodium content, anions such as phosphates, sulfates, and organic acids will increase the anion gap because these components replace bicarbonate.
2. *Increased* anion gap is associated with an increase in metabolic acid when there is an excessive production of metabolic acids as in
   (a) Alcoholic ketoacidosis
   (b) Diabetic ketoacidosis
   (c) Fasting and starvation
   (d) Ketogenic diets
   (e) Lactic acidosis
   (f) Salicylate, ethylene glycol (antifreeze), and methanol poisoning
3. *Increased* anion gap is also associated with decreased loss of metabolic acids as in renal failure
4. *Increased* bicarbonate loss with resulting normal anion gap is associated with
   (a) *Decreased* renal losses as in
       (1) Renal tubular acidosis
       (2) Use of acetazolamide
   (b) *Increased* chloride levels as in
       (1) Altered chloride reabsorption by the kidney
       (2) Parenteral hyperalimentation
       (3) Administration of sodium chloride and ammonium chloride
   (c) Loss of intestinal secretions as in
       (1) Diarrhea
       (2) Intestinal suction or fistula
       (3) Biliary fistula

TABLE 14-4.
Classification of Anion Gap Metabolic Alkalosis
(Hyperbicarbonatemia) on the Basis of Urinary Chloride Excretion

Saline-Responsive Urinary Chloride Excretion of Less Than 10 mEq/Day	Saline-Unresponsive Urinary Chloride Excretion of Less than 10 mEq/Day

1. Excess body bicarbonate content
  (a) Renal alkalosis
    Diuretic therapy
    Poorly reabsorbable anion therapy, such as carbenicillin, penicillin, sulfate, phosphate
    Posthypercapnia
  (b) Gastrointestinal alkalosis
    Gastric alkalosis
    Intestinal alkalosis such as chloride diarrhea
  (c) Exogenous alkali
    Baking soda
    Sodium citrate, lactate, gluconate, acetate
    Transfusions
    Antacids
2. Normal body bicarbonate content
  Contraction alkalosis—This means that the urinary loss of sodium chloride and water without bicarbonate loss will cause extracellular fluid contraction around an unchanged body content of alkali, resulting in hyperbicarbonatemia. This is especially important in persons with edema and persons who have excess body stores of water, sodium, bicarbonate, and chloride.
	1. Excess body bicarbonate content
	  (a) Renal alkalosis—normotensive conditions
	    Bartter's syndrome
	    Severe potassium depletion
	    Refeeding alkalosis
	    Hypercalcemia and hypoparathyroidism
	  (b) Hypertensive conditions—
	    Endogenous mineralocorticoids
	    Primary aldosteronism
	    Hyperreninism
	    Adrenal enzyme deficiency: 11- and 17-hydroxylase
	    Liddle syndrome
	  (c) Exogenous mineralocorticoids
	    Licorice
	    Carbenoxolone
	    Chewing tobacco

(After Narins RG et al: Diagnostic strategies in disorders of fluid, electrolyte, and acid-base homeostasis. Am J Med 72[3]:511, 1982)

Lactic Acid

Normal Values
0.5–2.2 mEq/L venous blood
0.5–1.6 mEq/L arterial blood

Background
Lactate is a product of carbohydrate metabolism. Lactic acid is produced during periods of anaerobic metabolism when cells do not receive adequate oxygen to allow conversion of fuel sources to carbon dioxide and water. Lactic acid will accumulate because of excess production of lactate and decreased removal of lactic acid from blood by liver.

Explanation of Test
This measurement contributes to the knowledge of acid–base volume in the body and is used to detect lactic acidosis in persons with underlying risk factors that predispose them to this imbalance, such as cardiovascular and renal disease. Lactate will be elevated in a variety of conditions in which hypoxia is present and in liver disease. Lactic acidosis can occur both in diabetics and nondiabetics, and it is an often fatal form of metabolic acidosis.

Procedure
A venous or arterial blood sample of at least 4 ml is obtained. The specimen must be brought to the laboratory immediately.

Clinical Implications
1. Values will be *increased* in
    (a) Lactic acidosis
    (b) Cardiac failure
    (c) Pulmonary failure
    (d) Hemorrhage
    (e) Diabetes
    (f) Shock
    (g) Liver disease
2. Lactic acidosis can be distinguished from ketoacidosis by the absence of severe ketosis and hyperglycemia.

Interfering Factors
Lactic acid levels normally rise during strenuous exercise when blood flow and oxygen cannot keep pace with increased needs of exercising muscle.

Clinical Alert

The presence of an unexplained fall in *p*H associated with a hypoxia-producing condition is reason to suspect lactic acidosis.

BIBLIOGRAPHY

Altose MD: The physiological basis of pulmonary function testing. Clin Symp 31(2):1–39, 1979

American Thoracic Society: Guidelines for bronchial inhalation challenges with pharmacologic and antigenic agents. ATS News, Spring:11–19, 1980

American Thoracic Society: Standardization of spirometry—1987 update. Am Rev Respir Dis 139:1285–1298, 1987

Anderson S: ABG's: Six easy steps to interpreting blood gases. Am J Nurs 90(8):42–45, August, 1990

Bass H: The flow-volume loop: Normal standards and abnormalities in chronic obstructive pulmonary disease. Chest 63:171–176, 1973

Berk JL, Sampliner JE: Handbook of Critical Care, 3rd ed. Boston, Little, Brown & Co, 1990

Boren H, Kory R, Snyder J: The Veterans Administration–Army cooperative study of pulmonary function: II—Lung volume and its subdivisions in normal men. Am J Med 41(1):96–114, 1966

Borrows B et al: Clinical usefulness of the single-breath pulmonary diffusing capacity test. Am Rev Respir Dis 84:789–806, 1961

Brust SA, Ross BB: Predicted values for closing volumes using a modified single-breath nitrogen test. Am Rev Respir Dis 107:744, 1973

Cherniack RM: Pulmonary Function Testing. Philadelphia, WB Saunders, 1977

Chusid EL: Diagnostic procedures in bronchopulmonary diseases. Hosp Pract 16(7):99–108, 1981

Clausen JL: Pulmonary Function Testing: Guidelines and Controversies. New York, Academic Press, 1982

Cohen S: Pulmonary function tests in patient care. Am J Nurs 80:1135–1161, 1980

Cropp G: The exercise bronchoprovocation test: Standardization of procedures and evaluation of response. J Allergy Clin Immunol 64:627–633, 1979

Eggleston P: Exercise challenge: Indications, techniques, and data analysis. J Allergy Clin Immunol 64:604–608, 1979

Ehrhardt S, Graham M: Pulse oximetry: An easy way to check oxygen saturation. Nursing '90 20(3):50–54, March 1990

Fishman AP: Assessment of Pulmonary Function. New York, McGraw-Hill, 1980

Forster RE et al: The Lung: Physiologic Basis of Pulmonary Function Tests, 3rd ed. Chicago, Year Book Medical Pub, 1986

Fraser RG, Pare JA: Organ Physiology: Structure and Function of the Lung, 2nd ed. Philadelphia, WB Saunders, 1977

Geschickter CF: The Lung in Health and Disease. Philadelphia, JB Lippincott, 1973

Gilb AF et al: Sensitivity of volume of isoflow in the detection of mild airway obstruction. Am Rev Respir Dis 112:401–405, 1975

Goldman HO, Becklake MR: Respiratory function tests: Normal values at median altitudes and the prediction of normal results. Am Rev Tuberculosis Pulm Dis 79:457, 1979

Guenter C, Welch MH (eds): Pulmonary Medicine, 2nd ed. Philadelphia, JB Lippincott, 1982

Halsted CH, Halsted JA (eds): The Laboratory in Clinical Medicine, 2nd ed. Philadelphia, WB Saunders, 1982

Isselbacher KJ et al (eds): Harrison's Principles of Internal Medicine, 11th ed. New York, McGraw–Hill, 1987

Jones NL: Exercise testing in pulmonary evaluation: Rationale, methods, and the normal respiratory response to exercise. N Engl J Med 293(11):541–544, 1975

Jones NL: Exercise testing in pulmonary evaluation clinical application. N Engl J Med 293(13):647–652, 1975

Kenasewitz GT: Pulmonary Function Testing Principles and Practice. New York, Churchill Livingstone, 1984

Kenney MR, Packa DR, Dunbar SB: AACN's Clinical Reference for Critical Care Nursing, 2nd ed. New York, McGraw–Hill, 1988

Keogh BA et al: Clinical significance of pulmonary function tests. Chest 78(6): 856–865, 1980

Miller WF et al.: Laboratory Evaluation of Pulmonary Function. Philadelphia, JB Lippincott, 1987

Morris JF, Koski A, Johnson LC: Spirometric Standards for Healthy Nonsmoking Adults. Am Rev Respir Dis 103:57–67, 1971

Ruppel G; Manual of Pulmonary Function Testing, 4th ed. St. Louis, CV Mosby, 1986

Schoenberg JB, Beck GJ, Bouhuys A: Growth and decay of pulmonary function in healthy blacks and whites. Respir Physiol 33:367–393, 1978

Shapiro BA, Harrison RA, Cane RD et al: Clinical Application of Blood Gases. Chicago, Year Book Medical Pub, 1989

Simmons DH: Current Pulmonology, vol 10. Chicago, Year Book Medical Publishers, 1989

Slonim NB, Hamilton LH: Respiratory Physiology, 4th ed. St. Louis, CV Mosby, 1981

Spyr J, Preach M: Pulse oximetry—understanding the concept and knowing the limits. RN 53(5):38–45, May, 1990

Victor LC, Chmielinski MA: Pulmonary function and exercise stress testing. Hosp Pract 17(7):125–132, 1982

West JB: Pulmonary Pathophysiology: The Essentials, 3rd ed. Baltimore, Williams & Wilkins, 1987

West JB: Respiratory Physiology, 3rd ed. Baltimore, Williams & Wilkins, 1985

Williams MH: Essentials of Pulmonary Medicine. Philadelphia, WB Saunders, 1982

Wilson AF: Pulmonary Functioning Testing: Indications and Interpretations. Orlando, Grune & Stratton, 1985

Woolf CR: The Clinical Core of Respiratory Medicine. Philadelphia, JB Lippincott, 1981

SPECIAL SYSTEM AND ORGAN FUNCTION STUDIES

Introduction

These special tests of the eye and of the nervous, cardiovascular, peripheral vascular, cerebrovascular, and muscle systems have been selected for discussion in this chapter because of their great importance in diagnosing alterations in the functions of these vital systems and organs.

Electroencephalography (EEG)

Normal Values
Normal, symmetric patterns of electrical brain activity in the range of alpha, 8 to 11 Hz (Hertz) (cycles per second)

Explanation of Test
This test measures and records electrical impulses from the cortex of the brain. Electrodes are placed outside the cranial vault to record the electrical manifestations of brain activity. This test is used to help diagnose epilepsy and as an aid in identifying brain tumors, abscesses, and subdural hematomas; to help diagnose cerebrovascular diseases, such as cerebral infarcts and intracranial hemorrhages; and to help diagnose cerebral diseases such as narcolepsy and Alzheimer's disease. It is common practice to use the EEG pattern along with other clinical procedures, drug levels, patient body temperature, and a thorough neurologic examination to determine electrocerebral silence. Recordings are obtained using guidelines as set by the American Electroneurodiagnostic Society. When this electrocerebral silence pattern is recorded and there is no chance of neurologic recovery, the patient may be considered brain dead despite the preservation of cardiovascular functions supported by mechanical respiration.

Procedure
1. An EEG can be done any time during the day.
2. The technician places electrodes in the form of small discs on the scalp, fastening them with skin glue or paste. Nineteen to 25 electrodes are attached according to an internationally accepted measurement called the *10–20 System*. This system correlates both standardization of electrode placement and anatomical structure of the brain. Conduction gel is placed in the electrode itself.
3. The patient sits in an easy chair or lies on a bed or couch.
4. The patient is instructed to keep the eyes closed and to relax.
5. Near the beginning of the examination, the patient may be asked to breathe deeply through the mouth 20 times a minute for 3 minutes. This hyperventilation may cause dizziness or numbness in hands or

feet, but it is nothing to be alarmed about. Rapid, shallow breathing contributes to alkalosis causing vasoconstriction, which may activate a seizure pattern.
6. A flashing light may be used over the face at frequencies of 1 to 30 times/second with the eyes opened or closed. This technique, called *photic stimulation*, may cause an abnormal discharge not otherwise recorded in the EEG.
7. Some patients may be sleep-deprived before the test to promote rest and sleep. Sleep is especially helpful in bringing out abnormalities, especially different forms of epilepsy.
8. The technician removes the discs after the test and removes the glue or paste from the scalp.
9. Total examining time is 1 hour 15 minutes.

Clinical Implications
1. Abnormal pattern readings will reveal generalized seizures (*e.g.*, grand mal and petit mal epilepsy), provided the EEG is recorded during the seizure. If a patient suspected of having epilepsy shows a normal EEG, the test may have to be repeated, with sleep deprivation or special electrodes.
    (a) The EEG is also abnormal during other types of seizure activity (*e.g.*, focal [psychomotor], infantile myoclonic, and Jacksonian seizures).
    (b) Between seizures, 20% of patients with petit mal epilepsy and 40% with grand mal epilepsy show a normal pattern.
    (c) The diagnosis of epilepsy can be made only by correlating the clinical history with the EEG abnormality, if one exists.
2. An EEG may often be normal in the presence of cerebral pathology.
    (a) However, most brain abscesses and glioblastomas cause EEG abnormalities.
    (b) Electroencephalographic changes due to cerebrovascular accidents depend on the size and location of the infarcts or hemorrhage.
    (c) Following a head injury, a series of EEGs may be helpful in identifying the prospect of epilepsy as a result of the trauma if a previous EEG is on record.
    (d) In dementia, the EEG may be either normal or abnormal.
    (e) In later stages of metabolic disease, the EEG will be abnormal; in the early stages, it will be normal.
3. The EEG is abnormal in most diseases in which there is an impairment of consciousness. The more profound the change in consciousness, the more abnormal the EEG pattern.

Interfering Factors
1. Sedative drugs and mild hypoglycemia may affect the normal EEG.
2. Oily hair or hair spray interferes with the placement of leads and a true tracing.

3. Artifacts may appear even in technically well done EEGs. Eye movements and body movements cause changes in the wave pattern and must be noted so that they will not be mistaken for brain waves.

Patient Preparation

1. Explain the purpose and procedure of the test. Some persons are very fearful of this test, even though it involves no pain or discomfort. Emphasize that it is not a test of thinking or intelligence, that no electrical impulses pass from the machine to the patient, and that the test has no relation to any type of shock treatment.
2. Food may be taken if the patient is sleep-deprived, but no coffee, tea, or cola is permitted within 8 hours of the test. Emphasize that food should be eaten to prevent hypoglycemia.
3. Smoking is usually allowed before the test.
4. Hair should be shampooed the evening before the test so that leads will remain firmly in place.
5. If a sleep study is ordered, an adult patient should sleep as little as possible the night before (up past midnight) so he will be tired enough to fall asleep during the test.
6. If a sleep-deprivation study is ordered for a child, call the diagnostic department for special instructions.

Patient Aftercare

1. The hair should be shampooed after the test to remove the substance used to fasten the discs. Oil can be of some help before the shampoo.
2. If the patient received a sedative during the test, allow him or her to rest with bedside rails in raised position.
3. Skin irritation may be present from the electrode application but resolves within a few hours.

Evoked Responses or Potentials

Normal Values

Normal waveform latencies are established by each individual laboratory because of varying factors such as instrument type and laboratory environment. Values vary between persons, in the same person over time, because of gender, height, and age.

Evoked Responses/Potentials

Auditory brain-stem response (ABR)
Visual-evoked response (VER)
Somatosensory-evoked response (SER)

Brain-stem auditory evoked potentials (BAEP): Absolute latency measured in milliseconds (msec) of the first five waveforms at a stimulation rate of 11 clicks/second sound

Wave	Mean	SD (Standard Deviation)
I	1.7	0.15
II	2.8	0.17
III	3.9	0.19
IV	5.1	0.24
V	5.7	0.25

Visual-evoked response (VER): Absolute latency measured in milliseconds of the first major positive peak (P_{100})

Wave	Mean	Range	SD
P_{100}	102.3	89–114	5.1

Explanation of Test

These tests use conventional EEG recording techniques with specific electrode placement for each procedure, along with computer data processing to evaluate electrophysiologic integrity of the auditory, visual, and sensory pathways. Somatosensory-evoked response (SER): Absolute latency of major waveforms measured in milliseconds at a stimulation rate of 5 impulses/second

Wave	Mean	SD
E.P.	9.7	0.7
A	11.8	0.7
B	13.7	0.8
II	11.3	0.8
III	13.9	0.9
N_2	19.1	0.8
P_2	22	1.2

Somatosensory-Evoked Response (SER)

This test is used in the assessment of patients with spinal cord lesions, stroke, and complaints of numbness and weakness of the extremities. It is done to study the conduction of impulses through the somatosensory pathway. Electrical stimuli are applied to the median or peroneal nerve at an intensity near that which produces thumb or foot twitches. With this procedure, it is possible to measure in milliseconds the time it takes for the current to travel along the nerve to the cortex of the brain. Somatosensory-evoked responses are also used to monitor the sensory pathway conduction during surgery to relieve spinal cord compression and/or ischemia, or scoliosis repair. A loss of the sensory potential can indicate impending cord damage.

Visual-Evoked Response (VER)

This test of visual pathway function is valuable in the diagnosis of lesions involving the optic nerves and optic tracts, multiple sclerosis, and other disorders. It is known that visual stimulation excites retinal pathways and initiates impulses that are conducted through the central visual path to the primary visual cortex. Fibers from this area project to the secondary visual cortical areas on the occipital convexity. Through this path, a visual stimulus to the eyes causes an electrical response in the occipital regions, which can be recorded with electrodes placed along the vertex and occipital lobes.

Auditory Brain-Stem Response (ABR)

Special recording and stimulating methods have been developed that permit recording of signals generated by subcortical structures in the auditory pathway. Stimulation of either ear evokes potentials that can reveal lesions in the brain stem involving the auditory pathway without affecting hearing. Evoked potentials of this type are also used to evaluate hearing in infants, children, and adults, which is called *electrical response audiometry.*

This study is also helpful in the evaluation of suspected peripheral hearing loss, cerebellopontine angle lesions, brain-stem tumors, infarcts, and multiple sclerosis. It is also useful in evaluating the mechanisms of coma as well as in monitoring the cause of disorders associated with coma.

Procedure

1. Electrodes that pick up a visually evoked response are placed on the scalp along the vertex and occipital lobes. The patient is asked to watch a checkerboard pattern flash for several minutes, first with one eye, then with the other.
2. Somatosensory-evoked responses are obtained from recordings of several pairs of pick-up electrodes. Electrical stimuli are applied to the median nerve at the wrist or the peroneal nerve at the knee with electrodes placed over the sensory cortex of the opposite hemisphere in the scalp. This procedure measures in milliseconds the time it takes for the current to travel along the nerve to the cortex of the brain.
3. Auditory brain-stem responses are obtained from scalp electrodes placed on the vertex and each earlobe. Stimuli consisting of clicking noises or tone bursts are delivered to one ear through earphones. Because sound waves delivered to one ear can be heard by the opposite ear, a continuous masking noise is simultaneously delivered to the opposite ear.

Clinical Implications

1. Abnormal visual-evoked responses (VERs) are associated with
   (a) Demyelinating disorders such as multiple sclerosis
   (b) Lesions of the optic nerves and eye (prechiasmal defects)
   (c) Lesions of the optic tract and visual cortex (postchiasmal defects)
   (d) Abnormal visual-evoked potentials may also be found in persons without a history of retrobulbar neuritis, optic atrophy, or visual field defects. However, many patients with proven damage to the postchiasmal visual path and known visual-field defects may have normal evoked potentials.
2. Abnormal SERs are associated with
   (a) Spinal cord lesions
   (b) Cerebrovascular accident
   (c) Multiple sclerosis
   (d) Cervical myelopathy
3. Abnormal auditory brain stem-evoked responses (ABRs) are associated with
   (a) Acoustic neuroma
   (b) Cerebrovascular accidents
   (c) Multiple sclerosis
   (d) Lesions affecting any part of the auditory nerve or brain-stem area

   Note: Some difficulty of interpreting brain stem-evoked potentials may arise in persons with peripheral hearing defects that alter the evoked potential results.

Patient Preparation

1. Explain the purpose and procedure of the test.
2. Hair should be shampooed before testing.

Patient Aftercare

Assist the patient in washing the hair (if so desired) to remove gels applied to the scalp. Also, be sure that gel is carefully washed from any other area of the body to be tested.

Cognitive Tests (Event-Related Potentials [ERPs])

Normal Values

No shift of P_3 components to longer latencies
ERP: absolute latency of P_3 waveform

Wave	Mean	SD
P_3	294	21

Explanation of Test

Event-related potentials are being used more frequently as objective measures of mental function in neurologic diseases that produce cognitive defects. These measurements use the method of auditory-evoked response testing (see p. 866) in which sound stimuli are presented through earphones. A rare tone is associated with a prominent endogenous P_3 component that reflects the differential cognitive processing of that tone. Although a systematic neurologic increase in P_3 component latency occurs as a function of increasing age in normal persons, in many instances of neurologic diseases producing dementia, the latency of the P_3 component has been reported to exceed substantially the normal age-matched value.

This test is useful in evaluating persons with dementia or decreased mental functioning. It is also helpful in differentiating persons with real organic defects in cognitive function from those who are unable to interact with the examiner because of motor or language defects and those who are unwilling to cooperate because of problems like depression or schizophrenia.

Procedure

1. The procedure is the same as that used in obtaining auditory brain stem responses (see p. 866).
2. Patients are asked to count the occurrences of rare tones.

Interfering Factors

Latency of P_3 component normally increases with age.

Clinical Implications

An increased or abnormal P_3 latency is associated with neurologic diseases producing dementia such as

1. Alzheimer's disease
2. Metabolic encephalopathy such as hypothyroidism and alcoholism with severe electrolyte disturbances
3. Brain tumor
4. Hydrocephalus

Patient Preparation

Explain the purpose and procedure of the test.

Brain Mapping (Computerized Topography)

Normal Values

Normal frequency signals presented as a color-coded map of electrical activity

Explanation of Test

Brain mapping uses traditional EEG data and unique computer digitization to display the diagnostic information as a topographic map of the brain. The computer analyzes EEG signals for amplitude and distribution of alpha, beta, theta, and delta frequencies and displays the analysis as a color map. Specific and/or *minute* abnormalities are enhanced, allowing comparison to normal data. The technology also maps evoked responses, permitting observation of persistent alteration in latency (delay in conduction) and cognitive function. This methodology is used in the assessment of patients with migraine headaches, episodes of vertigo or dizziness, persons who lose pieces of time, and some patients with generalized seizures, dementia of organic origin, ischemic abnormalities, and some psychiatric disorders. With this procedure, it is possible to localize a specific area of the brain that may be showing a generalized area of deficit in the conventional EEG. It is a helpful research aid in the evaluation of children to demonstrate areas possibly related to hyperactivity and dyslexia and of older adults with dementia and Alzheimer's disease.

Procedure

1. The patient should be rested and awake for the test so that no sleep signals appear (as indicators of beta activity).
2. A procedure similar to the conventional EEG is followed. Forty-two electrodes are placed on the scalp.
3. Prior to placement of the electrodes, the skin is cleansed with a special solution such as Omniprep. The solution is somewhat abrasive. The electrodes are connected with a paste or adhesive.
4. The patient sits in an easy chair and is instructed to keep the eyes closed to relax.
5. Total examining time is approximately 2 hours.

Interfering Factors

1. Tranquilizers may affect the outcome.
2. Oily hair or hair spray interferes with placement of electordes.
3. Eye and body movements cause changes in the signals and wave patterns.

Clinical Implications

Abnormal maps based upon signal analyses are compared with normal data and are indicative of

1. Area of focal seizure discharge in persons with generalized seizures
2. Area of focal irritation in persons with migraine
3. Area of ischemia
4. Area of dysfunction in dementia
5. Schizophrenia
6. Psychosis

Patient Preparation

1. Explain the purpose and procedure of the test. There are no known risks. Emphasize that electrical impulses pass only from the *patient* to the machine, not from the machine to the patient.
2. Food and fluids are permitted prior to testing but no coffee, tea, or caffeinated drinks are permitted within 8 hours of the test.
3. Hair should be clean before the test.
4. Advise the patient that no tranquilizers are to be taken prior to testing (how long). Other prescribed medications such as antihypertensives and insulin do not have to be discontinued, but notify the testing laboratory of what drugs the patient has taken.

Patient Aftercare

1. The residue from the conductor gel is removed by the technologist. The patient is advised to shampoo the hair after the test to remove the conductor gel completely.
2. There are no known after effects.

Electromyography, Electromyoneurogram (EMG)

Normal Values

1. Normal nerve conduction
2. Normal muscle action potential
   (a) On insertion
   (b) At rest
   (c) During minimum voluntary muscle contraction
   (d) During maximum voluntary muscle contraction

Explanation of Test

Electromyoneurography is the combined use of electromyography and electroneurography. These studies, done to detect neuromuscular abnormalities, measure nerve conduction and electrical properties of skeletal muscles. These tests, along with evaluation of range of motion, motor power, sensory defects, and reflexes, can differentiate between neuropathy and myopathy. The electromyogram is useful in defining the site and cause of muscle disorders such as myasthenia, muscular dystrophy, and myotonia as well as lesions involving the motor neurons in the anterior horn of the spinal cord. Electromyogram is helpful in localizing the site of peripheral nerve disorders such as radiculopathy and axonopathy. Skin and needle electrodes are used to measure and record electrical activity. Sound equivalents of electrical activity are heard over a loudspeaker and recorded. The tape can be played later and restudied as often as necessary.

Procedure
1. The test is done in a copper-lined room to screen out interference.
2. The patient lies and/or sits during the test.
3. A surface disk is applied to ground the patient. The muscles and nerves the examiner checks are dependent on the patient's signs and symptoms, history, and physical condition (certain nerves innervate specific muscles).
4. Instructions are given to relax (the examiner may massage certain muscles to get the patient to relax) and to contract certain muscles (*e.g.*, to point toes, when directed).
5. The test consists of two parts. The first test is done to determine *nerve conduction*.
   (a) The metal surface electrodes are coated with electrode paste and firmly fixed over the body part that is being tested. Electrodes may be taped to the involved areas. The metal electrode is placed over a specific nerve area and electrical current is passed through the patient. This will cause sensations directly proportional to the time involved.
   (b) The amplitude wave is read on an oscilloscope.
   (c) Electrical current leaves no mark but can cause an unusual and surprising sensation, not usually considered unpleasant. Measurement can be made of how fast and how well a nerve transmits messages. Nerves in the face, arms, or legs may be tested in this way.
6. The second test is done to determine *muscle potential.*
   (a) A monopolar electrode (½-in–3-in very fine needle) is inserted, and a pricking sensation may be felt as the needle pierces the skin. The needle is advanced into the muscle by increments. The examiner may move the needle around without removing it to see if readings change, or he or she may reinsert the needle in another muscle area.
   (b) The electrode causes no pain unless the end of the needle is near a terminal nerve; then it can cause considerable pain. Ten or more insertions may be made. No shocks are given because the needle detects the electricity normally present in muscle.
   (c) The examiner watches the oscilloscope for a normal wave and listens to a loudspeaker for a normal quiet sound at rest. A "machine-gun" popping sound or rattling sound like hail on a tin roof is normally heard when the patient is asked to contract the muscles.
   (d) If the patient complains of pain, the examiner removes the needle because pain yields false results.
   (e) Total examining time is 45 to 60 minutes if testing is confined to a single extremity, and up to 3 hours for more than one extremity. There is no completely "routine" EMG. The length of the test depends on the clinical problem.

Clinical Implications

Abnormal results are indicative of muscle or nerve disorders. Any spontaneous, involuntary electrical activity that occurs while the muscle is in a resting state, together with abnormal waveforms, is indicative of neuromuscular abnormality. Abnormal conduction velocity rates and terminal latency or slowing are associated with nerve disorders.

1. Diseases or disturbance of striated muscle fibers or cell membrane
   (a) Muscle fiber disorder such as muscular dystrophy
   (b) Cell membrane hyperirritability such as myotonia and myotic disorders such as polymyositis, hypocalcemia, thyrotoxicosis, tetanus, and rabies
   (c) Myasthenia
      (1) Myasthenia gravis
      (2) Cancer due to nonpituitary ACTH secretion by tumor
         (a) Bronchial cancer
         (b) Sarcoid
      (3) Deficiencies
         (a) Familial hypokalemia
         (b) McArdle's phosphorylase
      (4) Hyperadrenocorticism
      (5) Acetylcholene blockers
         (a) Curare
         (b) Botulism
         (c) Kanamycin
         (d) Snake venom
2. Disorders or diseases of lower motor neuron
   (a) Lesion involving motor neuron on anterior horn of spinal cord (myelopathy)
      (1) Tumor
      (2) Trauma
      (3) Syringomyelia
      (4) Juvenile muscular dystrophy
      (5) Congenital amyotonia
      (6) Anterior poliomyelitis
      (7) Amyotrophic lateral sclerosis
      (8) Peroneal muscular atrophy
   (b) Lesion involving nerve root (radiculopathy)
      (1) Guillain-Barré
      (2) Entrapment
         (a) Tumor
         (b) Trauma
         (c) Herniated disk
         (d) Hypertrophic spurs
         (e) Spinal stenosis

(c) Damage or disease to peripheral or axial nerve
  (1) Entrapment
    (a) Carpal and tarsal tunnel
    (b) Facial, ulnar, radial, and peroneal palsy
    (c) Neuralgia paresthetica
  (2) Endocrine
    (a) Hypothyroidism
    (b) Diabetes
  (3) Toxic
    (a) Heavy metals
    (b) Solvents
    (c) Antiamebicides
    (d) Chemotherapy
    (e) Antibiotics
(d) Early peripheral nerve degeneration and regeneration

Interfering Factors
1. Conduction can vary with age; conduction is normally decreased in the elderly.
2. Pain can yield false results.
3. Electrical activity from extraneous persons and objects can yield false results.
4. The test is ineffective in the presence of edema, hemorrhage, or thick subcutaneous fat.

Patient Preparation
1. Explain the purpose and procedure of the test. There is a risk of hematoma if the patient is on anticoagulant therapy.
2. Sedation or analgesia may be ordered.

Patient Aftercare
1. If the patient has experienced pain or is in pain, provide relief.
2. Provide restful, relaxing activities. The patient may be exhausted if the examination time is lengthy.

Clinical Alert

1. When ordering the test, provide the examiner with all available pertinent information. The more data given, the more precise will be the interpretation of findings.
2. Enzyme levels that reflect muscle activity (AST, LDH, CPK) must be determined before testing because EMG will cause misleading elevation of these enzymes for up to 10 days.
3. Although it is rare, hematomas may form at needle insertion sites. Notify the physician if this occurs.

Electronystagmogram (ENG)

Normal Values
Normal vestibular–ocular reflex
Nystagmus accompanying head turning is expected

Explanation of Test
This study aids in the differential diagnoses of lesions in the brain stem and cerebellum, and unilateral hearing loss of unknown origin, and helps identify the cause of vertigo or ringing in the ears. Evaluation of the vestibular system and muscles controlling eye movement is based on measurements of the nystagmus cycle. In health, the vestibular system maintains visual fixation during head movements through *nystagmus*, the involuntary back and forth eye movement cause by the initiation of the vestibular–ocular reflex.

Procedure
1. The test is usually done in a darkened room, with the patient sitting or lying on an examination table.
2. If there is was in the ears, it should be removed prior to testing.
3. Five electrodes are taped to the face in locations around the eye.
4. During the study, the patient is asked to look at different objects, to open and close the eyes, and to change position.
5. Near the end of the test, air is gently blown into the external ear canal, first on the affected side. Water may also be used to irrigate the ears during the test.
6. Total examining time is one hour.

Clinical Implications
Prolonged nystagmus following a head turn is abnormal and can be caused by lesions of the vestibular or ocular system.

1. Cerebellum disease
2. Brain-stem lesion
3. Peripheral lesion occurring in the elderly, head trauma, and middle ear disorders
4. Congenital disorders

Interfering Factors
1. Test results are altered by an inability of the patient to cooperate, by poor eyesight, blinking of the eyes, and poorly applied electrodes.
2. Anxiety of the patient and some medications such as central nervous system depressants and stimulants and antivertigo agents can be the cause of false-positive test results.

Patient Preparation
1. Explain the purpose and procedure of the test. There is no discomfort or shock associated with the recording. There are no known risks.
2. No face makeup should be applied prior to testing.
3. Advise that no heavy meal should be eaten before the test and all caffeine and alcoholic beverages should be avoided for at least 48 hours before the test.
4. In most cases, medications such as tranquilizers, stimulants, or antidizziness medications are withheld for 5 days. However, a withholding check should be discussed with the attending physician.

Clinical Alert
1. The test is contraindicated in persons with pacemakers.
2. Water irrigation should not be done in persons who have perforated eardrums. However, a fingercot may be inserted into the ear canal to protect the middle ear.

Patient Aftercare
1. Allow the patient to rest comfortably for an hour before returning to his home or hospital room.
2. Nausea, vertigo, and weakness may be present for some time after the test is completed.

Electro-oculography (EOG)

Normal Values
2

1.80–2 is probably normal; values vary with laboratory methods used; bright light will cause the ratio to be larger.

Explanation of Test
This test of retinal function is used in the study of suspected hereditary and acquired degeneration of the retina. As a measurement of retinal function, the test serves primarily to complement electroretinography (ERG) by determining the functional state of retinal pigment epithelium, as in retinitis pigmentosa. This test determines the electrical potential of the eye at rest in both darkness and light. Normally, the potential between the front and back of the eye should grow as light is increased.

Clinical Implications

1. A value of 1.60 to 1.79 is probably abnormal; 1.20 to 1.59 is definitely abnormal; less than 1.20 is flat, based on normal values reported above. The outcome is usually reported as normal or abnormal.
2. The EOG ratio decreases in most retinal degeneration such as retinitis pigmentosa; this sometimes parallels the decrease on the ERG examination.
3. In Best's disease (congenital macular degeneration), the EOG is abnormal, but the ERG is normal.
4. In retinopathy due to toxins such as antimalarial drugs, the EOG may show abnormalities earlier than the ERG.
5. Supernormal EOGs have been noted in albinism and aniridia in which the common factor seems to be chronic excessive light exposure with resultant retinal damage.

Procedure

1. The patient sits in the examining chair.
2. Skin electrodes are placed in the inner and outer canthi of the eye, and an instrument similar to a bowl is used for adaptation. The results are recorded on a polygraph unit.
3. Two procedures are carried out. First, the patient is tested for 15 minutes in total darkness, and eye movement through a known angle is measured. Second, with the integrating sphere lighted, the patient is asked to move the eyes through the same angle, and the electrical potential is recorded.
4. Total examining time is 30 minutes.

Patient Preparation

1. Explain the purpose and procedure of the test.
2. No discomfort will be experienced

Patient Aftercare

No special aftercare is needed.

Clinical Alert

If fluorescein angiography (FA) and EOG are both ordered, the EOG must be done first because the eye must be dilated for the FA but not for the EOG. However, when an ERG and an FA are performed on the same day, the FA should be done first to avoid corneal edema caused by the corneal electrode used in ERGs. The waiting time between FA and ERG should be at least 2 hours.

Electroretinography (ERG)

Normal Values
Normal A and B waves

Explanation of Test
This test is used in the study of hereditary and acquired disorders of the retina, including partial and total color blindness (achromatopia), night blindness, retinal degeneration, and detachment of the retina in cases in which the ophthalmoscopic view of the retina is prohibited by some opacity, such as vitreous hemorrhage, cataracts, or corneal opacity. When these disorders exclusively involve either the rod systems or the cone systems to a significant degree, the ERG shows corresponding abnormalities.

In this test, an electrode is placed on the eye to obtain the electrical response to light. When the eye is stimulated with a flash of light, the electrode will record electric change that can be displayed and recorded on an oscilloscope. This test is indicated when surgery is considered in cases of questionable retinal viability.

Clinical Implications
1. Changes in ERG are associated with
   (a) Diminished response in ischemic vascular disease
       (1) Arteriosclerosis
       (2) Giant cell arteritis
   (b) Siderosis (poisoning of the retina when copper is imbedded intraocularly). This is not associated with stainless steel foreign bodies.
   (c) Drugs such as chloroquine or quinine that produce retinal damage (decreased ERG response).
   (d) Retinal detachment
   (e) Opacities of ocular media
   (f) Decreased response
       (1) Vitamin A deficiency
       (2) Mucopolysaccharidosis
2. Diseases of the macula do not affect the standard ERG. Macular disorder can be detected using a focal ERG.

Procedure
1. Eyes are propped open during the procedure.
2. The patient may be sitting up or lying down.
3. Topical anesthetic eye drops are instilled.
4. Bipolar cotton wick electrodes saturated with saline rest on the cornea.
5. Two states of light adaptation are used to detect rod and cone disorders along with different wavelengths of light to separate rod

and cone function. Normally, the more intense the light, the greater the electrical response.
   (a) Room light
   (b) Room darkened for 20 minutes, then a white light is flashed
   (c) Bright flash (in cases of trauma when there is vitreous hemorrhage, a much more intense flash of light must be used)
6. In infants and small children who are being tested for a congenital abnormality, chloral hydrate or a general anesthetic may be used.
7. Total examining time is 1 hour.

Patient Preparation
1. Explain the purpose and procedure of the test.
2. No discomfort is experienced; the electrode may feel like an eyelash in the eye.

Patient Aftercare
1. Caution the patient not to rub his eyes for 1 hour after testing to prevent accidental corneal abrasion.
2. Usually, anesthetic effects disappear in about 20 minutes.

Tests of Eye Function

Fluorescein Angiography (FA)

Normal Values
Normal retinal vessels, normal retina, normal choroidal circulation as seen in color photographs

Explanation of Test
The purpose of this test is to detect vascular disorders of the retina that may be the cause of poor vision. Fluorescein, a contrast substance, is injected intravenously over a 3-minute time period. Films of the eye taken by a special camera are studied to detect the presence of retinal disorders.

Procedure
1. A series of three drops is given at 5-minute intervals to dilate the pupil of the eye.
   (a) Complete dilatation occurs within 30 minutes of giving the last drop.
   (b) When dilatation is complete, a series of color photographs of both eyes is taken.
2. The patient sits with the head immobilized in a special frame in front of a fundus camera and indirect ophthalmoscope.
3. Fluorescein dye is slowly injected intravenously; the brachial vein is the site usually chosen.

4. Another series of photographs is taken as the dye flows through the retinal blood vessels (a period of approximately 3 minutes).
5. A final series of photographs is taken 15 to 60 minutes after the injection.

Clinical Implications
Abnormal results reveal

1. Diabetic retinopathy
2. Aneurysm
3. Hemorrhagic macular degeneration
4. Diabetic neovascularization

Patient Preparation
1. Determine whether the patient has any known allergies to medications or contrast substance.
2. Instruct the patient about the purpose, procedure, and side effects of the test. A legal consent form must be signed.
3. Some persons experience nausea for a short period after the injection.
4. Inform the patient that eye drops may sting or cause a burning sensation as they are instilled.
5. Advise the patient that pre-examination films are often taken to familiarize him or her with bright lights, necessity of fixation, and other aspects of the procedure.

Patient Aftercare
1. Educate the patient about color changes in the skin (yellow) and urine (bright yellow or green) that may be apparent for 36 to 48 hours after the test.
2. Advise the patient to wear dark glasses and not to drive while his or her pupils remain dilated (4–8 hours). During this time, persons are unable to focus on nearby objects and react abnormally to changes in light intensity.

Electrocardiography (ECG or EKG) (With Brief Description of Vector Cardiogram)

Normal Values
Normal positive and negative deflections in an ECG record (Fig. 15–1). One cardiac cycle is represented by the P wave, QRS complex, and T wave. Additionally, a Y wave may be observed. This cycle is repeated continuously. P = atrial depolarization; QRS = ventricular depolarization; T = ventricular repolarization/resting stage between beats; U wave = nonspecific recovery afterpotentials (Table 15–1).

(*text continues on page 882*)

TABLE 15–1.

Normal Measurements and Ranges of Components of
P–Q–R–S–T–U Cycle*

	P Wave		PR Interval		Q Wave Q% of R	
	Amplitude	Width	0.12 sec – 0.20 sec		Width	Depth
	Maximum	Maximum			Less than 0.04 sec	QR ratio
	2.5 mm	0.10 sec				
L₁						15% of R wave
L₂						20% of R wave
L₃					Up to 0.08 sec	25% of R wave
ᴬVR					Up to 0.08 sec	
ᴬVL					Less than 0.04 sec	25% of R wave
ᴬVF						
V₁					Up to 0.08 sec	
V₂						
V₃					Less than 0.04 sec	
V₄						
V₅						
V₆						

* For practical purposes, these are the upper and lower limits of the normal ECG. However, there are "gray zones," and variation from these limits may not necessarily imply abnormality.

Table 15–1.

Normal Measurements and Ranges of Components of
P–Q–R–S–T–U Cycle* (*Continued*)

QRS Interval	R-Wave Amplitude	ST Segment	T-Wave Amplitude	U-Wave Amplitude/Width
0.10 sec	Maximum to minimum	1 mm	1mm–5 mm	1.5 mm 0.24 sec
	5 mm–16 mm	Above or below		
		1 mm elevation		
		↓	↓	
	Less than +4 mm		Except in this lead (T is neg)	
	5 mm–13 mm Transverse heart			
	5 mm–21 mm Vertical heart	1 mm elevation		
	5 mm–27 mm	1 mm–2 mm depression	13 mm	
↓ 0.11 sec				
0.11 sec		2 mm–4 mm elevation		
↓	↓		↓	↓

(Ritota MC: *Diagnostic Electrocardiography, 2nd ed. Philadelphia, JB Lippincott, 1977*)

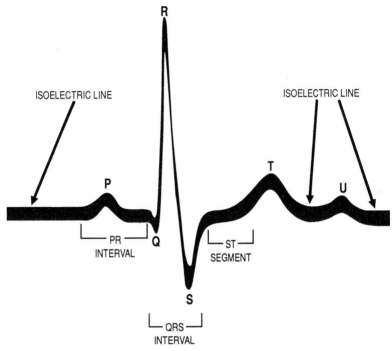

FIGURE 15–1.
Electrocardiographic components of the cardiac cycle. (After Phillips RE, Feeney MK: The Cardiac Rhythms, 3rd ed. Philadelphia, WB Saunders, 1990)

Mechanical contraction (systole) of a chamber follows its electrical depolarization. Muscular relaxation (diastole) follows chamber repolarization.

The paper grid permits measurement of height and depth and duration of complexes.

Waves

Capital letters refer to relatively large waves (over 5 mm), and small letters refer to relatively small waves (less than 5 mm).

1. The P wave is upright and represents *atrial* depolarization and the electrical activity associated with the original impulse from the sinus node and its subsequent spread through the atrial sinus.

    If P waves are present and of normal size, shape, and deflection, have normal conduction intervals to the ventricular complex, and demonstrate rhythmic timing variances between cycles, it can be assumed that the stimulus began in the sinoatrial node.

2. T_a wave is a deflection produced by atrial repolarization and is usually not seen in the 12-lead ECG.
3. The Q(q) wave is the first downward/negative deflection resulting from ventricular depolarization.
4. The R(r') wave is an upright/positive deflection resulting from ventricular depolarization.
5. The S(s') wave is the first downward/negative deflection that follows the first positive deflection.
6. The QS wave is a negative deflection that does not rise above the baseline.
7. The R^1 (r') wave is the second upward/positive deflection or the first positive/upward deflection during ventricular depolarization that follows the S wave. The negative deflection following the r' is termed the s'.
8. The T wave is a deflection produced by ventricular repolarization. There is a pause after the QRS complex, then a T wave appears. The T wave is a period of no cardiac activity, before the ventricles are again stimulated. It represents the recovery phase after contraction.
9. The U wave is a deflection (usually positive) following the T wave. It is thought to be caused by repolarization of Purkinje's (intraventricular) conduction system.

Intervals
1. The R–R interval is the distance between two successive R waves. In normal rhythms, the interval in seconds (or fractions of seconds) between two successive R waves, then divided into 60 seconds, will give the heart rate per minute.
2. The P–P interval will be the same as the R–R interval in normal sinus rhythm. The responsiveness of the sinus node to physiologic activity (exercise, rest, respiratory cycling) results in a rhythmic variance of P–P intervals.
3. The PR interval measures conduction tone and includes time for atrial depolarization and normal conduction delay in the atrioventricular node, and terminates with the onset of ventricular depolarization. It is the period from the start of the P wave to the beginning of the QRS complex. This interval represents the time taken for the impulse to traverse the atria and atrioventricular node and reach the ventricles and initiate ventricular depolarization.
4. The QRS interval is ventricular depolarization time and represents the electrical impulse as it travels from the atrioventricular node through the bundle branches to the Purkinje fibers and into the myocardial cells. Normal waves consist of an initial downward deflection (Q wave), a large upward deflection (R wave), and a second downward wave (S wave). It is measured from the onset of the Q wave (or R if no Q is visible) to the termination of the S wave.

Segments and Junctions

1. The PR segment is normally isoelectric and is that portion of the ECG tracing from the end of the P wave to the onset of the QRS complex.
2. The J junction is the point at which the QRS complex ends and the ST segment begins.
3. The ST segment is that part of the ECG from the J point to the onset of the T wave. Elevation or depression is determined by comparing its location with that portion of the baseline between the end of the T wave and the beginning of the P wave or when related to the PR segment. This segment represents the period between the completion of depolarization and onset of repolarization (recovery) of the ventricular muscles.
4. The TP segment is that portion of the ECG record between the end of the T wave and the beginning of the next P wave. It is usually isoelectric.

Voltage Measurements

1. Upright deflection voltage is measured from the upper part of the baseline to the peak of the wave.
2. Negative deflection voltage is measured from the lower portion of the baseline to the nadir of the wave.

Explanation of Test

An ECG is a recording of the electrical impulses that stimulate the heart to contract and is an indicator of dysfunctions that influence the conduction ability of the myocardium. The ECG is helpful in diagnosing the following: origins of and monitoring of pathologic rhythms; myocardial ischemia and infarction; atrial and ventricular hypertrophy; conduction delay of atrial, atrioventricular nodal, and ventricular electrical impulses; and pericarditis. It is also helpful in the diagnosis of systemic diseases that affect the heart; determination of effect of cardiac drugs, especially digitalis and antiarrhythmic agents; disturbances in electrolyte balance, especially potassium and calcium; and evaluation of cardiac pacemaker function.

The heart is unique among the muscles of the body in that it possesses the properties of automatic impulse formation and rhythmic contraction. Formation and conduction of these electrical impulses produces weak electrical current that spreads through the body. Each normal heart beat begins with an electrical impulse that originates in a specialized area of the right atrium called the sinus or sinoatrial node. This island of tissue serves as a battery for the heart and normally discharges an electrical force 60 to 100 times a minute in rhythmic fashion. Because the sinoatrial node controls the rate of the heart beat, it is designated as the pacemaker. (All areas of the myocardium have the potential ability to serve in this capacity, but they assume this role only under abnormal circumstances.) The original impulse is transmitted through the heart in an orderly path. When it reaches the muscles, contraction occurs. After contracting, the muscles rest and recover while the chambers fill with blood. The next impulse normally arrives when filling is complete and contraction again occurs. The combined periods of sequential atrial and ventricular contraction (depolarization) and recovery (repolarization) constitute the cardiac cycle.

Recording provides a continuous picture of the electrical activity during a cycle. Heart cells are charged or polarized in the resting state but when electrically stimulated, they depolarize and contract. The body fluid is an excellent conductor of electrical current. When the depolarization (stimulation) process sweeps in a wave across the cells of the myocardium, the electrical current generated is conducted to the body's surface where it is detected by special electrodes placed on the patient's limbs and chest. An ECG tracing also shows the voltage of the waves and the time duration of both waves and intervals. By studying the amplitude and time duration of the waves and intervals, disorders of impulse formation and conduction can be diagnosed.

Recording the Electrical Impulses

1. Because the electrical forces extend in several directions at the same time, a comprehensive view can be obtained only if the flow of current in different planes is recorded.
2. Twelve leads are used simultaneously.
   (a) Limb leads—I, II, III, AVL, AVF, AVR—record events in the frontal plane of the heart.
   (b) Chest leads—V_1, V_2, V_3, V_4, V_5, and V_6—record a horizontal view of the heart's electrical activity.
3. Occasionally, an esophageal lead, which is swallowed, is used to supply additional information.

ECG versus Vectorcardiogram

The vectorcardiogram, like the ECG, records the electrical forces of the heart. The major difference between these methods is the way in which these forces are displayed. A vectorcardiogram records a *three-dimensional* display of the heart's electrical activity, whereas the ECG shows activity in a *single plane.*

The three planes of the vectorcardiogram are as follows:

1. Frontal plane (combines the Y and X axes)
2. Sagittal plane (combines the Y and Z axes)
3. Horizontal plane (combines the X and Z axes)

Briefly, the two records of the heart's electrical activity may be compared as follows:

ECG	Vectorcardiogram
Records electrical forces as deflections on a scale	Depicts electrical forces as vector loops, thereby showing the *direction* of electrical activity
Recorded in the frontal and horizontal planes of the body	Recorded on the frontal, horizontal, and sagittal planes of the body
	The term *vector* is used to indicate the direction of electrical activity.

Clinical Implications of ECG

1. The ECG *does not* depict the actual mechanical state of the heart or function of the valves.
2. An ECG may be quite normal in the presence of heart disease unless the pathologic process disturbs the electrical forces.
3. Final conclusions from an ECG should be done only with a full knowledge of the clinical status of the patient.
4. Abnormalities of an ECG are categorized into five general areas:
   (a) Heart rate
   (b) Heart rhythm
   (c) Axis or position of the heart
   (d) Hypertrophy
   (e) Infarction/ischemia
      Certain specific abnormalities in these areas are typical of
      (1) Pathologic rhythms
      (2) Conduction system diseases
      (3) Myocardial ischemia
      (4) Myocardial infarction
      (5) Hypertrophy of the heart
      (6) Pulmonary infarction
      (7) Electrolyte changes in potassium, calcium, and magnesium
      (8) Pericarditis
      (9) Effects of drugs (*e.g.*, digitalis and quinidine)

Clinical Implications of Vectorcardiogram

1. The vectorcardiogram is more sensitive than the ECG in the diagnosis of myocardial infarction, but it is probably not more specific.
2. Vectorcardiography is more specific than the ECG in the assessment of hypertrophy or dilatation of the ventricles of the heart.
3. Intraventricular conduction abnormalities from a variety of causes can possibly be differentiated.

Clinical Considerations

1. If chest pain is experienced on a lead run, it should be noted on the involved ECG strip.

2. The presence of a pacemaker and whether or not a magnet was used in testing should be indicated.
3. Reproducibility of precardial lead placement should be ensured by proper positioning and by marking the position on the chest wall in ink when indicated.

Procedure

The following steps apply to both the ECG and the vectorcardiogram:

1. The patient is placed in a supine position on a table, bed, or couch. The recording can also be done during exercise or the patient can be ambulatory, in which case a Holter device is used for a continuous 24- to 48-hour recording.
2. The skin is prepared (including shaving if there is excess hair) by the application of contact paste or prejelled discs.
3. Electrodes are placed anywhere on the four extremities and on specific sites of the chest. The right leg is the ground.
4. The operator then records the ECG through machine setting.
5. The test may take only a few minutes or as long as 24 to 48 hours if a Holter recording has been ordered.

Interfering Factors

1. Race: ST elevation with T-wave inversion is more common in blacks, but disappears with maximal effort exercise.
2. Food intake: High carbohydrate content, especially, is associated with an intracellular shift of K potassium in association with intracellular glucose metabolism. Nondiagnostic ST depression and T wave inversion may occur.
3. Anxiety: Episodic anxiety and hyperventilation are associated with PR prolongation, sinus tachycardia, and ST depression with or without T-wave inversion. It may be due to an imbalance of autonomic nervous system input.
4. Deep respiration: Position of the heart in the chest becomes more vertical with deep inspiration and horizontal with deep expiration.
5. Exercise/movement: Strenuous exercise before the test can produce a misleading record. Muscle twitching by the patient can alter the record.
6. Position of heart within thoracic cage: There may be anatomic cardiac rotation in both horizontal and frontal planes.
7. Position of precardial leads: Inaccurate placement of the bipolar chest leads and the interchange of right and left arm and left leg electrodes will affect test results. In normal persons, lead reversal will produce the typical ECG findings of dextrocardia in frontal plane leads and can mimic a myocardial infarction pattern.

8. A leftward shift in the QRS axis occurs in conjunction with excess body weight, ascites, and pregnancy.
9. Age: At birth and infancy, there is hypertrophy of the right ventricle because, in the fetus, the right ventricle performs more work than the left ventricle. T-wave inversion in leads V_{1-3} persists into the second decade of life and into the third decade in blacks.
10. Sex: Slight ST segment depression is present in women.
11. Chest configuration and dextrocardia: In this congenital anomaly, the precordial leads must be recorded over the right side of the chest.
12. Many medications affect ECG results, such as severe drug overdose, especially when barbiturates are involved.
13. The serious effects of electrolyte imbalance on the ECG can be seen in clinical considerations of individual electrolytes (*e.g.*, potassium, on p. 286, and calcium):

Increased Ca^{2+}—prolonged PR
                      shortened QT
Decreased Ca^{2+}—prolonged QT alters electromechanical coupling

Patient Preparation

1. Explain the purpose and procedure of the test and the factors that interfere with an accurate test result, emphasizing that it is painless and that there is no current flow to the body. It must be kept in mind that a resting ECG (without stressing the heart) is no more than a one-minute record of the electrical activity of the heart.
2. The patient must be completely relaxed in order to ensure a satisfactory tracing.
3. Ideally, the person should be at rest for 15 minutes prior to ECG recording, with no recent meal, and no smoking for 30 minutes before testing.

Patient Aftercare

In patients with heart symptoms, it is important that the limitations of an ECG are recognized. A normal ECG does not rule out coronary artery disease or areas of ischemia in the heart. On the other hand, an abnormal ECG in and of itself does not signify heart disease.

It is most important that the patient does not become a cardiac "cripple" solely on the basis of an ECG. On the other hand, a person may receive unwarranted assurance of the absence of heart disease solely on the basis of the normal ECG. Patients need to know that the resting ECG is usually normal for patients with only angina and no other heart problems. It can, however, provide evidence of prior heart damage of which the person may not have been aware.

Clinical Alert

1. When an ECG shows changes indicating ischemia, injury, or infarction, these changes must be reported and acted upon immediately to increase myocardial blood supply and reduce oxygen demand.

    (a) When ECG changes representing stages of ischemia, injury, or necrosis are seen and symptoms of possible myocardial infarction appear, the first concern is to correct the imbalance between myocardial oxygen supply and demand.

      (1) Give ordered nitroglycerine to dilate blood vessels.
      (2) Sedate with narcotics to limit size of infarction.
      (3) Administer calcium channel blocks to relieve coronary spasm.
      (4) Start oxygen to increase supply of oxygen.
      (5) Give beta-blocking drugs to slow rapid heart rate.
      (6) Give antiarrhythmics to correct abnormal rhythms.
      (7) Give constant reassurance to reverse panic.

    (b) Monitoring for cardiac rhythm disturbances is essential. Lethal dysrhythmias (atrioventricular blocks) and ventricular tachyarrhythmias require immediate intervention.

2. Serious diagnostic error can be made if the ECG is not interpreted in the light of history and signs and symptoms.

3. When looking at the ECG interpretation of heart position, keep in mind that this refers to a pattern resulting from electrical spread of excitation. The electrical axis is not synonymous with the anatomic position of the heart.

Signal-averaged Electrocardiogram (SAE)

Normal Values
Normal QRS complexes and ST segments

Explanation of Test
The signal-averaged ECG (SAE) is a noninvasive, convenient, and relatively inexpensive tool used for the identification of patients at risk for malignant ventricular dysrhythmias. It has proved useful in stratifying risk of arrhythmia in select groups of high-risk patients, particularly

the post-myocardial infarction population. The SAE may be used as a precursor to electrophysiologic studies.

During the later phase of the QRS complex and ST segment, the myocardium produces high-frequency, low-amplitude signals termed *late potentials*. These late potentials have been noted to correlate with areas of delayed activation through the myocardium, a condition that produces reentrant forms of ventricular tachycardia. Myocardial disorders that may result in regions of delayed conduction include myocardial infarction, nonischemic dilated cardiomyopathy, left ventricular aneurysm, and some forms of healed ventricular incisions (*e.g.*, tetralogy of Fallot).

Indications
The SAEs are performed to evaluate the etiology of ventricular dysrhythmias.

1. Differentiation of reentrant from other forms of ventricular tachycardia
2. Precursor to electrophysiology studies

Procedure
A modification of body-surface ECG, the SAE uses computer processing techniques to provide signal averaging, amplification, and filtering of electrical potentials. Electrodes are placed on the abdomen and anterior and posterior thorax. The signals received are converted to a digital signal. A typical QRS complex is used as a template against which subsequent cycles are compared. Ectopic or noisy cycles are eliminated from evaluation. Typically, several hundred beats are averaged to analyze the late potential. The collection period is usually completed within 20 minutes. Optimal recordings are obtained if the patient is placed in a comfortable position, the patient is quiet during recording, electrodes are properly applied, and interference (*e.g.*, from other electrical equipment) is eliminated.

Interfering Factors
1. There is an increased time required for collection of beats to be analyzed with slow heart rates and frequent ventricular ectopics. Additionally, patient movement, including talking and restlessness due to pain or full bladder, delays obtaining adequate information.
2. Bundle branch block can interfere with averaging of impulses.
3. It does not provide information on efficacy of antiarrhythmic drug therapy.
4. Late potentials are not present in all patients with ventricular tachycardia.
5. Ventricular pacing prolongs ventricular activation time, thus obscuring late potentials (atrial pacing, even at rapid rates, does not alter late potentials).

Clinical Implications
1. Predictive value for ventricular tachycardia in patients who have had a myocardial infarction and patients with chronic coronary artery disease.
2. Late potentials are a stronger predictor of sudden death or sustained ventricular tachycardia than ventricular dysrhythmias on a 24-hour ambulatory recording.
3. Evidence that late potentials are associated with ventricular tachycardia is the finding that in successful antiarrhythmic surgery late potentials were abolished.
4. Patients with late potentials have an incidence of 17% of sustained ventricular tachycardia or sudden death (versus 1% incidence in patients without late potentials). The incidence is even greater when in conjunction with decreased ejection fraction.
5. It is used in screening of patients to determine those who should undergo electrophysiologic (EP) study for evaluation of risk of ventricular tachycardia.
6. It is useful in diagnosing unexplained syncope (later identified as ventricular tachycardia on EP study).

Holter Continuous ECG Monitoring

Normal Values
Normal sinus rhythm

Explanation of Test
Holter monitoring is a method of continuously recording the ECG on magnetic tape for prolonged periods of time. Twenty-four and 48 hours are the common recording durations. The tape recorder is a battery-powered device with very slow (3¾ in/min) tape speeds and is small enough to be carried on a strap over the shoulder or around the waist. Two ECG channels recorded simultaneously are graphic records of the electrical impulses that are generated by depolarization and recovery of the myocardium.

The Holter recorder is equipped with a digital clock, which is synchronized to the tape recorder, and this allows for accurate time marking. The patient carries a diary in which he or she enters any symptoms experienced during the monitoring period, his or her activity status, and the time at which the symptoms occurred. When a symptom occurs, the patient pushes an event-marker button on the recorder. This marks one of the channels for easy recognition during playback.

A 24-hour recording contains over 100,000 cardiac cycles. Playback and tape analysis are done at 60, 120, or 180 times real time. The tape may be rapidly analyzed by computers that can provide summaries of heart rates, frequency of premature atrial or ventricular complexes, coupling intervals, and other variations in pattern. Another method of scanning the tapes superimposes each QRS complex on the preceding complex. This makes any variations in the QRS contour become apparent, and arrhythmias are found in this way. In either method of scanning, segments of the tape recording can be reproduced on ECG paper. The diary the patient kept is also used to see if there is a correlation between symptoms and ECG findings. A report is then produced that provides ECG strips and a summary of arrhythmias that were found during the recording.

Indications for Holter Monitoring
Holter monitors are placed on patients for a variety of reasons.

1. They are used for documentation of a suspected rhythm disturbance. The recording, along with the diary the patient keeps, can be used to correlate rhythm disturbances with patient symptoms of syncope, palpitations, chest pain, lightheadedness, and unexplained dyspnea. If these symptoms have no obvious cause, a Holter recording can be used to detect the presence of unsuspected arrhythmias in patients, such as supraventricular and ventricular tachycardias, bradycardia-tachycardia in patients with sick sinus syndrome, and other ventricular and supraventricular arrhythmias.
2. The recording of the onset and termination of a rhythmic disturbance may provide insight into the electrophysiologic mechanisms responsible for the arrhythmia.
3. Pacemaker functioning can be checked.
4. The efficiency of antiarrhythmic therapy and lack of toxicity can be documented in a Holter report.

Procedure
1. The patient is placed in a supine position on a table.
2. The skin is prepared. This involves shaving the chest, if necessary, cleansing the skin with alcohol, and reddening the skin by rubbing it with gauze or similar rough material. These preparations are important for good electrode contact.
3. Electrodes are placed: two for each channel, and one ground. Electrodes are positioned over bony prominences. The two negative electrodes are placed on the manubrium, whereas their corresponding positive electrodes (for the two channels) are placed in the V_1 and V_5 positions.
4. Loose wires are taped down and everything is secured. The recorder is started and calibrated. The patient is then free to pursue all activities except bathing.

5. After the required (24 to 48 hours) amount of time, the recorder is stopped and the electrodes are removed from the patient's chest.
6. The tape is scanned by a technician.

Interfering Factors
1. Incomplete diary and/or event: Marker not pushed during symptoms
2. Interference caused either mechanically or by patient scratching electrode area

Clinical Implications
Abnormal results include

1. Rhythm disturbances such as
   (a) Supraventricular tachycardia
   (b) Ventricular tachycardia
   (c) Bradycardia–tachycardia in patients with sick sinus syndrome
   (d) Other ventricular and supraventricular abnormal rhythms
2. Hypoxic/ischemic changes

Phonocardiography

Normal Values
Normal heart sounds

Explanation of Test
This test graphically records the occurrence, timing, and length of sounds of the heart cycle. Heart murmurs can be both visualized and accurately timed. Sounds that originate in the heart and large vessels are recorded from the body's surface and correspond to what is heard through a stethoscope. This diagnostic technique involves the electronic detection, amplification, and recording of cardiac sounds. A specially designed microphone, placed on the patient's chest, picks up the low-frequency cardiac vibrations for amplification and recording. The phonocardiograph is recorded simultaneously with carotid pulse, ECG, and respiration.

Phonocardiography provides information about underlying hemodynamics that is not obtainable through physical examination. It also provides a permanent objective record of events with which subsequent comparison may be made. It is useful in detecting abnormalities in valvular function and can be used in conjunction with other cardiovascular monitoring techniques to assess specific portions of the cardiac cycle such as systolic ejection time and pre-ejection time. It is a valuable teaching aid.

Procedure
1. The test should be done in a quiet room.
2. The patient is placed on a table in a supine position with pillows under his or her head.
3. Electrocardiographic leads are placed on all four extremities, and standard lead two (2) is recorded throughout the procedure. A neck cuff for the indirect carotid pulse is secured in place and inflated to 15 to 20 mm Hg. Microphones (small, round, bell-like devices) for sound recording are placed over the pulmonary area and apex.
4. The patient is instructed to inhale deeply and to allow most of the air to escape from the lungs. At this point in expiration, the patient is instructed to suspend breathing for a few seconds without tensing the muscles. Then the patient is asked to breathe quietly through the mouth, and a recording is made.
5. The pulmonary area microphone is then removed and placed over the aortic area and a recording is made during held expiration.
6. Next, the neck cuff is removed and the patient's upper body is lowered to one pillow. The upper microphone is placed over the left sternal border in the fourth intercostal space, and a jugular pulse recording is made during held expiration.
7. The patient is turned on the left side and another recording is made.
8. Total examining time is about 30 minutes.

Clinical Implications
Phonocardiography can be used to augment, but not replace, auscultation.

Stress/Exercise Testing
(Graded Exercise Tolerance Test)

Normal Values
Negative when patient has no significant symptoms, arrhythmias, or other ECG abnormalities and when patient reaches 85% of maximum heart rate predicted for age and sex

Explanation of Test
This test measures the efficiency of the heart during a dynamic exercise stress period on a motor driven treadmill or ergometer. It is valuable in diagnosing ischemic heart disease and in investigating physiologic mechanisms underlying cardiac symptoms such as angina, dysrhythmias, inordinate rise in blood pressure, and functional valve incompetence. Exercise testing is also done to measure functional capacity for work, sport, or participation in a rehabilitation program, and to estimate response to medical or surgical treatment. Additionally, the func-

tion of physiologic responsive pacemakers (*e.g.*, upper rate limit) can be evaluated.

The systolic blood pressure normally increases with exercise, and the diastolic normally remains essentially unchanged. Stress exercise testing takes place in a controlled environment that requires a low temperature (68°) and low humidity.

Procedure

There are many different types of stress tests in use today. Most of them include the following steps:

1. Recording electrodes are placed on patient's chest (see description of ECG) and attached to a monitor. A blood pressure recording device is also used.
2. While the patient walks on a motor-driven treadmill or pedals an ergometer if walking is not possible, a computerized ECG and heart monitoring device records the performance. The patient walks at progressive speeds and elevations in an effort to increase heart rate and workload.
3. The ECG, heart rate, and blood pressure are recorded at rest. The patient is asked to report any symptoms such as chest pain or shortness of breath that are experienced during the test. Normal persons are symptom-free at submaximal efforts. At peak or maximal efforts, symptoms expected in normal persons are exhaustion, fatigue, and sometimes nausea or dizziness.
4. The patient is stressed in stages. Each stage consists of a predetermined level of the treadmill (in miles per hour) and an elevation of the treadmill (in percent grade).
5. The ECG, heart rate, and blood pressure are constantly monitored for any signs of abnormality and any unusual symptoms such as intolerable dyspnea, chest pain, and severe cramping (claudication) in the legs.
6. Usually, a 3-minute and 10-minute recovery stage are recorded while the patient is seated. The test is terminated if there are ECG abnormalities, fatigue, weakness, abnormal blood pressure changes, or intolerable symptoms.
7. Commonly used criteria for stopping a test include attainment of
   (a) Maximum possible performance
   (b) End point based on emergence of signs or symptoms indicative of a disease process
   (c) Predetermined end point such as 85% of age-related maximal heart rate, arbitrary work load (one that raises heart rate to 150), or diagnostic ECG change
8. Total examination time is about 30 minutes; however, the patient should plan to be in the laboratory for 1 to 1½ hours.

Clinical Implications

Abnormal responses to exercise testing include

1. Alterations in blood pressure such as
   (a) Failure of systolic pressure to rise
   (b) Progressive fall in systolic pressure
2. Alterations in heart rate such as
   (a) Excessive tachycardia
   (b) Bradycardia
3. Changes in ECG such as
   (a) Ischemic deviation of ST segments; can be depression or elevation
   (b) Dysrhythmia, ventricular tachycardia, multifocal ventricular premature contractions, atrial tachycardia, atrioventricular block greater than first degree
   (c) Failure of physiologic pacemakers to convert to atrioventricular block when upper rate limit is reached.
4. Ectopic rhythms, either ventricular or supraventricular, must be considered abnormal responses but not necessarily ischemic responses.
5. Ischemic ST-segment displacement greater than 0.1 mm of 80-msec duration or longer is the most common abnormality found. Men aged 40 to 59 who develop ST depression during exercise that is not present at rest have five times the risk of developing overt coronary heart disease as do men who do not develop ST depression.
6. Unusual symptoms such as
   (a) Anginal pain
   (b) Inappropriate breathlessness
   (c) Faintness, dizziness, lightheadedness, confusion
   (d) Claudication, leg pain
7. Unusual signs such as
   (a) Cyanosis, pallor, mottling of skin
   (b) Cold sweat, piloerection
   (c) Ataxia, glassy stare
   (d) Gallop heart sounds
   (e) Valvular regurgitative murmur
   (f) Abnormal cardiac impulse

Interfering Factors

Common causes of false-positive exercise ECG responses include

1. Left ventricular hypertrophy
2. Digitalis
3. ST-segment abnormality at rest
4. Hypertension
5. Valvular heart disease

6. Left bundle branch block
7. Anemia
8. Hypoxia
9. Vasoregulatory asthenia
10. Lown–Ganong–Levine syndrome

Patient Preparation

1. Explain the purpose and procedure of the test. No food, coffee, or cigarettes are allowed prior to testing. Water is allowed.
2. A legal consent form must be signed.
3. Have the patient wear flat walking shoes or tennis shoes; bedroom slippers are not suitable. Men should wear gym shorts or loose-fitting light trousers. Women should wear a bra, a short-sleeved blouse that buttons in front, and slacks, shorts, or pajama pants (no one-piece undergarments or panty hose).
4. Some medications should be discontinued before testing. Beta-adrenergic blocking agents such as propranolol should be reduced or tapered gradually before stopping. Check with the laboratory for specific protocols for digoxin, isordil, and other drugs.

Patient Aftercare

The patient should not leave the premises until the physician is satisfied that pretest baseline levels of heart rate, blood pressure, and ECG waveform have been met.

Clinical Alert

Stress/exercise testing can be risky for patients with chest pain of recent onset or attacks of angina several times a day. The test is usually not given to these patients at this time, but it may be rescheduled in 4 to 6 weeks.

Cardiac Catheterization and Angiography
(Angiocardiography, Coronary Arteriography)

Normal Values

Normal heart and coronary arteries
Normal pressure and cardiac output
Normal percentage of oxygen saturation

Explanation of Test

This is a method of studying and diagnosing defects in the chambers of the heart, its valves, and its vessels by inserting arterial and venous catheters carrying contrast material into the right and left sides of the heart. As the catheters are advanced, fluoroscopy and rapidly taken x-ray pictures projected on TV monitors show the action of the heart under study. The injected dye or contrast medium provides definition of the cardiac structures. Each coronary artery is filmed as well. An oscilloscope near the TV monitor shows the patient's heart rate, rhythm, and pressures.

Coronary arteriograms are highly useful in diagnosing heart disease, determining the extent of damage, diagnosing congenital abnormalities, identifying cardiac structure and function before surgery, and measuring pressures within heart chambers and great vessels. They are also useful in determining cardiac output (using contrast dilution, thermodilution, and Fick method), and obtaining blood samples directly from the heart to measure oxygen content of blood and oxygen saturation.

Cardiac catheterization with angiography is indicated in patients with angina, incapacitating chest pain, syncope, valvular and ischemic disease; in patients with cholesteremia and familial heart disease who are experiencing chest pain; in patients with abnormal resting or exercise ECGs; in patients who have had cardiac revascularization with recurring symptoms; in young patients with a history of coronary insufficiency and ventricular aneurysm; and in patients with coronary neurosis who can be assured that their arteries are normal. This test can be done in the acute stage of myocardial infarction, and, if necessary, the patient can be sent to surgery immediately.

Although it is an examination with some risks, it is highly accurate as a diagnostic technique.

Procedure

1. The test is usually done in a darkened room.
2. To decrease fear of the procedure, the patient is continuously told what is being done.
3. The patient lies on an x-ray table; ECG leads are attached to the chest. During the procedure, the patient will be turned from side to side and may be asked to exercise (optional) to evaluate heart changes of any kind during activity. Atrial pacing can also be done as part of a cardiac catheterization in persons who cannot walk (paraplegics) or cannot use a treadmill. In these instances there is a sequence of events in which the heart is stressed, a rest period follows, measurements are taken, the heart is paced again, and another rest period follows.
4. The catheterization procedure is done under sterile conditions. The skin is prepared with an antiseptic solution. A local anesthetic is injected before making small incisions for the insertion of the catheter into an artery and vein. (Incisions are not always made.) Catheters are gently pushed into the heart and great vessels.

5. The patient may be able to watch all procedures on a screen of brightened heart image with "instant replay"; usually the screens are placed so that the examiner can see them.
6. After x-ray films have been taken at all angles, catheters are removed and skin incisions (if any) are closed with a few stitches. A sterile pressure bandage is applied. The procedure takes about 1 hour, or a little longer if the patient is stressed with exercise or drugs.

Clinical Implications
1. Abnormal results are as follows:
    (a) Advancing catheters will reveal altered intracardiac pressures
    (b) Injecting contrast will reveal altered ventricular contractibility and blocked coronary arteries
    (c) Analyzing blood oxygen will confirm cardiac or arterial irregularities
2. Abnormal pressures are indicative of
    (a) Valve stenosis or insufficiency
    (b) Left and/or right ventricular failure
    (c) Idiopathic hypertrophic subaortic stenosis (IHHS)
    (d) Rheumatic fever
3. Abnormal blood oxygen samples are indicative of
    (a) Congenital or acquired shunting of blood
    (b) Septal defects
    (c) Leakage or abnormal sequential circulation of blood through the heart
4. When contrast is injected into the ventricles, abnormal size, bulging, ejection fractions, aneurysms of the heart, leaks, stenosis, and altered contractibility of the heart can be detected.
5. When contrast is injected into coronary arteries, abnormal circulation through coronary vessels can be detected.

Patient Preparation
1. Explain the purpose, procedure, benefits, and risks of the test. A legal permit must be signed before the examination. Ascertain allergies, especially the potential for a reaction to contrast components.
2. The patient should be fasting for at least 3 hours before testing. Check with the physician about administration of routine, scheduled medications such as cardiac drugs or insulin.
3. Analgesics, sedatives, or tranquilizers are administered before the examination.
4. Have the patient void before going to the catheterization laboratory.
5. Allow the patient to wear dentures.

6. The patient should be aware that he or she will be asked to breathe deeply and cough during the test, and that he or she will experience certain sensations that are common to the procedure.
   (a) Catheter insertion, through antecubital or groin sites, may produce significant sensations of pressure with introduction.
   (b) A slight shock (like hitting the "funny bone") might be felt if the nerve lying next to the artery is touched, and a tiny bump in the neck is experienced as the catheter is inserted and pushed through the artery into the chest. Neither of these sensations is very painful.
   (c) When contrast is injected, a pumping sensation (with palpitations and warm flashes) lasts 30 to 60 seconds. The injection causes skin vessels to vasodilate, and warm systemic blood rises to the skin surface, returning again as the heat fades.
   (d) Nausea, vomiting, headaches, and cough are side effects that some patients may experience.
   (e) Angina may occur with exercise or contrast injection. This is relieved with nitroglycerine or narcotics.

Patient Aftercare
1. Bed rest is maintained for 2 to 12 hours after the test. Time limits are based on the exact procedure used, the physician's desires, and patient status. Elevation of the head may be restricted to 20 degrees to 45 degrees. The patient may be allowed to turn from side to side. Encourage movement of uninvolved extremities.
2. Check vital signs and dressing for swelling or bleeding. Some discomfort at the puncture site can be expected.
3. Antibiotics may be administered before or after the examination to prevent infection.
4. Encourage fluids after testing.
5. Keep the affected extremity extended (not elevated) and immobilized with a sandbag to decrease discomfort and bleeding. Apply ice and/or a sandbag to the site, if ordered. Analgesics, if ordered, can be administered for pain at insertion sites.
6. Sutures, if used, are removed in 7 days.

Clinical Alert
1. This procedure is contraindicated in patients with gross cardiomegaly.
2. Complications that can occur include
   (a) Dysrhythmias
   (b) Allergic dye reactions (evidenced by urticaria, pruritus, and conjunctivitis)

   (c) Thrombophlebitis of cutdown vein
   (d) Infection at cutdown site
   (e) Pneumothorax
   (f) Hemopericardium
   (g) Embolism
   (h) Tears in liver, especially in infants and children (results from poor technique)
   (i) Excessive bleeding at the site
3. Notify attending physician if there is any increased bleeding, a drastic fall or increase in blood pressure, or a decrease in peripheral circulation.
4. When angiography is performed, the following equipment should always be available for complications:
   (a) Resuscitation equipment
   (b) DC defibrillator
   (c) External pacemaker
   (d) Electrocardiographic monitor
   (e) Cardiac drugs (epinephrine, norepinephrine, isoproterenol, lidocaine, bretylium, atropine)

Electrophysiology Procedure (EP; His Bundle Procedure)

Normal Values
Normal conduction intervals
Normal refractory periods
Normal recovery times
No arrhythmias induced

Explanation of Test
An electrophysiology procedure (EP) is an invasive test used in the diagnosis and treatment of ventricular arrhythmias; it is similar to cardiac catheterization. The difference lies in the fact that an EP study measures the electrical conduction system of the heart through solid electrode catheters instead of the open-lumen catheters used to measure pressures. The electrode catheters are almost always inserted into veins because of the greater risk in the arterial system. Using fluoroscopy as a guide, the catheters are advanced into the right atrium and the right ventricle. Besides an x-ray monitor that shows the location of the catheter, there is also a physiologic monitor that shows the patient's surface ECG leads as well as intracardiac electrograms from the catheters (Fig. 15–2).

FIGURE 15–2.
His bundle electrogram. Note electrophysiologic events are presented in relation to the surface electrocardiogram. (After Phillips RE, Feeney MK: The Cardiac Rhythms, 3rd ed. Philadelphia, WB Saunders, 1990)

An EP study is highly useful in diagnosing diseases of the heart's conduction system and to point the direction toward optimal treatment. Besides measuring control resting values for the patient, the electrode catheters are also used to pace the heart in an attempt to induce any arrhythmia that may be giving the patient problems. If the patient is on medication to control dysrhythmias, the EP study can determine how well the medication is working by how easily the arrhythmia can be induced. This is in contrast to the trial-and-error method in which there is no way to know that a particular drug is ineffective until that drug has failed.

An EP procedure is indicated for patients to differentiate disorders of impulse formation (supraventricular versus ventricular rhythms). Electrophysiology studies are also used to provide diagnostic insight into the etiology and mechanism of conduction disorders (atrioventricular block, bypass tracts). Electrophysiology studies are often used as a workup for syncope or sick sinus syndrome. Finally, EP studies are indicated in testing the effectiveness of an antiarrhythmic drug.

Procedure
1. The test is usually done in a darkened room.
2. To decrease fear of the procedure, the patient is continuously told what is beind done.
3. The patient lies on an x-ray table; ECG leads are attached to the chest.
4. The procedure is done under sterile conditions. The skin is prepared with an antiseptic solution. Usually one or two sites are chosen (right and/or left antecubital area, right and/or left groin). The sites chosen depend on where in the heart the catheters will have to be placed and also upon the patency and size of the patient's veins. A local anesthetic is injected into the skin before a needle is inserted into the vein. (An incision is usually not needed.) The catheters are gently pushed into the heart.
5. Baseline values are recorded. Some baseline values require pacing. (For example: sinus node recovery times require pacing the atrium until the sinus is fatigued and then measuring the time it takes to recover.)
6. After baseline values have been determined, pacing is used to induce arrhythmias. If a sustained arrhythmia is induced, an attempt will usually be made to terminate the arrhythmia by pacing. If the patient's cardiovascular system cannot compensate for the arrhythmia so that the patient starts to lose consciousness, an external cardioverter/defibrillator will be used to terminate the arrhythmia.
7. A quiet conversation is continuously held with the patient in order to assess his or her level of consciousness.
8. After the procedure, the catheters are removed and a sterile pressure bandage is applied (no stitches).
9. The procedure takes a minimum of 1 hour for a repeat study of drug effectiveness to a maximum of 4 hours to evaluate a complex arrhythmia such as the pre-excitation syndromes. Each drug has certain effects that must be anticipated during the loading phase—for example, hypotension with quinidine and procainamide and abdominal cramping with quinidine, and pain in vein used for phenytoin as well as a state of "happy drunkeness." Intravenous saline is used to support blood pressure.

Clinical Implications
Abnormal results of an EP procedure will reveal

1. Conduction intervals that are longer or shorter than normal
2. Refractory periods that are longer than normal

3. Recovery times that are prolonged
4. The induction of an arrhythmia that would not have been induced in a normal subject with an identical protocol

Abnormal results are indicative of

1. Long AH intervals indicate disease in the atrioventricular node if sympathetic and vagal influences have been eliminated.
2. Long HV intervals indicate disease in the His–Purkinje's system.
3. Prolonged sinus node recovery times indicate sinus node dysfunction, such as sick sinus syndrome.
4. Prolonged sinoatrial conduction times can indicate sinus exit block.
5. A wide or split His bundle deflection indicates that a His bundle lesion is present.
6. The induction of sustained ventricular tachycardia by using one or two premature stimuli confirms the diagnosis of recurrent ventricular tachycardia.

Patient Preparation
1. Explain the purpose and procedure of the test. A description of possible sensations that may be experienced, even more than procedural steps, will help to reduce anxiety. The patient should be aware that he or she might experience certain sensations that are common to the procedure.
   (a) A peculiar sensation in the arm and neck as the catheter is advanced. The sensation feels like a "bug crawling."
   (b) Palpitations or heart racing may be felt when the heart is paced.
   (c) Lightheadedness or dizziness may be experienced. This is not a common sensation to be ignored. The patient must tell the nurse or doctor any time he or she feels lightheaded or dizzy.
2. Obtain a legal, signed permit before the procedure. The patient needs to know the reason for the study and that there is a high degree of suspicion that he or she may be susceptible to a dangerous tachycardia. Patients who are not in full agreement that this method is the best approach to the patient's problem should not be tested. Be certain that the patient has been informed of the major risks and benefits of the study.
3. Blood samples for potassium level (and drug levels if the effectiveness of a drug is to be determined) are drawn.
4. A standard 12-lead EKG should be taken before the test.
5. Nothing can be consumed for at least 3 hours before testing.
6. Analgesics, sedatives, or tranquilizers are not usually given before the procedure, but *nothing* can be consumed for at least 3 hours before testing.
7. Have the patient void before going to the EP laboratory.
8. Allow the patient to wear dentures.

Patient Aftercare

1. Bed rest with no leg bending is maintained for 6 to 8 hours after the procedure.
2. Check vital signs, distal perfusion, and the insertion site for swelling or bleeding, every 15 minutes × 4, 30 minutes × 2, and every 1 hour × 2.
3. Keep the affected extremity extended (not elevated) to decrease discomfort and bleeding. Analgesics, if ordered, can be administered for pain at the insertion site.
4. Keep the head of bed elevated less than 45 degrees for 6 hours.
5. Encourage side-to-side turning and range of motion of uninvolved limbs.
6. Infection control. If an electrode catheter is left in place for sequential studies, it is sutured in place and covered with a sterile dressing. Scrub the site and length of the catheter with a povidone-iodine solution, dry with sterile sponges, and recover with a sterile dressing.

Clinical Alert

1. Contraindications: Although the unstable clinical setting of acute myocardial infarction may limit detailed and prolonged EP procedures, brief but clinical useful procedures can be safely performed.
2. Observe the patient for complications that can occur, which include
   (a) Hemorrhage, particularly from the femoral site when the femoral artery has been punctured
   (b) Thromboembolism: thrombosis at the puncture site or thromboembolism from the catheter
   (c) Phlebitis
   (d) Hemopericardium
   (e) Atrial fibrillation, usually transient
   (f) Ventricular fibrillation
3. Notify the attending physician if there is any bleeding, fall in blood pressure, a decrease in distal perfusion, or life-threatening arrhythmia. Be aware of drug studies carried out and monitor for effects of that pharmaceutical.
4. If the series of tests is successful, reinforce to the patient that, with compliance to prolonged drug therapy, there should be no recurrence of tachycardia.
5. When an adverse reaction to a drug is found, ECG monitoring is the major requirement for the elimination time of the drug.

Transesophageal Echocardiography (TEE)

Normal Values
Essentially normal position, size and movement of heart valves and heart chamber walls

Explanation of Test
This test allows optimal ultrasonic visualization of the heart when traditional transthoracic (noninvasive) echocardiography fails or proves nonconclusive. A miniaturized high-frequency ultrasound transducer is mounted on an endoscope and coupled with an ultrasound instrument to display and record the ultrasound images. Controls on the handle of the endoscope allow remote manipulation of the transducer tip. Various images of heart anatomy are displayed by rotating the tip of the instrument and by varying the depth of insertion.

Because the exam is somewhat uncomfortable for the patient, TEE is not appropriately for use as a screening test. Indications for TEE include

1. A suboptimal transthoracic echocardiogram, generally due to
   (a) Patient obesity
   (b) Trauma to the chest wall
   (c) Presence of chronic obstructive pulmonary disease
2. When results of traditional transthoracic echocardiography do not agree or correlate with clinical findings.

Procedure
1. The purpose and procedure, benefits and risks of the test are explained.
2. An informed consent must be signed.
3. The patient must be NPO for approximately 8 hours prior to the procedure to reduce the risk of aspiration.
4. Premedications such as analgesics or sedatives may be ordered. Check with laboratory for specific instructions.
5. A topical anesthetic is applied to the pharynx. A bite block is generally used to prevent accidental damage to the equipment.
6. The patient is placed in a left lateral decubitus position while the lubricated endoscopic instrument is inserted to a depth of 30 to 50 cm. The patient is asked to swallow in order to facilitate placement of the device.
7. Manipulation of the ultrasound transducer provides a number of image planes. Generally, scan time is limited to a maximum of 15 minutes.

Clinical Implications

Abnormal values help to diagnose

1. Heart valve diseases
2. Pericardial effusion
3. Congenital heart disease
4. Endocarditis
5. Intracardiac tumors or thrombi
6. Left ventricular dysfunction

Patient Preparation

Explain purpose and procedure of the test. See procedure items 1 through 4 listed on page 906.

Clinical Alert

This test is somewhat uncomfortable for the patient. Although risks of this procedure have not been extensively investigated in the United States, it is believed that the potential for complications is minimal when performed by an experienced operator.

NONINVASIVE VASCULAR TESTS

Noninvasive vascular diagnostic techniques provide anatomic and physiologic information about the arterial and venous vasculature. Several types of examinations can be used to establish vessel patency in order to localize obstruction, assess collateral circulation, and determine the need for angiography. These test results provide complementary data used to confirm diagnoses, predict the potential outcomes of therapeutic interventions, monitor therapy, and followup the progress of vascular disease. These noninvasive tests are usually done before invasive diagnostic procedures are attempted. Keep in mind, however, that the reported results and values of noninvasive vascular studies must be correlated with a thorough history and physical examination. These noninvasive tests are not meant to replace a proper assessment.

Because of the many different kinds of testing modalities in use, the caregiver needs to become familiar with those laboratory policies, results, and reports in use at their specific facility.

Blood flow studies can be grouped into three main categories: (1) tests for arterial disease, (2) tests for venous disease, (3) tests for extracranial cerebrovascular disease. The noninvasive tests are usually performed by trained vascular technologists. Testing methods incorporate

Doppler instruments, duplex scanners, spectral analyzers, and plethysmography techniques. (Doppler ultrasound is addressed in Chap. 13.)
Of these, duplex scanning is the most widely used noninvasive testing
method. It combines high-resolution and real-time imaging, together
with Doppler flow spectrum analyses. Real-time imaging permits
scanned vessels to be visualized on a screen as they function. The Doppler component measures and characterizes blood flow within these
vessels. Direction and velocity of blood flow are depicted on a traced
signal report (see Table 15–2). Color flow Doppler, known as angio-

TABLE 15–2.
Results of Methods Used in Arterial and Venous Duplex Scans

Arterial Evaluation Using Combined Modalities of Duplex Scans

Real-Time Imaging Component	Doppler Component	Diagnosis
Vessel lumen narrowed	Higher velocity of blood through stenotic vessel(s) Increased turbulence	Arterial stenosis
Unable to image vessel; thrombus noted in vessel	No Doppler flow	Arterial occlusion

Venous Evaluation Using Combined Modalities of Duplex Scans

Real-Time Imaging Component	Doppler Component	Diagnosis
Vein cannot be compressed; thrombus noted in vessel	No flow in vein, no variation with respiration; no venous flow augmentation when limb is compressed proximally or distally to the obstruction	Venous occlusion or deep venous obstruction
Flow is reversed; venous valves are incompetent	Venous flow reversed when limb is compressed proximal to the transducer	Vascular damage Vascular insufficiency

(Rudolph D: Duplex scanning. Am J Nurs: *123–124, April, 1990)*

dynography, provides a colored image rather than a grey-scale image and depicts the direction and the velocity of blood flow in varying shades of blue and red (see Chap. 13).

The duplex scan is useful, but not limited to, the following testing situations:

1. Scanning carotid arteries for the presence and location of plaques or stenosis in persons with asymptomatic cervical bruits, or who exhibit a history of cerebrovascular accident (strokes) or transient ischemic attacks
2. Obtaining measurements of localized dilation or aneurysms in the extremities (behind the knees)
3. Confirmation of suspected arterial stenosis in the arms and legs
4. Evaluation of arterial bypass grafts
5. Scanning arteries and veins for decreased blood flow, due to obstruction
6. Scanning abdominal arteries for evidence of rejection of renal transplants
7. Evaluation of arms and legs for deep vein thrombosis or venous insufficiency
8. Scanning for source of emboli in the presence of pulmonary embolism

Plethysmography techniques use various transducers to record volume dimensional changes of a finger, toe, arm, leg, eye, or other part of the body. Transducers can be categorized as impedance, air, water, and photo-electric.

Several tests can be done to detect peripheral artery disease. A listing follows (not all-inclusive).

Noninvasive Tests for Detecting Peripheral Artery Disease

Test	Normal or Expected Values
Arterial Doppler examination of upper and lower extremities	Multiphasic signal with prominent systolic component and one or more diastolic sounds
Limb pressures obtained with Doppler and calculated to obtain indexes	Ankle pressure equal to or greater than arm pressure
	Proximal thigh pressure of 20–60 mm Hg or more above arm pressure. Less than 20–30 mm Hg pressure gradient between adjacent levels of measurement in leg.

Test	Normal or Expected Values
Toe and finger pressures with photoplethysmography technique	Normal toe pressure of at least 80% of ankle pressure or greater; finger pressure usually 80% of wrist pressure or greater
Treadmill exercise to assess collateral circulation and functional impairment with or without ECG monitor; measurement of ankle pressure with a Doppler before and after treadmill exercise	No drop in ankle pressure; treadmill exercise test normal
Reactive hyperemia test—ankle pressure before and after 3-min application of proximal thigh cuff, using segmental pressure/Doppler technique	Ankle pressure after cuff release falls no more than 35% below preischemia value and returns to baseline within 1 min.
Duplex scannings	Widely patent artery without stenosis or plaque apparent (based upon waveform analysis and clear image)
Pulse volume recordings	Normal sympathetic vasoconstrictive reflex with attenuation of pulse amplitude in response to deep breath indicative of intact sympathetic vasomotor innervation

Clinical Alert

1. Measurement of ankle systolic pressure is the single most valuable noninvasive test for assessing the arterial circulation in the lower limb. An ankle brachial index of .005 with a characteristic triphasic arterial signal rules out arterial insufficiency as a cause for a leg ulcer. Venous ulcers have a greater chance of healing if the arterial inflow is normal.

2. The pressures help to identify obstructive disease involving the pedal arch and digital arteries. When ankle pressures are falsely elevated because of noncompressible calcified arteries, toe pressure measurement is necessary.

Abnormal test results may indicate various arterial diseases or arterial status such as the following:

1. Arteriosclerosis
2. Arterial insufficiency and digital ischemia

3. Diabetic ischemia differentiated from neuropathy
4. Reynaud's phenomenon/disease
5. Arterial reconstruction results
6. Healing potential for skin lesions or amputation sites
7. Acute embolic phenomena
8. Thoracic outlet syndrome
9. Vascular trauma
10. Vasculogenic impotence
11. Iatrogenic arterial injury
12. Aortic iliac arterial injury
13. Aneurysms or arterial dilations
14. Abdominal aortic aneurysms

Clinical Responsibilities for Peripheral Arterial Blood Flow Studies

Patient Preparation

1. Explain the purpose, method of testing, and benefits of the tests. Explain that there are no known risks. Emphasize that the examinations are painless.
2. Help the patient to relax. A tense and nervous patient may provide inaccurate readings.
3. If the patient is in pain, the pain should be controlled before the patient is tested.
4. Explain that studies must be performed at rest for baseline values.
5. Because nicotine constricts vessels, no smoking is permitted 2 hours prior to testing. Emphasize that all patients with arterial disease should discontinue smoking.

Clinical Alert

1. Tests cannot usually be successfully performed on a cold, cyanotic, pale, or waxen-appearing extremity because adequate blood flow may not be present.
2. Notify the technologist if the patient is in isolation. If the patient is too ill to be transported to the vascular laboratory, notify that department. Some tests can be done at bedside.
3. Diabetics can develop a medial artery calcification that reduces elasticity of vessels and eventually prohibits compression of these vessels.

Clinical Implications of Abnormal Ankle Brachial (ab) Index (A Peripheral Aterial Blood Flow Study)

Normal ankle pressures are the same or higher than the arm pressure. With peripheral vascular disease, a peripheral resistance (arterial obstruction) increases and ankle pressures decrease. Different levels of ischemia cause different symptoms, and the symptoms vary from patient to patient. Diabetes complicates the peripheral vascular problems. In such persons, ankle pressures are not always indicative of the severity of the problem.

0.96 and above—normal	No significant peripheral vascular occlusion in the legs at rest. If there is leg pain, other causes must be found.
0.85–0.95	Mild ischemia; usually mild or no symptoms; claudication after walking distances
0.51–0.84	Moderate ischemia. Persons usually contact healthcare system because of leg cramping after walking (*claudication*). Trophic skin changes become clinically evident.
0.26–0.50	Severe ischemia; increased claudication, decreased walk distance; may experience rest pain with dependent rubor as the values numbers decrease into the .30 category.
0.25 and below	Gangrene or ischemic ulcers are often present. For limb salvage, patient will need bypass or amputation.

Clinical Alert

In persons with ischemia or an ankle brachial index of .30 or less, caregivers must be careful to protect the foot because tissue breakdown can occur very rapidly. Pain medication must be administered promptly to these patients. Frequently, they are in too much pain to do self-care. Moreover, they cannot tolerate leg elevation. Many can hardly bear to stay in bed at night.

Noninvasive Tests for Detecting Peripheral Venous Disease

The primary modality for venous studies is duplex scanning (see p. 908). A listing of common noninvasive test modalities and normal or expected values follows (not all-inclusive).

Test	Normal or Expected Values
Venous Doppler assessment involves examination of veins in upper and lower extremities. Using a hand-held duplex Doppler and scanner, veins are studied at posterior tibial, popliteal, superficial, and femoral levels to detect presence of obstruction in the lower extremities; at the radial, brachial, axillary, and subclavian veins to rule out upper extremity deep venous obstructions.	Blood flow spontaneous and phasic with respiration in patent veins. Augmentation of Doppler signal with distal compression and proximal release maneuver in limb.
Plethysmographic studies determine venous outflow using various transducers. Studies are done to identify incompetent values in deep or superficial venous systems and to determine refilling of calf veins after exercise or manual compressions.	Normal venous refilling time (20 sec or above) and competent values

Abnormal test results may indicate various venous diseases or venous status such as the following:

1. Acute deep vein thrombosis
2. Postphlebotic syndrome
3. Superficial thrombophlebitis
4. Primary as differentiated from secondary varicose veins
5. Incompetent perforator
6. Source of emboli in pulmonary embolism

Clinical Responsibilities for Peripheral Venous Blood Flow Studies

Patient Preparation

1. Explain the purpose, method, benefits, and risks (none known) of the test.
2. Stress that no pain is involved in testing and no needles or catheters are inserted.
3. Use measures to promote relaxation. Tenseness will result in inaccurate outcomes.
4. Pain should be controlled before the patient goes to the testing department.

Clinical Alert

1. Notify the testing laboratory if the patient is in isolation.
2. Test can be done at bedside if assessment reveals the patient is too ill to transport.
3. A cold extremity and vasoconstriction inhibit the examination.

Noninvasive Tests for Detecting Extracranial Cerebrovascular Disease

Noninvasive vascular/direct need tests can establish the presence of cerebrovascular disease. High-risk stroke-prone patients, diabetics, and those with hypertension or cardiac disease can be screened for carotid vessel disorders.

Testing modalities include duplex scans and Doppler. A list of common, noninvasive modalities follows (not meant to be all-inclusive):

Testing Method	Normal or Expected Values
Duplex scan of carotid arteries shows presence or absence of plaque. Spectral analysis shows stenosis of artery.	A normal image similar to oblique view on contrast arteriogram of carotid artery bifurcation with no occlusion or calcification; nonturbulent arterial blood flow; absence of plaque and/or stenosis
Transcranial Doppler ultrasound evaluates the intracranial vessels by recording blood flow velocity measurements. It is used to detect arterial spasm, stenosis, and/or arteriovenous malformations with collateral pathways. A transducer probe, using conduction gel is placed temporally, transoccipitally, and transorbitally (over the eye) to transmit flow patterns.	Normal blood flow of intracranial arteries

Abnormal test results may indicate some of the following:

1. Extracranial occlusive disease with asymptomatic carotid bruits
2. Cause of amaurosis fugax (brief episode of total blackout of vision in one eye)
3. Plaques and vessel wall irregularities in carotid arteries

4. Cause of transient ischemic attacks
5. Upper extremity pulse deficits
6. Cerebrovascular accident
7. Reversible neurologic ischemic deficit; lasts longer than transient ischemic attack
8. Vertebrobasilar insufficiency
9. Arterial spasms
10. Intracranial arterial stenosis
11. Arteriovenous malformations and/or collateral pathways within the cranium

Clinical Responsibilities for Carotid Extracranial Cerebrovascular Blood Flow Studies

Patient Preparation

1. Explain the purpose of the test and that assessment of cerebral blood flow is based on an *indirect* evaluation of carotid artery blood flow. There are no known risks, except that in oculoplethysmography there is a 3% risk of conjunctival hemorrhagic irritation. Inform the patient that tests are painless.
2. Assess the range of motion or back problems. The patient must be able to remain on his or her back for the exam.
3. Help the patient to relax. A nervous patient may produce inaccurate test results.
4. Oculoplethysmograph examinations are not done on patients with lens implants, systolic blood pressure over 200, allergies to local anesthetic, history of detached retina, recent eye surgery, or infection.
5. The tests are painless. There is no physical preparation. However, psychological support may be necessary. Testing time is less than 30 minutes.

Clinical Alert

1. Some persons are not candidates for direct neck carotid study because of abnormal neck size (too large) and abnormal anatomy.
2. Notify the testing laboratory if the patient is in isolation, is confused, has dyspnea, or has back problems.

Clinical Implications of Abnormal Spectral and Duplex Scan Scores

1. Normal: 1%–15% reduction in diameter; not hemodynamically significant
2. Mild stenosis: 16%–49% reduction in diameter

3. Moderate stenosis: 50%–75% reduction in diameter; hemodynamic significance determined positive or negative by oculopneumoplethpmography
4. High-grade stenosis: >75% reduction in diameter
5. Significance of abnormal values depends on whether the patient shows symptoms. With evidence of stenosis, the findings are not clinically significant unless the stenosis is over 75%, even without stenosis.

MAGNETIC RESONANCE IMAGING (MR, NMR); MRI, MRF, MRS, AND MRA

Normal Values
Normal relaxation times, spin densities, flow velocities, and pulse and echo frequencies. These parameters are different for every type of test.

Explanation of Test
Magnetic resonance testing comprises several methodologies: MR imaging (MRI); MR blood flow scanning (MRF); and MR spectroscopy (MRS). Magnetic resonance imaging studies anatomic structures with differing water content. Magnetic resonance angiography (MRA) uses magnetic resonance imaging technique to study the vascular tree (likened to noninvasive angiography). Magnetic resonance blood flow scanning studies physiologic measurements, and MRS studies chemical components (Table 15–3).

These noninvasive methods of fluid-filled soft-tissue study, as well as the study of structural dynamics of molecules, produce cross-sectional images of the anatomy by placing patients in strong magnetic fields and bombarding them with radio waves. The super-conducting magnet circles around the body, causing the hydrogen nuclei in the body to align themselves to the magnetic field. The hydrogen nuclei emit their own signals, which are converted to computerized images. These images are based on body water content. The hydrogen atom is most commonly measured in these studies because it is the most abundant atom on the human body and has the highest sensitivity to nuclear resonance. Water is composed of hydrogen and oxygen, and human tissue is about 70% water.

The MR techniques are used primarily to image the body to differentiate diseased tissue from healthy tissue, to study the condition of blood vessels and determine blood flow, and, in proton basic spectroscopy, to evaluate pyruvate, phosphate, water, fat, and lactic acid metabolism. These studies are helpful in detecting ischemia and infarctions, in determining location of thrombi and viability of transplants, in following patient after administration of antineoplastic agents, and

TABLE 15–3.
Major Measurement Parameters of Magnetic Resonance Testing

Parameter	Measurement	Related To
Relaxation Times		
T_1 = longitudinal relaxation time	A time constant related to the interchange of energy between a spin and its environment	Tissue type such as muscle, brain, liver, spinal cord, and bone marrow
T_2 = transverse relaxation time	A time constant related to the interchange of energy between spins	
Flow and Perfusion		
Q = blood volume flow rate	Signals of blood flow and perfusion measured in milliliters per minute	Physiologic movement
Nuclear Density		
W = larmor frequency	A characteristic frequency at a given magnetic-field strength at which magnetic resonance occurs for a particular nucleus.	Tissue type such as cartelagic, soft tissue, heart, etc.
Proton Chemical Shifts		
	Concentration of specific molecular constituents	Concentrations of water, iron, sodium, etc.

in differentiating benign from malignant masses and degenerative brain diseases from psychiatric disorders. Magnetic resonance imaging has superior value in imaging the central nervous system, especially the brain. The gray matter in the brain has about 15% more water than white matter and can be differentiated in MRI. Other uses include cardiac evaluation; diagnosis of thrombi lesions; imaging of liver, brain, and spinal cord; and pelvic imaging. It may have potential for diagnosing Alzheimer's disease.

Procedure
Two procedures are in common use: body imaging and blood flow scanning.

Procedure for Body Imaging

1. The patient lies down on a narrow pallet that slides in and out of the cylindrical magnetic core.
2. If a head scan is done, a clear plastic cylinder containing antenna is placed around the head.
3. Local surface coil antennas are in use that improve the resolution to very restricted areas of the body, such as the knee and spine.
4. A monotonous clanging noise produced by the machine can be heard by the patient.
5. It is necessary for the patient to be completely still during imaging.
6. Total examining time is 60 to 90 minutes (10 to 60 minutes with fast imagers).

Procedure for Blood Flow Scanning of the Extremities

1. The patient will be lying down during the test and will remain as motionless as possible.
2. The limb to be examined is extended and rests on the system's examining table. Prior to testing, a finger plethysmograph is applied. Reference points on the leg are identified by a light marker: ankle, knee, and hip. The fingertips, wrist, and elbow are selected on the arm. These landmarks are stored by the computer system.
3. The examination table rotates to accommodate upper and lower extremities. The patient's limb is moved into and out of the flow cylinder during each extremity study.
4. If complete extremity studies (leg, arm, finger) are to be performed, usually the leg study will be done first.
5. Flow data are computed and projected on a graphics monitor and recorded on a computer-generated printout. Information is stored digitally for recordkeeping purposes and evaluation. Data can be recorded for a single vessel or for limb as a whole. To normalize for variations in limb size, limb circumference is measured every 5 cm and blood flow is measured in terms of milliliters per minute per 100 cc of distal tissue.
6. Flow monitoring data are acquired in 25 seconds for a single cross section of an extremity. A multiple cross-sectional study of both limbs requires about 30 minutes.

Interfering Factors

1. *Body Imaging*
   Respiratory motion causes severe artifacts in abdominal and thoracic imaging.
2. *Blood Flow Scanning in the Extremities*
   Unusually large legs or bulky casts may prevent access into the scanner.

Clinical Implications of Body Imaging
Changes in waveforms, signal intensity, and spectral peaks are associated with

1. Coronary occlusion
2. Myocardial infarction
3. Ischemia of cardiac and skeletal muscle and bone
4. Significant atherosclerosis
5. Ectopic thyroid tissue
6. Spinal lesions
7. Brain iron deposits in neurodegenerative disease
8. Cerebral infarcts, tumors, hemorrhages and vascular abnormalities
9. Anaerobic metabolism
10. Infection sites
11. Anatomic malformation of the vascular tree
12. Pelvic and urogenital lesions

Clinical Implications of Blood Flow Scanning
Changes in blood flow in the extremity are associated with

1. Anatomic malformations
2. Atherosclerosis
3. Aneurysm
4. Thrombus
5. Embolism
6. Bypass grafts
7. Endarterectomies
8. Endovascular procedures
9. Shunt placements

Clinical Alert

1. Contraindications to examination are pacemakers, surgical clips, metalic implants, neuro- or musculoskeletal stimulators, and patients on life-support equipment and infusion pumps.
2. Patients who are critically ill or medically unstable are not usually candidates for upper body or whole body scanning because it is impossible to monitor cardiac rhythm and other signs inside the scanner unless special equipment is available.
3. Pregnancy is usually a contraindication because the long-term effects of magnetization are not known at this time. Examination of extremities (MRF) using low magnetic fields, however, may be permitted.
4. Although MRI is a service offered by many radiology departments, it is not an x-ray. No radiation is involved in this technology.

Patient Preparation for Body Imaging

1. Explain the purpose, procedure, and risks. Major potential risks are tissue heating and heating of metallic prosthetic implants from absorption of energy. No adverse effects have been reported, the standard examination does not require contrast media, and there is no radiation risk. No tooth discomfort is felt in metal fillings.
2. Assess for contraindications to testing, and obtain a relevant history regarding implanted heart valves, surgical and aneurysm clips, and internal orthopedic screws and rods.
3. Help the patient to remove anything metal, such as dental bridges and appliances, credit cards, keys, hairclips, shoes, belts, jewelry, or clothing with metal fasteners.
4. Those who are to have body imaging may experience a closed-in feeling that can be avoided if the patient keeps his eyes closed during the entire test. Explain to these persons that it is better not to eat a large meal at least 1 hour before testing to reduce physiologic demands in the body and possible emesis that could occur in claustrophobic persons.
5. The patient should be helped to relax and remain as motionless as possible during testing.

Patient Preparation for Blood Flow Scanning

1. Patients who are having blood flow testing should abstain from alcohol, nicotine, caffeine, and iron prescription drugs, and testing should be done 2 hours after meals to avoid unexpected vasoconstrictions or dilation. No smoking should be permitted before the test. The patient is asked to rest supine 10 minutes before the test.
2. Same as 1, 2, 3, and 4 in body imaging and as appropriate for extremity to be scanned. It is much less restrictive than full body imaging. There are also fewer restrictions concerning metal in and on the patient.

Patient Aftercare

No special aftercare is needed.

Special Pediatric Considerations for MR Testing

Pediatric uses of MR testing are as follows:

1. Age, ability to understand and cooperate, physical condition, and reasons for testing must be considered
2. Body imaging. Most of adult information applies. Tranquilizers and modified restraints may be employed in selected cases.
3. Blood flow in extremities. Simple restraints may be used to restrict motion of arms or legs. No tranquilizers or sedatives may be given because blood flow will be affected.

Magnetic Resonance Angiography (MRA)

Normal Values
Standard spin echo pulse sequences in conjunction with electrocardiographic gating. Images are acquired in end diastole and end systole and electronically subtracted so that only the flow signals are displayed.

Explanation of Test
MRA creates a projection image that looks like a traditional x-ray-angiogram after injection of contrast media. Rapidly flowing blood normally produces little or no MR signal and generally appears dark, providing natural contrast between blood and vascular structures. For this reason, intravenous injection of a contrast material is *not* necessary for imaging the vascular system with magnetic resonance.

Procedure
1. Test is performed in the MRI department
2. Methodology is the same as that used in MRI and MRF and differences depend upon the examination site.

Clinical Implications
Abnormal test results such as magnified MR signals are associated with the following conditions:

1. Plaque hemorrhage
2. Content of arteriosclerotic plaque
3. Vascular malformations
4. Embolus
5. Thrombus
6. Stenosis/Occlusion
7. Infection
8. Graft/angioplasty/atrioventricular fistula patency
9. Arterial calcification

Patient Preparation
Same as for MRI and MRF. Depends upon examination site.

Patient Aftercare
Same as for MRI and MRF. Depends upon examination site.

Clinical Alert
Like MRI/MRF, the procedure depends upon body part to be examined.

BIBLIOGRAPHY

Bandyk D: Postoperative surveillance of infrainguinal bypass. Surg Clin North Am 70: 1990

Basmajiar JV: Muscles Alive: Their Functions Revealed by Electromyography, 4th ed. Baltimore, Williams & Wilkins, 1978

Berk JL, Sampliner JE (eds): Handbook of Critical Care, 3rd ed. Boston, Little, Brown & Co, 1990

Bernstein EF (ed): Noninvasive Diagnostic Techniques in Vascular Disease. St. Louis, CV Mosby, 1985

Boldridge D: Clinical significance of free floating venous thrombi. J Vas Surg II: 1990

Bushong SC: Magnetic Resonance Imaging. St. Louis, CV Mosby, 1988

Callow A: Current status of vascular grafts. Surg Clin North Am 62: 1982

Cohn ML: Low-frequency magnetic field technology: Quantifying spinal range of motion. Arch Physical Med Rehabil 70(6):455–457, June, 1989

Coburn KL, Hudson–Sullivan C, Hunaly J: High-tech maps of the brain. Am J Nurs 888(11):1500–1503, November, 1988

Dubin D: Rapid Interpretation of EKGs. Tampa, FL, C.O.V.E.R. Co., 1974

ECG: Rapid ECG Interpretation Patient Care Flow Charts. Darien, CT, Roche, Miller & Fink Corp, 1974

Edmonds JH: Electrocardiography in Urgent Situations. Philadelphia, Lea & Febiger, 1988

Ellestad MH: Stress Testing Principles and Practice, 2nd ed. Philadelphia, FA Davis, 1984

Fahey VA et al: Advances in diagnostic testing for vascular disease special studies. Cardiovasc Nurs 25(3):13–18, May/June, 1989

Flom B et al: Effects of preparatory information of a myleogram on patient's expectation and anxiety level. Patient Ed Counsel 14(20):115–126, October, 1989

Foster RR, Hunsberger MM, Anderson JJT: Family-Centered Nursing Care of Children. Philadelphia, WB Saunders, 1989

Gallen IR (ed): Noninvasive cardiac diagnosis. I. Med Clin North Am 64:1–146, 1980

Garrow IR: Indices of adiposity. Rev Clin Nutr 53(8):697–706, 1980

Greenspon AJ: Effects of atrial pacing on signal averaged ECG. Am Heart J 1:29–34, January 1990

Grossman W (ed): Cardiac Catheterization and Angiography, 2nd ed. Philadelphia, Lea & Febiger, 1980

Hagan AD, Demaria AN: Clinical Application of Two-Dimensional Echocardiography and Cardiac Doppler, 2nd ed. Boston, Little, Brown & Co, 1989

Hatle L, Angelson B: Doppler Ultrasound in Cardiology: Physical Principles and Applications. Philadelphia, Lea & Febiger, 1982

Heiken JP: Manual of Clinical Magnetic Resonance Imagery. New York, Raven Press, 1986

Holmes RL: Computer-assisted quanitation of coronary artery stenosis. Radiol Technol 60(1):37–41, September/October, 1988

Holt JA et al: Automated rapid assessment of surfactant and fetal lung maturity. Lab Med 21(6):359–362, June, 1990

Johnson EW (ed): Practical Electromyography, 4th ed. Baltimore, Williams & Wilkins, 1980

Jones NL, Campbell EJ: Clinical Exercise Testing, 2nd ed. Philadelphia, WB Saunders, 1982

Kinney MR, Packa DR, Dunbar SB: AACN's Clinical Reference for Critical-Care Nursing, 2nd ed. New York, McGraw–Hill, 1988

McCauley RGK: Pediatric imaging: Reassessing the clinical options. Diagn Imag: 82–91, March, 1986

Mannick J: Advances in Surgery, vol 19. Chicago, Year Book Medical Pub, 1986

March K: Transcranial Doppler sonography—Noninvasive monitoring of intracranial vasculature. J Neurosci 22(2):113–116, April, 1990

Milnor W: Hemodynamics. Baltimore, Williams & Wilkins, 1989

Monticco LM, Hill KM: EP studies: When they're called for, what they reveal. RN S2(2):54–55, February, 1989

Moser DK, Woo MA, Stevenson WG: Noninvasive identification of patients at risk for ventricular tachycardia with the signal-averaged electrocardiogram. AACN Clinical Issues in Critical-Care Nursing (1)1:79–86, May 1990

Niedermeyer E, Lopes da Silva F (eds): Electroencephalography: Basic Principles, Clinical Applications and Related Fields. Baltimore, Urban and Schwarzenberg, 1982

Phillips RE, Feeney MK: The Cardiac Rhythms: A Systematic Approach to Interpretation, 3rd ed. Philadelphia, WB Saunders, 1990

Plankey ED, Knohf J: Prep talk: What patients need to know about magnetic resonance imaging. Am J Nurs 90(1):27–28, January, 1990

Race GJ (ed): Laboratory methods/diagnostic procedures. In Spittell JA, Jr(ed): Practice of Medicine, Vol 2. Hagerstown, MD, Harper & Row, 1978

Raines J, Traad E: Noninvasive evaluation of peripheral vascular disease. Med Clin North Am 64(2):283–304, 1980

Robes RS, Cohen AM: Magnetic resonance imagery and spectroscopy in study of cardiovascular disease. J Vasc Surg 2:354, 1985

Rudolphi DM: Duplex scanning. Am J Nurs 123–124: April, 1990

Rutherford R: Vascular Surgery, 2nd ed. Philadelphia, WB Saunders, 1984

Schmitt DD, Towne JB: Magnetic resonance imaging and the vascular surgeon. In Haimovici's Vascular Surgery: Principles and Techniques. Norwalk, CT, Appleton and Lange, 1989

Schmitt DD: The Magnetic Resonance Imaging Scan: Patient Information Booklet. Washington, DC, National Institutes of Health, Clinical Centers Communications, 1987

Seaton D: The patient with peripheral arterial occlusive disease. Nurs Clin North Am 12: 1977

Shahrokhi F, Chiappi K, Young R: Pattern shift visual evoked responses. Arch Neurol 35(2):65–71, 1978

Spiegel MB: Electromyoneurography. Am Fam Physician 119–130: November 18, 1978

Squires N, Donchin E, Squires K et al: Biosensory stimulation: Inferring decision-related processes from the P300 component. J Exp Psychol (Hum Percept) 3:299–315, 1977

Stoner EK: Electromyography and nerve conduction studies. In Spittell JA, Jr (ed): Practice of Medicine, vol. 2. Hagerstown, MD, Harper & Row, 1978

Teasley D: Don't let cardiac catheterization strike fear in your patient's heart. Nursing 12(3):52–56, 1982

Tye TL et al: Transesophageal echocardiography. Journal of Diagnostic Medical Sonography 316–321, 1989

Weisberg J: Doppler today. Appl Radiol Nuclear Med 9(1):100–109, 1980

PRENATAL DIAGNOSIS AND TESTS OF FETAL WELL-BEING

Introduction

Tests in this chapter are used to monitor changes in the status of the maternal–fetal unit, to identify the fetus at risk for intrauterine asphyxia and, in the early diagnosis of infection, to identify genetic and biochemical disorders, together with all major anomalies. Tests done to predict normal fetal outcome and to identify the fetus at risk for asphyxia during labor are outlined in Table 16–1.

Fetal Biophysical Profile (FBP)

Explanation of Test
This test is used in the later stages of pregnancy to assess fetal well-being. The biophysical profile provides more information than the non-stress test and has better accuracy. The profile can identify the fetus that is suffering the effects of hypoxia and is therefore at risk of in utero distress or death.

The biophysical profile uses ultrasound imaging to evaluate five distinct parameters:

1. Evidence of cardiac acceleration with fetal motion (nonstress test)
2. Muscle tone
3. Fetal motion
4. Fetal respiration
5. Amount of amniotic fluid

Based on sonographic evidence during a typical 20- to 30-minute survey, each parameter is assigned a value of zero to two points (two is optimal). The maximum number of points obtainable is 10 points, indicating a normal test without evidence of fetal distress.

In addition, the biophysical profile provides the clinician with valuable information regarding the fetal size, position, and number, the placental location and grade, and evidence of specific fetal activities such as micturition and eye movements. In some laboratories, Doppler examinations are performed on the umbilical vessels to assess uterofetal blood flow.

Procedure
1. The purpose and procedure of the test is explained.
2. The patient lies on her back as for an obstetric sonogram. A coupling agent is applied to the skin of the lower abdomen. The ultrasound transducer is moved across the lower abdominal area in order to visualize the fetus and surrounding structures.
3. Examining time is generally 30 minutes.

TABLE 16–1.

Tests Done to Predict Normal Fetal Outcome and Identify Fetus at Risk for Intrauterine Asphyxia

Name of Test and Normal Values	Reason for Performing Test
Breast Stimulation Test (BST) Normal values: Reactive; negative Implies that placental support is adequate and that the fetus is probably able to tolerate the stress of labor should it begin within a week. There should be a low risk of intrauterine death due to hypoxia.	After 26 weeks' gestation, the nipples are stimulated to release oxytocin that causes uterine contractions similar to labor contractions.
Oxytoxic Challenge Test (OCT) Normal values: Reactive; negative Implies placental reserve is sufficient should labor begin within 1 wk	Intravenous oxytocin is administered to produce three good-quality contractions of at least 45 seconds each in 10 minutes, and the fetal heart rate is monitored for reaction to this stress. It is performed when a nonstress test is nonreactive or a BST is either positive or unsatisfactory.
Acoustic Stimulation Normal values: Reactive	Using an electronic fetal monitor and sound source on the maternal abdomen, an evaluation of fetal movement in response to stimulation is done.
Nonstress Test Normal values: Reactive; at least two episodes of fetal movement associated with a rise in fetal heart rate Provides a baseline status and implies an intact central and autonomic nervous system that are not being affected by intrauterine hypoxia	It determines fetus' ability to respond to environment by an increase in fetal heart rate associated with movement when not under the stress of labor

Clinical Implications

1. When the five major parameters of the biophysical profile are observable, this indicates a nondistressed fetus (10 points or a high score).
2. A low score indicates the presence of or potential for fetal distress.

Clinical Alert

A fetus that appears to lack evidence of respiration may simply be sleeping. The presence of rapid eye movements must be determined sonographically in order to assess the fetal state properly. If there is no eye movement and no respiration, the fetus is most likely asleep. If there is evidence of rapid eye movement and no evidence of breathing, the fetus is probably in distress.

Patient Preparation

The purpose and procedure of the test is explained.

Hormonal Testing

Normally, all steroid hormones increase in amount as pregnancy progresses. Serial testing is done to monitor a particular hormone over a period of time for a continuing rise in level. The significance of decreasing values indicates that the maternal-placental-fetal unit is not functioning well. The mother is not adversely affected by a decrease in steroids because the hormone level already exceeds her nonpregnant level. For the infant it is different. The infant is maintained in a closed environment, and can be quite susceptible to maternal system adjustments. Biochemical analyses of several hormones are used to monitor changes in the status of the maternal-fetal unit (see Chaps. 3 and 6).

1. In early pregnancy, human chorionic gonadotropin (HCG) provides evidence of a viable pregnancy.
2. The HCG, along with prolactin and the luteinizing hormone (LH), prolongs the life of the corpus luteum once the ovum is fertilized. The HCG stimulates the ovary for 6 to 8 weeks of pregnancy, prior to the placental synthesis of progesterone. Its function later in pregnancy is unknown.
3. Late in pregnancy, estriol and human placental lactogen (HPL) reflect fetal homeostasis.

Human placental lactogen is a protein hormone produced by the placenta. Testing of HPL only evaluates placental functioning. Blood testing of the mother usually begins after the 30th week and may be done weekly thereafter. A level of 1 μg/ml may be detected by 6 to 8 weeks of gestation. The level of HPL slowly increases throughout pregnancy, reaching a level of 7 μg/ml at term, and dropping abruptly to zero after delivery. A value of 4 μg/ml after 30 weeks of gestation is an indication of probable fetal distress. However, falsely high values are common.

Low HPL values indicate the need for further assessment with non-stress testing, and amniocentesis to corroborate results.

Fetoscopy

Explanation of Test
Fetoscopy is a technique for observing the fetus directly and obtaining a sample of fetal blood or skin. Fetoscopy permits direct visualization of the fetus in 2- to 4-cm segments so that developmental defects can be identified. A fetal blood sample permits the diagnosis of disorders such as hemophilia A and B that are not presentable by other means.

Procedure
1. Real-time ultrasound locates the area through which to insert a cannula and trocar transabdominally into the uterus.
2. Following insertion, an endoscope (fetoscope), consisting of a fiberoptic light source and self-focusing lens, is inserted into the desired part of the fetus for viewing and sampling.
3. Skin biopsies and blood samples may be obtained.

Clinical Alert
1. There is an increased risk of spontaneous abortions (5% to 10%) and of preterm delivery (10%).
2. It is offered only to those women who have a significant risk of producing a child with a birth defect that can be diagnosed only by fetoscopy.

Chorionic Villus Sampling (CVS)

Explanation of Test
Chorionic villus sampling is a new procedure that can provide very early diagnosis of fetal genetic or biochemical disorders. Chorionic villus sampling involves extracting a small amount of tissue from the villi of the chorion frondosum. This tissue is rapidly proliferating trophoblastic cells that ultimately form the placenta. Although not a part of the fetus, these villi cells are genetically identical to it.

Chorionic villus sampling differs from amniocentesis in several respects. In amniocentesis, the cells that are examined are desquamated fetal cells; CVS cells are viable and easier to culture. Consequently, karotyping can be performed on CVS cells much more rapidly, allowing for diagnosis in about 1 day—much quicker than for cells taken from amniotic fluid. In addition, CVS can be performed much earlier in pregnancy, typically at 7 to 11 menstrual weeks. Because amniocentesis is generally performed after 16 weeks with results available several weeks later, CVS has the advantage of providing first-trimester diagnosis. This is of particular value if the couple chooses to abort an affected fetus, as first trimester terminations are medically safer.

Chorionic villus sampling is performed to reveal chromosome abnormalities and metabolic or blood disorders of the fetus. However, CVS is *not* capable of measuring alpha$_1$-fetoprotein (AFP) levels, so it is unable to detect neural tube defects or any other disorders associated with elevated AFP levels.

Indications for CVS
1. Advanced maternal age (over 35 years)
2. Fetus at risk for detectable Mendelian disorders
3. Birth of previous child with evidence of chromosome abnormality
4. Parent with known structural chromosomal rearrangement

Procedure
1. The patient is asked to lie on her back while ultrasound is used to document fetal life and number and to localize trophoblastic tissue. The patient may be asked to fill or empty her bladder in order to optimize the sampling path. A bimanual pelvic exam is often performed concurrently with this preliminary ultrasound examination.
2. The patient is then asked to assume a lithotomy position. A sterile speculum is inserted.
3. The vagina is cleansed with an iodine-based antiseptic.
4. A flexible catheter with a stainless steel obturator is introduced into the vaginal canal, through the cervical canal, and into the area of the trophoblastic tissue. Ultrasound is used continuously for visualization of the course of the catheter.
5. A syringe is attached to the end of the catheter and negative pressure is used to extract approximately 5 cc of tissue.
6. The sample is immediately examined under a low-power microscope to determine if an adequate quantity and quality of tissue has been obtained.
7. Up to three passes of the catheter may be made, using a new, sterile catheter each time.
8. After sufficient tissue has been gathered, ultrasound is again used to monitor fetal viability.

Patient Preparation
1. Genetic counseling typically precedes any CVS procedure.
2. Explain the purpose, procedure, and risks of the test. Although CVS

is a relatively new technique, its complication rate is only slightly higher than that for amniocentesis.
3. A legal consent form must be signed by the patient and the father of the baby.
4. Have the patient drink four glasses of water about 1 hour prior to the exam. Advise the patient not to void.
5. Obtain baseline data on maternal vital signs and fetal heart rate.
6. Advise the patient that she may experience cramping as the catheter passes through the cervical canal.
7. Help the patient to relax.

Patient Aftercare
1. Monitor maternal vital signs and fetal heart rate every 15 minutes for the first hour after completion of the test.
2. Instruct the patient to notify her physician if she experiences abdominal pain or bleeding, elevated temperature, or chills.

Clinical Alert

1. At this time, CVS is not a routine alternative to amniocentesis. The safety of the CVS procedure is related to the experience and skill of the examiner. In experienced hands, the complication rate and fetal loss are only slightly greater than that for amniocentesis.
2. Transcervical CVS (as described previously) is difficult in patients with a fundal implantation site or an extremely retroflexed or anteflexed uterus. In these patients, a transabdominal approach similar to the technique used for amniocentesis is employed.
3. Chorionic villus sampling cannot be used to detect neural tube defects or any disorders associated with maternal serum.

AMNIOTIC FLUID STUDIES
Introduction

The origin of amniotic fluid is not completely understood, but it is believed to be primarily a product of fetal pulmonary secretions, urine, and metabolic products from the intestinal tract.

Initially, amniotic fluid is produced from the cells of the amniotic membrane, but later, most of it is derived from the maternal blood. The volume increases from about 30 ml at 2 weeks' gestation to 350 ml at 20 weeks' gestation. After 20 weeks, the volume ranges from 500 ml to 1000 ml. There is constant change in the amniotic fluid as a result of fluid movement in both directions through the placental membrane. Later in pregnancy, the fetus contributes to the volume of amniotic fluid by excretion of urine, and, by swallowing amniotic fluid, the fetus absorbs up to 400 ml every 24 hours through its gastrointestinal tract and bloodstream and by the umbilical arteries exchanged across the placenta. Some fluid probably is also absorbed in direct contact with the fetal surface of the placenta. Amniotic fluid contains cast-off cells from the fetus and resembles extracellular fluid in which undissolved material is suspended. Amniotic fluid is slightly alkaline and contains albumin, urea, uric acid, creatinine, lecithin, sphingomyelin, bilirubin, fat, fructose, epithelial cells, leukocytic enzymes, and lanugo hair.

Amniotic Fluid Analysis

When amniocentesis is advised early in pregnancy (15 to 18 weeks), it is for the purpose of studying the genetic makeup of the fetus and determining developmental abnormalities. Fetal cells are separated from the amniotic fluid by centrifugation and placed in tissue culture medium so that they can be grown and harvested for subsequent karyotyping to identify chromosome disorders. Testing in the third trimester is for the purpose of determining fetal age and well-being, studying blood groups, or detecting amnionitis.

Amniocentesis

Explanation of Test

Amniotic fluid for analysis is aspirated using a needle inserted through the abdominal and uterine walls into the amniotic sac. This method of prenatal diagnosis is preferably performed after the 15th week. By this time, the amniotic fluid level has expanded to 150 ml to supply an adequate specimen of 10 ml. It also appears to be the best time, based on uterine size and number of viable cells. If a determination of fetal maturity is to be made, it should be done after the 35th week of gestation.

Amniocentesis gives high-risk couples the opportunity to have healthy children, provided the parents are willing to terminate pregnancy in the event an abnormal fetus is detected. The test is used in the evaluation of hematologic disorders, fetal infections, inborn errors of metabolism, and in the determination of fetal sex for the purpose of diagnosing sex-linked disorders. It is *not* used to determine sex simply out of curiosity.

Identification of chromosomal abnormalities and neural tube defects such as anencephaly, encephalocele, spina bifida, and myelomeningocele can be done as can the estimation of fetal age, well-being, and pulmonary maturity.

The development of significant Rh antibody titers in the mother or a history of previous erythroblastosis is also an indication for amniocentesis.

High-Risk Parents Who Should Be Offered Prenatal Diagnosis
1. Women of advanced maternal age (35 or over) who are at risk for children with chromosome abnormality, especially trisomy 21 (at age 35 to 40, the risk for Down syndrome is 1% to 3%; at age 40 to 45, there is a 4% to 12% risk; and over age 45, the risk is 12% or greater)
2. Women who have previously borne a trisomic child, or who previously had a child with any kind of chromosome abnormality
3. Parents of previous child with spina bifida or anencephaly or family history of neural tube disorders
4. Couples in which either parent is a known carrier of a balanced translocation chromosome for Down syndrome
5. Couples in which both partners are carriers for a diagnosable metabolic or structural autosomal recessive disorder. Presently, over 70 inherited metabolic disorders can be diagnosed by amniotic fluid analysis.
6. Couples in which either partner or a previous child is affected with a diagnosable metabolic or structural dominant disorder
7. Women who are presumed carriers of a serious x-linked disorder
8. Couples and families whose medical history reveals mental retardation, ambiguous genitalia, parental exposure to environmental agents (drugs, irradiation, infections)
9. Couples and families whose medical history reveals multiple miscarriage or stillbirths, infertility
10. Anxiety about potential offspring

Clinical Implications
1. Elevated level of AFP is an indicator of possible neural tube defects. New evidence indicates that *decreased* levels of AFP are associated with fetal trisomy 21.
2. Creatinine levels are reduced in prematurity.
3. Increased and decreased total volume of amniotic fluid is associated with certain developmental arrests.
4. Increased bilirubin levels are associated with impending fetal death.
5. Color changes of fluid are associated with fetal distress and other disorders.
6. Sickle cell anemia and thalassemia can be detected by examination of fibroblast DNA obtained by amniocentesis.

7. X-linked disorders are not routinely diagnosable *in utero*. However, because they affect only men, the sex of the fetus may be determined in a woman who is a carrier of a deleterious x-linked gene, as in hemophilia or Duchenne's muscular dystrophy. In these cases, if desired, a male fetus may be aborted.

8. Cystic fibrosis

9. The presence of some of the over 100 detectable metabolic disorders. Examples of these are Tay–Sachs disease, Lesch–Nyhan syndrome, Hunter syndrome, Hurler syndrome, and various hemoglobinopathies. Hereditary metabolic disorders are caused by the absence of an enzyme due to a gene deletion, the alteration of an enzyme structure due to a gene mutation, or a mutation of the gene that regulates the synthesis of the enzyme. If the enzyme in question is expressed in amniotic fluid cells, it can be used potentially for prenatal diagnosis. An unaffected fetus would have normal levels of the enzyme, a clinically normal "carrier" of the mutant gene defect would have approximately half the enzyme level, and an *affected* fetus would have very small amounts or no enzyme levels.

10. For disorders in which an abnormal protein is not expressed in amniotic fluid cells, other test procedures are necessary, such as *DNA restriction endonuclease analysis.*

Interfering Factors

1. Fetal blood contamination can cause false-positive levels of AFP.
2. False-negative and false-positive errors in karyotyping occur.
3. Polyhydramnios may falsely lower bilirubin values by dilution.
4. Hemolysis of specimen can alter test results.
5. Oligohydramnios may increase falsely some values in amniotic fluid analysis, especially bilirubin, which can lead to error in predicting the clinical state of the fetus.

Procedure (in Combination With Ultrasound)

1. The patient is asked to lie on her back with arms behind her head to prevent touching the abdomen and the sterile field during the procedure.
2. Pre-tap ultrasound scanning is performed to assess fetal number, viability, and position. An appropriate pocket of amniotic fluid is localized. The tap site should be away from the fetus, the umbilical cord insertion, and any thick segment of placenta.
3. The skin is thoroughly cleansed with antiseptic solution such as Betadine. Sterile drapes are placed around the puncture site. A local anesthetic is injected slowly under the skin and then into the subcutaneous tissues.
4. A 3.5-inch spinal needle (20–22 gauge) with stylet is inserted through the abdominal wall into the amniotic sac. The fetus and,

when possible, the placenta are avoided. Continuous ultrasound surveillance will demonstrate if the fetus moves dangerously close to the needle, necessitating withdrawal.

5. After the stylet is removed, a syringe is attached to the needle so that a 20-ml to 30-ml specimen can be obtained. The first 0.5 ml of fluid is discarded in order to prevent contamination by maternal cells or blood.

6. An adhesive bandage is placed over the puncture site when aspiration is completed. Post-tap ultrasound scanning is used to confirm fetal viability.

7. The specimen is placed in a sterile brown or foil-covered silicone container that protects fluid from light and prevents breakdown of bilirubin. The container is labeled with the patient's name, date, and expected date of delivery or estimated weeks of gestation.

8. Amniotic fluid should be delivered to the laboratory immediately.

9. The actual procedure time is about 20 minutes. However, the laboratory work for genetic diagnoses takes at least 2 weeks and perhaps as long as 4 weeks to complete. Specimens done for fetal age, such as creatinine, take 1 to 2 hours; L/S and phosphotidyl glycerol take 3 to 4 hours; Gram stain to rule out infection takes ½ hour, and cultures take 24 to 48 hours.

10. The procedure may have to be repeated if no amniotic fluid is obtained or if there is failure of cell growth or negative culture.

11. Record the type of procedure done, date, time, name of physician performing the test, mother–fetal response, and disposition of specimen.

Patient Preparation

1. Genetic counseling that is elective, not mandatory, should include a discussion of the risk of having a genetically defective infant, risk of a positive test result, and problems (depression and guilt) resulting from a selective abortion. The father should be present for the counseling and be a partner in the decision-making process. In genetic counseling, persons must not be coerced into undergoing abortion or sterilization; this should be an individual choice.

2. Explain the purpose, procedure, and risks of the test.

3. A legal consent form must be signed by the patient and her husband.

4. Instruct the patient to void just before the test so that the bladder will be empty.

5. Obtain baseline data on maternal blood pressure, pulse, respiration and fetal heart rate. Monitor natal signs for 15 minutes.

6. The patient should be made aware of short-lived feelings of nausea, vertigo, and mild cramps that may occur during the procedure.

7. Help the patient to relax.

Patient Aftercare

1. Check blood pressure, pulse, respiration, and fetal heart tone every 15 minutes for the first half hour after completion of the test. Palpate the fundus to assess fetal and uterine activity.
2. Have the patient rest on her left side to counteract supine hypotension and to increase venous return and cardiac output.
3. Instruct the patient to notify her physician if she experiences amniotic fluid loss, signs of onset of labor, abdominal pain, bleeding, elevated temperature, chills, unusual fetal activity, or lack of movement.

Clinical Alert

1. Fetal loss is less than 0.5%. Repeat amniocentesis is necessary in 0.1% of all amniocentesis procedures.
2. Fetal complications include
   (a) Spontaneous abortion as a possible consequence of test
   (b) Injury to fetus (fetal puncture)
   (c) Hemorrhage
   (d) Infection
   (e) Rh sensitization if fetal blood enters mother's circulation
3. Maternal complications include
   (a) Hemorrhage   (b) Hematomas
4. This test is contraindicated in women with a history of premature labor or incompetent cervix and in the presence of *placenta previa* and *abruptio placentae*. If the amniotic fluid is bloody (blood is usually of maternal source), and if a significant number of fetal cells (Kleibauer Betke smear) are present in an Rh-negative mother, the use of human anti-D globulin (RhoGAM) should be considered. Some doctors prefer to administer RhoGAM to all Rh-negative mothers following amniocentesis, provided they are not already sensitized at that time.
5. Families should be counseled that prenatal diagnoses based on amniotic fluid assay are not infallible, and that sometimes results may not reflect the true fetal status. Amniocentesis cannot guarantee a normal child. It can only determine the presence or absence of specific disorders and within the limits of laboratory error. Some conditions cannot be determined by this method (*e.g.*, nonspecific mental retardation, cleft lip and palate, and PKU).
6. Excellent results from amniocentesis are possible only if the following safety factors are established:

(a) Gestation of 15 weeks or greater
(b) Ultrasound monitoring to locate suitable pools of amniotic fluid, to outline the placenta, to exclude the presence of multiple pregnancy, and to estimate maturity accurately. This is necessary for the correct interpretation of AFP levels in amniotic fluid and in maternal blood.
(c) Excellent amniocentesis technique
(d) Needle gauge of 20 or 22
(e) Not more than two needle insertions for one tap
(f) Anti-D immunoglobulin for Rh-negative women
7. The level of accuracy is 99.8% for cytogenetic analysis.
8. Techniques have been developed for performing amniocentesis in multiple gestation. Fluid must be aspirated from each individual sac followed by the administration of a small amount of contrast material. When the tap of the adjacent sac produces clear amniotic fluid, the clinician is assured that each fetus will be properly assessed.
9. An anterior placenta does not preclude the amniocentesis procedure. A thin portion of placenta can be traversed during amniocentesis with no apparent increase in post-amniocentesis complications.

Alpha$_1$-Fetoprotein (AFP)

Normal Values
Vary considerably depending on age of fetus and laboratory method. A peak is reached at 13 to 15 gestational weeks at 30 to 43 μg/ml; at 40 weeks, the value is 0.8 μg/ml.

Background
Alpha$_1$-fetoprotein (AFP) is synthesized by the embryonic liver and is the major protein (glycoprotein) in fetal serum. It resembles albumin in molecular weight, amino acid sequence, and immunologic characteristics. It is not detectable in normal persons after birth. Normally, a fetoprotein is a substance found in high levels in a developing fetus and in low levels in maternal serum and amniotic fluid.

Explanation of Test
This prenatal measurement of AFP in the amniotic fluid is used to diagnose neural tube defects (malformation of the central nervous system). In pregnancies in which the fetus has a neural tube defect, fetoprotein leaks into the amniotic fluid, causing elevated levels. Causes of

neural tube defect are not known, but a genetic component is assumed because there is an increased risk of recurrence. Neural tube defects are usually polygenic (multifactional) traits. In cases of anencephaly and open spina bifida, both maternal blood and amniotic fluid AFP levels are abnormal by the 18th week of gestation. In addition, measurement of AFP has been used as an indicator of fetal distress when it can be increased in both amniotic fluid and maternal serum. However, confirmation must come from further studies.

Clinical Implications
Increased levels are associated with

1. Neural tube defects such as anencephaly (100% reliable), encephalocele, spina bifida, and myelomeningocele (90% reliable).
2. Congenital Finnish nephrosis
3. Omphalocele
4. Turner syndrome with cystic hydromas
5. Obstructions of the gastrointestinal tract
6. Missed abortion
7. Fetal distress
8. Imminent or actual fetal death
9. Severe Rh immunization
10. Esophageal and duodenal atresia

Interfering Factors
1. Fetal blood contamination will cause increased levels.
2. Increased levels are associated with multiple pregnancies.
3. Some false positives (0.1% to 0.2%) are associated with fetal death, twins, or anomalies. Sometimes no explanation is available.

Clinical Alert

1. Any couple delivered of a child with a neural tube defect should be offered antenatal detection in future pregnancies. If one parent has spina bifida, the pregnancy should be monitored.
2. Cases of elevated AFP must be confirmed with high-resolution ultrasound.

Total Volume

Normal Values
Corrected level of amniotic fluid equals measured level of specific substance times actual volume divided by average volume.

Average volumes are approximately 350 ml at 15 weeks, 450 ml at 20 weeks, 750 ml at 25 weeks, 1500 ml at 30 and 35 weeks; volume then decreases to 1250 ml at term.

Explanation of Test

Measurement of the total volume of amniotic fluid is helpful in estimating the changes in total amounts of certain imported substances that circulate in the amniotic fluid such as bilirubin pigment, creatinine, and surface-active agents. Knowledge of total volume is important because marked changes in amniotic fluid can decrease the predictive value of serial concentration measurements of specific substances. This measurement is most important when the results of testing do not agree with the clinical picture.

Procedure

In the laboratory, a sample of amniotic fluid is studied using a solution of para-aminohippuric acid (PAH) for absorbency and dilution to calculate probable amniotic fluid volume in milliliters.

Clinical Implications

1. Increased amniotic fluid, over 2000 ml (polyhydramnios), is suggested by a total intrauterine volume greater than standard deviations above the mean for a given gestational age. It is estimated that 18% to 20% of fetuses with polyhydramnios will have congenital anomalies. Esophageal atresia and anencephaly are the two most common anomalies. The remainder of fetuses will have involvement secondary to Rh disease, diabetes, and unknown causes. Polyhydramnios is also associated with multiple births (*e.g.*, twins).
2. Oligohydramnios (reduction in the amount of amniotic fluid to under 300 ml) is suggested by a total intrauterine volume value of two standard deviations below the mean that is seen before the 25th week of gestation. A disturbance of kidney function due to renal agenesis or kidney atresia may cause oligohydramnios. After this time, premature rupture of membranes, intrauterine growth retardation, and post-term pregnancies are suspected causes of decreased amniotic fluid levels.

Clinical Alert

If either polyhydramnios or oligohydramnios is suspected, the fetus should be screened with ultrasound to detect the presence of structural anomalies.

Creatinine

Normal Values
1.5–2 mg/dl or greater indicates fetal maturity. Values are laboratory-dependent.

Background
Creatinine, a by-product of muscle metabolism in amniotic fluid, is a reflection of increased fetal muscle mass and the ability of the mature (glomerular filtrating system) kidney to excrete creatinine into the amniotic fluid. Amniotic creatinine increases progressively as pregnancy advances. The mother's blood creatinine should be known before the amniotic fluid creatinine value is interpreted.

Explanation of Test
Measurement of this substance is used as an indicator of fetal physical maturity and correlates reasonably well with pulmonary maturity. As pregnancy progresses, creatinine levels increase. A value of 2 mg/dl is accepted as an indication that pregnancy is 37 weeks or more. However, the use of this value alone to assess maturity is not advisable for several reasons. A high creatinine value may be a reflection of muscle mass in a fetus and does not necessarily indicate kidney maturity. For example, a macrosomatic fetus of a diabetic mother may have high creatinine levels due to increased muscle mass. In addition, a small, growth-retarded infant of a hypertensive mother may have low creatinine levels due to decreased muscle mass. Creatinine levels can be misleading if used without other data. As long as maternal blood creatinine levels are not elevated, measurement of amniotic creatinine has a certain degree of reliability when used in conjunction with other maturity studies.

Procedure
1. A 0.5-ml specimen of amniotic fluid is needed for this measurement.
2. Protect the specimen from direct light.

Clinical Implications
1. Decreased values are associated with prematurity and small, growth-retarded infants of hypertensive mothers, due to decreased muscle mass.
2. Creatinine levels lower than expected may be due to the following:
    (a) Gestation less advanced
    (b) Fetus smaller than normal
    (c) Fetal kidney abnormalities

Interfering Factors
1. There is a 5% false-positive rate.
2. Causes of elevated amniotic fluid creatinine not consistent with

gestational age include abnormal maternal creatinine, diabetes, and pre-eclampsia.

Lecithin/Sphingomyelin Ratio (L/S) (Surfactant Components)

Normal Values
Ratio of 2 : 1 or greater indicates pulmonary maturity, and 1 : 2 dilution on shake test indicates lung maturity.

Background
Lecithin and sphingomyelin have detergent gravity. These substances, produced by lung tissue, stabilize the neonatal alveoli and prevent their collapse on expiration and consequential atelectasis. Lecithin in amniotic fluid will be less than sphingomyelin until 26 weeks; at 30 to 32 weeks, the two lipids are about equal. At about 35 weeks, the amount of lecithin rises abruptly, but the sphingomyelin stays constant or decreases slightly.

Explanation of Test
The relationship of the phospholipids and surface-active agents, lecithin and sphingomyelin, is used as an index of fetal lung maturity. If early delivery is indicated due to conditions such as diabetes, premature rupture of membranes, maternal hypertension, placental insufficiency, or erythroblastosis, a measurement of the L/S ratio can be used to determine a mature fetal lung that might be expected to function properly at birth. Unfortunately, early delivery may be necessary for fetal welfare, but the result may be prematurity, pulmonary immaturity, and perinatal mortality. A measurement of the L/S ratio should also be performed on all repeat cesarean sections before the time of delivery to determine when fetal lungs are mature.

Clinical Implications
1. Decreased levels are often associated with pulmonary immaturity and respiratory distress syndrome (RDS).
2. An L/S ratio greater than 2 : 1 signifies fetal lung maturity, and the occurrence of RDS is extremely unlikely.
3. An L/S ratio of 1.5 to 1.9 : 1 indicates possible mild or moderate RDS.
4. An L/S ratio of 1 to 1.49 : 1 indicates immaturity of the fetal lungs with moderate to severe RDS.
5. An L/S ratio of less than 1 indicates severe RDS.

Clinical Alert

1. If the L/S ratio is less than 1.2 : 1, it is preferable to delay induced delivery until the lung has become more mature.

2. The maturation of the fetal lung appears to be regulated by a number of hormonal factors, some stimulatory and some possibly inhibitory. For this reason, hormones such as celestone will be given in 12-mg dosages for two doses and administered 12 to 18 hours apart in combination with other therapy in instances of premature labor.

3. Under certain conditions of acute and chronic stress, premature maturation of fetal lungs may be seen. Conditions in which one may see accelerated maturation of the lungs include
   (a) Premature rupture of the membranes. (Prolonged rupture of the membranes after 72 hours has an acute effect on lung maturation.)
   (b) Acute placental infarction
   (c) Placental insufficiency
   (d) Chronic *abruptio placentae*
   (e) Renal hypertensive disease due to degenerative forms of diabetes
   (f) Cardiovascular hypertensive disease in clients with history of drug abuse
   (g) Severe pregnancy-induced hypertension
   This accelerated maturation of the fetal lungs is thought to be a protective mechanism for preterm fetus if delivery actually does occur.

4. Delayed maturation of fetal lungs may be seen in
   (a) Infants born to mothers with class A, B, and C diabetes
   (b) Infants born to mothers with nonhypertensive glomerulonephritis.
   (c) Hydrops fetalis
   In these instances, no higher L/S ratio (3 : 1) may be necessary to ensure adequate lung maturity.

5. A lung profile of amniotic fluid to evaluate lung maturity looks for not only lecithin but also for two other phospholipids—phosphatidylglycerol (PG) or phosphatidylinositol (PI). Phosphatidylinositol increases in the amniotic fluid after 26 to 30 weeks, peaks at 35 to 36 weeks, and then decreases gradually. Phosphatidylglycerol appears after 35 weeks and continues to increase until term. Results are classified as positive PG or negative PG. The lung profile is a useful adjunct to

evaluating L/S ratio. It appears that lung maturity can be confirmed in most pregnancies, if the PG is present in conjunction with an L/S ratio of 2 : 1. The PG may provide stability that makes the infant less susceptible to respiratory distress syndrome when experiencing hypoglycemia, hypoxia, or hypothermia. More research is being done on using PI in the same manner as the PG. The PG measurement is especially useful in borderline cases and in class A, B, and C diabetes where pulmonary maturation is delayed.

Interfering Factors
1. High false-negative rates
2. Unpredictability or borderline values
3. Unpredictability of contaminated blood specimens
4. Occasional false-positive values associated with conditions such as Rh diseases, diabetes, and severe birth asphyxia

Shake Test

The shake test is a qualitative measurement of the amount of pulmonary surfactant contained in the amniotic fluid. It is quick and inexpensive. It is a bedside test of lung maturity and, in an obstetric emergency, an immediate decision can be made about delivery. The advantage of this functional test over the L/S ratio is that it can be performed easily by a physician, technician, or nurse, and results are highly reliable. The test is based on the ability of the surfactant in the amniotic fluid to form a complete ring of bubbles on the surface of the fluid in the presence of 95% ethanol. Exact amounts of 95% ethanol, isotonic saline, and amniotic fluid are shaken together for 15 seconds. The L/S ratio is normally not done when the shake test is positive because the shake test also indicates fetal maturity. A dilutionable table is available from which determinations can be made of various stages of lung maturity. There is a high false-negative rate but a low false-positive rate.

Foam Stability Index (FSI)

The FSI is similar to the shake test. In this test, 0.5 ml of amniotic fluid is added to various amounts of 95% ethanol. The sample is shaken and observed for foam, which indicates maturity. This test seems as reliable as the L/S ratio in normal pregnancy, and seems to have a lower false-positive rate than the shake test.

Fern Test

Normal Values
Positive test for amniotic fluid

Background
Fern production is the result of activity of electrolytes in the cervical glands under the control of estrogen. Close to term, amniotic fluid will show a typical fern pattern in the laboratory that is similar to that seen in cervical mucus, indicating a predominantly estrogen effect; urine will not produce any kind of fern pattern.

Explanation of Test
This study differentiates urine from amniotic fluid. It is done to determine whether the fluid passed by a woman is urine, or to test for prematurely ruptured membranes.

Procedure
1. A vaginal examination using a sterile speculum is done.
2. Only a few drops of fluid on a slide are necessary.

Clinical Implications
1. A positive test shows a fern pattern that is indicative of amniotic fluid.
2. A negative test shows no ferning or crystallization, indicating little or no estrogen effect.
3. If the specimen is urine, no fern pattern is seen.

Interfering Factors
Blood in the specimen inhibits fern formation.

Clinical Alert

Urine can also be differentiated from amniotic fluid when it is tested for the presence of urea and potassium. However, urine samples are usually detected by lack of AFP and by odor and appearance.

Color of Amniotic Fluid

Normal Values
Colorless or pale straw in color

Explanation of Test
Amniotic fluid specimens may vary in color from no color to a pale straw color. White particles of vernix caseosa from the skin of the fetus may be present, as well as lanugo hair. The color of the amniotic fluid changes in the presence of certain disorders such as missed abortion, chromosomally abnormal fetus, and fetus with anencephaly.

Procedure
Every specimen should be inspected for color change from normal.

Clinical Implications
1. Yellow is indicative of blood incompatibility and the presence of bile pigment released from red blood cell hemolysis.
2. Dark yellow aspirate indicates probable fetal involvement.
3. Red color indicates contamination with blood. In this instance, a determination must be made in the laboratory whether the source of the blood is from the mother or fetus. If the origin is from the fetus, a danger exists.
4. Green opaque fluid indicates contamination with meconium. Meconium is passed as a result of hyperperistalsis in response to a stressor that can be of a transient, one-time nature or of a more serious nature, such as hypoxia. A very good correlation is that the more meconium present, the more severe and immediate the stress. Additional assessments, such as amnioscopy and amniography, must be made to determine if the fetus is suffering ongoing episodes of hypoxia. Green color can also be suggestive of erythroblastosis but is not indicative of it.
5. Yellow-brown opaque fluid may indicate intrauterine death, although not necessarily from erythroblastosis.

Clinical Alert

1. Before the amniotic membranes have ruptured, color change and staining can be observed by amnioscopy. During this procedure, an amnioscope is placed in the vagina and against the fetal presenting part. The amniotic fluid is visualized through the amniotic membranes. Problems with amnioscopy include inadvertent rupturing of membranes, insufficient dilatation of the cervix and difficulty in inserting the amnioscope, intra-

uterine infection, and occasional difficulty in interpreting the color of the amniotic fluid. The test may also be difficult to perform if a patient is in active labor.

2. Meconium staining may also be observed when an amniocentesis is done. After the membranes have ruptured, meconium staining may be observed in the drainage from the vagina. Once meconium staining is identified, more assessments (such as fetal heart rate patterns) must be made before delivery is contemplated, to determine if the fetus is suffering ongoing episodes of hypoxia.

3. The presence of meconium in the amniotic fluid is normal in breech presentations.

Bilirubin Optical Density (ΔOD)

Normal Values
ΔOD of 0.02 or less is indicative of maturity
<0.28 mg/dl or a 1+ is normal or possibly slightly affected

Background
Bilirubin is a pigment that is acquired by the amniotic fluid during its circulation through the gastrointestinal tract. It is not excreted by the mother as is fetal serum bilirubin. Bilirubin may be found in amniotic fluid as early as the 12th week of pregnancy, and it reaches its highest concentration between 16 and 30 weeks of pregnancy. As the pregnancy continues, the amount of bilirubin progressively decreases, finally disappearing near term. Bilirubin is known to be increased in the amniotic fluid of erythroblastotic fetuses and fetuses with anencephaly and intestinal obstruction.

Explanation of Test
This measurement is used to monitor the condition of a fetus in a Rh_0-negative pregnant woman who has a rising anti-Rh_0 antibody titer. A rising titer is synonymous with Rh erythroblastosis fetalis or hemolytic disease of the newborn (HDN). This determination is usually not made before 20 to 24 weeks because no therapy is available to the fetus before that time. Close to term, the concentration of bilirubin pigment in the amniotic fluid will normally decrease in the absence of Rh sensitization.

Optical density is a laboratory method of measuring bilirubin and is reported as the deviation (Δ) or difference between the expected and plotted curves on a spectrophotometer. Optical density levels can be interpreted by realizing that a value of 0.1 ΔOD (deviation of optical density) corrected will correspond to approximately 0.14 mg/dl of bilirubin. The degree of hemolytic disease falls into three zones in testing.

1. If the optical density falls into zone 1 (low zone) at 28 to 31 weeks, the fetus will not be affected or will have very mild hemolytic disease.
2. If the optical density falls on zone 2 (mid zone), there is moderate involvement of the fetus. The age of the fetus and the trend in optical density indicate the necessity for intrauterine transfusion and premature delivery.
3. If the optical density falls into zone 3 (high zone), the fetus is severely affected and death is a possibility. In this case, a decision concerning delivery or intrauterine transfusion dependent on the age of the fetus should be made. After 32 to 33 weeks of gestation, early delivery and extrauterine treatment are preferred.

Procedure
1. Ten milliliters of amniotic fluid should be collected in a brown tube and then placed in a light-proof container.
2. Fluid should be sent to the laboratory immediately.
3. The specimen may be kept up to 24 hours in the refrigerator. It can be frozen if a longer time will elapse before analysis.
4. Avoid including any blood in the specimen. If initial aspiration produces a bloody fluid, the needle should be repositioned to obtain a specimen free of red cells. A bloody specimen must be examined at once before hemolysis occurs.

Clinical Implications
1. ΔOD greater than 0.04 is indicative of prematurity.
2. A value of 0.28 to 0.46 is 2+, zone 1, and the fetus is affected by hemolytic disease but is not in danger. Amniocentesis should be repeated in 2 to 3 weeks.
3. A value of 0.47 is 3+, zone 2, and the fetus is moderately affected and in danger. Amniocentesis is repeated frequently so a trend can be determined.
4. A value of 0.95 is 4+, zone 3, and indicates impending fetal death.

Interfering Factors
Blood in the specimen can be the source of inaccurate results.

Clinical Alert

1. Difficulty in the interpretation of this value occurs if the measurement is between 0.03 and 0.04 or if the bilirubin concentration unexpectedly decreases early in pregnancy.

2. If the bilirubin level fails to decline as expected or the level increases, this is an indication that the fetal condition is deteriorating.

Cytologic Examination of Fetal Cells for Maturity (Lipids)

Normal Values
Interpretive report

Explanation of Test
This determination of fetal maturity is done by staining fetal fat cells from the amniotic fluid with Nile blue sulfate. The fetus sheds cells during its intrauterine life. In the last weeks of pregnancy, the sebaceous glands begin to function, and the cells are sloughed into the amniotic fluid. These sebaceous cells contain lipid globules. The number of these fat cells increases as the fetus matures, and the percentage of these cells in the amniotic fluid gives an indication of gestational age.

Procedure
An amniotic fluid specimen is obtained and examined.

Clinical Implications
1. When the number of sebaceous cells is less than 2%, the prematurity rate is 85%.
2. If more than 20% of cells in the fluid stain orange, the infant should weigh at least 2500 g and have a gestational age of 35 weeks or greater.
3. If less than 10% of cells in the fluid stain orange, the gestational age is less than 35 weeks.

BIBLIOGRAPHY

Amenta JS, Silverman SA: Amniotic fluid, lecithin, phosphatidyl glycerol, L/S ratio, and foam stability test in predicting respiratory distress in the newborn. Clin Chem 79:52, 1983

Auvenshine MA, Enriquez MG: Maternity Nursing: Dimensions of Change. Belmont, CA, Wadsworth Publishing, 1985

Callen PW: Ultrasonography in Obstetrics and Gynecology. Philadelphia, WB Saunders, 1988

Copel JA et al: Contraction stress testing with nipple stimulation. J Reprod Med 30(6):465–470, June, 1985

Fleischer AC, James AE: Diagnostic Sonography Principles and Clinical Applications. Philadelphia, WB Saunders, 1989

Graham D, Jacques S, DeGeorges V: The role of ultrasound in the diagnosis and management of the obstetrical patient. J Obstet Gynecol Neonatal Nurs (12)5:307–312, September/October, 1983

Griffith–Kenney J: Contemporary Women's Health: A Nursing Approach. Menlo Park, CA, Addison–Wesley, 1986

Hagen–Ansert SL: Textbook of Diagnostic Ultrasonography. St. Louis, CV Mosby, 1989

Hill WC: Characteristics of uterine activity during the breast stimulation stress test. Obstet Gynecol 64(4):459–492, October, 1984

Hogge WA, Schonberg SA, Golbus MS: Prenatal Diagnosis by Chorionic Villus Sampling: Lessons of the First 600 Cases. New York, John Wiley & Sons, 1985

Hogge WA, Schonberg SA, Golbus MS: Chorionic villus sampling. J Obstet Gynecol Neonatal Nurs: January/February, 1986

Ladewig PA, London L, Olds B: Essentials of Maternal–Newborn Nursing. Menlo Park, CA, Addison–Wesley, 1986

MacMillen JB, Hale RW: Contraction stress testing with mammary self-stimulation. J Reprod Med 29(4):219–221, April, 1954

Manning FA, Lange IR, Morrison I et al: Fetal biophysical profile score and the non-stress test: A comparative trial. Obstet Gynecol 64:326, September, 1984

Platt LD, Eglinton GS, Sipes I et al: Further experience with the fetal biophysical profile. Obstet Gynecol 61:480, 1983

Ravel R: Clinical Laboratory Medicine, 5th ed. Chicago, Year Book Medical Pub, 1989

San Francisco General Hospital: Standardized Procedures for Nonstress, Oxytocin Challenge Test, and Breast Stimulation Tests in the Prenatal Testing Center. August/September, 1985

Vintzileos AM, Campbell WA, Ingardia CJ et al: The fetal biophysical profile and its predictive value. Obstet Gynecol 62:271, 1983

Wiedmeir SE et al: Tests for fetal well-being and distress. Lab Med 19(9):527–563, September, 1988

APPENDIX I:
EXAMPLES OF CONVERSIONS TO SYSTÈME INTERNATIONAL (SI) UNITS

Component	System	Present Reference Intervals	Present Unit	Conversion Factor	SI Reference Intervals	SI Unit Symbol
Alanine aminotransferase (ALT)	Serum	5–40	U/L	1.00	5–40	U/L
Albumin	Serum	3.9–5.0	mg/dl	10	39–50	g/L
Alkaline phosphatase	Serum	35–110	U/L	1.00	35–110	U/L
Aspartate aminotransferase (AST)	Serum	5–40	U/L	1.00	5–40	U/L
Bilirubin	Serum					
Direct		0–0.2	mg/dL	17.10	0–4	μmol/L
Total		0.1–1.2	mg/dL	17.10	2–20	μmol/L
Calcium	Serum	8.6–10.3	mg/dL	0.2495	2.15–2.57	mmol/L
Carbon dioxide, total	Serum	22–30	mEq/L	1.00	22–30	mmol/L
Chloride	Serum	98–108	mEq/L	1.00	98–108	mmol/L
Cholesterol	Serum					
Age < 29 yr		< 200	mg/dl	0.02586	< 5.15	mmol/L
30–39 yr		< 225	mg/dl	0.02586	< 5.80	mmol/L
40–49 yr		< 245	mg/dl	0.02586	< 6.35	mmol/L
> 50 yr		< 265	mg/dl	0.02586	< 6.85	mmol/L
Complete blood count	Blood					
Hematocrit						
Men		42–52	%	0.01	0.42–0.52	1
Women		37–47	%	0.01	0.37–0.47	1
Hemoglobin						
Men		14.0–18.0	g/dl	10.0	140–180	g/L
Women		12–16	g/dl	10.0	120–160	g/L

Red cell count						
Men		4.6–6.2 × 10^6	/mm^3	10^6	4.6–6.2 × 10^{12}/L	
Women		4.2–5.4 × 10^6	/mm^3	10^6	4.2–5.4 × 10^{12}/L	
White cell count		4.5–11.0 × 10^3	/mm^3	10^6	4.5–11.0 × 10^9/L	
Platelet count		150–300 × 10^3	/mm^3	10^6	150–300 × 10^9/L	
Cortisol	Serum					
8 AM		5–25	μg/dl	27.59	140–690	nmol/L
8 PM		3–13	μg/dl	27.59	80–360	nmol/L
Cortisol	Urine	20–90	μg/24 hr	2.759	55–250	nmol/24 hr
Creatine kinase	Serum					
High CK group (black men)		50–520	U/L	1.00	50–520	U/L
Intermediate CK group (nonblack men, black women)		35–345	U/L	1.00	35–345	U/L
Low CK group (nonblack women)		25–145	U/L	1.00	25–145	U/L
Creatinine kinase isoenzyme, MB fraction	Serum	> 5	%	0.01	> 0.05	1
Creatinine	Serum				35–115	μmol/L
Men		0.4–1.3 0.7–1.3	mg/dl mg/dl	88.40 88.40		
Women		0.4–1.1	mg/dl	88.40		
Digoxin, therapeutic	Serum	0.5–2.0	ng/ml	1.281	0.6–2.6	nmol/L
Erythrocyte indices	Blood					
Mean corpuscular volume (MCV)		80–100	microns^3	1.00	80–100	fL
Mean corpuscular hemoglobin (MCH)		27–31	pg	1.00	27–31	pg
Mean corpuscular hemoglobin concentration (MCHC)		32–36	%	0.01	0.32–0.36	1

(continued)

953

Component	System	Present Reference Intervals	Present Unit	Conversion Factor	SI Reference Intervals	SI Unit Symbol
Ferritin	Serum					
Men		29–438	ng/ml	1.00	29–438	μg/L
Women		9–219	ng/ml	1.00	9–219	μg/L
Folate	Serum	2.5–20.0	ng/ml	2.266	6–46	nmol/L
Follicle-stimulating hormone (FSH)	Serum					
Children		12 or <	mIU/ml	1.00	12 or <	IU/L
Men		2.0–10.0	mIU/ml	1.00	2.0–10.0	IU/L
Women, follicular		3.2–9.0	mIU/ml	1.00	3.2–9.0	IU/L
Women, midcycle		3.2–9.0	mIU/ml	1.00	3.2–9.0	IU/L
Women, luteal		2.0–6.2	mIU/ml	1.00	2.0–6.2	IU/L
Gases, arterial	Blood					
pO_2		80–95	mm Hg	0.1333	10.7–12.7	kPa
pCO_2		37–43	mm Hg	0.1333	4.9–5.7	kPa
Glucose	Serum	62–110	mg/dl	0.05551	3.4–6.1	mmol/L
Iron	Serum	50–160	μg/dl	0.1791	9–29	μmol/L
Iron-binding capacity	Serum					
TIBC		230–410	μg/dl	0.1791	41–73	μmol/L
Saturation		15–55	%	0.01	0.15–0.55	1
Lactic dehydrogenase	Serum	120–300	U/L	1.00	120–300	U/L
Luteinizing hormone	Serum					
Men		4.9–15.0	mIU/ml	1.00	4.9–15.0	IU/L
Women, follicular		5.0–25	mIU/ml	1.00	5.0–25	IU/L

Test	Specimen	Conventional range	Conventional units	Factor	SI range	SI units
Women, midcycle		43–145	mIU/ml	1.00	43–145	IU/L
Women, luteal		3.1–31	mIU/ml	1.00	3.1–31	IU/L
Magnesium	Serum	1.2–1.9	mEq/L	0.4114	0.50–0.78	mmol/L
Osmolality	Serum	278–300	mOsm/kg	1.00	278–300	mmol/kg
Osmolality	Urine	None defined	mOsm/kg	1.00	None defined	mmol/kg
Phenobarbital, therapeutic	Serum	15–40	μg/ml	4.306	65–175	μmol/L
Phenytoin, therapeutic	Serum	10–20	μg/ml	3.964	40–80	μmol/L
Phosphate (phosphorus, inorganic)	Serum	2.3–4.1	mg/dl	0.3229	0.75–1.35	mmol/L
Potassium	Serum	3.7–5.1	mEq/L	1.00	3.7–5.1	mmol/L
Protein, total	Serum	6.5–8.3	g/dl	10.0	65–83	g/L
Sodium	Serum	134–142	mEq/L	1.00	134–142	mmol/L
Theophylline, therapeutic	Serum	5–20	μg/ml	5.550	28–110	μmol/L
Thyroid-stimulating hormone (TSH)	Serum	0–5	μIU/ml	1.00	0–5	mIU/L
Thyroxine	Serum	4.5–13.2	μg/dl	12.87	58–170	nmol/L
T_3-uptake ratio	Serum	0.88–1.19	1	1.00	0.88–1.19	1
Tri-iodothyronine (T_3)	Serum	70–235	ng/ml	0.01536	1.1–3.6	nmol/L
Triglycerides	Serum	50–200	mg/dl	0.01129	0.55–2.25	mmol/L
Urate (uric acid) Men	Serum	2.9–8.5	mg/dl	59.48	170–510	μmol/L
Women		2.2–6.5	mg/dl	59.48	130–390	μmol/L
Urea nitrogen	Serum	6–25	mg/dl	0.3570	2.1–8.9	mmol/L
Vitamin B_{12}	Serum	250–1000	pg/ml	0.7378	180–740	pmol/L

(Blair ER et al (eds): *Damon Clinical Laboratories Handbook*. Lexi-Comp, Inc., Stow, Ohio 1989).

APPENDIX II: PRECAUTIONS TO PREVENT TRANSMISSION OF HUMAN IMMUNODEFICIENCY VIRUS

UNIVERSAL PRECAUTIONS

Because medical history and examination cannot reliably identify all patients infected with human immunodeficiency virus (HIV) or other blood-borne pathogens, blood and body-fluid precautions should be consistently used for *all* patients. This approach, previously recommended by the Centers for Disease Control and referred to as *universal blood and body-fluid precautions* or *universal precautions*, should be used in the care of *all* patients, especially those in emergency care settings in which the risk of blood exposure is increased and the infection status of the patient is usually unknown.

Barrier Precautions

All health-care workers should routinely use appropriate barrier precautions to prevent exposure of skin and mucous membranes when contact with blood or other body fluids of any patient is anticipated.

1. Gloves should be worn when touching blood and body fluids, mucous membranes, or nonintact skin of all patients, for handling items or surfaces soiled with blood or body fluids, and for performing venipuncture and other vascular access procedures.
2. Gloves should be changed after contact with each patient.
3. Masks and protective eyewear or face shields should be worn during procedures that are likely to generate droplets of blood or other body fluids to prevent exposure of mucous membranes of the mouth, nose, and eyes.
4. Gowns or aprons should be worn during procedures that are likely to generate splashes of blood or other body fluids.

Hand Washing

1. Hands and other skin surfaces should be washed immediately and thoroughly if contaminated with blood or other body fluids.
2. Hands should be washed immediately after gloves are removed.

Protection Against Injury

1. All health care workers should take precautions to prevent injuries caused by needles, scalpels, and other sharp instruments or devices
   (a) During procedures
   (b) When cleaning used instruments
   (c) During disposal of used needles
   (d) When handling sharp instruments after procedures
2. To prevent *needlestick injuries*, needles should not be recapped, purposely bent or broken by hand, removed from disposable syringes, or otherwise manipulated by hand.
3. After they are used, disposable syringes and needles, scalpel blades, and other sharp items should be placed in puncture-resistant containers for disposal. The puncture-resistant containers should be located as close as practical to the use area.
4. Large-bore reusable needles should be placed in a puncture-resistant container for transport to the reprocessing area.

Saliva

Although saliva has not been implicated in HIV transmission, to minimize the need for emergency mouth-to-mouth resuscitation, mouthpieces, resuscitation bags, or other ventilation devices should be available for use in areas in which the need for resuscitation is predictable.

Exudate

Health care workers who have exudative lesions or weeping dermatitis should refrain from all direct patient care and from handling patient-care equipment until the condition resolves.

Pregnancy

1. Pregnant health care workers are not known to be at greater risk of contracting HIV infection than health care workers who are not pregnant.
2. If a health-care worker develops HIV infection during pregnancy, the infant is at risk of infection resulting from perinatal transmission.
3. Because of this risk, pregnant health care workers should be especially familiar with and strictly adhere to precautions to minimize the risk of HIV transmission.

Isolation

1. Implementation of universal blood and body-fluid precautions for *all* patients eliminates the need for use of the isolation category of "blood and body-fluid precautions" previously recommended by the Centers for Disease Control for patients known or suspected to be infected with blood-borne pathogens.
2. Isolation precautions (*e.g.*, enteric, AFB) should be used as necessary if associated conditions, such as infectious diarrhea or tuberculosis, are diagnosed or suspected.

PRECAUTIONS FOR INVASIVE PROCEDURES

In this document, an invasive procedure is defined as surgical entry into tissues, cavities, or organs, or repair of major traumatic injuries.

1. In an operating or delivery room, emergency department, or outpatient setting, including both physicians' and dentists' offices
2. Cardiac catheterization and angiographic procedures
3. A vaginal or cesarean delivery or other invasive obstetric procedure during which bleeding may occur
4. The manipulation, cutting, or removal of any oral or perioral tissues, including tooth structure, during which bleeding occurs or the potential for bleeding exists

The universal blood and body-fluid precautions listed previously, combined with the precautions listed in the following section, should be the minimum precautions for *all* such invasive procedures.

Barrier Protection

1. All health care workers who participate in invasive procedures must routinely use appropriate barrier precautions to prevent skin and mucous membrane contact with blood and other body fluids of all patients.
2. Gloves and surgical masks must be worn for all invasive procedures.
3. Protective eyewear or face shields should be worn for procedures that commonly result in the generation of droplets, splashing of blood or other body fluids, or the generation of bone chips.
4. Gowns or aprons made of materials that provide an effective barrier should be worn during invasive procedures that are likely to result in the splashing of blood or other body fluids.
5. All health care workers who perform or assist in vaginal or cesarean deliveries should wear gloves and gowns when handling the placenta or the infant until blood and amniotic fluid have been removed from the infant's skin. They should also wear gloves during post-delivery care of the umbilical cord.
6. If a glove is torn or a needle stick or other injury occurs, the glove should be removed and a new glove used as promptly as patient safety permits. The needle or instrument involved in the incident should also be removed from the sterile field.

(OSHA Instruction CPL-2-2.44A, Office of Health Compliance Assistance.)

APPENDIX III: EXAMPLE OF CONSENT FOR HUMAN IMMUNODEFICIENCY VIRUS (HIV) ANTIBODY TESTING

I have asked or been asked to have my blood tested for antibodies to the HIV (Human Immunodeficiency Virus), the virus which causes AIDS. It has been explained to me that the test is for HIV infection. It is not a test for AIDS. If I do have antibodies to the virus (a POSITIVE test), this means that I have been infected with the virus. If I do not have antibodies (a NEGATIVE test) but am in a group of people who are at high risk for AIDS (people who have had multiple sex partners or who share needles when using drugs), this does not mean that I will not become infected in the future. In fact, I may already be infected but have not yet had time to develop antibodies.

I have been told that the blood tests for antibodies to the virus are not foolproof. In a small number of people, other things such as another virus or disease may wrongly cause a positive test. This is called a false positive test. It is also possible to have a false negative test. In this case, I do have the antibodies to the virus but the test did not show this. If the first test on my blood is positive, the test will be repeated. If positive again, a different test will be conducted. These tests will all be done on the blood taken after I sign this consent.

I have been told that HIV is spread through the blood from an infected person. It is also spread by having sex with an infected person. I understand that if my test is positive, I can spread the infection to others. I must not give blood or plasma or donate my organs or sperm if I am positive.

If I have a positive test, I should expalin this to any sexual partner. If I am unable to tell my spouse or any other sexual partner whom I have identified, my doctor or counselor may do so but only to protect their health.

If I have a positive test, my case may be reported to public health agencies. However, the public health staff may only use or give out that information for the public health purpose for which it was given. Otherwise, information about my HIV testing cannot be revealed to any-one outside the VA without my written permission, or, a court order, a medical emergency, for research, Congressional oversight, or audit purposes, or for medical treatment provided to me by the Armed Forces.

I have been told that the results of my test (positive or negative) will be in my medical record. I understand that any VA employee who improp-erly releases information about my HIV testing is subject to a fine. Even though I understand every effort will be made to protect the results of my test, I also understand that disclosure of a positive test result can lead to discrimination in housing, jobs and other areas in some communities.

I have been counseled about the HIV test and have been given a chance to ask questions. I understand that the test is voluntary and that I will still receive care from the VA if I refuse to have the test done.

Therefore, I give my permission for my blood to be tested for HIV antibodies.

_____   _____
PATIENT or LEGAL GUARDIAN   DATE

_____   _____
WITNESS   DATE

(Veterans Administration, Form 10-0121, Dec 1988)

APPENDIX IV
TABLE OF VITAMINS

| Substance Tested | Clinical Significance of Values | |
Reference Range (RR) and Critical Range (CR)	Increase	Decrease
Vitamin A		
Retinol (serum)	Excessive dietary intake and toxicity	Fat malabsorption syndrome
RR: 30–65 μg./dl. or 1.22–2.62 μ./mol./liter	Hyperlipemia	Steatorrhea
CR: <10 μg./dl. indicates severe deficiency	Hypercholesterolemia	Celiac disease
	Uncontrolled diabetes-mellitus	Liver disease
Carotene (serum)	Chronic nephritis	Protein–calorie malnutrition
RR: 48–200 mcg./dl.	Oral contraceptives	Febrile disease
50–300 μg./100 ml.	Pregnancy	Insufficient dietary intake
100–300 iu./100 ml.	Idiopathic hypercalcemia in infants	Hypothyroidism
	Amennorhea	Disseminated TB
	Carotenodermia	Carcinoid syndrome
		Very low protein
		Sterility
		Anemia
		Cystic fibrosis
		Sprue
		Short bowel syndrome
		Cirrhosis
		Viral hepatitis
		Kwashiorkor
		Nyctalopia (night blindness)
		Xerophthalmia
		Darier's disease
		Measles
		Oral contraceptives (carotene)

Substance Tested	Clinical Significance of Values	
Reference Range (RR) and Critical Range (CR)	Increase	Decrease

Vitamin B₁
Thiamine (Urine)
RR: >100 μg./24 hr.
        >377 nmol./d.

		Decrease
		Inadequate dietary intake
		Thyrotoxicosis
		Malabsorption syndrome
		Beriberi
		Liver disease
		Alcoholism
		Diuretic therapy
		Increased metabolic demands, *i.e.*, fever, exercise, pregnancy
		Peripheral neuropathy
		Wernicke's encephalopathy
		CHF
		Hyperthyroidism
		Pyruvate carboxylose deficiency
		Personality changes
		Depression
		Thiamine responsive BCK (Branched-chain ketoaciuria)
		High carbohydrate diet
		Renal-long term dialysis
		Nutritional polyneuropathy
		Photophobia

Vitamin B₂
Riboflavin (Urine)
*RR: 80–269 μg./g. or
      24–81 μmol./mol.*

		Decrease
		Insufficient dietary intake B₂
		Malabsorption syndrome
		Stress, neuropathy, dermatitis, pregnancy, hyperthyroidism, alcoholism, infections, malignancy, pellagra
		Depression
		Hypochondria
		Ariboflavinosis
		Oral–buccal
		Cavity lesions (Cheilosis, angular stomatitis)
		Normocytic anemia

(continued)

Substance Tested Reference Range (RR) and Critical Range (CR)	Clinical Significance of Values	
	Increase	Decrease
Vitamin B$_6$ (Pyridoxine) (Urine: Pyridoxal, Pyridoxamine) Measure xanthurenic acid after tryptophan challenge <50 mg./24 hrs. >100 mg./24 hrs. indicates B$_6$ deficiency (Plasma) *RR:* 3.6–18.0 ng./ml. or 14.6–72.8 nmol./liter	High supplemental doses Severe sensory neuropathy SGOT liver disease CHD muscular disease Serum GPT liver disease	Malnutrition Malabsorption Malignancy Kwashiorkor Pregnancy Oral contraceptives Uremia Neuritis Anemia: hypochromic; microcytic Chronic alcoholism Industrial exposure to hydrozene Pellagra Some drugs (Isoniazid and penicillamine) Infancy Abnormal brain wave patterns Convulsions
Vitamin C Ascorbic Acid (Plasma) *RR:* 0.6–2.0 mg./dl. or 34–114 μmol./liter Men lower than women; level decreases with age.	Excessive dietary intake or megadoses of vitamin Oxalic acid calculi	Insufficient dietary intake Pregnancy, esp. postpartum Anemia (possibly) Infection and fever Scurvy Stress Smokers Impaired iron absorption Duodenal ulcers Postoperative state Exposure to cold Trauma Oral contraceptives Parenteral hyperalimentation Elderly Lactation Diabetes Cancer Corticosteroid therapy Hodgkin's disease Active rheumatic fever Tuberculosis Petechiae Aversion to work Depression Social introversion Hypochondria

Substance Tested	Clinical Significance of Values	
Reference Range (RR) and Critical Range (CR)	Increase	Decrease

Vitamin D (Cholecalciferol)

(Serum) 25-Hydroxy, D_3 and 1–25 Dihydroxy, D_3 Metabolite: 25-$(OH)D_3$ RR: Winter: 14–42 ng./ml. or 37.4–199.7 nmol./liter Summer: 15–80 ng./ml. or 34.9–104.8 nmol./liter Most active form: Metabolite 1,25-$(OH)_2D_3$ RR: 24–45 pg./ml. or 60–180 pmol./liter	1,25 DHCC Vitamin D-dependent rickets Type II Primary hyperparathyroidism Sarcoidosis Vitamin D_3 25-hydroxycholecalciferol Malabsorption syndrome Steatorrhea Nontropical sprue Cirrhosis and biliary cirrhosis Osteomalacia Winter without sufficient sunlight Hypervitaminosis D Calcium renal calculi	Inadequate dietary intake Hepatic disorders Malabsorption diseases Biliary and portal cirrhosis Thyrotoxicosis Dietary and anticonvulsant osteomalacia 1,25-$(OH)_2D_3$ Chronic renal failure Osteomalacia (tumor induced) Pseudohypoparathyroidism Hyperthyroidism Some drugs Adolescents needing insulin Vitamin D-dependent rickets Type I Hypoparathyroidism Pseudohypoparathyroidism Premature infants Postmenopausal osteoporosis Uremia Surgical removal of kidneys

Vitamin E

Tocopheral (serum) RR: 0.5–2.0 mg./dl. or 11.6–46.4 μmol./liter	Increased dietary intake or increased vitamin E supplement	Fat malabsorption diseases Premature infants Protein–calorie malnourishment Acanthocytosis Vitamin E deficiency Hemolytic anemia Diet high in unsaturated fatty acids A-beta lipoproteinemia Glutathione synthetase deficiency Cystic fibrosis Biliary atresia Wernicke's encephalopathy Fibrocystic breast disease RLF (retrolenta fibroplasia)

(continued)

Substance Tested	Clinical Significance of Values	
Reference Range (RR) and Critical Range (CR)	*Increase*	*Decrease*

Vitamin K (phylloquinone menaquinone)

RR: Serum: prothrombin time: normal indirect	Increased dietary intake or administered vitamin K preparations Premature infant—hyperbilirubinemia following parenteral vitamin K Kernicterus	Coagulation disorders due to faulty formation of Factors II, VII, IX, and X Conditions that limit absorption or synthesis of vitamin K (obstructive jaundice, pancreatic disease, colitis, antibacterial therapy, salicylates), mineral oil Hemorrhagic disease of newborn (HDN) Infants with diarrhea, esp. breast fed Cystic fibrosis

APPENDIX V
TABLE OF TRACE MINERALS

Substance Tested

Specimen Needed,
Reference Range (RR)
and Critical Range (CR)   **Clinical Significance of Values**

Aluminum
(Serum)
RR: 0.4 μg./dl. or 0.15 umol./
liter

Increase: excessive occupational exposure,
lung diseases, Shaver's disease (abrasives
from aluminum oxide)
Toxicity not seen normally, except in renal
failure, when aluminum-containing antacids
are used; long-term intermittent dialysis

Antimony
(Urine [24 hr./100 ml.])
RR: <50 mcg./liter
CR: >1 mg./liter

Increase: excessive occupational exposure (ore
mining, bronze, ceramic)

Arsenic
(Blood [20 ml.])
(Urine [24 hr./50 ml.])
(Hair [0.5 g.])
(Nails)
RR Blood: <3 mcg./100 ml.
RR Urine: <100 mcg./liter/d.
CR Urine: >850 mcg./liter/d.
RR Hair: <65 mcg./100 g.
CR Hair: >100 μg./100 g.
RR Nails: 90–180 μg./100g.

Increase: accidental or intentional poisoning.
Excessive occupational exposure (ceramics,
agriculture)

Beryllium
(Urine [24 hr.])
RR: 0.05 μg./d.
CR: >20 μg./liter or >2.22
μmol./liter

Increase: excessive occupational exposure
(metal extraction, refinery, rocket base,
nuclear plants, extensive coal burning).
Acute lung irritation, pneumonitis, beryl-
liosis, secondary polycythemia

Substance Tested	
Specimen Needed, Reference Range (RR) and Critical Range (CR)	**Clinical Significance of Values**

Bismuth

(Urine [24 hr.])
RR: <20 µg./liter or
    <95.7 nmol./liter
RR: Plasma: <1.0 µg./dl. or
    <47.9 nmol./liter

Increase: excessive occupational exposure to cosmetic disinfectant, pigment, and solder resulting in osteosclerosis

Boron

(Blood [4 ml. serum])
RR: 1 mg./dl.
CR: 10 to 20 mg./dl.
(Urine [24 hr./5 ml.])
RR: 0.3 mg./dl.

Increase: excessive occupational exposure (glass, soap, fireproofing). Accidental ingestion of boric acid or boric salts

Cadmium

(Blood [1 ml.])
RR: 0.1–0.5 µg./dl. or
    0.89–4.45 nmol./liter
CR: 10–300 µg./dl. or
    0.89–26.70 mol./liter
RR: 10–580 mcg./liter (after exposure) 20 mcg./liter (without exposure)

Increase: (tissue) in prostatic and renal cancer; (urine) in hypertension, industrial exposure; (blood) poisoning from foods prepared in cadmium-lined vessel, inhaling of cadmium fumes, hypertension, and softened drinking water

Chromium

(Blood [Serum])
RR: 14 ng./ml. or
    2.7 nmol./liter
(Urine)
RR: 0.8 µg./d. or
    15.4 nmol./d.
(Hair)
RR: 0.21 ± 0.14 µg./g. or
    4.0 ± 2.7 nmol./g.

Increase: industrial overexposure to the metal, such as in tanning, electroplating and steel making. High levels normal at birth—previous (recent) radioactive tests with chromium may affect test results. Ingestion of excess chromium in drinking water
Decrease: impaired ability to metabolize glucose suggested as causal factor in pregnancy, diabetic children; hair decreased in diabetics. Stress, acute infectious disease, congestive heart failure (CHD)

Cobalt—Part of Vitamin B$_{12}$

(Blood [Serum—metal-free container])
RR: 0.12–0.20 µg./dl. or
    20.4–33.9 nmol./liter

Increase: excessive ingestion of beer containing cobalt as a stabilizer; dermatitis and red blood cell disease from industrial exposure with inhalation of cobalt dust; goitrogenic effect after prolonged consumption of cobaltous chloride
Decrease: insufficient dietary intake and hematopoiesis imbalance

Substance Tested

Copper

(Blood [Serum or
plasma—metal-free
container])
RR: men: 70–140 μg./dl. or
10.99–21.98 μmol./liter
women: 85–155 μg./dl. or
12.56–24.34 μmol./liter
(Urine [24 hr.])
RR: 15–30 μg./24 hr. or
0.24–0.47 μmol./liter

Increase (Serum): leukemia, hemochromatosis, myocardial infarction, rheumatoid arthritis, biliary cirrhosis of liver, typhoid fever, Hodgkin's, pellagra, tuberculosis, anemia (megaloblastic and aplastic) thalassemia, brain infarction, ankylosing spondylitis, hypo- and hyperthyroidism, collagen diseases, complications of renal dialysis and neonatal transfusions, cancer of bone, GI system, lung, breast and cervix

Pregnancy (last trimester), oral contraceptives, ovarian hyperfunction, viral hepatitis, gastric cancer, pulmonary cancer, pernicious anemia, Buerger's disease, lupus erythematosis, trauma

Decrease: Wilson's disease, nephroses, hypoproteinemia, sprue, Menkes' syndrome, some iron-deficiency diseases, burns, chronic ischemic heart disease, ACTH or prednisone Rx of leukemia

Other decreases: Infancy, long term total parenteral nutrition (TPN), antacids, zinc supplementation, ovarian hypofunction, TPN, cystic fibrosis, protein losing enteropathy, kwashiorkor, small bowel disease, scleroderma, porphyria, lymphangiectasia, sickle cell anemia.

Increase (Urine): Wilson's disease, chronic active hepatitis, biliary cirrhosis, rheumatoid arthritis, proteinuria

Decrease: protein malnutrition

Cyanide

(Blood [5 ml.])
RR: 0.004 mg./liter or 0.15
μmol./liter (nonsmokers)
CR: >0.1 mg./liter or >3.84
μmol./liter

Increase: industrial exposure (pesticides, metallurgy). Inhalation of hydrocyonic acid and fumes from burning nitrogen-containing products. Ingestion of salts, some fruit seeds and laetrile

Fluoride

(Blood [5 ml.])
RR: 0.01–0.20 mg./liter or
0.5–10.5 μmol./liter
(Urine [10 ml.])
RR: 0.2–1.1 mg./liter or
10.5–57.9 μmol./liter
CR: 4.0–5.0 mg./liter or
2.10.4–263.0 μmol./liter

Increase: excessive industrial and insecticide exposure (aluminum, yeast, welding, fertilizers); possibly elevated with fluoride treatment for osteoporosis; prolonged use of water with a high natural fluorine content of 20–80 mg./day

(continued)

Substance Tested

Specimen Needed, Reference Range (RR) and Critical Range (CR)	Clinical Significance of Values

Gold

(Blood [<10 μg./dl. or <0.51 μmol./liter])
Therapeutic: 38–500 μg./dl. or 1.93–25.40 μmol./liter

Increase: rheumatoid arthritis if gold sodium thiomalate given

Iron

(Blood [3 ml.])
RR: (diagnostic)
Men: 50–160 μ./dl. or 8.95–28.64 μmol./liter
Women: 40–150 μg./dl. or 7.16–26.85 μmol./liter
CR: 280–2550 μg./dl. or 50.12–456.5 μmol./liter
Serious Iron Poisoning: >1800 μg./dl. or >322.2 μmol./liter

Increase: pernicious anemia, aplastic and hemolytic anemia, hemochromatosis, B_6 deficiency, thalassemia, acute hepatitis, repeated transfusions, nephritis, excessive iron therapy
Iron overload from dietary iron (supplements/iron cooking pot), oral contraceptives
Decrease: iron-deficiency anemia, acute and chronic infection, cancer, postoperatively, kwashiorkor, remission of pernicious anemia; hemorrhagic anemia, hypothyroidism, vitamin C deficiency, bacterial endocarditis, nephrotic syndrome, sports anemia. (*See Chapter 2 for complete explanation of iron testing*)

Lead

(Blood [2 ml.])
RR: <30 μg./dl. or 1.45 μmol./liter (children)
<40 μg./dl. or 1.93 μmol./liter (unexposed adults)
<60 μg./dl. or <2.90 μmol./liter (accepted industrial exposure)
CR: >100 mg./dl. or >4.83
(Urine [24 hr.])
RR: <80 μg./liter or <0.39 μmol./liter
<120 μg.//liter or 0.58 μmol./liter (accepted industrial exposure)

Increase: industrial exposure plumbism, peripheral neuropathy (wrist drop), dietary ingestion (contaminated cans, improperly glazed ceramics, drinking water)

Manganese

(Blood [15 ml.])
RR: 0.4–1.14 μg./dl. or 73–255 nmol./liter
(Hair)
0.23 ± 0.11 μg. or 4.2 ± 2.0 μmol./kg.

Increase: industrial exposure (drugs, welding, glass, ceramics), estrogens, acute hepatitis, myocardial infarction
Decrease: deficient dietary intake. High calcium and phosphorous dietary intake interferes with manganese absorption; reproduction dysfunction, abnormal bone formation, impaired glucose tolerance

Substance Tested

Specimen Needed, Reference Range (RR) and Critical Range (CR)	Clinical Significance of Values

Mercury

(Urine [24 hr.])
RR: <20 μg./liter or
    <0.1 μmol./liter
CR: >150 μg./liter or
    >0.75 μmol./liter
(Blood [5 ml.])
RR: <5 μg./dl. or
    <0.25 μmol./liter
(Hair)
Approximately 300× blood
level

Increase: industrial exposure (agriculture, amalgams and dyes); excessive therapeutic intake; Minamata disease (CNS), methylmercury from contaminated fish/acid rain

Nickel

(Urine [24 hr.])
RR: Men: 2.6 ± 1.3 μg./dl. or
    44.2 ± 22.1 μmol./dl.
    Women: 2.2 ± 0.8 μg./
    dl. or 37.4 ± 13.6
    nmol./dl.
(Blood [metal-free container])
RR: Men: 0.45 ± 0.14 μg./dl.
    or 76.5 ± 23.8 nmol./
    liter
    Women: 0.53 ± 0.11
    μg./dl. or 90.1 ± 18.7
    nmol./liter

Increase: industrial and environmental exposure (incl. electroplating, ceramics, magnets, spark plugs, paints, stainless steel, enamels, batteries, glass and alloys); after myocardial infarction
Decrease: hepatic cirrhosis, chronic anemia

Selenium

(Urine [24 hr.—metal-free container])
RR: 10–100 μg./liter or
    0.13–1.27 μmol./liter
CR: >400 μg./liter or
    >5.08 μmol./liter

Increase: industrial exposure (glass, developing films, paints, dyes, electronic equipment, fungicides, rubber and semiconductors); selenium supplementation
Decrease: anemia, Keshan disease, TPN, cardiomyopathy, Kaschin–Beck disease, cirrhosis, acrodermatitis enteropathica, chronic renal failure, neuronal ceroid lipofuscinosis, kwashiorkor

Silica

(Lung Tissue [10 g.])
RR: 0.2% of dry weight lung
    tissue

Increase: industrial exposure (clay, cement, and mining)

Silver

(Serum [metal-free container])
RR: 0.21 ± 0.15 μg./dl. or
    19.47 ± 13.90 nmol./
    liter

Increase: industrial exposure (associated with argyria [bluish-gray skin]). Silver salts are used as bacteriostatics and antiseptics

(continued)

Substance Tested

*Specimen Needed,
Reference Range (RR)
and Critical Range (CR)* | **Clinical Significance of Values**

Thallium

(Blood [metal-free container])
RR: 0.5 μg./dl. or 24.5 nmol./liter
CR: 10–800 μg./dl. or 0.5–39.1 μmol./liter
(Urine [metal-free container])
RR: <2.0 μg./liter or <9.78 nmol./liter
CR: 1.0–2.0 mg./liter or 4.9–97.8 μmol./liter

Increase: industrial exposure (diamonds, dyes, and optical glass, rodentocides). Used in medications, cosmetics and pesticides

Zinc

(Serum)
RR: 55–150 μg./dl. or 10.7–22.9 μmol./liter
(Urine [24 hr.])
CR: >800 μg./d. or >12.2 μmol./d.
(Hair cut close to scalp in 2–5 cm lengths)
RR: 216 ± 87 μg/g (ISD) or 3.30 ± 1.33 μmol/g (ISD)

Serum Increase: coronary heart disease, arteriosclerosis, osteosarcoma, inhalation of zinc oxide (industrial exposure)
Serum Decrease: Tuberculosis, metastatic cancer to liver, sprue, thalassemia major, acute M.I., acute infection, alcoholic cirrhosis, hypogonal dwarfism, leukemia, lymphoma, pernicious anemia, Danboldt syndrome, and typhoid fever; dietary intake (TPN, vegetarianism), acrodermatitis enteropathica, oral contraceptives, anemia (decreased hemoglobin production), nyctalopia (night blindness), fever (increased WBC), abnormal glucose tolerance/decreased insulin concentration, iron deficiency, emotional disorders
Urine Increase: Hyperparathyroidism
Urine Decrease: Hypogonadal dwarfism
Hair Decrease: Diabetes, celiac disease, protein malnutrition

REFERENCES FOR
Appendix I (Table of Vitamins)
Appendix II (Table of Trace Minerals)

Cornatzer WE: Role of Nutrition in Health and Disease. Springfield, IL, Charles C. Thomas, 1989

Education Department, National Livestock and Meat Board: Iron in Human Nutrition. Chicago, National Livestock and Meat Board, 1990

Guthrie H: Introductory Nutrition, 7th ed. St. Louis, CV Mosby, 1989

Hussey G, Klein M: A randomized, controlled trial of vitamin A in children with severe measles. N Engl J Med 323 (3):160–164, 1990

Kanarek R, Marks–Kaufman R: Nutrition and Behavior—New Perspectives. New York, Van Nostrand Reinhold, 1991

Rolfes SR, De Bruyne LK: Nutrition prior to conception. In Whitney EN (ed): Life Span Nutrition—Conception Through Life. St. Paul, West Publishing Co, 1990

Subcommittee on the Tenth Edition of the RDAs: Recommended Dietary Allowances, 10th ed. Washington, DC, National Academy Press, 1989

Walker AF ed: Applied Human Nutrition for Food Scientists and Home Economists. New York, Van Nostrand Reinhold, 1990

Wardlaw G, Insel P: Perspectives in Nutrition. St. Louis, CV Mosby, 1990

Whitney E, Cataldo CB, Rolfes SR: Understanding Normal and Clinical Nutrition, 3rd ed. St. Paul, West Publishing Co, 1991

Zeman F: Clinical Nutrition and Dietetics. New York, Macmillan, 1991

INDEX

The letter *f* after a page number indicates a figure; *t* following a page number indicates tabular material.